Cardiac Electrophysiology: Computational Modeling of the Heart

Cardiac Electrophysiology: Computational Modeling of the Heart

Editor: Ashton Peterson

AMERICAN
MEDICAL PUBLISHERS
www.americanmedicalpublishers.com

AMERICAN
MEDICAL PUBLISHERS
www.americanmedicalpublishers.com

Cataloging-in-Publication Data

Cardiac electrophysiology : computational modeling of the heart / edited by Ashton Peterson.
p. cm.
Includes bibliographical references and index.
ISBN 978-1-63927-959-3
1. Electrocardiography. 2. Electrophysiology. 3. Heart--Electric properties.
4. Heart--Diseases. 5. Arrhythmia. 6. Heart conduction system. 7. Cardiology.
I. Peterson, Ashton.
RC683.5.E5 C37 2023
616.120 754 7--dc23

American Medical Publishers,
41 Flatbush Avenue,
1st Floor, New York,
NY 11217, USA

ISBN 978-1-63927-959-3 (Hardback)

Contents

Preface

Cardiac electrophysiology is referred to as the science of describing, identifying and managing the electrical processes of the heart. The electrical system of the heart generates impulses that regulate the frequency of heartbeats. Electrophysiology studies are conducted to assess various arrhythmias, evaluate irregular electrocardiograms, and design treatments based on the assessment. There are several risks and complications associated with these diagnostic procedures such as heart attack, infection or bleeding, stroke, blood clots in the lungs or legs, and damage to the blood vessels or heart valves. Cardiac electrophysiology is occasionally carried out to estimate the risk of sudden cardiac death. There are various treatments of these conditions, which includes cardioverter-defibrillators, medicines, catheter ablation, pacemakers and other interventions. This book provides comprehensive insights on cardiac electrophysiology. It explores all the important aspects of computational modeling of the heart in the modern day. The readers would gain knowledge that would broaden their perspective in this area of study.

This book has been the outcome of endless efforts put in by authors and researchers on various issues and topics within the field. The book is a comprehensive collection of significant researches that are addressed in a variety of chapters. It will surely enhance the knowledge of the field among readers across the globe.

It gives us an immense pleasure to thank our researchers and authors for their efforts to submit their piece of writing before the deadlines. Finally in the end, I would like to thank my family and colleagues who have been a great source of inspiration and support.

Editor

1

Optimization of Lead Placement in the Right Ventricle During Cardiac Resynchronization Therapy

Edison F. Carpio[1], *Juan F. Gomez*[1], *Rafael Sebastian*[2], *Alejandro Lopez-Perez*[1], *Eduardo Castellanos*[3], *Jesus Almendral*[3], *Jose M. Ferrero*[1] *and Beatriz Trenor*[1*]

[1] Centre for Research and Innovation in Bioengineering (Ci2B), Universitat Politècnica de València, Valencia, Spain, [2] Computational Multiscale Simulation Lab (CoMMLab), Department of Computer Science, Universitat de València, Valencia, Spain, [3] Electrophysiology Laboratory and Arrhythmia Unit, Grupo HM Hospitales, Hospital Monteprincipe, University CEU-San Pablo, Madrid, Spain

***Correspondence:**
Beatriz Trenor
btrenor@eln.upv.es

Patients suffering from heart failure and left bundle branch block show electrical ventricular dyssynchrony causing an abnormal blood pumping. Cardiac resynchronization therapy (CRT) is recommended for these patients. Patients with positive therapy response normally present QRS shortening and an increased left ventricle (LV) ejection fraction. However, around one third do not respond favorably. Therefore, optimal location of pacing leads, timing delays between leads and/or choosing related biomarkers is crucial to achieve the best possible degree of ventricular synchrony during CRT application. In this study, computational modeling is used to predict the optimal location and delay of pacing leads to improve CRT response. We use a 3D electrophysiological computational model of the heart and torso to get insight into the changes in the activation patterns obtained when the heart is paced from different regions and for different atrioventricular and interventricular delays. The model represents a heart with left bundle branch block and heart failure, and allows a detailed and accurate analysis of the electrical changes observed simultaneously in the myocardium and in the QRS complex computed in the precordial leads. Computational simulations were performed using a modified version of the O'Hara et al. action potential model, the most recent mathematical model developed for human ventricular electrophysiology. The optimal location for the pacing leads was determined by QRS maximal reduction. Additionally, the influence of Purkinje system on CRT response was assessed and correlation analysis between several parameters of the QRS was made. Simulation results showed that the right ventricle (RV) upper septum near the outflow tract is an alternative location to the RV apical lead. Furthermore, LV endocardial pacing provided better results as compared to epicardial stimulation. Finally, the time to reach the 90% of the QRS area was a good predictor of the instant at which 90% of the ventricular tissue was activated. Thus, the time to reach the 90% of the QRS area is suggested as an additional index to assess CRT effectiveness to improve biventricular synchrony.

Keywords: cardiac resynchronization therapy, heart failure, LBBB, computational modeling, QRS duration, optimization

INTRODUCTION

Heart failure (HF) constitutes a major public health problem worldwide and much attention has been paid to the understanding of the arrhythmogenic mechanisms in the failing heart induced by the structural, electrical, and metabolic remodeling. Heart failure is also characterized by a compromised ventricular contraction, which is fundamental for an optimal cardiac function. Lack of synchrony in heart contraction is worsened when the failing heart is also affected by left bundle branch block (LBBB). These patients present electrical and mechanical ventricular dyssynchrony causing pump dysfunction, reduced functional capacity, and myocardial remodeling. In particular, LBBB is associated with delayed contraction of the left ventricle (LV), reduced ventricular performance and widening of the QRS complex.

The relative QRS duration (QRSd) provides a powerful prognostic value for patients with HF and is a primary indicator of eligibility for cardiac resynchronization therapy (CRT). CRT helps to reduce mortality and morbidity associated with HF (Abraham et al., 2002; Cleland et al., 2005). Recent studies have also concluded that patients with LBBB are more likely to respond to CRT than those with right bundle branch block (RBBB) or nonspecific interventricular conduction delays (IVCDs) (Zareba et al., 2011).

During CRT, two synchronized electrical stimuli are usually delivered to reduce ventricular dyssynchrony. One stimulation lead is usually placed on the apex of the right ventricle (RV), and the other one on the epicardium of the LV lateral wall. Patients with positive therapy response present QRS shortening and an increased LV ejection fraction (LVEF) (Bonakdar et al., 2009; Zhang et al., 2015; Coppola et al., 2016). However, around one third of the patients do not respond favorably to this therapy (Linde et al., 2012; Bertaglia et al., 2017) and implantation issues, such as perforation of the RV apex, have been observed.

Optimal location of pacing leads is crucial to achieve the best degree of ventricular synchrony. LV lead position has been recognized as an important determinant for response to CRT since the initial development of this therapy (Singh et al., 2011; Crozier et al., 2016; Lee et al., 2017). Experimental studies and computational models (Lopez-Perez et al., 2015) have been used to optimize LV lead location. In current guidelines (Brignole et al., 2013), the LV posterior-lateral wall is the recommended LV region for CRT application. Several studies have reported the beneficial results of pacing from the lateral region of the LV (Rossillo et al., 2004). However, there are still several open questions.

First, as suggested by Zanon et al. the ideal LV lead placement should be the latest electrical intrinsic activated region (Zanon et al., 2014), typically the postero-lateral wall (Sipal et al., 2018). This location provided the maximum increase in contractility, expressed as the highest value of the first derivative of LV pressure over time (LV dP/dt_{max}). However, the electromechanical modeling study by Pluijmert et al. (2016) determined that in fascicular block conditions the latest activated area did not provide the maximum response in contractility. A different criterion suggested in the literature is to place the LV lead in the site corresponding to the shortest QRS registered. Nevertheless, simulation studies that apply this last non-invasive criterion (Miri et al., 2009a,b) estimated QRSd through calculation of the total ventricular activation time (TAT), a parameter not easily accessible in clinical or even experimental settings. In addition, studies such as Potse et al. (2012) have observed that biventricular pacing did not change QRS duration but reduced total ventricular activation time when the stimulation was applied in one point of the LV free wall.

Second, there is controversy about whether a higher degree of synchrony can be achieved by stimulating from points in the RV other than the apex (Da Costa et al., 2013; Pastore et al., 2013). Third, individualized programming of the atrioventricular delay (AVD) and interventricular delay (VVD) intervals is not typically performed in most patients in the normal clinical practice, and it has been primarily reserved for non CRT responders (Gras et al., 2009). The largest trials studying CRT used various methods to optimize these intervals, most frequently based on echocardiography and intracardiac electrogram interval measurements, but unequivocal proof of the benefit brought by optimization is still lacking (Abraham et al., 2010; Krum et al., 2012; Brugada et al., 2014). Echocardiography presents inherent variability of results and is highly operator dependent. Optimization based on intracardiac electrogram intervals has not proved yet to be of clear benefit above arbitrary atrioventricular interval (Ulč and Vančura, 2013). Another optimization method based on the surface ECG uses fusion with intrinsic conduction and avoids echocardiographic atrioventricular and biventricular optimization (Arbelo et al., 2014). Applying this method Arbelo et al. determined that electrocardiographic optimization improved invasive LV dP/dt_{max}. Similarly, randomized studies demonstrated that electrocardiographic optimization had superior LV remodeling at 6-month follow up although survival was not different, compared with optimization by echocardiography (Bertini et al., 2008; Tamborero et al., 2011). All these results suggest that minimizing QRSd could be used as a non-invasive method to optimize CRT.

In this study, we used a 3D biophysical model of the heart and torso to optimize pacing leads location, AVD, and VVD settings during CRT procedure, based on the shortest QRS duration measured on the torso surface. Results were compared with other optimization criteria. This analysis was used to define an electrical biomarker that relates the optimal lead configuration with the observed surface electrocardiogram signals.

Abbreviations: AV, atrioventricular; AVD, atrioventricular delay; BiV, biventricular; CRT, cardiac resynchronization therapy; CV, conduction velocity; dV/dt_{max}, maximum upstroke velocity; FEM, finite element method; HF, heart failure; LBBB, left bundle branch block; LV, left ventricle; LV dP/dt_{max}, LV pressure rise; LVEF, LV ejection fraction; LVLED, LV lead electrical delay; PMJ, Purkinje myocardial junction; PS, Purkinje system; QRSa, QRS area; QRSd, QRS duration; RV, right ventricle; TAT, total ventricular activation time; t_{90}, time to 90% of the ventricular activation; t_{90}QRSa, time to 90% of the QRS area; VVD, interventricular delay.

METHODS

Anatomical Model

A 3D biventricular model of the heart was built from segmentation of a DE-MRI images stack. The cardiac DE-MRI was acquired from the Hospital Clinic Universitari de Valencia (Valencia, Spain). Regarding the ethical considerations, the protocol was approved by the Ethics Committee for Clinical Research of the Hospital Clinic Universitari de Valencia, which certifies that the present study was conducted in accordance with the recommendations gathered in the Declaration of Helsinki, originally adopted by the General Assembly of the World Medical Association in 1964, and in its subsequent revisions. Furthermore, the patient, who underwent the standard clinical protocol, gave written informed consent for the use of his anonymized clinical data in this study.

Manual image segmentation was performed using Seg3D software (Scientific Computing and Imaging Institute, University of Utah, USA) (Seg3D, 2013), including papillary muscles and main endocardial trabeculations (**Figure 1A**). From the segmented DE-MRI stack, a surface model of the ventricles was generated and subsequently meshed using MeshGems-Hexa (Distene S.A.S., Bruyeres-le-Chatel, France), obtaining a hexahedra-based volume mesh comprised of 4 million nodes (vertices) and 3.71 million elements, with an average edge length of 0.4 mm (see **Supplementary Material** for further detailed information). Transmural heterogeneity (**Figure 1B**) was defined by three different transmural layers for endocardial (blue), midmyocardial (green), and epicardial (red) cells within the volume mesh of our ventricular model, spanning 17, 41, and 42% of ventricular wall thickness, respectively (Sicouri and Antzelevitch, 1991; Sicouri et al., 1994; Desk et al., 1998).

To include the anisotropy of the cardiac muscle through fibers orientation (**Figure 1C**), we implemented Streeter's rule-based method (Streeter, 1979) modeled by the set of equations described in Sebastian et al. (2009) defining the helix (α_h) and transmural (α_t) angles. In papillary muscles and endocardial trabeculations, fibers are known to be aligned parallel to the longitudinal axis of those anatomical structures (Greenbaum et al., 1981). In order to reproduce such configuration, we performed the topological skeletonization of the volume mesh to extract the medial axes of each one of those structures, what enabled to properly assign the fiber orientation. Finally, we performed a Gaussian smoothing with a 3D kernel to soften abrupt transitions in fibers direction between the myocardial wall and the papillary muscles and trabeculations.

A Purkinje system (PS) network (**Figures 1D,E**) was developed based on a stochastic grown method (Sebastian et al., 2013) formed by linear elements. The RV section was composed of two main branches, one descending to the apex, and another extending to the surroundings of the moderator band, with several subdivisions. The LV section was formed by three main branches with several subdivisions: one descending to the apex toward the papillary muscles of the lateral wall, another one to the anterior wall, and the last one to the posterior wall. The location of the PMJs that start the endocardial activation from the main PS branches was optimized to obtain a typical ECG wave morphology in the precordial leads. Purkinje-Myocardial junctions (PMJs) conductivity were adjusted to allow retrograde and anterograde electrical propagation. A total of 1391 PMJ were distributed across the RV and LV.

The biventricular mesh was fit into a human torso mesh (Ferrer et al., 2015) to be able to properly solve the forward problem in electrophysiology and simulate the electrocardiogram (ECG) (**Figure 1F**). The torso dataset was obtained from the online open repository at the Center for Integrative Biomedical Computing (CBIC) from University of Utah (MacLeod et al., 1991). The torso volume mesh was made of tetrahedral elements of 0.5 mm spatial resolution. Note that the problem of passive propagation of extracellular potentials, i.e., only diffusion without reaction component, does not require such a fine spatial resolution outside the heart domain (Prassl et al., 2009); for this reason, the torso mesh is highly refined only in the region where it intersects with the ventricles (see **Supplementary Material** for complementary description).

Electrophysiological Model

O'Hara et al. (2011) model is the most recent action potential model developed for human ventricular electrophysiology. Our simulations were conducted using a modified version of this model to achieve realistic conduction velocity and electrical propagation in 3D ventricular tissue. For this reason, the original fast sodium current (I_{Na}) formulation was modified. Firstly, the steady state inactivation (h_{ss} and j_{ss}) and activation (m_{ss}) gates were changed as in Passini et al. (2016) and Mora et al. (2017), respectively. Secondly, the time constant of the inactivation gates was modified as in Dutta et al. (2017). Finally, the sodium conductance (G_{Na}) was decreased to 23% of its original value to obtain approximately a maximum upstroke velocity (dV/dt_{max}) of 260 V/ms as in the original O'Hara et al. (2011) model. Furthermore, the late sodium current (I_{NaL}) conductance (G_{NaL}) was duplicated to maintain the relationship between I_{NaL} and peak I_{Na} observed in voltage-clamp experiments as described in Mora et al. (2017). All these changes are detailed in the **Supplementary Material** together with the action potential (**Figure S1**) obtained with the original and modified O'Hara et al. models. The action potential model for Purkinje cells developed by Stewart et al. (2009) was used in the cardiac conduction system.

The electrical propagation through the ventricles was calculated by solving the monodomain equation (Equation 1) using ELVIRA FEM software (Heidenreich et al., 2010),

$$\nabla \cdot (\mathbf{D}\nabla V_m) = C_m \frac{\partial V_m}{\partial t} + I_{ion} + I_{stim} \tag{1}$$

where $\mathbf{D}$ is the equivalent conductivity tensor, V_m the transmembrane potential field, C_m the cell membrane capacitance, I_{ion} the transmembrane ionic current and I_{stim} the transmembrane stimulation current.

The ECG was simulated by solving the extracellular potential φ_e from the equation

$$\nabla \cdot ([D_i + D_e]\,\nabla \varphi_e) = -\nabla \cdot (D_i \nabla V_m) \tag{2}$$

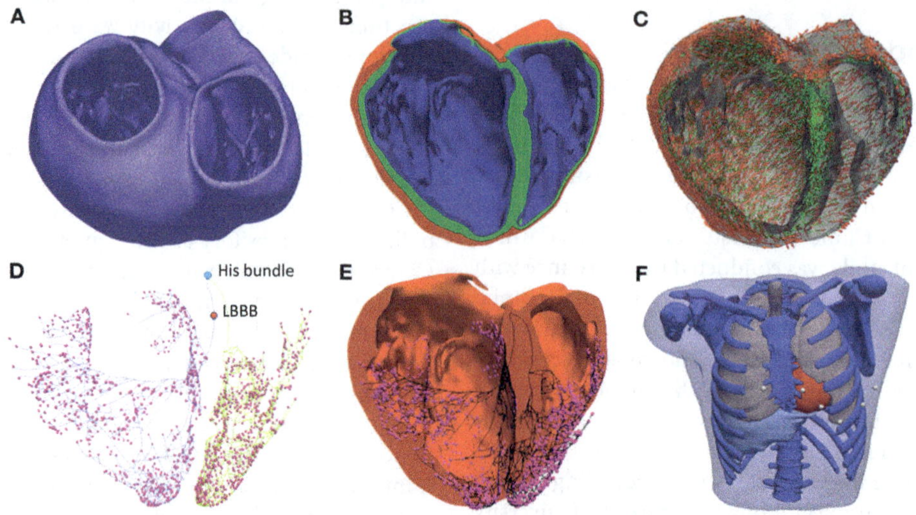

FIGURE 1 | Anatomical model. **(A)** Biventricular hexahedral mesh of a segmented human heart. **(B)** Model color-coded to show the assignment of the elements to the different cellular model in order to model the transmural heterogeneity: endocardial cells (blue), midmyocardial cells (green) and epicardial cells (red). **(C)** Arrows indicating the principal myofiber orientation of epicardial (red) and midmyocardial (green) cells. **(D)** Purkinje System (PS), including three main LV branches (posterior, septal, anterior) and RV main brunches (septal and anterior). Purkinje-Junctions are represented as magenta spheres. His Bundle, and the location of the LBBB are labeled in the model. **(E)** PS (black) coupled to the biventricular model. **(F)** Torso model with the biventricular mesh embedded (red) and precordial leads location (white).

where D_i and D_e are the volume-average conductivity tensors of the intra and extracellular domains, respectively (Potse et al., 2006). The reaction-diffusion simulation was run on the biventricular mesh. The right-hand side of Equation (2) was evaluated on this fine mesh and then interpolated on the coarser torso mesh. The extracellular potential φ_e was solved on the coarser mesh. The precordial ECG leads were then computed by extracting the extracellular potential at the electrode locations taking into account the Wilson terminal, as in clinical practice (see **Supplementary Material**).

In order to establish the conductivities that will define the conduction velocities (CV) in the heart domain, we performed a set of test simulations on a 3D slab model (20 × 20 × 6 mm) composed of regular hexahedral elements (voxels) with an edge length of 0.4 mm, matching the average length in the ventricular model. As a result, we set the conductivity values to 0.5 S/m and 0.1 S/m for longitudinal (σ_L) and transversal (σ_T) conductivity, respectively. This resulted in a CV of 0.61 m/s along the fiber direction and of 0.29 m/s in transverse direction. These values are consistent with experimental measurements in human ventricles (Taggart et al., 2000).

CV in the PS was adjusted to 2.5 m/s (Durrer et al., 1970; Dux-santoy et al., 2012). The electrical propagation in the torso mesh was considered isotropic and specific conductivities were assigned to each organ: (i) myocardium (4.589 mS/cm), (ii) bones (0.200 mS/cm), (iii) liver (0.277 mS/cm), (iv) lungs (0.389 mS/cm), (v) muscle (2.390 mS/cm), and (vi) blood (7.0 mS/cm) based on several experimental studies (Roth, 1992; Bradley et al., 1997; Keller et al., 2010).

Pathological Model

To simulate LBBB, an electrical block was generated on the left section of the PS before the bifurcation into three sub-branches by imposing null conductivity in two linear elements (see **Figure 1D**). HF condition was modeled by a reduction of 50% in CV, in accordance with protein connexin43 (Cx43) reduction observed in failing tissue (Coronel et al., 2013). The decrease and lateralization of this protein is associated with reduced longitudinal conduction velocity (Ai and Pogwizd, 2005; Akar et al., 2007; Wang and Hill, 2010).

Stimulation Protocols

For the present study a 3D anatomical model of the ventricles was generated, which does not include the geometry of the atria. Therefore, the intrinsic activation from the sinoatrial node was simulated by applying an electrical stimulus to the His bundle, either in healthy or HF + LBBB conditions (see **Figure 1D**). CRT leads were modeled as 0.5 mm^3 cubes injecting a transmembrane current of 400 $\mu A/\mu F$ in amplitude (see Equation 1). Four scenarios of CRT pacing were defined for HF + LBBB conditions with different combinations of atrioventricular delay (AVD) and interventricular delay (VVD) for each lead location configuration (AVD = 100 ms, VVD = 0 ms; AVD = 100 ms, VVD = 30 ms; AVD = 140 ms, VVD = 0 ms; AVD = 140 ms, VVD = 30 ms).

AVD is the time delay between the instant of initial activation of the sinoatrial node (external or intrinsic stimulation) and the instant of time of external CRT stimulation of the ventricles. To set the value of AVD in our simulations, several considerations were taken into account. Firstly, the typical duration of PR interval observed in LBBB patients is 200 ms (Rickard et al., 2017), which is the time that takes the initial atrial stimulation to spread through the atria (100 ms), plus the time delay in the atrioventricular (AV) node (80 ms) (Prinzen et al., 2017), plus the propagation time from the His bundle through Purkinje system to finally reach the first activation site of the ventricles (20 ms approximately). Secondly, our model does not include the atria or the AV node as mentioned before, so that the intrinsic activation was simulated by stimulating His bundle, which is included in our 3D model.

In our simulations, different AVDs could be simulated by changing the stimulation time of the His bundle (coming from the intrinsic activation of the atria). Thus, an AVD of 100 ms was modeled by applying an electrical stimulus to the His bundle of 80 ms after ventricular leads activation. Indeed, when we applied the external CRT ventricular stimulation, 100 ms after initial activation of the sinoatrial node (AVD of 100 ms), this intrinsic activation had reached the atrial side of the AV node (this takes 100 ms) and needed still 80 ms to reach His bundle (delay needed in the AV node). In the case of an AVD of 140 ms, the electrical stimulus in the His bundle was applied 40 ms after ventricular leads activation. Indeed, when we applied the external CRT ventricular stimulation, 140 ms after initial activation of the sinoatrial node, this intrinsic activation had reached the AV node in 100 and 40 ms of delay in the AV have also elapsed, the stimulus needed 40 ms more to reach the His bundle, and this is why we stimulated the His bundle 40 ms after the ventricles. Additionally, VVD was set to 0 ms (stimulation in both ventricles simultaneously) and 30 ms (the RV was stimulated 30 ms after the LV), according to the time ranges used in clinical practice (Brignole et al., 2013; Urbanek et al., 2017).

Leads Location

The RV septal wall is an alternative location for the RV pacing lead in CRT. In this study, three different locations for the RV pacing lead were tested based on medical protocols and research works (Da Costa et al., 2013; Pastore et al., 2013). The RV septal electrode was placed in the apex (RVapex), middle septal region (RVmid) or upper region near the outflow tract (RVupper) (**Figure 2A**).

For the LV pacing lead location, the LV free wall was divided into three different regions (Singh et al., 2011; Dou et al., 2012): anterior, lateral, and posterior (**Figure 2B**). In addition, each region was divided into three segments: apical, mid-cavity, and basal, leading to a set of nine segments for the LV free wall as illustrated in **Figure 2C** as in Singh et al. (2011). The LV pacing lead was placed in the middle of each segment, both in the epicardial (**Figure 2C**) and endocardial wall (**Figure 2D**) to represent and simplify the different possible positions of the electrode within the same region, due to variety of veins configurations observed in CRT patients.

To summarize, we have a total of 54 lead location configurations obtained by combination of the three RV lead locations with 18 LV lead locations (9 epicardial and 9 endocardial) for the application of the CRT protocol.

QRS Measurements

QRS complex was computed in the precordial leads location on the torso surface for each CRT configuration and QRSd was measured using an algorithm implemented in Matlab software (Mathworks Inc., Natick, MA, USA). This algorithm determines the beginning and end of the QRS complex based on the first and second derivate of the electrocardiographic signal (see **Figure S2**). The QRS onset was calculated applying a threshold in the first derivate to determine a change in the slope. To estimate the end of QRS complex, additional signal processing was required as baseline was not reached in most CRT configurations. A time interval after the QRS complex was set based on the 95% of the accumulated area under the curve of the second derivate, and the end of the signal. To set the end of the QRS, the lowest value of the first derivate was used within this interval (see **Supplementary Material** for details). Once the beginning and end of QRS complex were determined for each precordial lead, the QRSd was calculated as the time interval between the onset beginning and the latest end of the QRS among all leads (Surawicz et al., 2009). This is the recommended criterion by the American Heart Association, the American College of Cardiology Foundation, and the Heart Rhythm Society (AHA/ACC/HRS). The total activation time (TAT) of the ventricular mesh was estimated as the time interval between the first and last depolarized node mesh above a threshold of −10 mV.

Correlation Analysis

Shortest QRSd was the criterion applied to evaluate the optimal location of the LV lead for different positions of the pacing lead in the RV. However, the total activation time (TAT), QRS area (QRSa) and the time to 90% of activated tissue (t_{90}) are other important parameters that have been used to evaluate CRT response. For this reason, three linear correlations between these parameters were performed using Pearson correlation method. Values of $p < 0.05$ were considered statistically significant. Values for the analysis are shown in **Tables S1–S5**.

RESULTS

Model Validation

Simulated ventricular activation maps for non-pathological and HF conditions with LBBB (HF + LBBB) are shown in **Figure 3A**. In healthy conditions, the electrical impulse traveled from the bundle of His to the first activation point in the LV endocardium in approximately 20 ms. RV activation started 10 ms after the onset of LV activation (Durrer et al., 1970). The computed time until all the ventricular tissue was depolarized (total activation time or TAT) was approximately 103 ms, in accordance with human data (Boukens et al., 2014). The outflow tract and the posterobasal area were the last activated regions in the RV, while the latest areas depolarized in the LV were the anterior mid and basal regions.

Under HF + LBBB conditions, activation began in the RV endocardium and reached the LV endocardium in the apical septal region after 46 ms from the onset of the RV depolarization. This is in agreement with the data recorded experimentally by Auricchio et al. (2004). The last activated region in the LV was the lateral wall in accordance with the study of Mafi Rad et al.

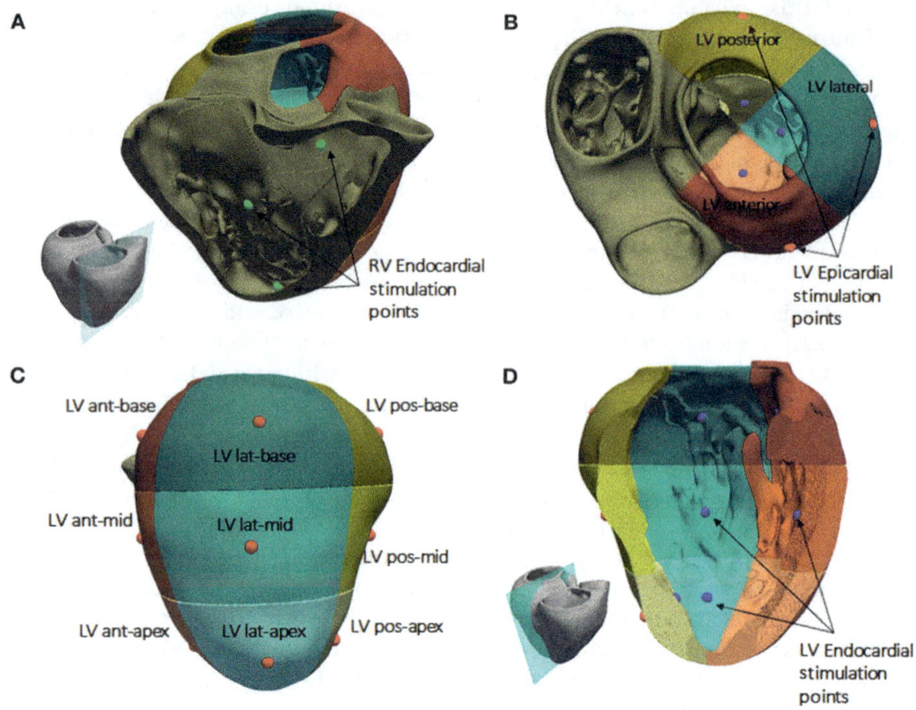

FIGURE 2 | Heart subdivisions and stimulation points for CRT protocol. **(A)** RV septal endocardial stimulation points tested (green). **(B)** Left ventricular (LV) free wall region divided into three regions: posterior (yellow), anterior (brown), and lateral (green). **(C)** Subdivisions of the three LV free wall regions into nine segments. Epicardial stimulation points tested in the middle of each segment (red dots). **(D)** Endocardial stimulation points tested in the LV free wall (blue dots).

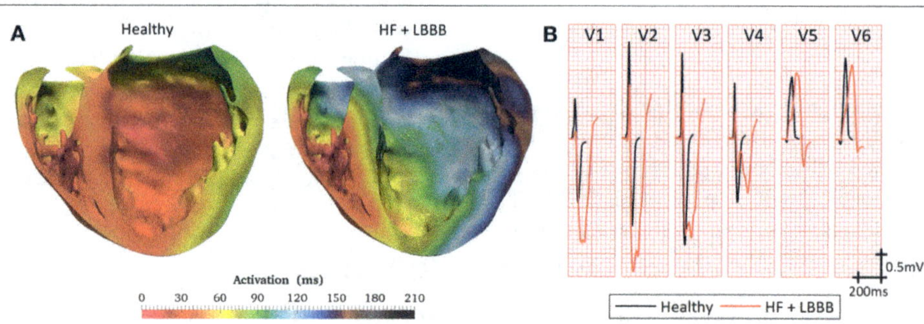

FIGURE 3 | Model validation. **(A)** Cross section of biventricular model showing color coded local activation maps of a healthy (left) and pathological heartbeat (right). **(B)** Precordial leads signals recorded on torso surface.

(2014). Additionally, the TAT was increased in 104% compared to a healthy heart.

Figure 3B shows the computed QRS complexes in the precordial leads for simulations in a healthy heart and under HF + LBBB conditions. For non-pathological conditions, QRS duration (QRSd) was 93 ms, while in HF + LBBB QRSd was increased to 190 ms. Both values are within experimental ranges (Spragg et al., 2010; Tian et al., 2017). Additionally, QRS complexes in HF + LBBB simulations present an rS pattern (small R wave followed by a bigger S wave) (Sweeney et al., 2014) in leads V1 and V2 and a mid-QRS notching in several leads. These observations are in agreement with the criteria proposed by Strauss et al. (2011) to define complete LBBB.

QRS Duration During CRT

A total of 54 electrode placement configurations with four different delays (two AVD and two VVD configurations) settings were tested for the CRT simulations. QRSd values are shown in **Table S1**.

Figure 4 compares the simulated QRS complexes in a scenario with HF + LBBB before (red traces) and after (green traces) the application of the CRT protocol. The optimal configurations in terms of shortest QRSd for the RV lead placement tested (apex, mid septum, and upper septum) are shown in the different rows. Epicardial vs. endocardial LV lead stimulation for those configurations are shown in columns.

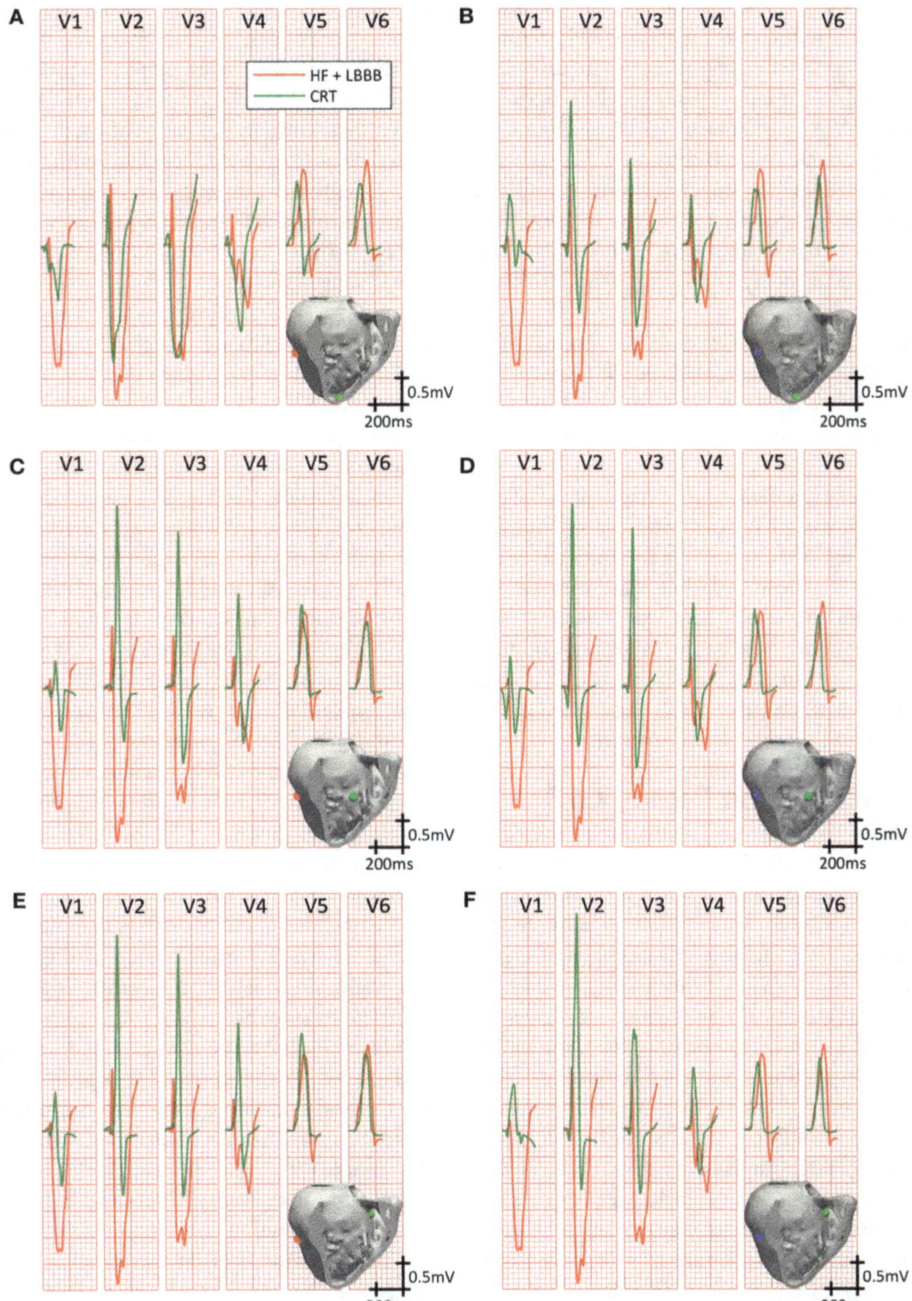

FIGURE 4 | Precordial leads signals on CRT. QRS complexes in the precordial leads under HF + LBBB conditions, before (red trace) and after (green trace) the application of the best CRT configurations (shorter QRSd). Three different locations for the RV pacing lead were tested: RV apex with epicardial **(A)** and endocardial **(B)** LV lead stimulation; RV mid septum with epicardial **(C)** and endocardial **(D)** LV lead stimulation; and RV upper septum with epicardial **(E)** and endocardial **(F)** LV lead stimulation. Stimulation points are shown in light green inside the insets for the RV lead, and in blue and red for the LV endocardial and epicardial lead, respectively.

Firstly, we analyzed the optimal lead placement. The shortest QRSd among all configurations tested was obtained when the RV lead was placed in the upper septum near the outflow track (third row). Furthermore, for all RV lead placement the optimal location of the LV lead, both in the epicardium and endocardium, was the LV mid posterior wall.

Secondly, we analyzed the effect of the delay between pacing leads and intrinsic activation in a fixed location. The best configurations for the RV lead placed in the apex are depicted in the first row. QRSd was reduced from 172 ms (**Figure 4A**) to 157 ms (**Figure 4B**), but bigger reductions were obtained for different intrinsic and pacing delays (AVD = 140 ms, VVD = 0 ms; AVD = 100 ms, VVD = 30 ms, respectively).

When the RV lead was located in the middle of the septum (second row), the QRSd was reduced from 161 ms (**Figure 4C**) to 146 ms (**Figure 4D**) for optimal configurations. In this case, these results were obtained for different pacing delays between leads but the same AVD (AVD = 140 ms and VVD = 30 ms vs. AVD = 140 ms and VVD = 0 ms, respectively).

If the RV lead was placed in the upper septum, the QRSd was reduced from 149 ms (**Figure 4E**) to 143 ms (**Figure 4F**). However, in this case both configurations were achieved with the same intrinsic and biventricular delay (AVD = 140 ms, VVD = 30 ms).

Finally, the influence of LV epicardial vs. endocardial pacing was assessed. QRSd was decreased in all cases after CRT application, but the reduction was greater for LV leads placed in the endocardium (column 2) compared to epicardium (column 1).

Summarizing, the optimal location in terms of shortest QRSd was obtained when the RV lead was placed in the upper septum and the LV lead was located in the mid posterior wall region. Once the optimal lead location was selected for both RV and LV leads, the shortest QRSd was measured for different intrinsic and biventricular delays, without highlighting a particular optimal setting. Finally, the shortest QRSd was obtained in all configurations when the LV lead was placed in the endocardium compared with those in the epicardium.

Ventricular Activation Time During CRT

Another helpful parameter to assess CRT outcome is the total activation time (TAT) of the ventricles. This parameter is not directly accessible in clinical practice during CRT procedures, but simulations can provide additional information to achieve the ideal configuration. Ideally, within normal physiological ranges, the shorter the QRS the shorter TAT, leading to an increase in ventricular synchrony. In **Figure 5**, the percentage of activated ventricular tissue is shown as a function of time for the healthy heart, under HF + LBBB conditions, and for the optimal CRT configurations (as a function of RV location), which are shown in **Figure 4**. Under HF + LBBB conditions (red trace), the electrical impulse spreads throughout the ventricles much slower (gradual slope) than in the healthy heart (black trace) or in CRT (green trace) configurations, completing ventricular activation after 210 ms. For CRT simulations, the rate of activated tissue was initially low, but increased rapidly to reach rates similar to those observed in healthy cases. This was especially noticeable when the LV lead was located in the epicardium (first column) and the RV lead was located in the mid and upper septum (**Figures 4C,E**, respectively). These results can be explained because of several factors. Firstly, the configuration of the PS and the PMJ distribution strongly affects the initial spread of the wavefront. Given the PS RV morphology, i.e., two main branches, one descending to the apex and another growing around the moderator band (**Figure 1D**), when the RV lead was located in the apex, the electrical stimulus entered fast in the PS (around 5 ms) and propagated to remote areas faster than through the myocardium (see **Video 1**, CRT). However, it took around 40 ms to retrogradely enter in the PS when the RV lead was located in the mid septal region, and around 90 ms when the RV lead was in the upper septum. For this reason, it took 75 ms to activate initially only 10% of the myocardium. Secondly, stimulation in the epicardial layer took longer to reach PMJ locations. Thirdly, the stimulation delay between both ventricles (VVD) also affected the initial slope of cardiac activation. Nevertheless, after 70 ms for the endocardial configurations (second column) and 125 ms for the epicardial ones the percentage of activated tissue during CRT application was higher than the percentage of HF + LBBB conditions. Moreover, during the final phase of ventricular activation, the rising rate was considerably reduced. Indeed, the electrical impulse took between 26 and 54 ms (15% to 26% of the TAT) to activate the last 10% of the ventricular tissue.

Finally, after applying the CRT protocol, the TAT was decreased by 15, 14, 12, 15, 19, 22%, with respect to HF + LBBB conditions, as shown in **Figures 5A–F**, respectively. The locations of the pacing leads for the shorter QRS complexes coincided with the locations of the electrodes for the shorter TAT. However, when VVD and AVD were modified, the shortest QRS did not match the shortest TAT, which means that QRSd and TAT are not totally correlated. In addition, the difficulty in QRS measurement at the beginning and end of the signals has to be considered.

In clinical practice, a shorter QRSd is one of the standard criteria used to evaluate CRT response. However, both non-responder and responder patients show a reduction in QRSd after CRT application (Molhoek et al., 2004; Elhakam Elzoghby et al., 2017). Therefore, an additional indicator would be useful for a better perception of CRT benefit. As shown in **Figure 5**, TAT could be strongly modified by the initial rate of activation, as well as by the last activation interval. To avoid this, we analyzed the time elapsed to 90% of ventricular activation (t_{90}), (**Figure 6**). This parameter allows us to determine which configuration leads to a faster activation of most of the ventricular tissue, thus decreasing electrical dyssynchrony.

Figure 6 shows t_{90} values for a configuration with the RV lead placed in the apex, mid septum, and upper septum, and the LV lead located in the epicardium (**Figures 6A–C**), and the same RV configurations with the LV located in the endocardium (**Figures 6D–F**). The different delays applied between the His Bundle and CRT leads (AVD) and between the RV and LV leads (VVD) are shown in columns.

The optimal location of the LV pacing lead, both in the epicardium and endocardium, changed during CRT application for each of the pacing lead locations in the RV. However, the optimal AVD and VVD were the same in all cases, 140 and 0 ms (third column), respectively.

On the one hand, when AVD was modified (column 1 vs. column 3 and column 2 vs. column 4) similar results were obtained, except when the RV lead was located in the upper septum area. The electrical propagation of the intrinsic stimulus contributed to decrease t_{90} (7% reduction) for an AVD of 140 ms. On the other hand, when VVD was increased (column 1 vs. column 2 and column 3 vs. column 4) t_{90} increased up to 19% for all the RV lead locations.

When the RV lead was located in the apex, the optimal location of the LV lead in the epicardium was the LV anterior wall at basal level (**Figure 6A**). For the same RV lead location,

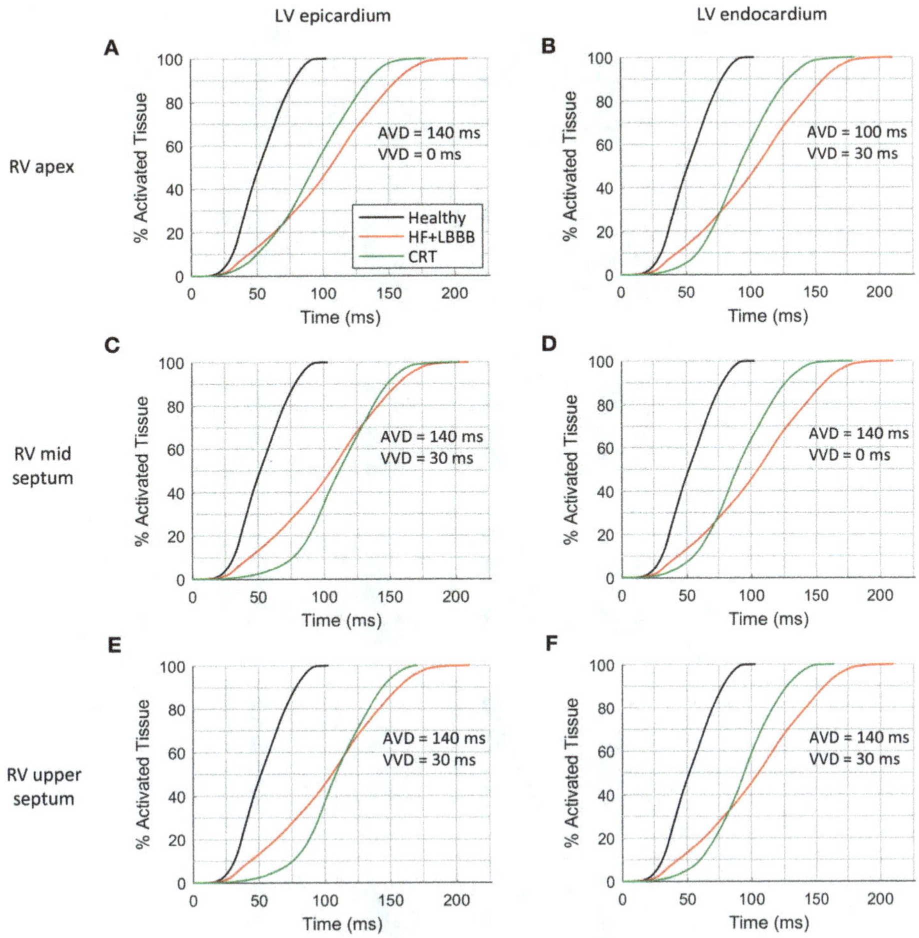

FIGURE 5 | Cumulative frequency histograms of the normalized percentage of activated tissue. The curves correspond to healthy (black), HF + LBBB (red) and CRT (green) scenarios. The best CRT configurations (shortest QRSd) for the three locations of the RV lead were tested: RV apex with epicardial **(A)** and endocardial **(B)** LV lead stimulation; RV mid septum with epicardial **(C)** and endocardial **(D)** LV lead stimulation; and RV upper septum with epicardial **(E)** and endocardial **(F)** LV lead stimulation.

the optimal LV lead location in the endocardium was the LV posterior wall at mid-cavity level (**Figure 6D**). Changing the RV lead location to mid septum, the optimal LV lead location in the epicardium was the LV mid lateral wall, while the optimal LV lead location in the endocardium was the LV mid posterior wall (**Figures 6B,E**, respectively).

Finally, for the RV lead location in the upper septum, the optimal placement of the LV pacing lead in the epicardium was in the LV mid lateral wall, while the optimal placement of the LV lead in the endocardium was the apex of the LV lateral wall (**Figures 6C,F**, respectively). **Table 1** summarizes the optimal placement of the LV lead for a faster activation of 90% of the ventricular tissue. The optimal locations calculated are not in agreement with the optimal RV lead location determined based on a shorter QRSd in most cases. This result suggests the hypothesis that the shortest QRSd does not necessarily imply the fastest ventricular activation of 90% of the ventricular muscle.

Correlation Between Ventricular Activation and QRS

To better highlight the relationship between QRSd and TAT, a correlation analysis was carried out (**Figure 7A**). Results showed an elliptical distribution of data with a moderate positive linear relationship, statistically significant ($R = 0.78$ and $p < 0.05$). This moderate correlation could justify the difference between the optimal AVD and VVD values for the simulations with a shortest QRSd and with a shortest TAT.

A similar correlation analysis was made between area of the QRS (QRSa) and TAT (**Figure 7B**). We first calculated the QRSa for the average signal of the six precordial leads, between the beginning and end values determined during the measurement of the QRSd. The results of the correlation show a scattering distribution of data with a statistically non-significant p-value ($R = -0.12$ and $p = 0.076$). Thus, a linear relationship between QRSa and TAT was not observed in this study.

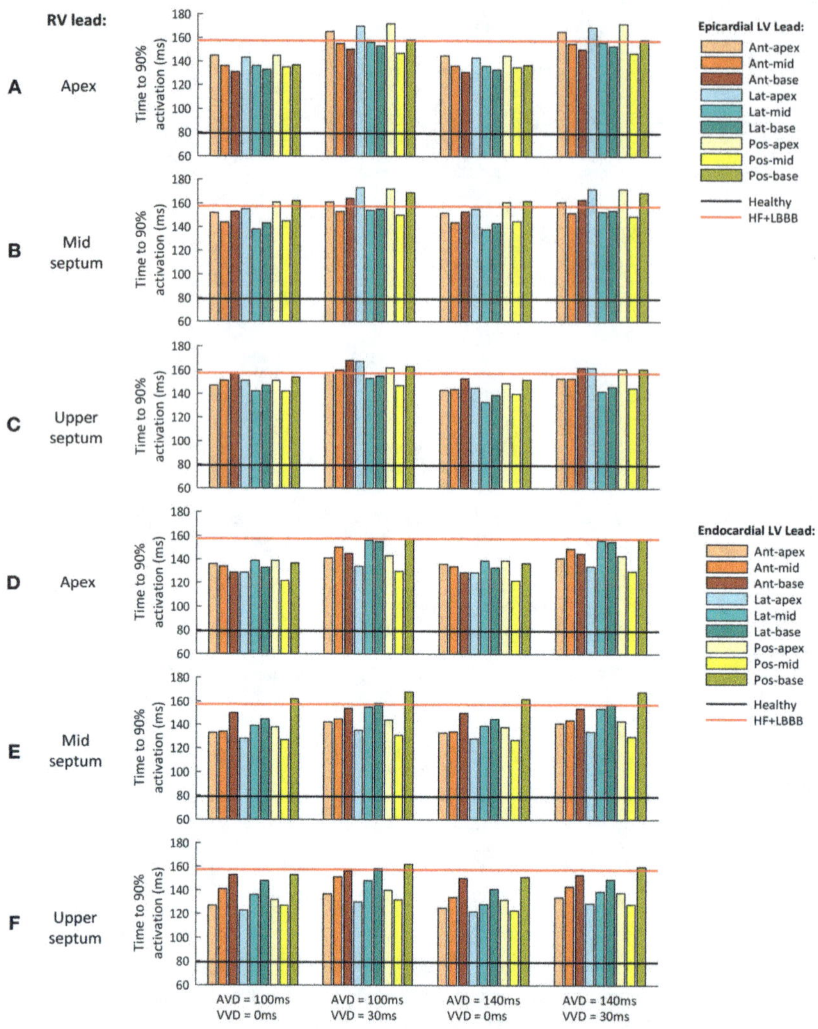

FIGURE 6 | Time to 90% of ventricular activation for the different CRT configuration delays assessed. **(A–C)** Epicardial LV lead stimulation for the three RV lead location tested: **(A)** RV apex, **(B)** RV mid septum and **(C)** RV upper septum. **(D–F)** Endocardial LV lead stimulation for the three RV lead location tested: **(D)** RV apex, **(E)** RV mid septum and **(F)** RV upper septum. The three LV regions (anterior, lateral and posterior walls) are shown in different color brightness (red, blue and yellow). The values for healthy and HF + LBBB configurations are depicted in black and red lines respectively.

Finally, when correlating the curves of percentage of activated tissue and percentage of QRS area as a function of time, a direct relationship between both variables was observed. **Figure 7C** shows the correlation between time to 90% of QRSa (t_{90}QRSa) and time to 90% of the ventricular activation (t_{90}) for each CRT simulations. A significant correlation with a high linear dependence was observed ($R = 0.94$ and $P < 0.05$). Simulations with shorter t_{90}QRSa correspond to the simulations with shorter t_{90}. Therefore, a new biomarker based on time up to 90% of the QRS area can be used as an indicator of electrical synchrony.

DISCUSSION

In this study, biophysical 3D multiscale simulations were conducted to assess alternative locations of the RV lead for a better CRT response in LBBB HF patients. The major findings of this study can be summarized as follows: (i) the optimal leads location based on shortest QRS criterion was the RV upper septum and the LV mid posterior region minimizing also TAT; (ii) for the optimal lead location, the delay configuration leading to the shortest QRSd was AVD = 140 ms, VVD = 30 ms. However, the AVD and VVD setting leading to the shortest TAT was different, suggesting that minimizing QRSd is a good criterion to select leads location but not to select the pacing delay; iii) the time to 90% of the QRS area (t_{90}QRSa) was a good predictor of the instant at which 90% of the ventricular tissue had been activated (t_{90}). This indicator could be used in clinical trials to complement QRSd criterion to select the optimal delay of the pacing leads to obtain a faster ventricular activation of most of the ventricular muscle.

Optimal Lead Location

The location of the optimal pacing site varies significantly between patients, so that a strategy of individualized LV lead placement is required to maximize the benefit of CRT (Derval

TABLE 1 | Optimal placement of the LV lead on CRT.

Criterion	RV lead	LV lead	AVD (ms)	VVD (ms)
LV EPICARDIAL STIMULATION				
Shortest QRS duration	Apex	Posterior - mid	140	0
	Mid septum	Posterior - mid	140	30
	Upper septum	Posterior - mid	140	30
Shortest TAT	Apex	Posterior - mid	140	0
	Mid septum	Posterior - mid	140	0
	Upper septum	Posterior - mid	140	0
Faster activation of 90% of the ventricular tissue	Apex	Anterior - base	140	0
	Mid septum	Lateral - mid	140	0
	Upper septum	Lateral - mid	140	0
LV ENDOCARDIAL STIMULATION				
Shortest QRS duration	Apex	Posterior - mid	100	30
	Mid septum	Posterior - mid	140	0
	Upper septum	Posterior - mid	140	30
Shortest TAT	Apex	Posterior - mid	140	0
	Mid septum	Posterior - mid	140	0
	Upper septum	Posterior - mid	140	0
Faster activation of 90% of the ventricular tissue	Apex	Posterior - mid	140	0
	Mid septum	Posterior - mid	140	0
	Upper septum	Lateral - apex	140	0

TAT, total activation time; AVD, atrioventricular delay; VVD, interventricular delay.

et al., 2010; Spragg et al., 2010). The apex for permanent LV pacing should be avoided, as this location has been associated with poor outcomes in studies such as MADIT-CRT (Yoshikawa et al., 2010; Singh et al., 2011). The experimental study PATH-CHF I suggested that the mid lateral left ventricular site for the LV lead may show greater acute benefit in patients with LBBB (Auricchio et al., 1999). In general, a lateral or posterior vein is the desired location for achieving optimal hemodynamic support as this is usually the site of most delayed activation of the left ventricular wall in patients with LBBB (Stellbrink et al., 2000; Singh et al., 2006).

Our simulation results suggested the upper area of the RV septum as the optimal position for the RV lead, in agreement with some experimental (Muto et al., 2007; Flevari et al., 2009; Cano et al., 2010; Da Costa et al., 2013) and simulation (Miri et al., 2009a) studies. The study of Leclerq and coworkers (Leclercq et al., 2016) demonstrates that septal and apical RV pacing in CRT have a similar clinical outcome and similar LV reverse remodeling after 6 months of therapy. However, other studies (Victor et al., 2006) reported the shortest QRSd for RV septum pacing but not a better CRT response (similar LVEF at 6 months). This highlights the need of additional indicators to determine the optimal placement of the pacing leads.

In the present simulation study the most delayed activation area was located in the anterior basal LV region in the HF + LBBB configuration under intrinsic activation. We also assessed the latest activated area of the LV, when only RV stimulation was applied. If the RV lead was placed in the apex, the anterior basal LV area was activated the latest. However, the LV lateral wall was the latest activated area when the RV lead was located either in the middle or upper septal regions (see **Figure S3**).

The study of Zanon et al. (2014) determined that the LV lead location in the latest activated site was predictive of the maximum increase in contractility (LV $dP/dt_{\max}$). On the other hand, in the recent study of Sipal and coworkers (Sipal et al., 2018), comparing the clinical benefits of LV lead implantation guided by the shortest BiV-paced QRSd using surface ECG and with the standard unguided CRT, there was a significantly higher rate (85 vs. 50%, $p = 0.02$) of response (>15% reduction in LV end-systolic volume) to CRT as well as a shorter QRSd ($p < 0.001$) and a greater QRS shortening for the surface ECG guided group. Furthermore, the optimal site for LV lead placement was the posterior and posterolateral region, in agreement with our simulations. For all RV lead locations tested in our study, when the LV lead was placed in the latest activated area of the LV, none of those configurations led to the shortest QRSd.

In our study, we also showed that when pacing in the latest electrically activated area of the LV, that area did not provide the shortest TAT. Similar results were observed in the simulation study by Pluijmert et al. (2016). In that work, the authors found that the LV pacing region that provided the maximum acute hemodynamic response, located near the latest activated area, did not lead to the largest reduction of TAT during biventricular stimulation. Even stimulating regions leading to the largest reduction of TAT showed poor increase of hemodynamic response. However, other studies have found a positive correlation between acute hemodynamic response and TAT reduction (Crozier et al., 2016). The optimal method to place the LV pacing lead is thus object of controversy: while several studies support that pacing in the latest activated area leads to better hemodynamic response, others consider the criterion of maximal reduction in QRSd as the best choice.

Optimal Delay Between Pacing Leads

Optimization of AVD and VVD is crucial during CRT application. A longer inter-lead electrical delay was associated with more pronounced LV reverse remodeling in CRT patients with a presumed optimal LV lead position concordant or adjacent to the latest mechanically activated non-scarred segment (Sommer et al., 2018).

In clinical practice this value should be specifically set for each patient, although optimization is rarely performed in the real practice. The largest trials studying CRT used various methods to optimize these intervals, most frequently based on echocardiography and intracardiac electrogram interval measurement, but unequivocal proof of the benefit brought by optimization is still lacking (Abraham et al., 2010; Krum et al., 2012; Brugada et al., 2014). Echocardiography presents inherent variability of results and is highly operator dependent (Gras et al., 2009). Optimization based on intracardiac electrogram intervals has not proved yet to be of clear benefit above arbitrary AV interval (Ulč and Vančura, 2013). Multisite pacing has shown favorable results, although it is technically complex (Cazeau et al., 2001). A less time-consuming and easier optimization method

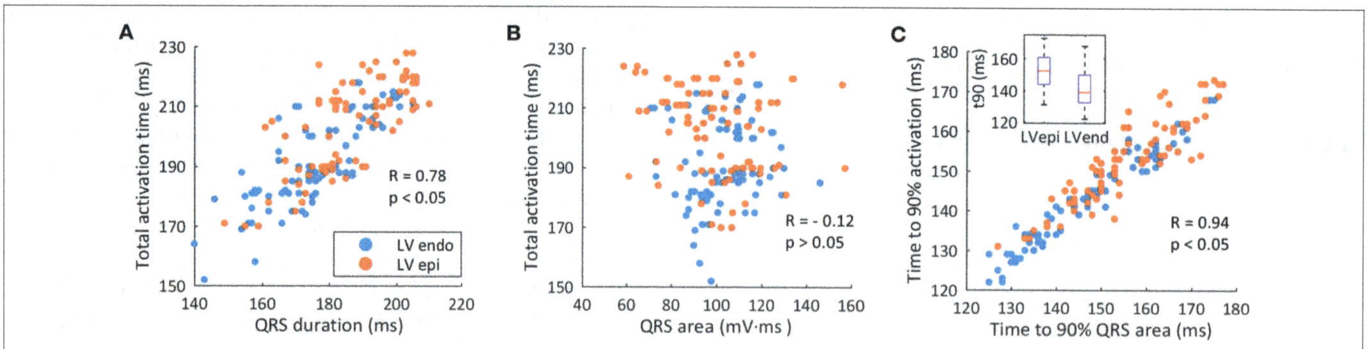

FIGURE 7 | Correlation between ventricular activation and QRS. **(A)** Correlation between QRS duration and TAT (red circles show LV epicardial leads, blue circles show LV endocardial leads). **(B)** Correlation between the QRS area and TAT. **(C)** Correlation between t_{90}QRSa and t_{90}.

might enable a more systematic optimization of the AVD and VVD at routine follow-up visits in all recipients of CRT systems.

The morphology of the PS clearly determined in our study the influence of AVD. When the RV lead was placed in the apex, the intrinsic activation of the His bundle found the majority of the Purkinje network already depolarized via retrograde conduction. However, if the RV lead was placed in the middle septum or closer to the outflow tract, further from any possible entrance to the cardiac conduction system, the intrinsic depolarization wavefront spread faster to the myocardium than the wavefront generated through the CRT leads, leading to a reduction in TAT. Some experimental studies (Prinzen and Peschar, 2002) support the idea that PS may not allow retrograde conduction in LBBB patients due to structural damage, or if allowed, reduced conduction velocity would be observed in LV PS sections, neglecting the influence of PS. Whether the rest of the LV branches are able to conduct retrogradely (Huang et al., 2017) or other areas of the Purkinje network deteriorate, as HF evolves, remains unknown. Experimental studies have measured a strong reduction in septal conduction velocity during LBBB when HF was advanced compare to acute LBBB (Strik et al., 2013). In that case, the simulation results of this study should be considered with caution. Although new methodologies are arising to better describe the PS (Lee et al., 2014; Barber et al., 2018). The lack of technology to characterize the PS in a patient specific manner, limits the optimal configuration for CRT.

Traditional CRT pacing mode does not promote ventricular activation through conduction system from the sinoatrial node. The lack of enough information on the chronic effects of the fusion leads (intrinsic stimulation combined with external pacing) and this method is avoided, setting the shortest AVD based on echocardiography (Barold et al., 2008). In our study, a fusion between the intrinsic activation and biventricular (BiV) pacing for the optimal CRT configuration (pacing lead location and delays) was assessed. Several experimental works support this procedure (Van Gelder et al., 2005; Vatasescu et al., 2009; Arbelo et al., 2014; Guo et al., 2015). Guo et al. determined that congestive heart failure patients with BiV pacing + intrinsic activation presented improvement in cardiac function and quality of life (Guo et al., 2015). Meanwhile, Vatasescu and coworkers observed that BiV pacing fused with intrinsic activation might increase the rate of structural responders (Vatasescu et al., 2009).

Biophysical models of the heart have been used to optimize AVD, VVD and lead location during CRT simulation (Miri et al., 2008, 2009a,b; Pluijmert et al., 2016; Lee et al., 2017). QRSd, estimated as the difference between the time of the first and last activated cardiac cell (or TAT), have been used as one optimization criterion by Miri and coworkers. In our study, the optimal LV lead location based on the shortest QRSd (calculated in the ECG signal) was similar to the region with shortest TAT (see **Table 1**). However, VVD value that produced the shortest QRSd did not match with the VVD that produced the shortest TAT, which means that QRSd and TAT are not totally correlated. A simulation study by Potse et al. (2012) support this result. The authors observed that biventricular pacing did not change QRS duration but reduced total ventricular activation time when the LV stimulation was applied in one point of the LV free wall.

Indicators to Evaluate CRT Outcome

The Echocardiography Guided Cardiac Resynchronization Therapy (EchoCRT) study further reinforced the importance of QRSd over mechanical dyssynchrony as the most important indicator for CRT responses (Ruschitzka et al., 2013). Other studies have proposed indexes based on QRS measurements. Van Gelder et al. (2009) showed a relation between the Q-LV interval (the interval from Q wave to intrinsic deflection on the LV EGM) and the acute hemodynamic effect on optimized biventricular stimulation. A longer Q-LV interval predicted a greater increase in LV pressure rise (LVdP/dt_{max}) and vice versa. Normalizing the QLV by QRS duration, termed LV lead electrical delay (LVLED), was also shown to correlate with Doppler-derived dP/dt values. LVLED greater than or equal to 50 % was associated with significantly greater reductions in all-cause death or HF hospitalization at 12 months of follow-up in patients with non-ischemic cardiomyopathy (Singh et al., 2006).

Our simulations show that the difference in QRSd was significant when the LV was paced in different sites and for a fixed placement of RV. However, these differences in QRSd were decreased when adjusting the delay between leads in a fixed location for both leads (see **Table S1**). Thus, the shortest QRSd predicted precisely the region in the LV subdomains that produced the shortest TAT for the three locations of the RV lead tested, leading to an increase in ventricular synchrony. However, this index could not determine the pacing delay configuration between leads that allows to obtain the shortest TAT. There is no consensus on how QRS should be accurately measured, and therefore small differences are expected between methods (De Pooter et al., 2016). In our study, the optimal QRSd obtained after CRT application supposed a 20% reduction of the QRSd. This result is in agreement with the study of Elhakam Elzoghby et al. (2017), where 180 patients under heart failure conditions and LBBB were studied, and similar reductions were obtained. Other studies obtained lower QRS reduction values, namely 17 and 12%, for CRT responders in Molhoek et al. (2004) and Pitzalis et al. (2002) studies, respectively.

The assessment of interventricular dyssynchrony was done analyzing the TAT. Our results showed that a shorter duration of the QRS complex is moderately correlated with a shorter TAT (**Figure 7A**). The narrowest QRS complex predicted the optimal location of the stimulation leads but not the optimal value of the VVD. In this way, the t_{90} index selected correctly the best delay configuration to provide the fastest activation of the majority of the heart. In several configurations, TAT value was exactly the same (see **Table S2**), but t_{90} discerned the shortest order of activation. Thus, the shortest QRSd predicted the location for the optimal leads placement, but t_{90} predicted the best pacing delay with the shortest TAT. We hypothesized that setting the pacing delay properly with this new index could improve CRT non-responders rate.

Other simulation studies have assessed the evolution of TAT during CRT (Romero et al., 2010; Potse et al., 2012) focused on the assessment of the LV intraventricular delay. The recent study of Tomassoni (2016) showed how CRT response assessment is highly variable depending on the criteria used to define the response. QRS width has been shown to correlate well with interventricular dyssynchrony but unfortunately this has poor accuracy for detecting intraventricular dyssynchrony. As a result, it is estimated that only 70% of patients with LBBB have echocardiographic evidence of mechanical dyssynchrony (Bleeker et al., 2004). The role of mechanical dyssynchrony for improving patient selection for CRT remains controversial. The multicenter, nonrandomized Predictors of Response to CRT (PROSPECT) study evaluated the ability of 12 echocardiographic indices of dyssynchrony to predict CRT responses at 6 months (Chung et al., 2008). These indices provided only modest sensitivity and specificity, and researchers reported large variability in quantification of dyssynchrony. Mechanical dyssynchrony has also been used to select CRT candidates with a narrow QRS duration $\leq$ 120 ms, with limited success in randomized multicenter studies. In this line, mechanical response generated by electrical excitation (excitation-contraction coupling) could be different depending on the heart region (Gurev et al., 2010). Multiple simulation studies have addressed CRT from different perspectives. The recent work of Lee et al. (2018) organized and summarized the state of the art of computational modeling for CRT.

To our knowledge, and given the benefits of using a model where all variables are accessible, our study is the first to systematically explore the correlation between the activated portion of tissue (less accessible in clinical practice) and the QRS complex in the torso surface. Thus, we found that an index based on time to 90% of the QRS area (t_{90}QRSa) is a good predictor of the instant at which 90% of the ventricular tissue has been activated (t_{90}). This indicator could be used in clinical trials to complement QRSd measurements in defining the optimal location and delay of the pacing leads to produce faster ventricular activation of most of the ventricular muscle.

Epicardial vs. Endocardial Pacing

Although LV epicardial stimulation decreased QRS width in most cases, a greater reduction was observed for endocardial pacing. The study conducted by Spragg et al. (2010) showed that CRT administered at the optimal site of the LV endocardium was more effective than stimulation through an electrode in the coronary sinus. There is evidence to suggest that endocardial stimulation yields to more natural transmural activation patterns and a better response for CRT patients (Prinzen et al., 2009; Bordachar et al., 2010; Behar et al., 2016). In this line, new devices that allow endocardial pacing and single lead stimulation (Sperzel et al., 2015) coordinated with intrinsic activation will provide new possibilities.

The better results obtained with endocardial pacing are strongly influenced by PS. As PMJs are located in the endocardial surface, the wavefront generated for the LV lead gets into the Purkinje conduction system retrogradely and spreads faster to other inactivated areas (see **Video 2**, RETROGRADE). Thus, knowing the distribution and location of PMJ, as well as the conduction system morphology is a determinant factor for CRT improvement.

Limitations

CRT was analyzed only from an electrical point of view in our study. Mechanical behavior based on echocardiography is a common alternative to assess hemodynamic response, although this method is time-consuming and the optimal measurements remain unclear. Simulation studies including the mechanical behavior would be certainly enlightening.

In this study, a particular heart geometry and PS were assessed. The inclusion or not of the moderator band (which may be very patient-specific) may affect QRSd and TAT measurements, especially when pacing on the RV upper septal area. Although our results have been compared to other related studies, the specific findings observed in this study should be carefully validated against clinical studies and complemented with a set of computational models of different patients. In addition, two isolated stimuli were employed to assess CRT efficiency. The development of strategies that allow multi-site pacing should be taken into account in future studies. Additionally, the incorporation of levels of HF in different ventricular areas could modify simulation results.

CONCLUSION

In conclusion, our study showed that the optimal location for the RV lead in CRT site as an alternative to RV apex, is the upper septum close to the outflow tract, based on the shortest QRSd criterion. Furthermore, LV endocardial pacing leads improve CRT outcome, with respect to epicardial stimulation, and areas with a higher density of PMJ are suggested for better CRT response.

CRT optimization based only on the shortest QRSd criterion may not be totally effective to reach the maximum TAT reduction, or to optimize biventricular pacing delay. However, a biomarker based on minimizing the value of t_{90} (time elapsed to 90% of ventricular activation) could be used to determine the optimal VVD value. The time to reach the 90% of the QRS area (t_{90}QRSa) is related to the time at which 90% of the ventricles are already activated (t_{90}). Thus, t_{90}QRSa is suggested as an additional index to assess CRT effectiveness to improve biventricular synchrony.

AUTHOR CONTRIBUTIONS

EFC, EC, JA, JF, and BT contributed to the conception and design of study. AL-P created the anatomical model and Purkinje system was developed by RS and JG. Computational simulations were performed by EFC and JG. The analysis/interpretation of results was performed by EFC, JG, RS, and BT. All authors contributed to draft the manuscript and all authors revised and approved the submitted version.

REFERENCES

Abraham, W. T., Fisher, W. G., Smith, A. L., Delurgio, D. B., Leon, A. R., Loh, E., et al. (2002). Cardiac resynchronization in chronic heart failure. *N. Engl. J. Med.* 346, 1845–1853. doi: 10.1056/NEJMoa013168

Abraham, W. T., Gras, D., Yu, C. M., Guzzo, L., and Gupta, M. S. (2010). Rationale and design of a randomized clinical trial to assess the safety and efficacy of frequent optimization of cardiac resynchronization therapy: the Frequent Optimization Study Using the QuickOpt Method (FREEDOM) trial. *Am. Heart J.* 159, 944–948.e1. doi: 10.1016/j.ahj.2010.02.034

Ai, X., and Pogwizd, S. M. (2005). Connexin 43 downregulation and dephosphorylation in nonischemic heart failure is associated with enhanced colocalized protein phosphatase type 2A. *Circ. Res.* 96, 54–63 doi: 10.1161/01.RES.0000152325.07495.5a

Akar, F. G., Nass, R. D., Hahn, S., Cingolani, E., Shah, M., Hesketh, G. G., et al. (2007). Dynamic changes in conduction velocity and gap junction properties during development of pacing-induced heart failure. *Am. J. Physiol. Hear. Circ. Physiol.* 293, H1223–H1230. doi: 10.1152/ajpheart.00079.2007

Arbelo, E., Jos', J., Josémar', J., Tolosana, J., Penela, D., Borr'as, R., et al. (2014). Cardiac resynchronization therapy, electrocardiogram, fusion, optimization. *J. Cardiovasc. Electrophysiol.* 25, 283–292. doi: 10.1111/jce.12322

Auricchio, A., Fantoni, C., Regoli, F., Carbucicchio, C., Goette, A., Geller, C., et al. (2004). Characterization of left ventricular activation in patients with heart failure and left bundle-branch block. *Circulation* 109, 1133–1139. doi: 10.1161/01.CIR.0000118502.91105.F6

Auricchio, A., Klein, H., Tockman, B., Sack, S., Stellbrink, C., Neuzner, J., et al. (1999). Transvenous biventricular pacing for heart failure: can the obstacles be overcome. *Am. J. Cardiol.* 83, 136D–142D. doi: 10.1016/S0002-9149(98)01015-7

Barber, F., García-Fernández, I., Lozano, M., and Sebastian, R. (2018). Automatic estimation of Purkinje-Myocardial junction hot-spots from noisy endocardial samples: a simulation study. *Int. J. Numer. Method. Biomed. Eng.* 34, 1–15. doi: 10.1002/cnm.2988

Barold, S. S., Ilercil, A., and Herweg, B. (2008). Echocardiographic optimization of the atrioventricular and interventricular intervals during cardiac resynchronization. *Europace* 10 (Suppl. 3), iii88–iii95. doi: 10.1093/europace/eun220

Behar, J. M., Jackson, T., Hyde, E., Claridge, S., Gill, J., Bostock, J., et al. (2016). optimized left ventricular endocardial stimulation is superior to optimized epicardial stimulation in ischemic patients with poor response to cardiac resynchronization therapy: a combined magnetic resonance imaging, electroanatomic contact mapping, and hemodynamic study to target endocardial lead placement. *JACC Clin. Electrophysiol.* 2, 799–809. doi: 10.1016/j.jacep.2016.04.006.

Bertaglia, E., Migliore, F., Baritussio, A., De Simone, A., Reggiani, A., Pecora, D., et al. (2017). Stricter criteria for left bundle branch block diagnosis do not improve response to CRT. *PACE - Pacing Clin. Electrophysiol.* 40, 850–856. doi: 10.1111/pace.13104

Bertini, M., Ziacchi, M., Biffi, M., Martignani, C., Saporito, D., Valzania, C., et al. (2008). Interventricular delay interval optimization in cardiac resynchronization therapy guided by echocardiography versus guided by electrocardiographic QRS interval width. *Am. J. Cardiol.* 102, 1373–1377. doi: 10.1016/j.amjcard.2008.07.015

Bleeker, G. B., Schalij, M. J., Molhoek, S. G., Verwey, H. F., Holman, E. R., Boersma, E., et al. (2004). Relationship between QRS duration and left ventricular dyssynchrony in patients with end-stage heart failure. *J. Cardiovasc. Electrophysiol.* 102, 1373–1377. 15, 544–549. doi: 10.1046/j.1540-8167.2004.03604.x

Bonakdar, H. R., Jorat, M. V., Fazelifar, A. F., Alizadeh, A., Givtaj, N., Sameie, N., et al. (2009). Prediction of response to cardiac resynchronization therapy using simple electrocardiographic and echocardiographic tools. *Europace* 11, 1330–1337. doi: 10.1093/europace/eup258

Bordachar, P., Derval, N., Ploux, S., Garrigue, S., Ritter, P., Haissaguerre, M., et al. (2010). Left ventricular endocardial stimulation for severe heart failure. *J. Am. Coll. Cardiol.* 56, 747–753. doi: 10.1016/j.jacc.2010.04.038

Boukens, B. J., Rivaud, M. R., Rentschler, S., and Coronel, R. (2014). Misinterpretation of the mouse ECG: "Musing the waves of Mus musculus." *J. Physiol.* 592, 4613–26. doi: 10.1113/jphysiol.2014.279380

Bradley, C. P., Pullan, A. J., and Hunter, P. J. (1997). Geometric modeling of the human torso using cubic hermite elements. *Ann. Biomed. Eng.* 25, 96–11. doi: 10.1007/BF02738542

Brignole, M., Auricchio, A., Baron-Esquivias, G., Bordachar, P., Boriani, G., Breithardt, O.-A., et al. (2013). 2013 ESC Guidelines on cardiac pacing and cardiac resynchronization therapy: the task force on cardiac pacing and resynchronization therapy of the European Society of Cardiology (ESC). Developed in collaboration with the european heart rhythm association. *Eur. Heart J.* 34, 2281–2329. doi: 10.1093/eurheartj/eht150

Brugada, J., Brachmann, J., Delnoy, P. P., Padeletti, L., Reynolds, D., Ritter, P., et al. (2014). Automatic optimization of cardiac resynchronization therapy using SonR - rationale and design of the clinical trial of the sonrtip lead and automatic AV-VV optimization algorithm in the paradym RF SonR CRT-D (RESPOND CRT) trial. *Am. Heart J.* 167, 429–436. doi: 10.1016/j.ahj.2013.12.007

Cano, O., Osca, J., Sancho-Tello, M. J., Sánchez, J. M., Ortiz, V., Castro, J. E., et al. (2010). Comparison of effectiveness of right ventricular septal pacing versus right ventricular apical pacing. *Am. J. Cardiol.* 105, 1426–1432. doi: 10.1016/j.amjcard.2010.01.004

Cazeau, S., Leclercq, C., Lavergne, T., Walker, S., Varma, C., Linde, C., et al. (2001). Effects of multisite biventricular pacing in patients with heart failure and intraventricular conduction delay. *N. Engl. J. Med.* 344, 873–880. doi: 10.1056/NEJM200103223441202

Chung, E. S., Leon, A. R., Tavazzi, L., Sun, J. P., Nihoyannopoulos, P., Merlino, J., et al. (2008). Results of the predictors of response to crt (prospect) trial. *Circulation* 117, 2608–2616. doi: 10.1161/CIRCULATIONAHA.107.743120

Cleland, J. G. F., Daubert, J.-C., Erdmann, E., Freemantle, N., Gras, D., Kappenberger, L., et al. (2005). *The Effect of Cardiac Resynchronization on Morbidity and Mortality in Heart Failure*. Available online at: www.nejm

Coppola, G., Ciaramitaro, G., Stabile, G., DOnofrio, A., Palmisano, P., Carità, P., et al. (2016). Magnitude of QRS duration reduction after biventricular pacing identifies responders to cardiac resynchronization therapy. *Int. J. Cardiol.* 221, 450–455. doi: 10.1016/j.ijcard.2016.06.203

Coronel, R., Wilders, R., Verkerk, A. O., Wiegerinck, R. F., Benoist, D., and Bernus, O. (2013). Electrophysiological changes in heart failure and their implications for arrhythmogenesis. *Biochim. Biophys. Acta* 1832, 2432–2441. doi: 10.1016/j.bbadis.2013.04.002

Crozier, A., Blazevic, B., Lamata, P., Plank, G., Ginks, M., Duckett, S., et al. (2016). The relative role of patient physiology and device optimisation in cardiac resynchronisation therapy: a computational modelling study. *J. Mol. Cell. Cardiol.* 96, 93–100. doi: 10.1016/j.yjmcc.2015.10.026

Da Costa, A., Gabriel, L., Romeyer-Bouchard, C., Géraldine, B., Gate-Martinet, A., Laurence, B., et al. (2013). Focus on right ventricular outflow tract septal pacing. *Arch. Cardiovasc. Dis.* 106, 394–403. doi: 10.1016/j.acvd.2012.08.005

De Pooter, J., El Haddad, M., Timmers, L., Van Heuverswyn, F., Jordaens, L., Duytschaever, M., et al. (2016). Different methods to measure QRS duration in CRT patients: impact on the predictive value of QRS duration parameters. *Ann. Noninvasive Electrocardiol.* 21, 305–315. doi: 10.1111/anec.12313

Derval, N., Steendijk, P., Gula, L. J., Deplagne, A., Laborderie, J., Sacher, F., et al. (2010). Optimizing hemodynamics in heart failure patients by systematic screening of left ventricular pacing sites. The lateral left ventricular wall and the coronary sinus are rarely the best sites. *J. Am. Coll. Cardiol.* 55, 566–575. doi: 10.1016/j.jacc.2009.08.045

Desk, R., Williams, L., and Health, K. (1998). *Characteristics and Distribution of M Cells in Arterially*. Available online at: http://ahajournals.org

Dou, J., Xia, L., Deng, D., Zang, Y., Shou, G., Bustos, C., et al. (2012). A study of mechanical optimization strategy for cardiac resynchronization therapy based on an electromechanical model. *Comput. Math. Methods Med.* 2012:948781. doi: 10.1155/2012/948781

Durrer, D., van Dam, R. T., Freud, G. E., Janse, M. J., Meijler, F. L., and Arzbaecher, R. C. (1970). Total excitation of the isolated human heart. *Circulation* 41, 899–912. doi: 10.1161/01.CIR.41.6.899

Dutta, S., Mincholé, A., Quinn, T. A., and Rodriguez, B. (2017). Electrophysiological properties of computational human ventricular cell action potential models under acute ischemic conditions. *Prog. Biophys. Mol. Biol.* 129, 40–52. doi: 10.1016/j.pbiomolbio.2017.02.007

Dux-santoy, L., Rodriguez, J. F., Sebastian, R., Saiz, J., Ferrero, J. M., Val, D., et al. (2012). "Biophysical modelling of bundle branch reentry initiation and maintenance," in *2012 Computing in Cardiology* (Krakow), 221–224.

Elhakam Elzoghby, I. A., Attia, I., Azab, A., Hammouda, M. E. A. (2017). Impact of cardiac resynchronization therapy on heart failure patients: experience from one center. *Arch. Med.* 9, 1–7. doi: 10.21767/1989-5216.1000232

Ferrer, A., Sebastián, R., Sánchez-Quintana, D., Rodríguez, J. F., Godoy, E. J., Martínez, L., et al. (2015). Detailed anatomical and electrophysiological models of human atria and torso for the simulation of atrial activation. *PLoS ONE* 10:e0141573. doi: 10.1371/journal.pone.0141573

Flevari, P., Leftheriotis, D., Fountoulaki, K., Panou, F., Rigopoulos, A. G., Paraskevaidis, I., et al. (2009). Long-term nonoutflow septal versus apical right ventricular pacing: Relation to left ventricular dyssynchrony. *PACE - Pacing Clin. Electrophysiol.* 32, 354–362. doi: 10.1111/j.1540-8159.2008.02244.x

Gras, D., Gupta, M. S., Boulogne, E., Guzzo, L., and Abraham, W. T. (2009). Optimization of AV and VV delays in the real-world CRT patient population: an international survey on current clinical practice. *PACE - Pacing Clin. Electrophysiol.* 32 (Suppl. 1), S236–S239. doi: 10.1111/j.1540-8159.2008.02294.x

Greenbaum, R. A., Ho, S. Y., Gibson, D. G., Becker, A. E., and Anderson, R. H. (1981). Left ventricular fibre architecture in man. *Heart* 45, 248–263. doi: 10.1136/hrt.45.3.248

Guo, T., Li, R., Zhang, L., Luo, Z., Zhao, L., Yang, J., et al. (2015). Biventricular pacing with ventricular fusion by intrinsic activation in cardiac resynchronization therapy. *Int. Heart J.* 56, 293–297. doi: 10.1536/ihj.14-260

Gurev, V., Constantino, J., Rice, J. J., and Trayanova, N. A. (2010). Distribution of electromechanical delay in the heart: insights from a three-dimensional electromechanical model. *Biophys. J.* 99, 745–754. doi: 10.1016/j.bpj.2010.05.028

Heidenreich, E. A, Ferrero, J. M., Doblaré, M., and Rodríguez, J. F. (2010). Adaptive macro finite elements for the numerical solution of monodomain equations in cardiac electrophysiology. *Ann. Biomed. Eng.* 38, 2331–2345. doi: 10.1007/s10439-010-9997-2

Huang, W., Su, L., Wu, S., Xu, L., and Xiao, F. (2017). Case report a novel pacing strategy with low and stable output : pacing the left bundle branch immediately beyond the conduction block. *Can. J. Cardiol.* 33, 1736.e1–1736.e3. doi: 10.1016/j.cjca.2017.09.013

Keller, D. U., Weber, F. M., Seemann, G., and Dössel, O. (2010). Ranking the influence of tissue conductivities on forward-calculated ecgs. *IEEE Trans. Biomed. Eng.* 57, 1568–1576. doi: 10.1109/TBME.2010.2046485

Krum, H., Lemke, B., Birnie, D., Lee, K. L. F., Aonuma, K., Starling, R. C., et al. (2012). A novel algorithm for individualized cardiac resynchronization therapy: rationale and design of the adaptive cardiac resynchronization therapy trial. *Am. Heart J.* 163, 747–752.e1. doi: 10.1016/j.ahj.2012.02.007

Leclercq, C., Sadoul, N., Mont, L., Defaye, P., Osca, J., Mouton, E., et al. (2016). Comparison of right ventricular septal pacing and right ventricular apical pacing in patients receiving cardiac resynchronization therapy defibrillators: the SEPTAL CRT study. *Eur. Heart J.* 37, 473–483. doi: 10.1093/eurheartj/ehv422

Lee, A. W., Crozier, A., Hyde, E. R., Lamata, P., Truong, M., Sohal, M., et al. (2017). Biophysical modeling to determine the optimization of left ventricular pacing site and AV/VV delays in the acute and chronic phase of cardiac resynchronization therapy. *J. Cardiovasc. Electrophysiol.* 28, 208–215. doi: 10.1111/jce.13134

Lee, A. W. C., Costa, C. M., Strocchi, M., Rinaldi, C. A., and Niederer, S. A. (2018). Computational modeling for cardiac resynchronization therapy. *J. Cardiovasc. Transl. Res.* 11, 92–108. doi: 10.1007/s12265-017-9779-4

Lee, H., Park, J. H., Seo, I., Park, S. H., and Kim, S. (2014). Improved application of the electrophoretic tissue clearing technology, CLARITY, to intact solid organs including brain, pancreas, liver, kidney, lung, and intestine. *BMC Dev. Biol.* 14:48. doi: 10.1186/s12861-014-0048-3

Linde, C., Ellenbogen, K., and McAlister, F. A. (2012). Cardiac resynchronization therapy (CRT): Clinical trials, guidelines, and target populations. *Hear. Rhythm.* 9(8 Suppl), S3–S13. doi: 10.1016/j.hrthm.2012.04.026

Lopez-Perez, A., Sebastian, R., and Ferrero, J. M. (2015). Three-dimensional cardiac computational modelling: methods, features and applications. *Biomed. Eng. Online* 14:35. doi: 10.1186/s12938-015-0033-5

MacLeod, R. S., Johnson, C. R., and Ershler, P. R. (1991). Construction of an inhomogeneous model of the human torso for use in computational electrocardiography. *Proc. Annu. Conf. Eng. Med. Biol.* 13, 688–689.

Mafi Rad, M., Blaauw, Y., Dinh, T., Pison, L., Crijns, H. J., Prinzen, F. W., et al. (2014). Different regions of latest electrical activation during left bundle-branch block and right ventricular pacing in cardiac resynchronization therapy patients determined by coronary venous electro-anatomic mapping. *Eur. J. Heart Fail.* 16, 1214–1222. doi: 10.1002/ejhf.178

Miri, R., Graf, I. M., and DÖssel, O. (2009a). Efficiency of timing delays and electrode positions in optimization of biventricular pacing: a simulation study. *IEEE Trans. Biomed. Eng.* 56, 2573–2582. doi: 10.1109/TBME.2009.2027692

Miri, R., Reumann, M., Farina, D., and Dössel, O. (2009b). Concurrent optimization of timing delays and electrode positioning in biventricular pacing based on a computer heart model assuming 17 left ventricular segments. *Biomed. Tech.* 54, 55–65. doi: 10.1515/BMT.2009.013

Miri, R., Reumann, M., Keller, D. U. J., Farina, D., and Dossel, O. (2008). "Comparison of the electrophysiologically based optimization methods with different pacing parameters in patient undergoing resynchronization treatment," in *2008 30th Annual International Conference of the IEEE Engineering in Medicine and Biology Society* (Vancouver, BC).

Molhoek, S. G., VAN Erven, L., Bootsma, M., Steendijk, P., Van Der Wall, E. E., et al. (2004). QRS duration and shortening to predict clinical response to cardiac resynchronization therapy in patients with end-stage heart failure. *Pacing Clin. Electrophysiol.* 27, 308–313. doi: 10.1111/j.1540-8159.2004.00433.x

Mora, M. T., Ferrero, J. M., Romero, L., and Trenor, B. (2017). Sensitivity analysis revealing the effect of modulating ionic mechanisms on calcium dynamics in simulated human heart failure. *PLoS ONE* 12:e0187739. doi: 10.1371/journal.pone.0187739

Muto, C., Ottaviano, L., Canciello, M., Carreras, G., Calvanese, R., Ascione, L., et al. (2007). Effect of pacing the right ventricular mid-septum tract in patients with permanent atrial fibrillation and low ejection fraction. *J. Cardiovasc. Electrophysiol.* 18, 1032–1036. doi: 10.1111/j.1540-8167.2007.00914.x

O'Hara, T., Virág, L., Varró, A., and Rudy, Y. (2011). Simulation of the undiseased human cardiac ventricular action potential: model formulation and experimental validation. *PLoS Comput. Biol.* 7:e1002061. doi: 10.1371/journal.pcbi.1002061

Passini, E., Mincholé, A., Coppini, R., Cerbai, E., Rodriguez, B., Severi, S., et al. (2016). Mechanisms of pro-arrhythmic abnormalities in ventricular repolarisation and anti-arrhythmic therapies in human hypertrophic cardiomyopathy. *J. Mol. Cell. Cardiol.* 96, 72–81. doi: 10.1016/j.yjmcc.2015.09.003

Pastore, G., Zanon, F., Baracca, E., Rigatelli, G., Corbucci, G., Mazza, A., et al. (2013). How can we identify the optimal pacing site in the right ventricular septum? A simplified method applicable during the standard implanting procedure. *Am. J. Cardiovasc. Dis.* 3, 264–272.

Pitzalis, M. V., Iacoviello, M., Romito, R., Massari, F., Rizzon, B., Luzzi, G., et al. (2002). Cardiac resynchronization therapy tailored by echocardiographic evaluation of ventricular asynchrony. *J. Am. Coll. Cardiol.* 40, 1615–1622. doi: 10.1016/S0735-1097(02)02337-9

Pluijmert, M., Bovendeerd, P. H. M., Lumens, J., Vernooy, K., Prinzen, F. W., and Delhaas, T. (2016). New insights from a computational model on the relation between pacing site and CRT response. *Europace* 18, iv94–iv103. doi: 10.1093/europace/euw355

Potse, M., Dubé, B., Richer, J., Vinet, A., and Gulrajani, R. M. (2006). A comparison of monodomain and bidomain reaction-diffusion models for action potential propagation in the human heart. *IEEE Trans. Biomed. Eng.* 53(12 Pt. 1), 2425–2435. doi: 10.1109/TBME.2006.880875

Potse, M., Krause, D., Bacharova, L., Krause, R., Prinzen, F. W., and Auricchio, A. (2012). Similarities and differences between electrocardiogram signs of left bundle-branch block and left-ventricular uncoupling. *Europace* 14(Suppl. 5), v33–v39. doi: 10.1093/europace/eus272

Prassl, A. J., Kickinger, F., Ahammer, H., Grau, V., Schneider, J. E., Hofer, E., et al. (2009). Automatically generated, anatomically accurate meshes for cardiac electrophysiology problems. *IEEE Trans. Biomed. Eng.* 56, 1318–1330. doi: 10.1109/TBME.2009.2014243

Prinzen, F. W., and Peschar, M. (2002). Relation between the pacing induced sequence of activation and left ventricular pump function in animals. *PACE - Pacing Clin. Electrophysiol.* 25, 484–498. doi: 10.1046/j.1460-9592.2002.00484.x

Prinzen, F. W., Van Deursen, C., Van Geldorp, I. E., Rademakers, L. M., Van Hunnik, A., Kuiper, M., et al. (2009). Left ventricular endocardial pacing improves resynchronization therapy in canine left bundle-branch hearts. *Circ. Arrhythmia Electrophysiol.* 2, 580–587. doi: 10.1161/CIRCEP.108.846022

Prinzen, F. W., Vernooy, K., Lumens, J., and Auricchio, A. (2017). "Physiology of cardiac pacing and resynchronization," in *Clinical Cardiac Pacing, Defibrillation and Resynchronization Therapy*, eds K. A. Ellenbogen, B. L. Wilkoff, G. N. Kay, C.-P. Lau, and A. Auricchio (Philadelphia, PA: Elsevier), 213–248. doi: 10.1016/B978-0-323-37804-8.00007-9

Rickard, J., Karim, M., Baranowski, B., Cantillon, D., Spragg, D., Tang, W. H. W., et al. (2017). Effect of PR interval prolongation on long-term outcomes in patients with left bundle branch block vs non-left bundle branch block morphologies undergoing cardiac resynchronization therapy. *Hear. Rhythm.* 14, 1523–1528. doi: 10.1016/j.hrthm.2017.05.028

Romero, D., Sebastian, R., Bijnens, B. H., Zimmerman, V., Boyle, P. M., Vigmond, E. J., et al. (2010). Effects of the purkinje system and cardiac geometry on biventricular pacing: a model study. *Ann. Biomed. Eng.* 38, 1388–1398. doi: 10.1007/s10439-010-9926-4

Rossillo, A., Verma, A., Saad, E. B., Corrado, A., Gasparini, G., Marrouche, N. F., et al. (2004). Impact of coronary sinus lead position on biventricular pacing: mortality and echocardiographic evaluation during long-term follow-up. *J. Cardiovasc. Electrophysiol.* 15, 1120–1125. doi: 10.1046/j.1540-8167.2004.04089.x

Roth, B. J. (1992). How the anisotropy of the intracellular and extracellular conductivities influences stimulation of cardiac muscle. *J. Math. Biol.* 30, 633–646. doi: 10.1007/BF00175610

Ruschitzka, F., Abraham, W. T., Singh, J. P., Bax, J. J., Borer, J. S., Brugada, J., et al. (2013). Cardiac-resynchronization therapy in heart failure with a narrow QRS complex. *N. Engl. J. Med.* 369, 1395–1405. doi: 10.1056/NEJMoa1306687

Sebastian, R., Zimmerman, V., Romero, D., Sanchez-Quintana, D., and Frangi, A. F. (2013). Characterization and modeling of the peripheral cardiac conduction system. *IEEE Trans. Med. Imaging.* 32, 45–55. doi: 10.1109/TMI.2012.2221474

Sebastian, R., Zimmerman, V., Sukno, F., Bijnens, B. B., and Frangi, A. F. (2009). Cardiac modelling for pathophysiology research and clinical applications. The need for an automated pipeline. *IFMBE Proc.* 25, 2207–2210. doi: 10.1007/978-3-642-03882-2_586

Sicouri, S., and Antzelevitch, C. (1991). A subpopulation of cells with unique electrophysiological properties in the deep subepicardium of the canine ventricle. *M cell. Circ. Res.* 68, 1729–1741. doi: 10.1161/01.RES.68.6.1729

Sicouri, S., Fish, J., and Antzelevitch, C. (1994). Distribution of m-cells in the canine ventricle. *J Cardiovasc.* 5, 824–837. doi: 10.1111/j.1540-8167.1994.tb01121.x

Singh, J. P., Fan, D., Heist, E. K., Alabiad, C. R., Taub, C., Reddy, V., et al. (2006). Left ventricular lead electrical delay predicts response to cardiac resynchronization therapy. *Hear. Rhythm* 3, 1285–1292. doi: 10.1016/j.hrthm.2006.07.034

Singh, J. P., Klein, H. U., Huang, D. T., Reek, S., Kuniss, M., Quesada, A., et al. (2011). Left ventricular lead position and clinical outcome in the multicenter automatic defibrillator implantation trial-cardiac resynchronization therapy (MADIT-CRT) trial. *Circulation* 123, 1159–1166. doi: 10.1161/CIRCULATIONAHA.110.000646

Sipal, A., Bozyel, S., Aktaş, M., and Akbulut, T., Argan, O., Çelikyurt, U., et al. (2018). Surface electrogram-guided left ventricular lead placement improves response to cardiac resynchronization therapy. *Anatol. J. Cardiol.* 19, 184–191. doi: 10.14744/AnatolJCardiol.2018.09216

Sommer, A., Kronborg, M. B., Nørgaard, B. L., Stephansen, C., Poulsen, S. H., Kristensen, J., et al. (2018). Longer inter-lead electrical delay is associated with response to cardiac resynchronization therapy in patients with presumed optimal left ventricular lead position. *Eurospace* 20, 1–8. doi: 10.1093/europace/eux384

Sperzel, J., Burri, H., Gras, D., Tjong, F. V. Y., Knops, R. E., Hindricks, G., et al. (2015). State of the art of leadless pacing. *Europace* 17, 1508–1513. doi: 10.1093/europace/euv096

Spragg, D. D., Dong, J., Fetics, B. J., Helm, R., Marine, J. E., Cheng, A., et al. (2010). Optimal left ventricular endocardial pacing sites for cardiac resynchronization therapy in patients with ischemic cardiomyopathy. *J. Am. Coll. Cardiol.* 56, 774–781. doi: 10.1016/j.jacc.2010.06.014

Stellbrink, C., Auricchio, A., Butter, C., Sack, S., Vogt, J., Böcker, D., et al. (2000). Pacing therapies in congestive heart failure II study. *Am. J. Cardiol.* 86, K138–K143. doi: 10.1016/S0002-9149(00)01298-4

Stewart, P., Aslanidi, O. V., Noble, D., Noble, P. J., Boyett, M. R., and Zhang, H. (2009). Mathematical models of the electrical action potential of Purkinje fibre cells. *Philos. Trans. A Math. Phys. Eng. Sci.* 367, 2225–2255. doi: 10.1098/rsta.2008.0283

Strauss, D. G., Selvester, R. H., and Wagner, G. S. (2011). Defining left bundle branch block in the era of cardiac resynchronization therapy. *Am. J. Cardiol.* 107, 927–934. doi: 10.1016/j.amjcard.2010.11.010

Streeter, D. G. (1979). "Morphology and fiber geometry of the heart," in *The Cardiovascular System*, Vol. 1, ed R. Berne (Bethesda, USA: American Physiological Society). 61–112.

Strik, M., Van Deursen, C. J. M., Van Middendorp, L. B., Van Hunnik, A., Kuiper, M., Auricchio, A., et al. (2013). Transseptal conduction as an important determinant for cardiac resynchronization therapy, as revealed by extensive electrical mapping in the dyssynchronous canine heart. *Circ. Arrhythmia Electrophysiol.* 6, 682–689. doi: 10.1161/CIRCEP.111.000028

Surawicz, B., Childers, R., Deal, B. J., and Gettes, L. S. (2009). AHA/ACCF/HRS recommendations for the standardization and interpretation of the electrocardiogram. Part III: intraventricular conduction disturbances a scientific statement from the american heart association electrocardiography and arrhythmias committee, council on clinical cardiology; the american college of cardiology foundation; and the heart rhythm society. *J. Am. Coll. Cardiol.* 53, 976–981. doi: 10.1016/j.jacc.2008.12.013

Sweeney, M. O., Hellkamp, A. S., Van Bommel, R. J., Schalij, M. J., Jan Willem Borleffs, C., and Bax, J. J. (2014). QRS fusion complex analysis using wave interference to predict reverse remodeling during cardiac resynchronization therapy. *Hear. Rhythm.* 11, 806-813. doi: 10.1016/j.hrthm.2014.01.021

Taggart, P., Sutton, P. M., Opthof, T., Coronel, R., Trimlett, R., Pugsley, W., et al. (2000). Inhomogeneous transmural conduction during early ischaemia in patients with coronary artery disease. *J. Mol. Cell. Cardiol.* 32, 621–630. doi: 10.1006/jmcc.2000.1105

Tamborero, D., Vidal, B., Tolosana, J. M., Sitges, M., Berruezo, A., Silva, E., et al. (2011). Electrocardiographic versus echocardiographic optimization of the interventricular pacing delay in patients undergoing cardiac resynchronization therapy. *J. Cardiovasc. Electrophysiol.* 22, 1129–1134. doi: 10.1111/j.1540-8167.2011.02085.x

Tian, Y., Zhang, Y., Yan, Q., Mao, J., Dong, J., Ma, C., et al. (2017). Fragmented QRS complex in healthy adults: prevalence, characteristics, mechanisms, and clinical implications. *Int. J. Hear. Rhythm* 2, 34–39. doi: 10.4103/2352-4197.208459

Tomassoni, G. (2016). How to define cardiac resynchronization therapy response. *J. Innov. Card. Rhythm Manag.* 35, 777–780. doi: 10.1002/clc.22043

Ulč, I., and Vančura, V. (2013). Optimization of pacing intervals in cardiac resynchronization therapy. *Cor Vasa* 55, e403–e410. doi: 10.1016/j.crvasa.2013.06.001

Urbanek, B., Kaczmarek, K., Klimczak, A., Ruta, J., Chudzik, M., Piestrzeniewicz, K., et al. (2017). Potential benefit of optimizing atrioventricular and interventricular delays in patients with cardiac resynchronization therapy. *Indian J. Med. Res.* 146, 71–77. doi: 10.4103/ijmr.IJMR_1560_14

Van Gelder, B. M., Bracke, F. A., Meijer, A., and Pijls, N. H. J. (2005). The hemodynamic effect of intrinsic conduction during left ventricular pacing as compared to biventricular pacing. *J. Am. Coll. Cardiol.* 46, 2305–2310. doi: 10.1016/j.jacc.2005.02.098

Van Gelder, B. M., Meijer, A., and Bracke, F. A. (2009). Timing of the left ventricular electrogram and acute hemodynamic changes during implant of cardiac resynchronization therapy devices. *PACE - Pacing Clin. Electrophysiol.* 32 (Suppl. 1), S94–S97. doi: 10.1111/j.1540-8159.2008.02262.x

Vatasescu, R., Berruezo, A., Mont, L., Tamborero, D., Sitges, M., Silva, E., et al. (2009). Midterm "super-response" to cardiac resynchronization therapy by biventricular pacing with fusion: insights from electro-anatomical mapping. *Europace* 11, 1675–1682. doi: 10.1093/europace/eup333

Victor, F., Mabo, P., Mansour, H., Pavin, D., Kabalu, G., Place, C., et al. (2006). A randomized comparison of permanent septal versus apical right ventricular pacing: short-term results. *J. Cardiovasc. Electrophysiol.* 17, 238–242. doi: 10.1111/j.1540-8167.2006.00358.x

Wang, Y., and Hill, J. A. (2010). Electrophysiological remodeling in heart failure. *J. Mol. Cell. Cardiol.* 48, 619–632. doi: 10.1016/j.yjmcc.2010.01.009

Yoshikawa, H., Suzuki, M., Tezuka, N., Otsuka, T., and Sugi, K. (2010). Differences in left ventricular dyssynchrony between high septal pacing and apical pacing in patients with normal left ventricular systolic function. *J. Cardiol.* 56, 44–50. doi: 10.1016/j.jjcc.2010.02.002

Zanon, F., Baracca, E., Pastore, G., Fraccaro, C., Roncon, L., Aggio, S., et al. (2014). Determination of the longest intrapatient left ventricular electrical delay may predict acute hemodynamic improvement in patients after cardiac resynchronization therapy. *Circ. Arrhythmia Electrophysiol.* 7, 377–383. doi: 10.1161/CIRCEP.113.000850

Zareba, W., Klein, H., Cygankiewicz, I., Hall, W. J., McNitt, S., Brown, M., et al. (2011). Effectiveness of cardiac resynchronization therapy by QRS morphology in the multicenter automatic defibrillator implantation trial-cardiac resynchronization therapy (MADIT-CRT). *Circulation* 123, 1061–1072. doi: 10.1161/CIRCULATIONAHA.110.960898

Zhang, J., Zhang, Y., Zhou, X., Li, J., Li, Y., Zhang, Y., et al. (2015). QRS duration shortening predicts left ventricular reverse remodelling in patients with dilated cardiomyopathy after cardiac resynchronization therapy. *Acta Cardiol.* 70, 307–313. doi: 10.1080/AC.70.3.3080635

2

Personalized Cardiac Computational Models: From Clinical Data to Simulation of Infarct-Related Ventricular Tachycardia

Alejandro Lopez-Perez [1], Rafael Sebastian [2], M. Izquierdo [3,4], Ricardo Ruiz [3,4], Martin Bishop [5] and Jose M. Ferrero [1]*

[1] Center for Research and Innovation in Bioengineering (Ci2B), Universitat Politècnica de València, Valencia, Spain, [2] Computational Multiscale Simulation Lab (CoMMLab), Universitat de València, Valencia, Spain, [3] INCLIVA Health Research Institute, Valencia, Spain, [4] Arrhythmia Unit, Cardiology Department, Hospital Clínico Universitario de Valencia, Valencia, Spain, [5] Division of Imaging Sciences & Biomedical Engineering, Department of Biomedical Engineering, King's College London, London, United Kingdom

***Correspondence:**
Alejandro Lopez-Perez
alopez@ci2b.upv.es

In the chronic stage of myocardial infarction, a significant number of patients develop life-threatening ventricular tachycardias (VT) due to the arrhythmogenic nature of the remodeled myocardium. Radiofrequency ablation (RFA) is a common procedure to isolate reentry pathways across the infarct scar that are responsible for VT. Unfortunately, this strategy show relatively low success rates; up to 50% of patients experience recurrent VT after the procedure. In the last decade, intensive research in the field of computational cardiac electrophysiology (EP) has demonstrated the ability of three-dimensional (3D) cardiac computational models to perform *in-silico* EP studies. However, the personalization and modeling of certain key components remain challenging, particularly in the case of the infarct border zone (BZ). In this study, we used a clinical dataset from a patient with a history of infarct-related VT to build an image-based 3D ventricular model aimed at computational simulation of cardiac EP, including detailed *patient-specific* cardiac anatomy and infarct scar geometry. We modeled the BZ in eight different ways by combining the presence or absence of electrical remodeling with four different levels of image-based patchy fibrosis (0, 10, 20, and 30%). A 3D torso model was also constructed to compute the ECG. *Patient-specific* sinus activation patterns were simulated and validated against the patient's ECG. Subsequently, the pacing protocol used to induce reentrant VTs in the EP laboratory was reproduced *in-silico*. The clinical VT was induced with different versions of the model and from different pacing points, thus identifying the slow conducting channel responsible for such VT. Finally, the real patient's ECG recorded during VT episodes was used to validate our simulation results and to assess different strategies to model the BZ. Our study showed that reduced conduction velocities and heterogeneity in action potential duration in the BZ are the main factors in promoting reentrant activity.

Either electrical remodeling or fibrosis in a degree of at least 30% in the BZ were required to initiate VT. Moreover, this proof-of-concept study confirms the feasibility of developing 3D computational models for cardiac EP able to reproduce cardiac activation in sinus rhythm and during VT, using exclusively non-invasive clinical data.

Keywords: myocardial infarction (MI), ventricular tachycardia (VT), border zone (BZ), electrical remodeling (ER), fibrosis, slow conducting channel (SCC), computational simulation, radiofrequency ablation (RFA)

INTRODUCTION

Cardiovascular disease is the leading cause of both morbidity and mortality worldwide, with ischemic heart disease being the most common cause among them (Nowbar et al., 2014; Abubakar et al., 2015). Months or even years after suffering from a myocardial infarction (MI), when the healing process is complete and the MI has reached the chronic stage (van den Borne et al., 2010; Daskalopoulos et al., 2012), a significant number of patients develop potentially lethal ventricular tachycardias (VT) due to the arrhythmogenic nature of remodeled tissue (Lazzara and Scherlag, 1984; de Bakker et al., 1993; Nguyen et al., 2014). Infarct-related VTs are commonly associated with the so-called *slow conducting channels* (SCC), also known as *isthmuses*, which are pathways composed of surviving myocytes across the infarct scar that are responsible for the initiation and maintenance of reentrant activity, usually leading to monomorphic VTs (de Bakker et al., 1988; Aliot et al., 2009). Moreover, SCC are closely related to the *border zone* (BZ) (also termed *gray zone* or *peri-infarct zone*), a region constituting the transition between infarct scar and healthy myocardium that comprises altered but still viable tissue surrounding the dense fibrotic scar (infarct scar) resulted from the healing of MI. Several studies have described the BZ as a region of slowed conduction composed of surviving but remodeled myocytes with infiltration of bundles of patchy fibrosis extending from the core of compact fibrosis (infarct scar), which results in a highly arrhythmogenic tissue (de Bakker et al., 1993; Rohr, 2012; Rutherford et al., 2012; Nguyen et al., 2014).

At present, cardiac delayed enhancement-MRI (DE-MRI) is commonly used to explore the infarcted area pre-operatively, since it enables *in-vivo* evaluation of the tissue damaged by MI (i.e., scar and BZ) due to the hyper-enhancement of the infarcted region in the images (Kim et al., 1999a; Fieno et al., 2000; Doltra et al., 2013). In fact, it is currently considered as the gold-standard test for *in-vivo* assessment of scar and myocardial viability after MI in clinical settings (Jamiel et al., 2017; Patel et al., 2017). Cardiac DE-MRI provides a substrate characterization after MI that has shown close correlation with histopathological analyzes (Kim et al., 1999a; Fieno et al., 2000; Wagner et al., 2003; Amado et al., 2004), allowing to differentiate between scar and BZ. The usefulness of MRI-based substrate characterization and SCCs delineation for planning and guiding ablation procedures aimed at infarct-related VTs has been tested in numerous studies (Ashikaga et al., 2007; Andreu et al., 2011, 2015, 2017; Perez-David et al., 2011; Wijnmaalen et al., 2011; Fernández-Armenta et al., 2013; Soto-Iglesias et al., 2016; Yamashita et al., 2016).

Radiofrequency ablation (RFA) is a common procedure to interrupt reentrant circuits through SCC responsible for VTs related to chronic MI (Stevenson et al., 1993; de Chillou et al., 2002; Wilber, 2008; Berruezo et al., 2015; Baldinger et al., 2016). As part of the electrophysiological (EP) study immediately prior to RFA in patients with infarct-related VT, interventional cardiologists try to induce the clinical VT originally undergone by the patient by means of pacing protocols applied at selected sites of myocardium. A positive induction of monomorphic VT is assumed as an evidence of the presence of at least one SCC responsible for the VT (Pedersen et al., 2014; Priori et al., 2015). In such a case, the SCC is ablated to block the propagation through the reentrant circuit, thus avoiding the reentry and, consequently, the VT. However, these procedures are invasive, risky and very time-consuming. Moreover, they show a relatively low success rate, as up to 50% of patients develop recurrent VT after the RFA procedure (Gerstenfeld, 2013; Yokokawa et al., 2013; Baldinger et al., 2016).

Electroanatomical mapping (EAM) systems (Ben-Haim et al., 1996; Gepstein et al., 1997), are commonly employed in the EP laboratory to guide RFA procedures aimed at assessing both atrial (Calkins et al., 2012) and ventricular arrhythmias (Aliot et al., 2009; Priori et al., 2015), due to its ability to integrate spatial 3D and EP information recorded by the catheter. In the case of infarct-related VTs, EAM systems are considered as a helpful tool to identify SCCs as RFA targets based on the abnormal features of electrograms (EGM) in such regions (Gardner et al., 1985; Bogun et al., 2005), especially when clinical VT is unmappable due to non-inducibility or hemodynamic instability (Marchlinski et al., 2000; Aliot et al., 2009; Priori et al., 2015).

In contrast to EAM systems, an alternative non-invasive approach for pre-operative characterization of target substrate and planning of RFA procedures is the use of 3D computational models able to simulate cardiac EP accurately. Such an approach has the potential to help physicians to better understand and predict the underlying mechanisms of a wide variety of cardiac disorders, as well as in therapy planning and management of those diseases (Vigmond et al., 2009; Smith et al., 2011; Trayanova et al., 2012, 2017; Krueger et al., 2013; Trayanova and Boyle, 2013; Lopez-Perez et al., 2015; Arevalo et al., 2016). Although such *in-silico* approaches show significant potential, a number of important questions related to the necessary level of detail required by the model remain unanswered. In particular, the specific manner in which the microscopic structural and functional remodeling, known to be present in the infarct BZ, is represented in these macroscopic clinical models, and the subsequent implications of these specific choices in the initiation and the sustenance of reentrant VT events, has yet to be fully investigated. Related to this, the degree of model personalization necessary for accurate simulation of *patient-specific* VT episodes is also a matter of debate; for example, the requirement of only personalized anatomy (from images), or whether the inclusion of functional personalization (from ECG or EAM data, for instance) should also be an essential feature in model construction. Full exploration of these effects is often limited by clinical data availability.

The main goal of this project is to develop a pipeline for performing personalized *in-silico* EP studies able to aid electrophysiologists in surgical planning of RFA procedures aimed at infarct-related VTs. For this purpose, we first evaluate the feasibility of building image-based 3D *patient-specific* models of ventricles and torso of chronically infarcted patients, as well as the capability of such models to reproduce patients' cardiac EP during VT episodes by computational simulation, including simulated ECGs aiming to compare them with patients' clinical recordings. Here we present a feasibility case study, building computational 3D models of ventricles and torso that are exclusively based on non-invasive high-resolution clinical data. The ventricular model includes personalized and detailed 3D geometry of both cardiac anatomy and the heterogeneous remodeling resulting from the MI healing process (infarct scar and BZ), since both factors seem to be essential to identify SCCs as RFA targets by means of *in-silico* EP studies. Additionally, as part of the EP modeling associated with our pipeline, we explore the impact on VT inducibility and VT features of different modeling strategies for the BZ, in which we include electrical remodeling (ER) and structural remodeling in the form of different densities of image-based patchy fibrosis in order to assess the arrhythmogenic effects of those factors, both separately and in combination.

MATERIALS AND METHODS

Clinical Data

In this work, we used a set of clinical data from a 58-year-old male patient referred for a RFA procedure aimed at finishing a monomorphic VT related to a large chronic MI, which extended over seven out of the 17 segments of the left ventricle (LV) model of the American Heart Association (AHA). Myocardial regions that appear affected in the DE-MRI were basal and medial segments of both inferoseptal and inferolateral walls and all segments of the inferior wall (basal, mid, and apical), which correlates with an occlusion of the right coronary artery (Ortiz-Pérez et al., 2008). The patient suffered the acute MI 11 years before the clinical VT episode related to the MI. The clinical dataset includes: clinical high-resolution cardiac DE-MRI, whole thorax MRI, EAMs recorded via CARTO system (Biosense Webster, Inc., Diamond Bar, CA, USA) (Gepstein et al., 1997) and 12-lead ECG signals recorded during the RFA procedure both in sinus rhythm and during VT episodes induced by pacing. Importantly, all those data were not specifically generated for research purposes, but they were collected in a clinical environment as part of its daily routine.

Cardiac DE-MRI was acquired by a MRI scanner Magnetom Avanto 1.5T (Siemens Healthcare, Erlangen, Germany) using a phased-array body surface coil, about 15 min after the administration of the gadolinium-based contrast MultiHance (gadobenate dimeglumine, 529 mg/ml) (Bracco Diagnostics Inc., Monroe Township, New Jersey, USA). The acquisition was synchronized with both ECG (ECG-gated) and breathing (navigator-gated), imaging the heart at the end-diastolic phase of cardiac cycle (trigger delay = 685 ms, for a nominal R-R interval of 928 ms along the acquisition). The DE-MRI stack comprised 96 slices of 256 × 256 pixels encompassing the whole heart (ventricles and atria), with a pixel size of 1.4 × 1.4 mm and a slice thickness of 1.4 mm, thus resulting in isotropic voxel.

In vivo EP data were recorded by CARTO 3 system using the *NaviStar ThermoCool* ablation catheter with 3.5 mm saline-irrigated tip (Abdelwahab and Sapp, 2007). A pressure sensor placed at catheter tip ensured the proper contact between the catheter and the myocardial wall. A total of 847 points were registered: 315 from LV endocardium, 78 from right ventricle (RV) endocardium and 454 from epicardium.

Regarding the ethical considerations, the protocol was approved by the *Ethics Committee for Clinical Research of the Hospital Clinic Universitari de Valencia* (Valencia, Spain), which certifies that the present study was conducted in accordance with the recommendations gathered in the Declaration of Helsinki, originally adopted by the General Assembly of the World Medical Association in 1964, and in its subsequent revisions. Furthermore, the patient, who underwent the standard clinical protocol, gave written informed consent for the use of his anonymized clinical data in this study.

3D *Patient-Specific* Ventricular Model

Anatomical Model

We generated the 3D *patient-specific* bi-ventricular model by segmenting the short-axis slices from the cardiac DE-MRI using Seg3D software (Scientific Computing and Imaging Institute, University of Utah, USA) (Seg3D, 2013). We did it manually to perform a highly detailed segmentation of whole ventricles, including papillary muscles and main endocardial trabeculations (see **Figures 1A,B**). An expert radiologist in cardiac imaging checked all segmentations in order to ensure the fidelity of the 3D reconstruction of the *patient-specific* anatomy. From the segmented DE-MRI stack, we generated a surface model of ventricles that we carefully checked with Blender (Blender Foundation, Amsterdam, The Netherlands) to refine and correct defects in the mesh at the local level after applying a global smoothing. Then, using the surface model as a template, we performed a volume meshing with MeshGems-Hexa (Distene S.A.S., Bruyeres-le-Chatel, France), obtaining a hexahedra-based volume mesh comprised by 4 million nodes (vertices) and 3.71 million elements, with an average edge length of 0.4 mm.

To include the anisotropy of the cardiac muscle, we implemented Streeter's rule-based method (Streeter et al., 1969) modeled by the set of equations described in Sebastian et al. (2009), defining the helix (α_h) and transmural (α_t) angles (see **Figure 1D**) for every hexahedral mesh element, based on the apex-base relative distance and transmural depth of its position

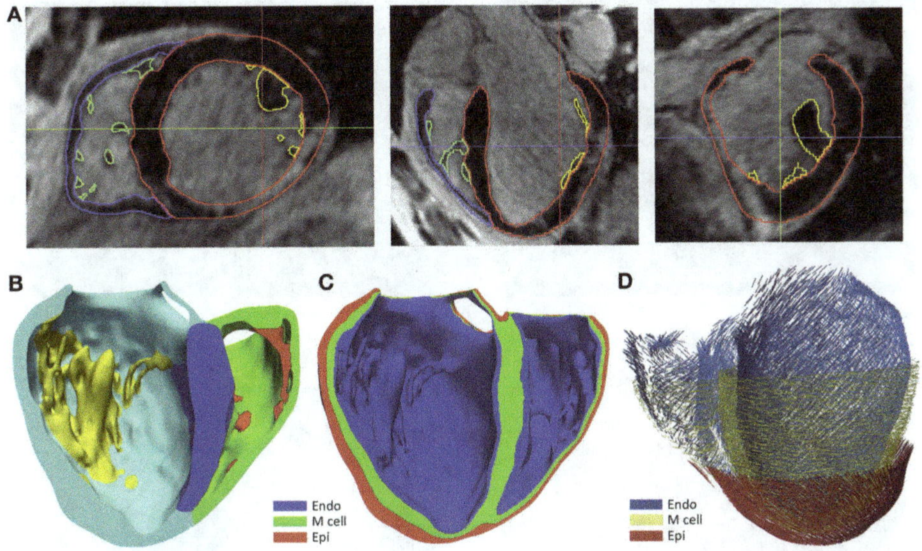

FIGURE 1 | (A) Manual segmentation process of cardiac DE-MRI performed with Seg3D, displaying three slices corresponding to the standard cardiac planes: short-axis (*left*), four-chamber plane (*center*) and long-axis showing the LV (*right*). (Note that in those views the LV appears on the right side and the RV on the left). Contours highlighted in distinct colors show: LV myocardium including the septum (*red*), RV myocardium (*blue*) and papillary muscles and endocardial trabeculations of LV (*yellow*) and RV (*green*). **(B)** Posterior view of a coronal cross-section (four-chamber plane) of the hexahedra-based FEM volume mesh of the 3D *patient-specific* ventricular model. Various cardiac regions are labeled with different colors: septum (*blue*), LV free wall (*cyan*), RV free wall (*green*) and papillary muscles and main endocardial trabeculations of LV (*yellow*) and RV (*red*). **(C)** Transmural heterogeneity of ventricular myocardium, showing the distribution of the three different kinds of ventricular myocytes: endo-, mid- (M cells), and epicardial cells. **(D)** Left antero-lateral view of the 3D ventricular model displaying a representation of cardiac fibers orientation at different wall depths (endocardium, mid-myocardium, and epicardium).

within the 3D model. We first applied this method to the whole LV myocardium (including septum) and then to RV free wall. In papillary muscles and endocardial trabeculations, fibers are known to be aligned parallel to the longitudinal axis of those anatomical structures (Greenbaum et al., 1981). In order to reproduce such configuration, we performed the topological skeletonization of the volume mesh to extract the medial axes of each one of those structures, what enabled to properly assign the fiber orientation within them. Finally, we performed a Gaussian smoothing with a 3D kernel to soften abrupt transitions in fibers direction between the myocardial wall and the papillary muscles and trabeculations, as well as at the RV free wall-septum junctions.

Infarct Scar and Border Zone

We generated 3D representations of the geometry of the infarct scar and BZ by segmenting the slices of the cardiac DE-MRI by means of a custom implementation of the so-called *standard deviation* (SD) *method* (Kim et al., 1999a). Briefly, we divided the segmented LV myocardium into two sub-regions (healthy and infarcted) (see **Figure 2A**), based on the pixel intensity levels (i.e., gray levels). Within the infarcted region, we classified every pixel as dense fibrotic scar (intensity levels higher than mean+3 × SD of healthy myocardium), BZ (levels between mean+2 × SD and mean+3 × SD) or healthy tissue (values under mean+2 × SD) (Kim et al., 1999a; Fieno et al., 2000; Kolipaka et al., 2005; Yan, 2006; Perez-David et al., 2011). Finally, we mapped the scar and BZ into the volume mesh of the 3D ventricular model, labeling every hexahedron in the 3D model as healthy, scar or BZ depending on its position relative to the surfaces representing the infarct scar and the whole MI (see **Figure 2B**).

In an attempt to reproduce the structural remodeling within the BZ (patchy fibrosis) based on our clinical data, we first mapped the intensity levels of the DE-MRI into the volume mesh of our 3D ventricular model (**Figure 3A**). Since the DE-MRI voxels (isotropic voxels with edge length of 1.4 mm) were larger than FEM mesh elements (hexahedra with average edge length of 0.4 mm), the intensity level corresponding to each DE-MRI voxel was assigned to several FEM elements that might comprise up to 64 hexahedra. We then generated different levels of fibrosis (10, 20, and 30%) within the BZ based on that information mapped from the DE-MRI (see **Figure 3**). Among the elements of the volume mesh previously labeled as BZ, we defined as fibrotic those ones associated with the highest intensity levels, in an amount depending on the desired fibrosis level. Thus, we labeled as fibrotic a percentage of elements belonging to the BZ that matched the specified level of patchy fibrosis.

As shown in **Figure 3**, our approach of image-based generation of different fibrosis levels within the BZ resulted in clusters of fibrotic tissue. This method produced a distribution that may be classified as patchy fibrosis, defined as a mixture of bundles of myocardial tissue and fibrotic tissue (de Jong et al., 2011).

CARTO Data Reannotation and Integration

Local activation times (LAT) annotations were automatically determined by the *Confidense* module of CARTO system. First, we discarded all points with peak-to-peak amplitude under

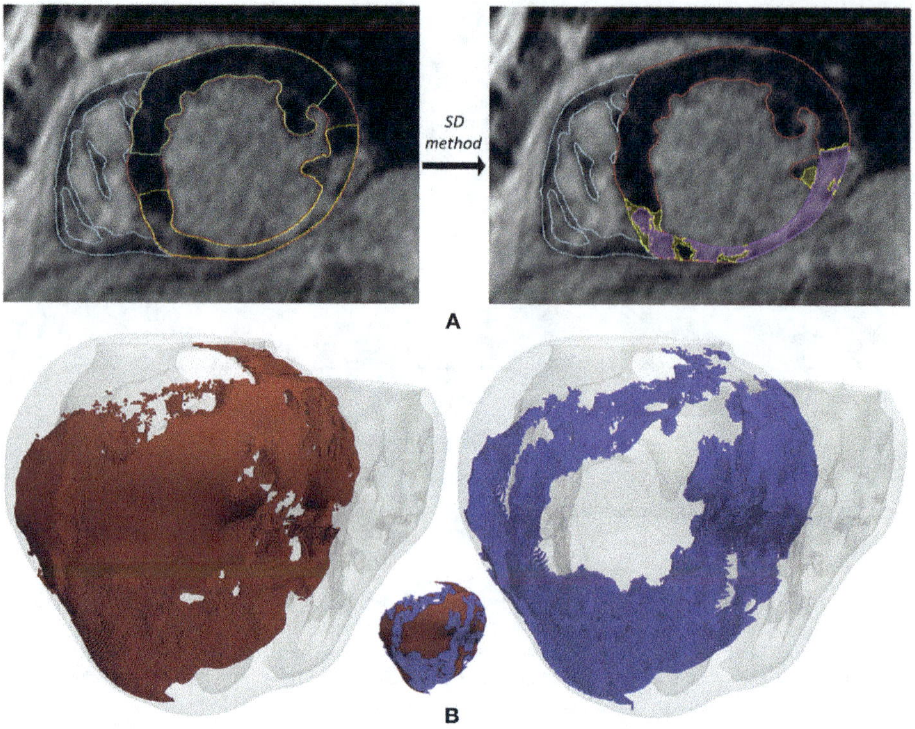

FIGURE 2 | (A) Segmentation process from short-axis DE-MRI slices of the heterogeneous remodeling caused by MI, including infarct scar and BZ. Left panel shows the first step that involves the manual delineation of remote ROI (region-of-interest) (*green*) and infarcted ROI (*yellow*) within the LV myocardium ROI (*red*), also displaying the RV myocardium ROI (*cyan*). Right panel shows the segmentation for infarct scar (*purple*) and BZ (*yellow*) resulting from the application within the infarcted ROI of thresholds determined by SD method from the remote ROI of each slice. **(B)** 3D representation of the MI reconstructed from DE-MRI images, showing posterior views of the 3D surface model of ventricles (rendered with transparency) along with those hexahedral elements of volume mesh labeled as infarct scar (*red*) and BZ (*blue*).

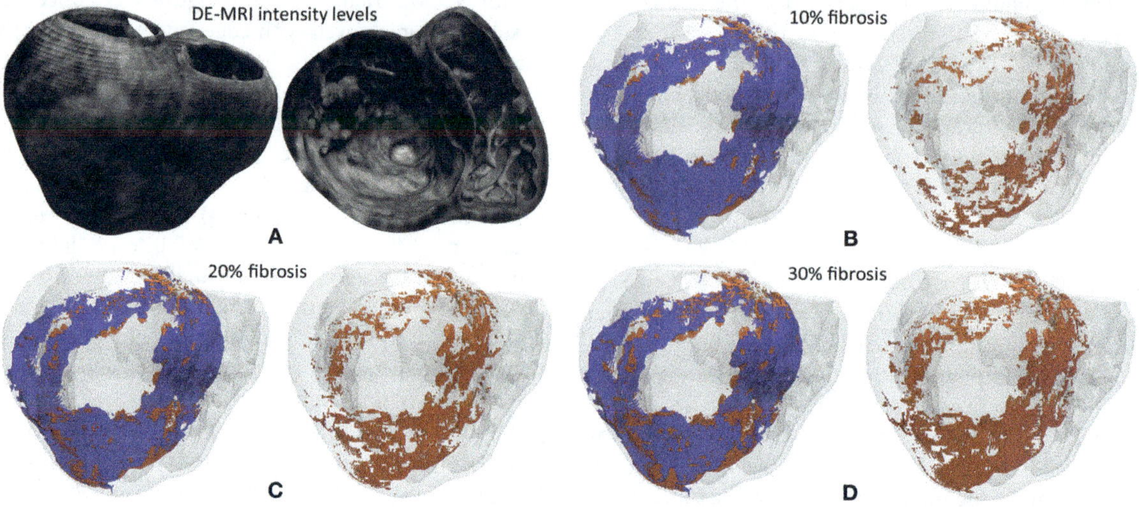

FIGURE 3 | (A) Gray intensity levels from DE-MRI mapped into the hexahedral volume mesh of the 3D ventricular model, showing a postero-basal view of the whole model (*left*) and a basal view of a cross-section in the short-axis plane (*right*). The next three panels show the 3D fibrosis distribution resulting from the introduction of several degrees of structural remodeling within the BZ: **(B)** 10%, **(C)** 20%, and **(D)** 30% patchy fibrosis. All those panels show a posterior view of the 3D surface model of ventricles (rendered with transparency) together with those hexahedral elements labeled as BZ (*blue*) and fibrosis (*orange*) extracted from the volume mesh of ventricular model. In each panel there is an image showing both the BZ and fibrosis (*left*) and another one only displaying the fibrotic elements (*right*).

0.5 mV in distal bipolar EGM (M1-M2), as they are considered as non-excitable tissue corresponding to the dense fibrotic scar (Marchlinski et al., 2000; Soejima et al., 2002). For the remaining EGMs, those acquired on healthy tissue were revised by a custom code for LAT re-annotation. We chose the deflection of distal bipolar signal closest to the point of maximum negative slope in distal unipolar signal as the activation time (Spach et al., 1979; Paul et al., 1990; Stevenson and Soejima, 2005), which showed good agreement with annotations determined by the *Confidense* module in most cases. However, such criterion is not reliable for points showing noisy and fragmented signals, typically located at the BZ surrounding the infarct scar (Aliot et al., 2009). In those cases, we placed LAT annotations manually under the close supervision of a well-trained electrophysiologist, who also reviewed LAT annotations for healthy EGMs. Furthermore, we discarded those points whose LAT value showed a poor spatio-temporal coherence with their closest neighbors. After this process, only 385 out of the 847 CARTO measurement points were preserved: 84 for LV endocardium, 49 for RV endocardium and 252 for epicardium.

We had three surfaces generated by the CARTO system, including both acquired and interpolated data: LV endocardium, RV endocardium and epicardium (**Figure 4A**). Epicardial mapping was performed by accessing pericardial space through percutaneous (non-surgical) transthoracic subxiphoid approach by means of puncture using an epidural needle (Brugada et al., 2003; Sosa and Scanavacca, 2005; Tedrow and Stevenson, 2009; Yamada, 2014), following the access procedure originally described by Sosa et al. (1996, 2000). We applied a rigid transformation using the ICP (iterative closest point) algorithm (Besl and McKay, 1992), to align those three CARTO surface meshes to our 3D *patient-specific* ventricular model. Then, we projected all measurement points from each CARTO mesh to the closest surface node of our ventricular model, in terms of Euclidean distance. Thus, we obtained all CARTO measurement points (those preserved after the checking process) mapped onto the external surface of our 3D bi-ventricular model (see **Figure 4B**). The earliest activated region was located on the septal region of the LV endocardium at mid-apical level and, the latest activated on the epicardial surface within the BZ near the scar.

3D Torso Model

The whole torso MRI stack was acquired in the coronal plane with a slice thickness of 10 mm. We roughly segmented the main organs (lungs, liver, heart) and structures (bones, body contour, blood pools, great vessels) using Seg3D software. The resolution of the torso MRI hampered a detailed reconstruction of some important structures, so we used the reconstructed parts of the model as landmarks to fit a detailed torso model previously developed (Ferrer et al., 2015) by means of a linear transformation. Next, we replaced the ventricles in the fitted detailed torso model by our *patient-specific* model and removed any intersections between our ventricular model and surrounding organs (see **Figure 5A**). Finally, we used TetGen (Si and Gärtner, 2005) to mesh the torso volume with tetrahedra, which resulted in 1.26 million nodes and 7.38 million elements organs (see **Figure 5B**). The average edge length was of 0.55 mm. Note that the problem of passive propagation of extracellular potentials, i.e., only diffusion without reaction component, does not require such a fine spatial resolution outside the heart domain (Prassl et al., 2009); for this reason, the mesh is highly refined only in the region of the ventricles, as shown in **Figure 5B**.

Electrophysiological Modeling

Healthy Myocardium

For healthy myocardium, we used the ten Tusscher model of human ventricular action potential (AP) (ten Tusscher and Panfilov, 2006), considering the transmural heterogeneity of the ventricular myocardium (Drouin et al., 1995; Antzelevitch et al., 1999). We defined three different transmural layers for endocardial, mid myocardial (M cells) and epicardial myocytes within the volume mesh of our ventricular model, spanning 17, 41, and 42% of ventricular wall thickness, respectively (see **Figure 1C**). These values were estimated from the data reported by several experimental studies (Sicouri and Antzelevitch, 1991; Sicouri et al., 1994; Yan et al., 1998).

In order to establish the conductivities that will define the conduction velocities (CV), we performed a set of test simulations on a 3D slab model (20 × 20 × 6 mm) composed of regular hexahedral elements (voxels) with an edge length of 0.4 mm, matching the average length in the ventricular model. As a result, we set the conductivity values to 0.24 S/m and 0.0456 S/m for longitudinal (σ_L) and transversal (σ_T) conductivity, respectively. This resulted in a CV of 0.68 m/s along the fiber direction and of 0.26 m/s in transverse direction. These values are consistent with the experimental measurements in human ventricles (Taggart et al., 2000).

Infarct Scar and Border Zone

We considered the infarct scar as a non-excitable tissue mainly composed of collagen, so we modeled it as an electrical insulator. To do so, we defined an internal boundary in our 3D model and imposed no-flux boundary condition at the interface between the scar and surrounding tissue, which mostly corresponded to the BZ.

To include the ER in the BZ, we modified the ten Tusscher model (ten Tusscher and Panfilov, 2006) by introducing reductions in the maximum conductance of certain ionic channels, as reported from several patch-clamp experiments with cells of epicardial BZs from canine hearts. According to those data, I_{Na} was reduced to 38% of its normal value (Pu and Boyden, 1997), I_{CaL} to 31% (Dun et al., 2004) and I_{Kr} and I_{Ks} to 30 and 20% (Jiang et al., 2000), respectively. At the tissue level, we reduced the conductivity parameters in the BZ to 0.05 S/m and 0.01 S/m for longitudinal (σ_L) and transversal (σ_T) conductivity, respectively. Importantly, we used the same conductivity values for the BZ for those versions of the model including fibrosis and ER and for those ones including only fibrosis in the BZ. Hence, we set reduced conductivities at tissue level for the BZ in all versions of the ventricular model regardless of whether or not it included ER at the ionic level. CVs measured on a 3D slab model using the remodeled version of ten Tusscher model were 0.17 m/s in the longitudinal direction and 0.065 m/s in the transverse directions, corresponding to a reduction of around 75% with respect to the

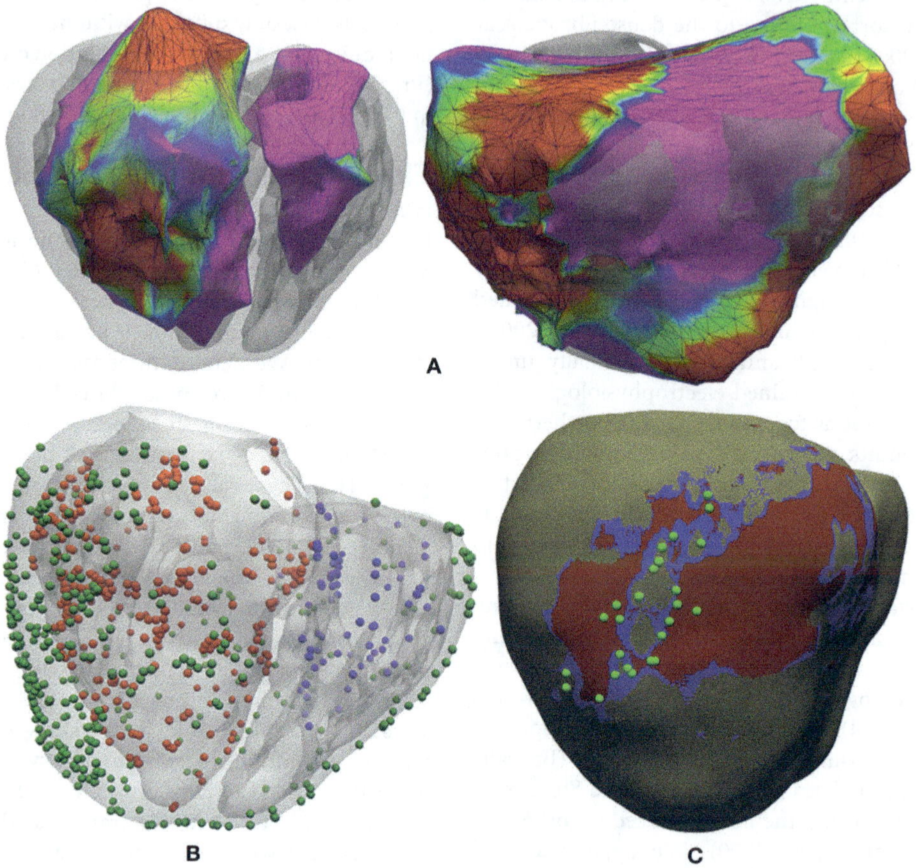

FIGURE 4 | Registration process between CARTO surface meshes and the 3D ventricular model. **(A)** Two posterior views of the 3D surface model of ventricles rendered with transparency, showing registered CARTO surfaces for both endocardia (*left*) and epicardium (*right*). **(B)** CARTO measurement points projected onto the 3D model with colored spheres representing CARTO points recorded from LV endocardium (*red*), RV endocardium (*blue*), and epicardium (*green*). **(C)** Postero-lateral view of the 3D ventricular model showing a possible epicardial SCC mainly composed of BZ (*blue*) intermingled with some thin patches of healthy tissue at epicardial level (*beige*) and completely surrounded by infarct scar (*red*), closely matching the location of projected CARTO points tagged during the RFA procedure as candidates to be part of a SCC (*green spheres*) according to the features of their EGMs.

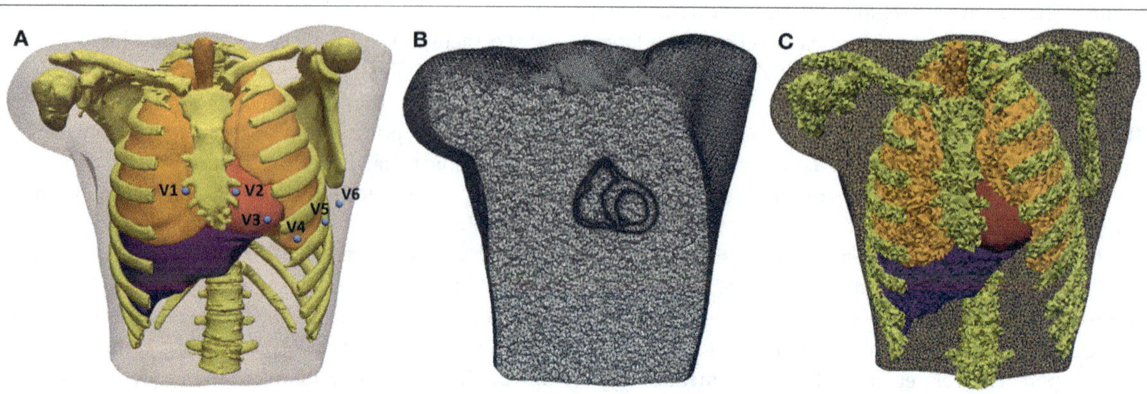

FIGURE 5 | 3D Torso model. **(A)** Anterior view of the torso model, showing the 3D surfaces that represents all organs and tissues included (bones, lungs, liver, ventricles, atria, and blood pools of four cardiac chambers). Blue spheres represent the location of virtual electrodes corresponding to precordial leads for ECG computation, placed in its standard positions. **(B)** Coronal cross-section of volume mesh of the 3D torso model, showing the edges of tetrahedral elements that are highly refined in the region of ventricles. **(C)** Labeled volume mesh. Different colors indicate to which organ or anatomical structure each tetrahedral element belongs as a result of the labeling process of volume mesh: lungs (*orange*), bones (*yellow*), liver (*purple*), and ventricles (*red*).

CVs in healthy tissue. Conductivities for BZ in combination with the original ten Tusscher model yielded CVs of 0.225 m/s and 0.09 m/s for longitudinal and transverse directions, respectively, which means a reduction of around 65%.

For fibrosis within the BZ, we used the MacCannell model for human ventricular fibroblast (MacCannell et al., 2007). At tissue level, we considered fibrotic tissue as isotropic and set its conductivity to 0.1 S/m; a reduction of 60% with respect to the longitudinal conductivity in healthy myocardium. Fibrotic tissue behaves as a passive conductor that only enables electrotonic conduction (passive propagation), rapidly leading to blocks due to the attenuation of propagated potentials. Since the conductivity value set for fibrosis affects the coupling between myocytes and fibroblasts, it defines the magnitude of the electrotonic load exerted by the fibroblasts over the adjacent myocytes (MacCannell et al., 2007), with fibroblasts acting as electrical sinks along plateau and repolarization phases, while behaving as electrical sources during resting state (Jacquemet, 2006; Miragoli et al., 2006; Xie et al., 2009; Rohr, 2012; Gomez et al., 2014; Trayanova et al., 2014; Mahoney et al., 2016; Zeigler et al., 2016). This electrotonic interaction between myocytes and fibroblasts can cause a considerable impact on electrical conduction at tissue and organ level depending on fibroblast density, as will be observed in our simulation results.

Electrical Modeling of the Torso

We automatically labeled every tetrahedral element of the volume mesh as belonging to a given organ. The 3D torso model included bones, lungs, liver, whole heart (ventricles and atria) and blood pools of all cardiac chambers organs (see **Figure 5C**). As in Ferrer et al. (2015), conductivity values assigned to different organs and tissues were taken from the literature (MacLeod et al., 1991; Gabriel et al., 1996; Klepfer et al., 1997; Bradley et al., 2000; Bressler and Ding, 2006). We considered isotropic propagation for all organs and tissues of our 3D torso model, except for the ventricular myocardium where we preserved the anisotropy imposed by the orientation of cardiac fibers. As in Klepfer et al. (1997), for the space not covered by any organ or anatomical structure we set a conductivity of 0.239 S/m calculated as the average of the conductivities for the other tissues, including the skeletal muscle that was not considered as a specific region in our torso model. Finally, to simulate ECG signals we defined virtual electrodes on the surface of torso model corresponding to the precordial leads, which were placed in their standard positions (see **Figure 5A**).

Computational Simulations

Simulations at the Organ Level

All simulations at the organ level were performed on eight different versions of our 3D *patient-specific* ventricular model, generated by combining the presence or absence of ER in the BZ with four different levels of image-based patchy fibrosis (0, 10, 20, and 30%), as detailed in **Table 1**. Thereby, we could independently assess the arrhythmogenic effect of the structural remodeling (fibrosis) and ER within the BZ, as well as the combination of both factors. We also performed some additional simulations with the model with ER and 10% fibrosis (model #6), aiming to study the effect of changing the conductivities within the BZ. We tested two new sets of values (0.12–0.03 S/m and 0.22–0.0485 S/m for longitudinal-transversal conductivities), which in combination with our remodeled version of the ten Tusscher model, respectively, resulted in CVs in the BZ reduced by 50 and 25% with respect to the CVs for healthy tissue.

To perform the simulations at the organ level, we used the software ELVIRA (Heidenreich et al., 2010), a FEM solver specifically developed for solving the anisotropic reaction-diffusion equation of the monodomain model for cardiac EP (Roth, 1988). For the numerical solution of our simulations, we applied the conjugate gradient method with an integration time step of 0.02 ms, using implicit integration for the parabolic partial differential equation of monodomain model and explicit integration with adaptive time stepping for the systems of ordinary differential equations associated with the ionic models.

Stabilization of myocyte-fibroblast coupling

Adjacent myocytes and fibroblasts are known to interact by coupling and signaling between them in both healthy and diseased myocardium (Kohl and Gourdie, 2014; Mahoney et al., 2016; Ongstad and Kohl, 2016). Electrotonic interaction induces changes in myocytes coupled to fibroblasts, such as elevation of resting potential (i.e., less negative) and APD shortening as a consequence of the effect of fibroblasts as electrical sinks (MacCannell et al., 2007; Zeigler et al., 2016). Thus, we needed to stabilize the myocyte-fibroblast electrotonic couplings as a first step in our simulation pipeline to let those interactions reach the steady state. For all models including any fibrosis level (10, 20, or 30%), first we performed a 1 s simulation without any stimulus. After an initial stabilization that caused a multi-foci ectopic-like activation, myocyte-fibroblast couplings remained stable in absence of stimulation (see **Video S1**), so the final state of those simulations would later serve as a starting point for the following ones in our simulation pipeline.

Simulation of the ECG

To obtain ECG signals on the body surface, we used an approximation of the bidomain model (Geselowitz and Miller, 1983) to compute the extracellular potentials across the torso volume. This approximation, described elsewhere (Keller et al., 2010) and recently used in other works (Ferrer-Albero et al., 2017; Martinez-Mateu et al., 2018), comprises several steps. First, transmembrane potentials, previously computed by simulation at the organ level using the solver ELVIRA as explained above, were interpolated from the ventricular model to the nodes of torso model corresponding to the ventricular myocardium. Then, solving the passive term (only diffusion) of the bidomain approach we obtained the extracellular potentials in the ventricles from the interpolated transmembrane voltages. Finally, applying Dirichlet boundary conditions at the ventricles-torso interface and Neumann-type conditions at the torso surface, the extracellular potentials were computed by using the FEM method to solve a Laplace equation over the volume mesh of 3D torso model. To obtain the numerical solution of the problem, we used the conjugate gradient method with the incomplete Cholesky decomposition as a pre-conditioner. (See

TABLE 1 | Different versions of the computational model of ventricles according to the kind of remodeling included in the BZ (ER and/or fibrosis) and results of *in-silico* VT inducibility tests performed with CVs in BZ reduced by 75% with respect to the healthy tissue.

Model version	Fibrosis in BZ (%)	ER in BZ	Pacing site		
			endo#1	***epi#1***	***epi#2***
#1	0	NO	no VT	no VT	no VT
#2	10		no VT	no VT	no VT
#3	20		no VT	no VT	no VT
#4	30		no VT	S3–290 ms 510 ms–117 bpm	no VT
#5	0	YES	no VT	S2–360 ms 506 ms–118 bpm	no VT
#6	10		S3–370 ms 526 ms–114 bpm	S2–360 ms 526 ms–114 bpm	no VT
#7	20		S3–370 ms 520 ms–115 bpm	S2–360 ms 520 ms–115 bpm	no VT
#8	30		no VT	no VT	no VT

In the cases of positive VT induction, we specify the premature stimulus (S2 or S3) responsible for the unidirectional block triggering the reentrant VT and its CI, as well as the BCL and heart rate associated with the VT.

Supplementary Material for more details about the method used to compute simulated ECGs).

RESULTS

3D Ventricular Model

As well as including *patient-specific* cardiac anatomy, our 3D ventricular model also integrated personalized geometry of heterogeneous remodeling caused by MI, differentiating between infarct scar and BZ that comprised 16 and 8.5% of the volume of LV myocardium, respectively. Importantly, 3D reconstruction of the MI remodeling from DE-MRI revealed the presence, at the epicardial level, of an isthmus mainly composed of BZ intermingled with several thin patches of healthy tissue that was surrounded by dense scar. Both the shape and features of this structure match the definition of a SCC representing a potential substrate for reentrant VT (de Bakker et al., 1988; Fernández-Armenta et al., 2013). Moreover, as observed in **Figure 4C**, integration of CARTO data onto the 3D model showed good agreement between the epicardial isthmus and a set of CARTO points labeled during the RFA procedure as candidates to be part of a SCC due to the characteristics of its bipolar EGMs (low voltage, fractionated and split signals, late and isolated potentials, etc.) (de Chillou et al., 2002; Bogun et al., 2005). The image-based *patient-specific* 3D model of infarcted ventricles developed in this work, as well as the 3D torso model, are both publicly available at http://commlab.uv.es/repository/.

Electrophysiological Modeling of the Border Zone

ER in the BZ, represented by our modified version of ten Tusscher model, resulted in a decrease of upstroke velocity and maximum amplitude of AP mainly caused by the downregulation of I_{Na}, as well as an increase in AP duration (APD) relative to the normal values due to the reduction of repolarizing potassium currents I_{Kr} and I_{Ks}. As observed in **Figure 6**, the main effect of the applied changes is the prolongation of the APD, which affects both a single isolated cell and a cell embedded in a 3D remodeled tissue in a similar degree. **Table S1** summarizes a quantitative analysis of the changes in several AP key biomarkers resulting from the modifications included in the ten Tusscher model for ER in the BZ, for both isolated and embedded cell.

Computational Simulations

Sinus Rhythm Simulation

We reproduced the patient's ECG in sinus rhythm using computational simulation, in order to test and validate our 3D *patient-specific* model. Since we had the endocardial EAMs for both ventricles, we used that information to generate a *patient-specific* stimulation sequence aiming to reproduce the patient's sinus activation pattern accurately. We used a total of 133 manually-checked endocardial CARTO points (84 for LV and 49 for RV) mapped onto the endocardial surfaces to create that personalized sinus stimulation sequence. We used those mapped points as stimulation sites, applying a stimulus at each one of them in the time instant given by the checked LAT value associated with the corresponding endocardial CARTO point. The endocardial CARTO point with the earliest LAT was the first stimulated site (at $t = 0$ ms) and the rest of points were sequentially stimulated until reaching the latest activated point (highest LAT value) according to recorded EAMs (see **Figure S1**). To perform these simulations of sinus rhythm, we took the final state of the stabilization step (myocyte-fibroblast coupling) as starting point ($t = 0$ ms). Then, we applied the CARTO-derived endocardial stimulation sequence to simulate six heartbeats at a basic cycle length (BCL) of 800 ms, thus matching the patient's heart rate in sinus rhythm (75 bpm) during the RFA procedure, which was measured from the ECG recordings included in CARTO data. Note that only the sixth beat was used to simulate the ECG signals in the 3D torso model for a single heartbeat in order to compare those signals to patient's recordings.

The activation map corresponding to sinus rhythm simulated with model #6 (with ER and 10% fibrosis in BZ) is displayed **Figure 7**. As observed, most of the ventricular tissue is already activated in around 140 ms. However, certain regions of the BZ

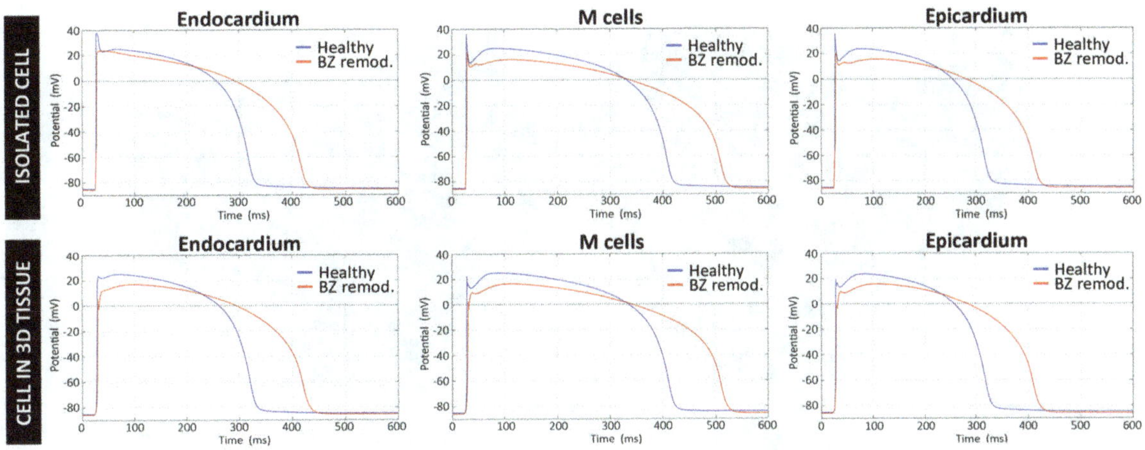

FIGURE 6 | Comparison between APs generated by the original version of ten Tusscher model (ten Tusscher and Panfilov, 2006), used in our simulations for healthy myocardium, and APs resulting from our modified version of such model for the remodeled BZ. Upper row shows APs from a simulation with a single isolated cell, after stabilizing the model at a BCL of 800 ms, while the lower row displays APs obtained for a cell embedded in a 3D tissue (i.e., surrounded by other cells and electrically coupled to them) exclusively composed of remodeled myocytes.

show a very late activation, especially the epicardial isthmus (see **Figure 7D**), where activation lasts up to 289 ms. Activation maps for this CARTO-derived sinus rhythm are very similar for all versions of the ventricular model. The only remarkable difference is the time that the tissue corresponding to the BZ takes to be fully activated, ranging from 243 ms for model *#1* (no ER and no fibrosis in BZ) to 296 ms for model *#8* (with ER and 30% fibrosis in BZ). Both factors slow down the activation of the BZ, with ER causing delays longer than fibrosis.

Figure 8 shows APD maps for four different versions of the ventricular model, depicting the repolarization dispersion (or APD heterogeneity) generated by both the ER and the presence of fibrosis in the BZ. The inclusion of ER in the BZ creates regions with longer APDs, while the presence of 10% image-based patchy fibrosis causes the opposite effect (APD shortening) in certain regions of the BZ. Thus, the combination of both factors increases the dispersion in the repolarization pattern, which may result in a higher arrhythmogenicity. For APD maps with 20% and 30% fibrosis in BZ, see **Figure S2**.

The comparison between the real and simulated ECG (at the precordial leads) for all versions of the ventricular model including ER in the BZ is shown in **Figure 9**. The inclusion or absence of ER in BZ did not have an important impact on the simulated ECG in sinus rhythm (see **Figure S3** for simulated ECGs with models without ER in BZ). Conversely, the presence of fibrosis in the BZ caused a deviation of the ST segment that matched that observed in the real ECG (see elevation in V1 and depression in V5 and V6, for instance). Furthermore, simulated QRS complex width and polarity was remarkably similar to the patient's one, with a signal correlation over 80%, except for V2 and V3 leads for which correlation was around 70%. The most important difference was the repolarization phase, since simulated ECGs showed a delayed T wave with respect to patient's one. Neither ER nor fibrosis in BZ appeared to have an important impact on repolarization, with only a slight effect on T wave magnitude depending on fibrosis level.

In-silico VT Induction

The final goal of our simulation pipeline was to reproduce the clinical VT *in-silico* in order to study its mechanisms and to identify reentry circuits responsible for the VT as ablation targets. Among CARTO points projected onto the 3D model, we chose two locations tagged as pacing sites in the actual procedure and replicated the same programmed electrical stimulation (PES) protocol applied by the electrophysiologists in the EP laboratory. First tested pacing site (*endo#1*) was located on the LV endocardium (**Figure 10**, green sphere), while the second one (*epi#1*) was on the LV posterior epicardial wall below the apical side of the MI (**Figure 10**, red sphere). Aiming to explore the influence of pacing location, we included an additional point (*epi#2*) located on the LV epicardial posterior wall, over the basal side of the MI (**Figure 10**, blue sphere).

Starting from the steady-state after the stabilization in sinus rhythm, we paced the ventricles from each pacing site (one at a time) with a train of six stimuli delivered with a BCL of 600 ms (S1 phase), followed by a single stimulus (S2 phase) coupled at 400 ms after the last S1. If it failed to induce VT, we reduced the S2 coupling interval (CI) in steps of 10 ms until reaching positive VT induction or propagation block at pacing site. In the latter case, when VT was non-inducible by a single S2 stimulus, we repeated the PES protocol adding another premature stimulus (S3 phase) after the S2 phase, with both S2 and S3 stimuli coupled at the same CI. We followed that protocol for the eight model versions (**Table 1**) and the three pacing sites (**Figure 10**). **Table 1** summarizes the results of all those *in-silico* tests of VT inducibility. Focusing on VT simulations at the organ level, such results show that our pipeline was able to replicate the outcomes of the VT inducibility tests performed in the EP laboratory. We achieved positive VT induction with several versions of the ventricular model from the two pacing sites (*endo#1* and *epi#1*) that succeeded in the real EP study. On the contrary, pacing site *epi#2* (not tested in the clinic) could not trigger VT on any model version.

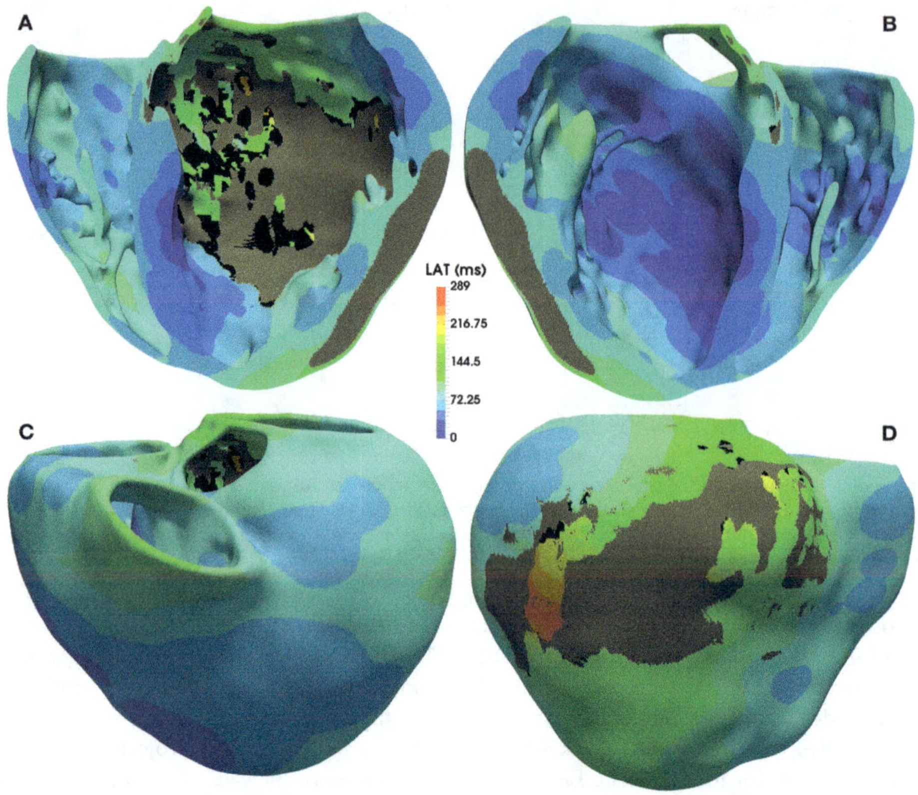

FIGURE 7 | Activation map for CARTO-derived sinus activation, corresponding to the sixth heartbeat simulated with the ventricular model with ER and 10% fibrosis in BZ (model *#6*). Top row shows an anterior **(A)** and a posterior **(B)** view of a coronal cross-section (four-chamber plane) of the ventricular model, showing the activation on the endocardial surfaces. Bottom row also displays anterior **(C)** and posterior **(D)** views of the whole model, showing the activation at epicardial level. Black regions correspond to not activated tissue (not depolarized) due to fibrosis accumulation. Gray region represents the infarct scar, modeled as non-conducting tissue.

Regardless the pacing site, all induced VTs showed a common mechanism characterized by a unidirectional block at the lower side (the most apical end) of the epicardial SCC previously described, consequently leading to reentry through its upper side (the most basal end). **Figures 11A–E** displays potential maps at different times, showing the propagation patterns generated by the S2 stimulus that gives rise to the unidirectional block and, subsequently, to the onset of the VT due to reentry. Such epicardial SCC enabled the perpetuation of the reentrant activity, showing a clockwise macroreentrant propagation pattern with the wavefront entering the SCC through its upper end and leaving it through the lower one (see **Figure 11F**), what triggered a self-sustained monomorphic VT with a BCL of 526 ms (114 bpm) on model *#6* (see **Video S2**).

In our model, the presence of ER in the BZ was necessary in three out of four configurations allowing positive VT induction (models *#5–7*). The only configuration providing positive VT induction without ER (model *#4*) required the highest fibrosis level (30%) in the BZ among tested ones, together with a CI for S2–S3 phases significantly shorter than that of cases including ER in BZ (see **Table 1**). Concerning pacing site *epi#2* that we added to those tested in the real EP study, the VT test was negative in all model versions, since the applied PES protocol never managed to induce unidirectional block at either of the ends of the epicardial SCC (see **Video S3**). Model *#8* was a special case, as it is the only configuration that always led to bidirectional block at the lower end of the epicardial SCC regardless both the pacing site and the CI for S2–S3 phases, blocking the propagation even in the S1 phase (see **Video S4**).

Figure 12 shows APD maps for three different versions of the ventricular model, exhibiting considerable repolarization dispersion caused by either ER or fibrosis in the BZ, as already observed in sinus activation (see **Figure 8** and **Figure S2**). Those maps, resulting from the propagation of the last stimulus of S1 phase, differ significantly between them, although sharing a common feature. All of them present regions of longer APDs (compared to the rest of BZ tissue) at both ends of the epicardial SCC that supports the reentrant activity. This effect seems more marked at the lower side of the SCC, where the unidirectional block that triggers the reentry occurs, especially in those models including ER in the BZ (**Figures 12B,C**). It is probably caused by a deeper impact of source-sink mismatches because of the narrower funnel shape of the lower end of the SCC compared to the upper one.

Following the premise of only including non-invasive clinical data in our pipeline, we obtained the simulated ECGs for all successful VT induction using the torso model in order to assess

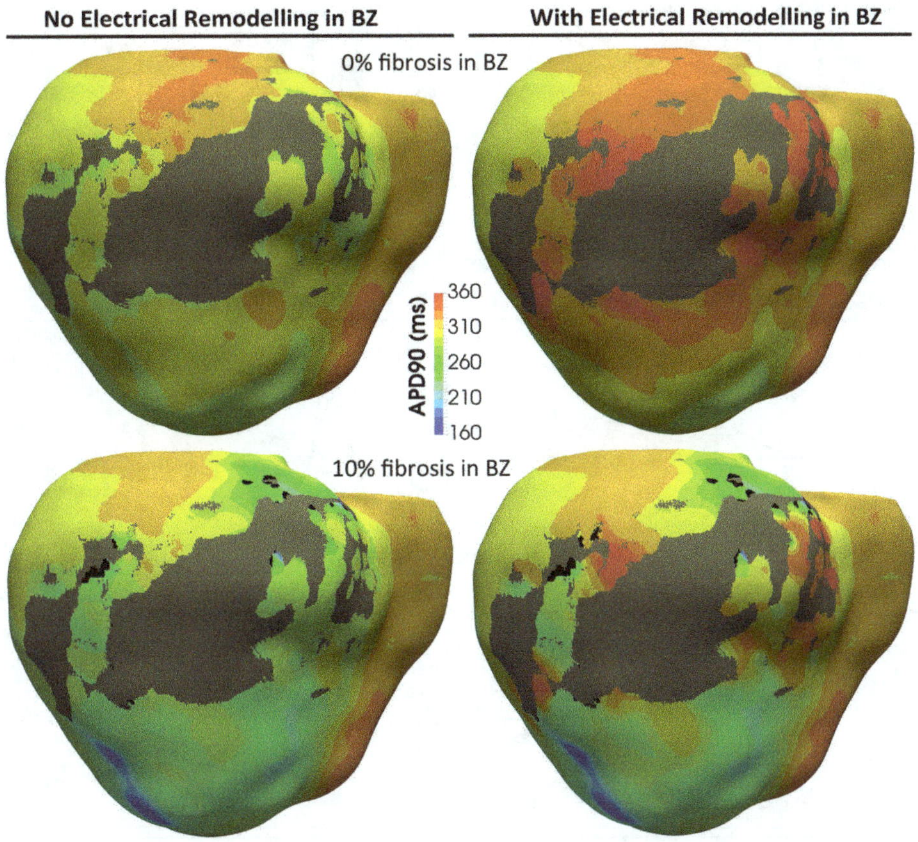

FIGURE 8 | APD maps showing the epicardial surface of the posterior wall of the ventricular model, exhibiting the differences in repolarization patterns during simulated sinus rhythm for the four versions of the model resulting from the combination of absence and presence of ER with no fibrosis and with 10% image-based patchy fibrosis in the BZ. Those maps correspond to the sixth heartbeat simulated from the CARTO-derived activation pattern at a BCL of 800 ms (75 bpm). As observed, both the ER and the presence of patchy fibrosis in the BZ affects the APDs in the BZ, creating repolarization dispersion around the infarct scar. (see **Supplementary Material** for APD maps with 20 and 30% fibrosis in the BZ).

the matching between the *in-silico* induced and the clinical VT by comparing both ECGs. The frequency of reentry around the scar was faster in the patient (BCL=340 ms, 175 bpm) than in the simulations (BCL = 506–526 ms, 114–118 bpm) (see **Table 1**), probably due to differences in CVs mainly in the BZ including the SCC. It is noteworthy that CVs, as well as APDs, were not personalized but based on population data. Aiming to compare the morphology of precordial leads, we removed the frequency variability by resampling a simulated ECG and overlapped it to the patient's ECG. **Figure 13** shows such comparison, where it is clearly appreciated that both morphologies present a high degree of correlation, with the simulated ECG following every signal deflection in the real signals in all precordial leads. Only lead V2 showed an enlarged amplitude in the simulated case in one of the sections of the signal. Hence, as in the case of sinus activation, V2 shows the most considerable differences with respect to the patient's ECG, along with V3 to a lesser extent. All configurations that managed to induce VT showed the same reentrant pattern depicted in **Figure 11F**, therefore resulting in highly similar ECGs, just revealing subtle differences in VT frequency, as observed in **Figure 13** and detailed in **Table 1**.

After analyzing our simulation results, given the significant difference in frequency between clinical and simulated VT (175 vs. 115 bpm), we chose model *#6* and pacing site *epi#1* to perform some additional tests aiming to study the influence of different CVs in the BZ on VT features and its related mechanisms. With CVs reduced by 25% with respect to healthy tissue, the result for VT induction was negative, since unidirectional block never happened (see **Video S5**), reaching propagation fail at pacing site at CI of 290 ms. In contrast, the test with CVs reduced by 50% resulted in a positive VT induction, triggered again by unidirectional block at the lower side of the epicardial SCC, due to S2–S3 stimuli with 320 ms for CI. Such interval is notably shorter than the successful CI in the case of CVs reduced in 75% (see **Table 1**), in which VT furthermore resulted from a single S2 stimulus. Regarding the simulated ECG, the morphology of the monomorphic VT did not exhibit significant variations. However, the acceleration of the reentrant activity due to increased CVs in the BZ led to a considerably shorter BCL

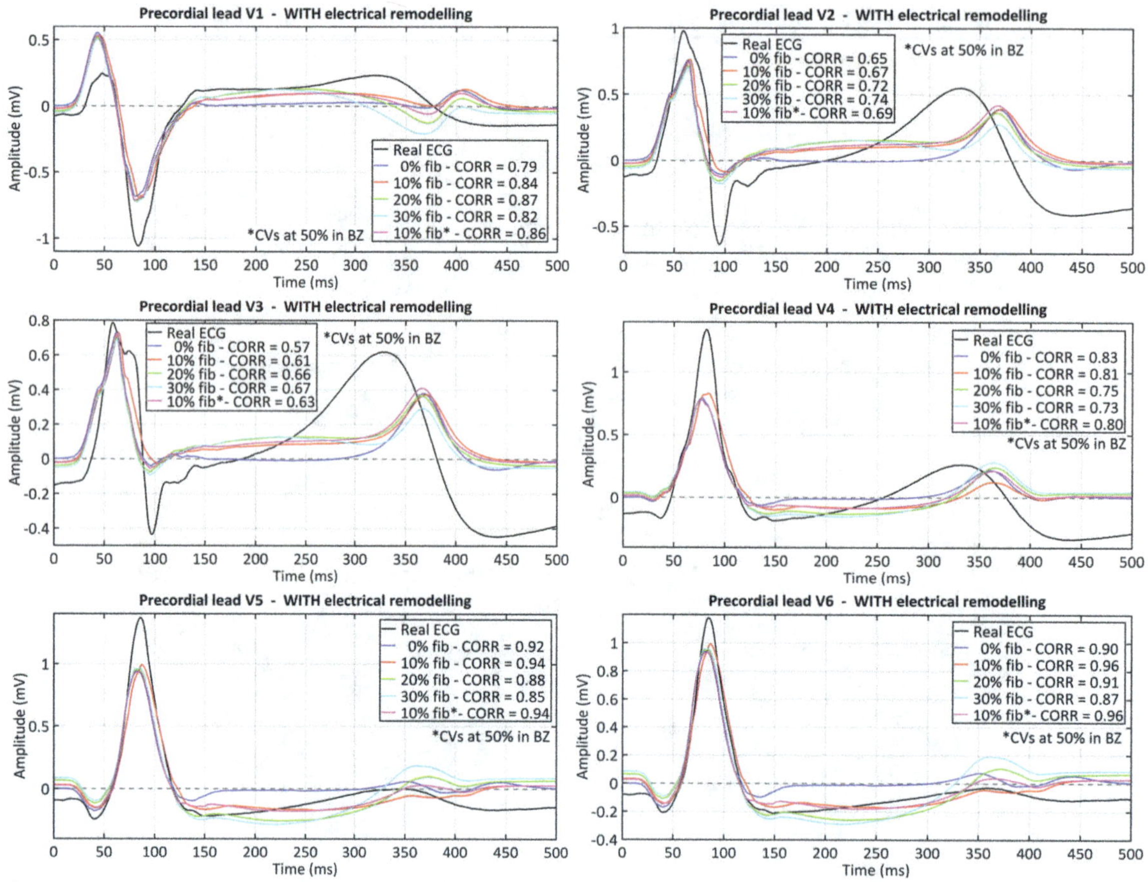

FIGURE 9 | Comparison between real and simulated ECG signals recorded at precordial leads in sinus rhythm. These plots display the ECG simulated with all model versions including ER (models #5–8), combined with the four tested levels of image-based patchy fibrosis in the BZ. The ECG for the model version with ER, 10% fibrosis and the CVs reduced by 50% in BZ (10% fib*), instead of 75%, is also represented. Correlation coefficients (CORR) are included in the plots legend. Those signals were obtained by propagating through the 3D torso model the sixth heartbeat simulated from the CARTO-derived sinus activation pattern at a BCL of 800 ms (75 bpm). (see **Supplementary Material** for simulated ECGs with model versions without ER in the BZ).

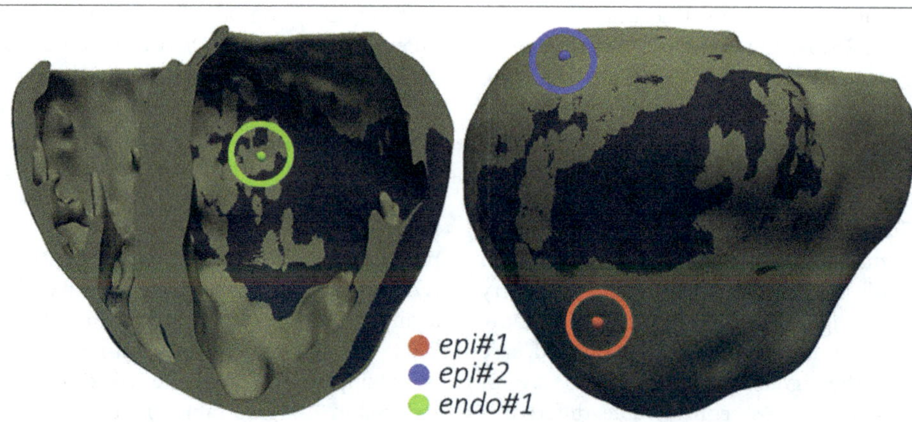

FIGURE 10 | Pacing sites for the application of PES protocols aiming to test VT inducibility by computational simulation. The dark gray region represents the infarct scar.

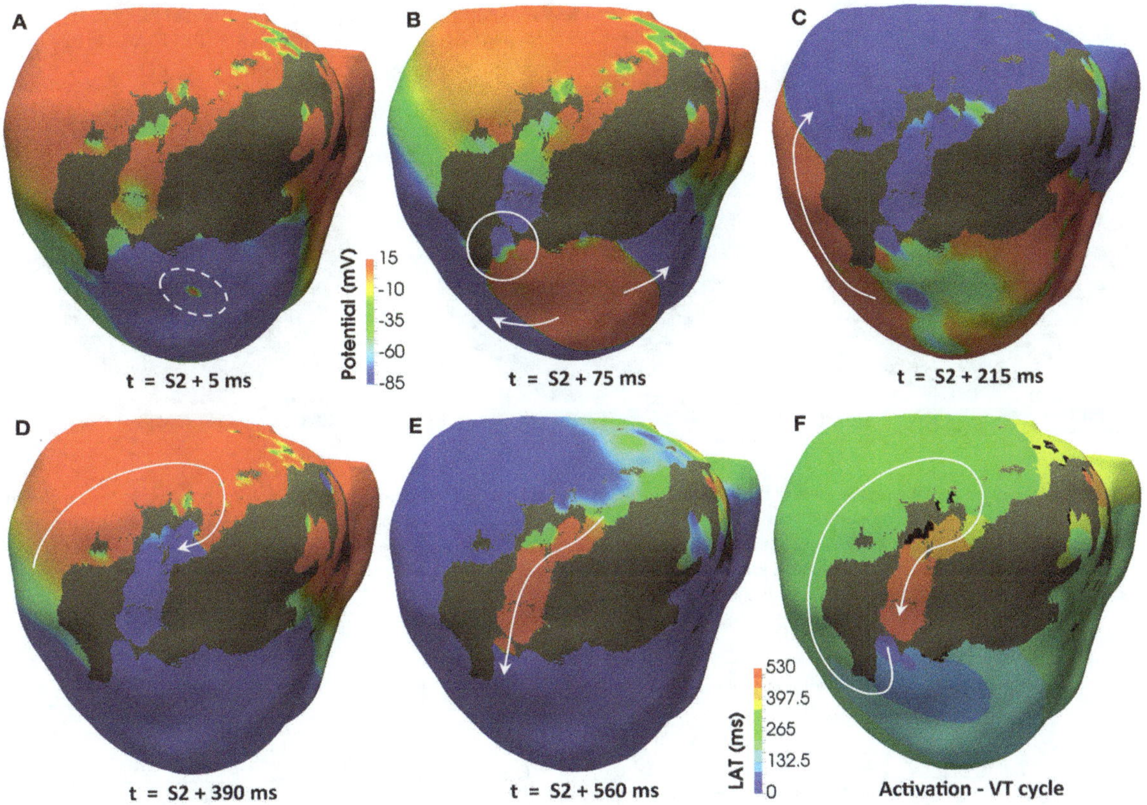

FIGURE 11 | Reentrant monomorphic VT induced *in-silico* by PES protocol. Posterior views of the 3D ventricular model displaying potential maps at different time instants of the PES protocol from pacing site *epi#1* leading to positive VT induction on the model #6 (ER and 10% fibrosis in BZ). Non-excitable scar is represented in gray color. White arrows indicate direction of the depolarization wavefront. **(A)** Only one premature stimulus (S2) was delivered at a CI of 360 ms. **(B)** The wavefront generated by S2 stimulus causes a functional propagation block at the lower side of the epicardial isthmus (see white circle). **(C)** The wavefront continues propagating around the infarct scar, but not through the epicardial isthmus due to the functional block caused by S2 stimulus. **(D)** The wavefront reaches the upper side of the epicardial isthmus after propagating all around the infarct scar. **(E)** The wavefront enters through the upper side of the epicardial isthmus, propagating across the channel until leaving it through its lower side (unidirectional block) to propagate again around the scar, giving rise to a reentrant activity leading to a self-sustained monomorphic VT. **(F)** Activation map of a cycle of the induced VT, confirming that the epicardial isthmus constitutes a SCC acting as structural substrate for this infarct-related VT.

(425 ms, 141 bpm) (see **Figure 13**), closer to that of the clinical VT but still a 20% slower (175 vs. 141 bpm).

DISCUSSION

3D Modeling

In this study, we have built a detailed image-based 3D cardiac model that faithfully reproduces the *patient-specific* anatomy and function of the ventricles of a given subject (see **Figure 1**) from non-invasive clinical data, reaching a high level of anatomical detail. In contrast, fiber orientation and transmural EP heterogeneity were included based on population data. Unlike ours, most previous 3D ventricular models ignore papillary muscles and endocardial trabeculations, especially those based on *in-vivo* clinical images. Subtlety and high inter-subject variability of endocardial structures add difficulty to the already challenging task of segmenting *in-vivo* cardiac datasets. In our particular case, since the reentrant circuit is entirely confined at the epicardial level, neither papillary muscles nor trabeculations appear to have any impact on VT mechanisms. However, significant influence of some endocardial structures (e.g., moderator band in RV) on activation patterns has been observed both experimentally (Durrer et al., 1970) and by computational simulation (Bishop et al., 2010), as well as their potential role in the VT features (Kim et al., 1999b; Bogun et al., 2008; Walton et al., 2018). Further investigations with large cohorts of patients are required to assess the convenience of systematically including endocardial details in *patient-specific* models devoted to infarct-related VT simulations.

An essential element of our model was the anatomical and functional modeling of the infarcted region. We based our *patient-specific* anatomical MI model on cardiac DE-MRI (see **Figure 2**), which is the current gold-standard technique for *in-vivo* assessment of myocardial ischemic injury in clinical environments (Jamiel et al., 2017; Patel et al., 2017). Moreover, DE-MRI is a routine imaging technique recommended for infarcted patients referred for RFA procedures (Pedersen et al., 2014; Priori et al., 2015), so it satisfies our requisite of exclusively using non-invasive clinical data. DE-MRI enables

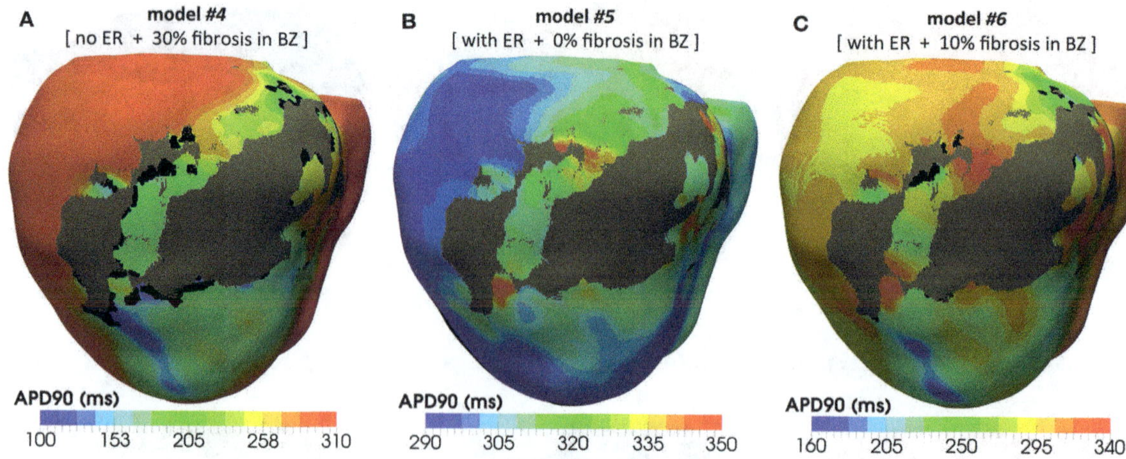

FIGURE 12 | APD maps resulting from the propagation of the last stimulus of the S1 phase triggered from pacing point *epi#1*. These maps correspond to three out of the four different versions of the ventricular model that enabled positive VT induction in *in-silico* tests: **(A)** model *#4* (no ER and 30% fibrosis), **(B)** model *#5* (with ER and 0% fibrosis), and **(C)** model *#6* (with ER and 10% fibrosis). All of them show repolarization dispersion in the BZ surrounding the infarct scar, with a region of longer APDs at both ends of the epicardial SCC, especially at the lower side where the unidirectional propagation block that triggers the reentrant activity occurs. Black regions correspond to not activated tissue due to fibrosis accumulation.

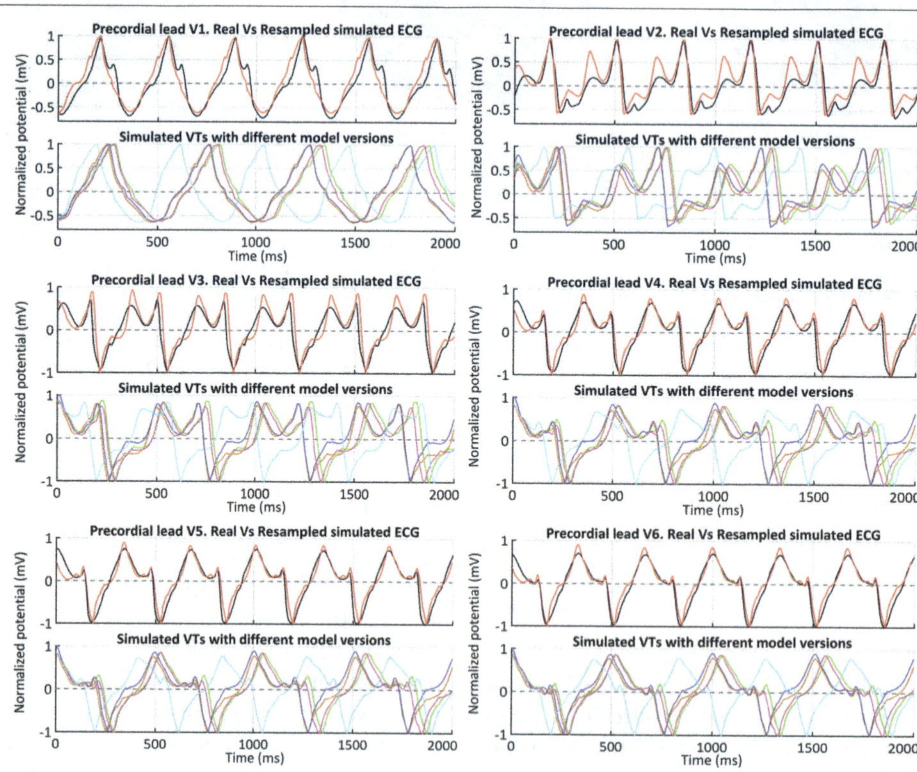

FIGURE 13 | ECGs during clinical VT. Comparison between real (*black*) and simulated ECGs with different model versions for *in-silico* induced VT. Simulated ECGs correspond to all model versions that enabled a positive VT induction: models *#4* (*orange*), *#5* (*blue*), *#6* (*green*) and *#7* (*magenta*). The ECG for model *#6* (ER and 10% fibrosis in BZ) with the CVs reduced by 50% (instead of 75%) is also represented (*cyan*). Together with the patient's ECG (*black*), a resampled version of the ECG obtained with model *#6* and CVs reduced by 75% in BZ is displayed (*red*) to ease a visual comparison of the waveform of both signals.

the segmentation of the MI differentiating between infarct scar and BZ, that is crucial in order to study infarct-related VT mechanisms by computational simulation (Ringenberg et al., 2014; Ukwatta et al., 2016). Nonetheless, the proper definition of both types of tissue from *in-vivo* clinical DE-MRI images remains controversial (especially for the BZ), something that has given rise to a great variety of methods for this problem (Karim et al., 2016).

Electrophysiological Modeling

Although it is not a completely acellular tissue (Sun et al., 2002; Rog-Zielinska et al., 2016), the infarct scar is mainly composed of extracellular matrix (collagen) (Cleutjens et al., 1999; van den Borne et al., 2010; Daskalopoulos et al., 2012). However, there is no representation for the extracellular space in the monodomain model. In such a case, a passive model (cellular level) combined with a low conductivity (tissue level) could be used to account for a slight electrotonic load caused by the scar (Ringenberg et al., 2014; Deng et al., 2015). We performed some initial tests assigning the MacCannell model to the scar region, as done in McDowell et al. (2011). When we computed the ECG, the signals showed considerable distortion caused by strong gradients resulting from the presence of such a large region (the scar occupies the 16% of LV in our model) that practically remained at resting potential across the simulations. This unwanted "side effect" would be critical for this work, since simulating the ECG properly is a key goal in order to compare our results to a real patient's recordings. Hence, we decided to disregard the potential electrotonic effect of the scar and modeled it as an electrical insulator by imposing no-flux boundary condition, as done in many other studies (Relan et al., 2011; Rantner et al., 2012; Arevalo et al., 2013, 2016; Ashikaga et al., 2013).

A few simulation studies focused on infarct-related VTs have also included fibrosis within the BZ. Some authors have randomly included fibrosis, either diffuse fibrosis modeled as an electrically passive tissue in a 3D model of rabbit ventricles (McDowell et al., 2011) or as micro-regions (patches) of non-conducting scarred tissue in a 3D canine model (Arevalo et al., 2013). Similarly, a very recent work included randomly generated patterns of non-conducting fibrotic tissue within the BZ in a model of infarcted rabbit ventricles (Campos et al., 2018). Another study faithfully reproduced fibrosis distribution in the BZ by means of highly detailed 3D models of wedge samples resulting from the reconstruction of high-resolution histological sections of infarcted rat hearts, considering it as non-conducting dense fibrotic tissue (Rutherford et al., 2012).

The gadolinium-based contrast agent used in DE-MRI is not specific for fibrosis, so the hyper-enhancement is assumed to be caused by its distribution through the extracellular space (Moon et al., 2004; Mewton et al., 2011), which is expanded in fibrotic regions resulting from the healing of MI (Hein and Schaper, 2001; Daskalopoulos et al., 2012; Seidel et al., 2016). Experimental observations based on histological sections have witnessed the presence of fibrosis infiltrated within the BZ (de Bakker et al., 1988; Smith et al., 1991; Rutherford et al., 2012; Tschabrunn et al., 2016), mainly showing the appearance of patchy/interstitial fibrosis. Importantly, this is considered the most arrhythmogenic kind of structural remodeling. Patchy fibrosis increases the susceptibility to unidirectional blocks due to source-sink mismatches and slows down conduction because of propagation delays caused by the tortuous pathways that the wavefront has to take, also leading to EGM fragmentation due to impaired activation (de Bakker et al., 2005; de Jong et al., 2011; Nguyen et al., 2014; Dhanjal et al., 2017). According to histological observations, it is widely assumed that voxels showing intermediate intensity levels in DE-MRI images, usually classified as BZ, correspond to a mixture of myocytes and fibrotic tissue (Hsu et al., 2006; Schuleri et al., 2009; Varga-Szemes et al., 2016). Consequently, we assumed that voxels in the BZ showing the highest intensity levels in the images probably correspond to pieces of myocardium having a high percentage of fibrotic tissue. Here, the intensity level of each DE-MRI voxel was mapped into a cluster of hexahedral elements in the volume mesh of ventricular model. This, along with the fact that the brightest voxels in the BZ are usually surrounded by others with similar intensities, makes our image-based method to generate patches within the BZ (see **Figure 3**), resulting in a pattern of patchy fibrosis similar to that observed in histological examinations (Schuleri et al., 2009; Rutherford et al., 2012). Finally, we defined image-based fibrosis up to 30% of the BZ (represented by the MacCannell model), since larger levels generated fibrotic barriers completely blocking the electrical propagation inside the epicardial SCC responsible for the VT, as for instance in the case of model *#8* described above. A recent study used a similar approach to include realistic fibrosis patterns based on DE-MRI images, although in that case the aim was to assess the influence of several strategies of fibrosis modeling on atrial fibrillation dynamics using a 3D model of human left atrium (Roney et al., 2016).

Regarding myocyte-fibroblast coupling, there is experimental evidence of the existence of this kind of heterocellular coupling via gap junctions in the remodeled myocardium resulting from MI (Camelliti et al., 2004; Schwab et al., 2013; Mahoney et al., 2016), as well as by tunneling nanotubes (Quinn et al., 2016). However, there is a lack of experimental studies focused on the characterization of myocyte-fibroblast coupling in the BZ of chronic MIs in terms of density and distribution of functional gap junctions connecting both types of cells (Ongstad and Kohl, 2016). Hence, magnitude and anisotropy of the electrotonic load caused by myocyte-fibroblast coupling in the BZ remain undetermined. Finally, we decided to consider this influence by means of a fibroblast model (MacCannell et al., 2007) and a conductivity value set for fibrotic tissue that mainly affects the myocyte-fibroblast coupling within the BZ by modulating the electrotonic interaction between both cell types.

Besides fibrosis, we also considered the ER in the viable but altered myocardium corresponding to the BZ that surrounds the infarct scar. However, it must be noted that all changes affecting ionic channels considered for the BZ are based on experiments with cells harvested from epicardial BZ of canine hearts (Pu and Boyden, 1997; Jiang et al., 2000; Dun et al., 2004). As recently discussed elsewhere (Connolly and Bishop, 2016), it is unclear to what extent such data are representative of the ER in BZ of human hearts. The presence of epicardial collateral circulation in canine hearts, not present in humans, is known to influence the formation of the epicardial BZ in dogs (Ursell et al., 1985; Schaper et al., 1988), which could give rise to functional differences with respect to the surviving myocytes in human BZ. On the other hand, all of those experimental studies (Pu and Boyden, 1997; Jiang et al., 2000; Dun et al., 2004) were performed a few days after the coronary occlusion, still in the healing phase of the MI rather than in its chronic stage (see Mendonca Costa et al., 2018 for a recent review). Nevertheless, these data have been widely used in previous studies (McDowell et al., 2011; Rantner et al., 2012; Arevalo et al., 2013; Ashikaga et al., 2013; Ringenberg et al., 2014; Deng et al., 2015; Hill et al., 2016) due to the lack of experimental data for ER in the BZ of chronically infarcted human hearts.

Our simulation results showed that VT inducibility was strongly related to slow conduction and APD heterogeneity in the BZ (including the SCC). Slow conduction in BZ is widely considered as a key factor in promoting reentry through SCC crossing the infarct scar, as it allows the working myocardium at the other side to recover its excitability before the arrival of the wavefront coming from the channel (Lazzara and Scherlag, 1984; de Bakker et al., 1993; Nguyen et al., 2014). However, the underlying mechanisms of this reduction in CVs still remain unclear, leading to a lack of consensus on the proper way to model it computationally. Some authors have reduced drastically only the transversal CV (McDowell et al., 2011; Deng et al., 2015). This approach could represent the severe reduction measured in gap junctional conductance in canine BZs only in the transverse direction (Yao et al., 2003) and/or the loss of side-to-side coupling between adjacent layers of myocytes due to the isolating effect of infiltrated fibrotic tissue (Spach and Boineau, 1997). Rutherford *et al.* managed to induce reentry in wedge models of infarcted myocardium due to the propagation delays exclusively caused by dense fibrosis (collagen) infiltrated within the BZ (Rutherford et al., 2012). Downregulation and lateralization of connexin 43 (i.e., gap junctions) have been also reported in the BZ (Smith et al., 1991; Severs et al., 2008). Downregulation of connexin 43 could result in an isotropic reduction of CV and its lateralization would exacerbate this effect in the longitudinal direction while keeping or even increasing transversal CV. Nonetheless, part of lateralized gap junctions of remodeled cardiomyocytes in the BZ are thought to be non-functional (Matsushita et al., 1999). Regarding tissue architecture, both DTI (diffusion tensor imaging) (Wu et al., 2006; Winklhofer et al., 2014) and histological preparations (Rutherford et al., 2012; Tschabrunn et al., 2016) have revealed fiber disarray within the BZ that consequently involves alterations in tissue anisotropy. Conversely, a recent study based on very high-resolution DTI observed good preservation of normal fiber orientation patterns in chronically infarcted regions of porcine and human hearts (Pashakhanloo et al., 2017). In conclusion, the slowed conduction in the BZ seems to derive from a complex combination of structural, electrical and gap junction remodeling that is not well-understood yet (de Bakker, 2017). In our case, aiming to reproduce macroscopically the global effect of all those combined factors affecting the propagation and promoting the reentrant activity, and in addition to the image-based patchy fibrosis, we imposed an isotropic reduction of CVs in the BZ as recently done by others (Ringenberg et al., 2014; Hill et al., 2016), testing reductions of 75, 50, and 25% for both longitudinal and transversal CVs with respect to the healthy myocardium.

Sinus Rhythm Simulation

Regarding the personalization of cardiac activation, other authors have exploited EAMs to personalize electrical propagation in simplified models by adapting the so-called apparent conductivities (Chinchapatnam et al., 2008; Relan et al., 2011; Chen et al., 2016). Since we excluded invasively recorded data from our pipeline, we just benefited from CARTO data to validate the full 3D model (ventricles-torso set) in sinus rhythm by means of the simulated ECG resulting from the activation pattern provided by endocardial EAMs. The main limitations of EAMs are the lack of accurate automatic tools to fit the data to a 3D model and to annotate LATs, especially in regions showing pathological EGMs due to the presence of fibrosis and scarred tissue. The myocardium affected by the MI (scar and BZ) is the most thoroughly mapped region aiming to find SCCs across the scar as potential substrates for reentry (Soejima et al., 2002; Baldinger et al., 2016; Pokorney et al., 2016). However, in that region most of EGMs show low amplitude and/or very fragmented signals (Gardner et al., 1985; Bogun et al., 2005; Aliot et al., 2009). That is why we had to exclude such a large amount of CARTO points: 462 points removed out of 847 included in the original CARTO data. In this regard, new multi-array catheters, such as *PentaRay* for CARTO system (Biosense Webster, Inc., Diamond Bar, CA, USA) or *IntellaMap Orion* for Rhythmia system (Boston Scientific, Marlborough, MA, USA) (Mantziari et al., 2015), are currently helping to acquire less noisy and much denser maps. Despite current limitations, including the uncertainty in LAT annotations, our whole-body level approach allowed obtaining ECGs in sinus rhythm where precordial leads showed a good signal correlation with real ECGs (between 80 and 96% for V1, V4, V5, and V6), as well as a similar R-wave progression (see **Figure 9**). This, along with the good agreement in QRS complex duration, indicates that chosen values for CVs in healthy myocardium and for conductivities of organs and structures in torso model are within a proper range. Moreover, the coincidence in T wave polarity between real and simulated ECGs (except for V1) suggests an appropriate definition of transmural layers, since transmural heterogeneity is known to have a great influence on the repolarization phase in organ-level simulations (Okada et al., 2011; Perotti et al., 2015). As observed in **Figure 9**, simulated signals for V2 and V3 are the leads that show most notable differences compared to real ECG, not only in the repolarization phase but also in QRS complex, as real ECG shows a prominent negative S wave that simulations could not properly reproduce. This might be partially caused by the fact that in the EP laboratory a pad for defibrillation shocks is usually fixed on the left side of patient's chest, forcing the relocation of V2 and (sometimes) V3 electrodes away from their standard positions. Hence, since we placed the virtual electrodes for simulated ECG on the standard position of precordial leads (see **Figure 5**), this is likely to be an important error source specifically affecting V2 and V3. Moreover, considering that V2 and V3 were also the most different signals obtained from simulated VTs compared to the real ECG (see **Figure 13**), it seems highly probable that V2 and V3 electrodes were not placed in its standard positions in the EP laboratory. In conclusion, we consider this reproduction of the patient's ECG for sinus activation is an important step for the validation of our pipeline, even though it is usually omitted in other studies that also aim for planning of RFA interventions.

In-silico VT Induction

The results of our simulation pipeline for *in-silico* tests of VT inducibility suggest that, in the presence of a SCC with slowed conduction, a key factor to cause a unidirectional block able to trigger a reentrant VT is the repolarization dispersion due to APD heterogeneity, as observed in **Figure 12**. In models *#5–7* such APD heterogeneity (see **Figures 12B,C**) comes from the increased APD associated with the ER in the BZ (see **Figure 6**), even causing permanent blocks when combined with high fibrosis levels (model *#8*). Nevertheless, in model *#4*, the APD heterogeneity responsible for the unidirectional block is exclusively caused by the presence of patchy fibrosis within the BZ, which by contrast gives rise to patches of tissue with decreased APD because of myocyte-fibroblast interactions (**Figure 12A**). This explains the need of a shorter CI to induce VT in model *#4* compared to those versions including ER in the BZ (see **Table 1**). On the other hand, the complete failure of pacing site *epi#2*, along with the fact that models *#4* and *#5* allowed positive VT induction from *epi#1* but not from *endo#1*, gives evidence of the important influence of the location of pacing sites on the result of VT inducibility tests and even on the morphology of induced VTs. If PES protocol delivered from *epi#2* had been able to cause a unidirectional block at the upper end of the epicardial SCC, for instance, the morphology of the resulting monomorphic VT would have been different. In such a case, macroreentry would show a counterclockwise propagation pattern that, consequently, would alter the morphology of the ECG during the VT episode. Nonetheless, not only the location of pacing sites but also the geometry of the SCC seems to have an essential role in VT mechanisms, what might be the reason for which in our model propagation blocks occur at the lower side of the SCC but never at the upper one. In our case, the lower end of the SCC is narrower than the upper (see **Figure 11**), which makes it more prone to functional propagation blocks due to source-sink mismatches caused by abrupt changes in the geometry of excitable tissue (Connolly et al., 2015; Ciaccio et al., 2018). With respect to the tests performed with different conductivities, simulation results confirm the great impact of CVs in the BZ both on the initiation mechanisms and on the frequency of infarct-related reentrant VTs.

Therefore, according to our simulation results, derived from a unique MI geometry, the most influential factors in promoting reentrant infarct-related VTs are the reduction of CVs and APD heterogeneity (repolarization dispersion) in the BZ, either caused by ER (model *#5*) or by the presence of fibrosis (model *#4*), as well as by the combination of both kinds of remodeling (structural and ER) (models *#6–7*). However, our results suggest that arrhythmogenicity is more strongly correlated with ER than with fibrosis in the BZ. Only in one case (model *#4* paced from point *epi#1*) we managed to induce VT in the absence of ER, requiring a high fibrosis level (30%) to create an APD heterogeneity enough to promote a unidirectional propagation block (**Figure 12A**), in combination with a shorter CI for premature stimulus. This is in agreement with that observed in Arevalo et al. (2013) and recently discussed in Trayanova et al. (2017), whose authors concluded that the presence of fibrosis in the BZ is not a necessary element in order to predict reentrant circuits by means of cardiac computational models, as long as ER in BZ is considered. Focusing on model versions including ER (models *#5–8*), moderate levels of patchy fibrosis in the BZ are thought to facilitate the initiation of VTs, as in the case of models *#6* (10%) and *#7* (20%) paced from point *endo#1* (see **Video S6**). However, elevated levels appear to prevent from VT mechanisms, as observed in model *#8* (30%), where the formation of a permanent bidirectional block avoids the self-sustained reentry and, consequently, the VT. This matches the conclusions reached in McDowell et al. (2011), where the authors observed an increased risk of infarct-related VTs for intermediate levels of diffuse fibrosis randomly distributed within the BZ, as well as a protective role against VT derived from higher levels. Hence, our approach of image-based patchy fibrosis seems to have a similar impact on infarct-related VT mechanisms.

Although the morphology of the signals of simulated ECG is highly similar to that of clinical VT (only V2 and V3 show notable differences, probably due to inaccurate electrode location) (see **Figure 13**), the BCL of *in-silico* induced reentry is larger than the patient's one, thus resulting in a slower VT. We think it is due to differences in CVs in the BZ and, consequently, in the epicardial SCC supporting the reentry, where the model is likely to conduct slower than the real case. When we increased CVs in the BZ up to 75% with respect to healthy tissue (i.e., a reduction of 25%), we could not induce VT because premature stimuli (S2–S3) stopped propagating at a CI too short to produce the functional block at the SCC entrance. The faster the propagation, the shorter the CI needed to generate a wavefront able to reach the SCC entrance within the time window in which its tissue is vulnerable to functional blocks. On the other hand, in the simulated ECGs in sinus rhythm we observed a delayed repolarization with respect to the patient's ECG (**Figure 9**), something that suggests that APDs in our model are larger than the patient's ones. We did not include the personalization of any parameter relative to cardiac EP in the design of our pipeline. However, we hypothesize that the choice of an ionic model with a basal APD shorter than ten Tusscher's one probably might allow inducing a reentry with a shorter CI for premature stimuli in spite of relatively high CVs in the BZ, triggering a reentry with a shorter BCL and, thus, a faster VT. Hence, we believe that including in our pipeline a coarse personalization of the APD based on the features of patient's ECG in sinus rhythm, as well as for CVs in healthy myocardium, could improve the performance of our approach. Although there are a few precedents in this regard (Relan et al., 2011; Chen et al., 2016; Gillette et al., 2018), further studies should be conducted in order to test such hypothesis.

As in this work, the ability to reproduce infarct-related VTs by means of image-based human cardiac computational models has been demonstrated in a number of previous studies (Relan et al., 2011; Ashikaga et al., 2013; Ringenberg et al., 2014; Arevalo et al., 2016; Chen et al., 2016; Deng et al., 2016; Prakosa et al., 2018). Concerning the global performance of our particular approach, we have been able to reproduce patient's ECG both in sinus rhythm and in clinical VT with good fidelity, considering that cardiac EP and myocardial architecture were not personalized. When PES protocols produce positive VT induction in the EP laboratory, electrophysiologists usually compare the resulting ECG to that registered during clinical VT episodes as a method to discern whether both VTs match or not, what helps in the process of choosing optimal ablation targets. Therefore, our pipeline completely based on non-invasive clinical data has the potential to replicate such process *in-silico*, such that it might become a helpful tool in therapy planning prior to RFA procedures aimed at finishing infarct-related VTs.

Limitations

The major limitation of our work derives from the fact that it relies on only one case. Thus, this work must be considered as a proof-of-concept study that shows promising, yet preliminary results. Hence, further studies including a larger number of patients should be conducted in order to improve and validate our pipeline, as well as to strengthen our conclusions.

Some features of the 3D ventricular model were not personalized. Myocardial architecture, for instance, was generated by means of a rule-based approach based on population data. The only alternative is the use of DTI (Hsu et al., 1998; Scollan et al., 1998; Holmes et al., 2000), although *in-vivo* cardiac DTI remains highly challenging because of the artifacts caused by cardiac motion. However, some studies have compared simulation results performed on 3D ventricular models using rule-based methods and *ex-vivo* DTI (Bishop et al., 2009; Bayer et al., 2012), finding only minor differences in electrical patterns at global level, what confirms the validity and robustness of rule-based approaches for simulations of cardiac EP.

Currently, the electrical propagation through ventricular myocardium is known to be characterized by three distinct conductivities in longitudinal, transverse (within myocardial sheets) and normal (along transmural direction) axes (Hooks, 2007; Caldwell et al., 2009). Recent computational studies have shown the impact on propagation patterns that might result from considering such full electrical anisotropy, both in simulations at organ level in healthy ventricles (Johnston et al., 2016) and in simplified models of cardiac tissue under diseased conditions (Johnston et al., 2018). Instead, we considered a unique conductivity for all directions perpendicular to myocyte longitudinal axis, as it has been commonly assumed in most of the 3D computational studies of cardiac EP so far. Hence, the incorporation of full anisotropy to the cardiac EP modeling of our pipeline might be one of the future improvements, as well as the study of its influence on infarct-related VT inducibility.

We did not incorporate the cardiac conduction system in our ventricular model, although it was not expected to have a significant impact on the infarct-related VT mechanisms that we aimed to study in this work. Considering the longer APD of Purkinje cells and the delay at the Purkinje-myocardial junctions, the kind of VTs simulated in this study could not have been mediated by the Purkinje system. In any case, currently there is no *in-vivo* imaging modality capable of providing information about the *patient-specific* geometry of Purkinje network. There are a few recent studies proposing approaches to infer models of conduction system from endocardial EAMs (Vergara et al., 2014; Palamara et al., 2015; Barber et al., 2017), yet it would break our requisite of only using non-invasive clinical data collected prior to the RFA procedure. Then, the only alternative would be to include a synthetic Purkinje model. Nevertheless, in such a case it would be impossible to assess to what extent the impact on simulation results of that artificial Purkinje network (if any) would be faithfully replicating the influence of the patient's conduction system in such scenario.

The poor quality of the anatomical whole-torso MRI hampered the construction of a *patient-specific* torso model, forcing us to reuse and adapt an existing one. However, given the results yielded for simulated ECGs, it does not appear to have been an important drawback, at least in this particular case.

CONCLUSIONS

Our 3D *patient-specific* model of the ventricles exclusively built from clinical data, in spite of avoiding the personalization of cardiac EP (based on population data), was able to reproduce the morphology of the clinical monomorphic VT suffered by the patient in the simulated ECGs. Furthermore, this allowed identification within the 3D model of the SCC responsible for the reentrant activity, matching the ablation target chosen by the experts in the RFA procedure that successfully eliminated VT inducibility in the patient. Hence, we have given a proof of the feasibility of developing 3D *patient-specific* computational models from clinical data aimed at simulation of the cardiac EP, with the potential to become a powerful tool for surgical planning. This approach could help to improve the currently low success rate of RFA procedures as well as to shorten surgery duration and, consequently, decrease the risk to the patient. It must be highlighted the great importance of the personalization of both cardiac anatomy and MI geometry from *in-vivo* high-resolution images to accurately locate reentry pathways as ablation targets by *in-silico* EP studies.

From the functional perspective, the computational modeling of the BZ remains a complex task due to the lack of experimental data from human hearts. In our study, the determinant aspects were the reduction of CVs and APD heterogeneity, which could be caused by ER in the BZ, a large amount of patchy fibrosis (30%) or a combination of both factors. The most arrhythmogenic versions of our ventricular model were those that combined the ER with intermediate fibrosis levels (10 and 20%) in the BZ. Such configurations generate an important repolarization dispersion (APD heterogeneity) around the infarct scar, especially in the vicinity of both terminal ends of the epicardial SCC, making the model more prone to the onset of reentrant activity due to functional unidirectional blocks in the channel.

Several challenging issues are still hampering the introduction of cardiac computational models as a common tool in clinical environments, such as the automatic and accurate reconstruction of *patient-specific* anatomy and infarct geometry from *in-vivo* images, especially from MRI modalities. Another important drawback is the current high cost of 3D computational simulations of cardiac EP at organ and body levels, whose computational burden demands the use of high-performance computational resources and long computing times.

AUTHOR CONTRIBUTIONS

AL-P, RS, MI, and JF jointly conceived this work and assessed the results. AL-P built the 3D models and performed the computational simulations for this work, all of this with the priceless help and close supervision from RS and JF. AL-P and RS wrote the manuscript. MI and RR collected and provided clinical data used in this work and gave valuable advice on the interpretation of electrophysiological data. MI checked the annotations of electrophysiological data and supervised this work, providing it with a clinical perspective. MB provided valuable advice on electrophysiological modeling issues, participated in the critical discussion of the results and contributed to the writing of the manuscript. All authors have read and approved the final version of the manuscript.

ACKNOWLEDGMENTS

Authors are very grateful to María P. López-Lereu and José V. Monmeneu, from the Unit of Cardiac Imaging of ERESA (Valencia, Spain), for the acquisition of the cardiac MRI datasets that were used in this work.

REFERENCES

Abdelwahab, A., and Sapp, J. L. (2007). NaviStar ThermoCool catheter for ventricular tachycardia. *Expert Rev. Med. Devices* 4, 307–314. doi: 10.1586/17434440.4.3.307

Abubakar, I. I., Tillmann, T., and Banerjee, A. (2015). Global, regional, and national age-sex specific all-cause and cause-specific mortality for 240 causes of death, 1990–2013: a systematic analysis for the Global Burden of Disease Study 2013. *Lancet* 385, 117–171. doi: 10.1016/S0140-6736(14)61682-2

Aliot, E. M., Stevenson, W. G., Almendral-Garrote, J. M., Bogun, F., Calkins, C. H., Delacretaz, E., et al. (2009). EHRA/HRS expert consensus on catheter ablation of ventricular arrhythmias: developed in a partnership with the European Heart Rhythm Association (EHRA), a registered branch of the European Society of Cardiology (ESC), and the Heart Rhythm Society (HRS); i. *Europace* 11, 771–817. doi: 10.1093/europace/eup098

Amado, L. C., Gerber, B. L., Gupta, S. N., Rettmann, D. W., Szarf, G., Schock, R., et al. (2004). Accurate and objective infarct sizing by contrast-enhanced magnetic resonance imaging in a canine myocardial infarction model. *J. Am. Coll. Cardiol.* 44, 2383–2389. doi: 10.1016/j.jacc.2004.09.020

Andreu, D., Berruezo, A., Ortiz-Pérez, J. T., Silva, E., Mont, L., Borràs, R., et al. (2011). Integration of 3D electroanatomic maps and magnetic resonance scar characterization into the navigation system to guide ventricular tachycardia ablation. *Circ. Arrhythmia Electrophysiol.* 4, 674–683. doi: 10.1161/CIRCEP.111.961946

Andreu, D., Ortiz-Pérez, J. T., Fernández-Armenta, J., Guiu, E., Acosta, J., Prat-González, S., et al. (2015). 3D delayed-enhanced magnetic resonance sequences improve conducting channel delineation prior to ventricular tachycardia ablation. *EP Eur.* 17, 938–945. doi: 10.1093/europace/euu310

Andreu, D., Penela, D., Acosta, J., Fernández-Armenta, J., Perea, R. J., Soto-Iglesias, D., et al. (2017). Cardiac magnetic resonance–aided scar dechanneling: influence on acute and long-term outcomes. *Hear. Rhythm* 14, 1121–1128. doi: 10.1016/j.hrthm.2017.05.018

Antzelevitch, C., Shimizu, W., Yan, G. X., Sicouri, S., Weissenburger, J., Nesterenko, V. V., et al. (1999). The M cell: its contribution to the ECG and to normal and abnormal electrical function of the heart. *J. Cardiovasc. Electrophysiol.* 10, 1124–1152. doi: 10.1111/j.1540-8167.1999.tb00287.x

Arevalo, H., Plank, G., Helm, P., Halperin, H., and Trayanova, N. (2013). Tachycardia in post-infarction hearts: insights from 3D image-based ventricular models. *PLoS ONE* 8:e68872. doi: 10.1371/journal.pone.0068872

Arevalo, H. J., Vadakkumpadan, F., Guallar, E., Jebb, A., Malamas, P., Wu, K. C., et al. (2016). Arrhythmia risk stratification of patients after myocardial infarction using personalized heart models. *Nat. Commun.* 7:11437. doi: 10.1038/ncomms11437

Ashikaga, H., Arevalo, H., Vadakkumpadan, F., Blake, R. C., Bayer, J. D., Nazarian, S., et al. (2013). Feasibility of image-based simulation to estimate ablation target in human ventricular arrhythmia. *Hear. Rhythm* 10, 1109–1116. doi: 10.1016/j.hrthm.2013.04.015

Ashikaga, H., Sasano, T., Dong, J., Zviman, M. M., Evers, R., Hopenfeld, B., et al. (2007). Magnetic resonance based anatomical analysis of scar-related ventricular tachycardia: implications for catheter ablation. *Circ. Res.* 101, 939–947. doi: 10.1161/CIRCRESAHA.107.158980

Baldinger, S. H., Stevenson, W. G., and John, R. M. (2016). Ablation of ischemic ventricular tachycardia: evidence, techniques, results, and future directions. *Curr. Opin. Cardiol.* 31, 29–36. doi: 10.1097/HCO.0000000000000237

Barber, F., Lozano, M., García-Fernández, I., and Sebastián, R. (2017). Inverse estimation of terminal connections in the cardiac conduction system. *Math. Methods Appl.* Sci. 41, 2340–2349. doi: 10.1002/mma.4280

Bayer, J. D., Blake, R. C., Plank, G., and Trayanova, N. A. (2012). A novel rule-based algorithm for assigning myocardial fiber orientation to computational heart models. *Ann. Biomed. Eng.* 40, 2243–2254. doi: 10.1007/s10439-012-0593-5

Ben-Haim, S. A., Osadchy, D., Scnuster, I., Gepstein, L., Hayam, G., and Josephson, M. E. (1996). Nonfluoroscopic, *in vivo* navigation and mapping technology. *Nat. Med.* 2, 1393–1395. doi: 10.1038/nm1296-1393

Berruezo, A., Fernandez-Armenta, J., Andreu, D., Penela, D., Herczku, C., Evertz, R., et al. (2015). Scar dechanneling: new method for scar-related left ventricular tachycardia substrate ablation. *Circ. Arrhythmia Electrophysiol.* 8, 326–336. doi: 10.1161/CIRCEP.114.002386

Besl, P. J., and McKay, N. D. (1992). A method for registration of 3-D shapes. *IEEE Trans. Pattern Anal. Mach. Intell.* 14, 239–256. doi: 10.1109/34.121791

Bishop, M. J., Hales, P., Plank, G., Gavaghan, D. J., Scheider, J., and Grau, V. (2009). "Comparison of rule-based and DTMRI-derived fibre architecture in a whole rat ventricular computational model," in *Functional Imaging and Modeling of the Heart-FIMH 2009, LNCS 5528*, eds N. Ayache, H. Delingette, and M. Sermesant (Nice; Berlin; Heidelberg: Springer), 87–96.

Bishop, M. J., Plank, G., Burton, R. A. B., Schneider, J. E., Gavaghan, D. J., Grau, V., et al. (2010). Development of an anatomically detailed MRI-derived rabbit ventricular model and assessment of its impact on simulations of electrophysiological function. *Am. J. Physiol. Heart Circ. Physiol.* 298, H699–H718. doi: 10.1152/ajpheart.00606.2009

Bogun, F., Desjardins, B., Crawford, T., Good, E., Jongnarangsin, K., Oral, H., et al. (2008). Post-infarction ventricular arrhythmias originating in papillary muscles. *J. Am. Coll. Cardiol.* 51, 1794–1802. doi: 10.1016/j.jacc.2008.01.046

Bogun, F., Krishnan, S., Siddiqui, M., Good, E., Marine, J. E., Schuger, C., et al. (2005). Electrogram characteristics in postinfarction ventricular tachycardia: effect of infarct age. *J. Am. Coll. Cardiol.* 46, 667–674. doi: 10.1016/j.jacc.2005.01.064

Bradley, C. P., Pullan, A. J., and Hunter, P. J. (2000). Effects of material properties and geometry on electrocardiographic forward simulations. *Ann. Biomed. Eng.* 28, 721–741. doi: 10.1114/1.1289467

Bressler, S. L., and Ding, M. (2006). "Event-related potentials," in *Wiley Encyclopedia of Biomedical Engineering*, ed M. Akay (Hoboken, NJ: John Wiley and Sons, Inc.), 1–8.

Brugada, J., Berruezo, A., Cuesta, A., Osca, J., Chueca, E., Fosch, X., et al. (2003). Nonsurgical transthoracic epicardial radiofrequency ablation. *J. Am. Coll. Cardiol.* 41, 2036–2043. doi: 10.1016/S0735-1097(03)00398-X

Caldwell, B. J., Trew, M. L., Sands, G. B., Hooks, D. A., LeGrice, I. J., and Smaill, B. H. (2009). Three distinct directions of intramural activation reveal nonuniform side-to-side electrical coupling of ventricular myocytes. *Circ. Arrhythmia Electrophysiol.* 2, 433–440. doi: 10.1161/CIRCEP.108.830133

Calkins, H., Kuck, K. H., Cappato, R., Brugada, J., Camm, A. J., Chen, S.-A., et al. (2012). 2012 HRS/EHRA/ECAS expert consensus statement on catheter and surgical ablation of atrial fibrillation: recommendations for patient selection, procedural techniques, patient management and follow-up, definitions, endpoints, and research trial design. *Europace* 14, 528–606. doi: 10.1093/europace/eus027

Camelliti, P., Devlin, G. P., Matthews, K. G., Kohl, P., and Green, C. R. (2004). Spatially and temporally distinct expression of fibroblast connexins after sheep ventricular infarction. *Cardiovasc. Res.* 62, 415–425. doi: 10.1016/j.cardiores.2004.01.027

Campos, F. O., Shiferaw, Y., Weber dos Santos, R., Plank, G., and Bishop, M. J. (2018). Microscopic isthmuses and fibrosis within the border zone of infarcted hearts promote calcium-mediated ectopy and conduction block. *Front. Phys.* 6, 1–14. doi: 10.3389/fphy.2018.00057

Chen, Z., Cabrera-Lozoya, R., Relan, J., Sohal, M., Shetty, A., Karim, R., et al. (2016). Biophysical modeling predicts ventricular tachycardia inducibility and circuit morphology: a combined clinical validation and computer modeling approach. *J. Cardiovasc. Electrophysiol.* 27, 851–860. doi: 10.1111/jce.12991

Chinchapatnam, P., Rhode, K. S., Ginks, M., Rinaldi, C. A., Lambiase, P., Razavi, R., et al. (2008). Model-based imaging of cardiac apparent conductivity and local conduction velocity for diagnosis and planning of therapy. *IEEE Trans. Med. Imaging* 27, 1631–1642. doi: 10.1109/TMI.2008.2004644

Ciaccio, E. J., Coromilas, J., Wit, A. L., Peters, N. S., and Garan, H. (2018). Source-sink mismatch causing functional conduction block in re-entrant ventricular tachycardia. *JACC Clin. Electrophysiol.* 4, 1–16. doi: 10.1016/j.jacep.2017.08.019

Cleutjens, J. P., Blankesteijn, W. M., Daemen, M. J., and Smits, J. F. (1999). The infarcted myocardium: simply dead tissue, or a lively target for therapeutic interventions. *Cardiovasc. Res.* 44, 232–241. doi: 10.1016/S0008-6363(99)00212-6

Connolly, A., Trew, M. L., Smaill, B. H., Plank, G., and Bishop, M. J. (2015). Local gradients in electrotonic loading modulate the local effective refractory period: implications for arrhythmogenesis in the infarct border zone. *IEEE Trans. Biomed. Eng.* 62, 2251–2259. doi: 10.1109/TBME.2015.2421296

Connolly, A. J., and Bishop, M. J. (2016). Computational representations of myocardial infarct scars and implications for arrhythmogenesis. *Clin. Med. Insights Cardiol.* 10:27. doi: 10.4137/CMC.S39708

Daskalopoulos, E. P., Janssen, B. J., and Blankesteijn, W. M. (2012). Myofibroblasts in the infarct area: concepts and challenges. *Microsc. Microanal.* 18, 35–49. doi: 10.1017/S143192761101227X

de Bakker, J. M., van Capelle, F. J., Janse, M. J., Tasseron, S., Vermeulen, J. T., de Jonge, N., et al. (1993). Slow conduction in the infarcted human heart. "Zigzag" course of activation. *Circulation* 88, 915–926. doi: 10.1161/01.CIR.88.3.915

de Bakker, J. M., van Capelle, F. J., Janse, M. J., Wilde, A. A., Coronel, R., Becker, A. E., et al. (1988). Reentry as a cause of ventricular tachycardia in patients with chronic ischemic heart disease: electrophysiologic and anatomic correlation. *Circulation* 77, 589–606. doi: 10.1161/01.CIR.77.3.589

de Bakker, J. M. T. (2017). Do myofibroblasts represent a hidden factor for impaired conduction and tachyarrhythmia in post-myocardial infarction? *JACC Clin. Electrophysiol.* 3, 715–717. doi: 10.1016/j.jacep.2017.01.007

de Bakker, J. M. T., Stein, M., and van Rijen, H. V. M. (2005). Three-dimensional anatomic structure as substrate for ventricular tachycardia/ventricular fibrillation. *Hear. Rhythm* 2, 777–779. doi: 10.1016/j.hrthm.2005.03.022

de Chillou, C., Lacroix, D., Klug, D., Magnin-Poull, I., Marquié, C., Messier, M., et al. (2002). Isthmus characteristics of reentrant ventricular tachycardia after myocardial infarction. *Circulation* 105, 726–731. doi: 10.1161/hc0602.103675

de Jong, S., van Veen, T., B., van Rijen, H. V. M., and de Bakker, J. M. T. (2011). Fibrosis and cardiac arrhythmias. *J. Cardiovasc. Pharmacol.* 57, 630–638. doi: 10.1097/FJC.0b013e318207a35f

Deng, D., Arevalo, H., Pashakhanloo, F., Prakosa, A., Ashikaga, H., McVeigh, E., et al. (2015). Accuracy of prediction of infarct-related arrhythmic circuits from image-based models reconstructed from low and high resolution MRI. *Front. Physiol.* 6:282. doi: 10.3389/fphys.2015.00282

Deng, D., Arevalo, H. J., Prakosa, A., Callans, D. J., and Trayanova, N. A. (2016). A feasibility study of arrhythmia risk prediction in patients with myocardial infarction and preserved ejection fraction. *Europace* 18, iv60–iv66. doi: 10.1093/europace/euw351

Dhanjal, T. S., Lellouche, N., von Ruhland, C. J., Abehsira, G., Edwards, D. H., Dubois-Randé, J.-L., et al. (2017). Massive accumulation of myofibroblasts in the critical isthmus is associated with ventricular tachycardia inducibility in post-infarct swine heart. *JACC Clin. Electrophysiol.* 3, 703–714. doi: 10.1016/j.jacep.2016.11.010

Doltra, A., Amundsen, B., Gebker, R., Fleck, E., and Kelle, S. (2013). Emerging concepts for myocardial late gadolinium enhancement MRI. *Curr. Cardiol. Rev.* 9, 185–190. doi: 10.2174/1573403X113099990030

Drouin, E., Charpentier, F., Gauthier, C., Laurent, K., and Le Marec, H. (1995). Electrophysiologic characteristics of cells spanning the left ventricular wall of human heart: Evidence for presence of M cells. *J. Am. Coll. Cardiol.* 26, 185–192. doi: 10.1016/0735-1097(95)00167-X

Dun, W., Baba, S., Yagi, T., and Boyden, P. A. (2004). Dynamic remodeling of K+ and Ca2+ currents in cells that survived in the epicardial border zone of canine healed infarcted heart. *AJP Hear. Circ. Physiol.* 287, H1046–H1054. doi: 10.1152/ajpheart.00082.2004

Durrer, D., Van Dam, R. T., Freud, G. E., Janse, M. J., Meijler, F. L., and Arzbaecher, R. C. (1970). Total excitation of the isolated human heart. *Circulation* 41, 899–912. doi: 10.1161/01.CIR.41.6.899

Fernández-Armenta, J., Berruezo, A., Andreu, D., Camara, O., Silva, E., Serra, L., et al. (2013). Three-dimensional architecture of scar and conducting channels based on high resolution ce-CMR: insights for ventricular tachycardia ablation. *Circ. Arrhythmia Electrophysiol.* 6, 528–537. doi: 10.1161/CIRCEP.113.000264

Ferrer, A., Sebastián, R., Sánchez-Quintana, D., Rodríguez, J. F., Godoy, E. J., Martínez, L., et al. (2015). Detailed anatomical and electrophysiological models of human atria and torso for the simulation of atrial activation. *PLoS ONE* 10:e0141573. doi: 10.1371/journal.pone.0141573

Ferrer-Albero, A., Godoy, E. J., Lozano, M., Martínez-Mateu, L., Atienza, F., Saiz, J., et al. (2017). Non-invasive localization of atrial ectopic beats by using simulated body surface P-wave integral maps. *PLoS ONE* 12:e0181263. doi: 10.1371/journal.pone.0181263

Fieno, D. S., Kim, R. J., Chen, E., Lomasney, J. W., Klocke, F. J., and Judd, R. M. (2000). Contrast-enhanced magnetic resonance imaging of myocardium at risk: distinction between reversible and irreversible injury throughout infarct healing. *J. Am. Coll. Cardiol.* 36, 1985–1991. doi: 10.1016/S0735-1097(00)00958-X

Gabriel, S., Lau, R. W., and Gabriel, C. (1996). The dielectric properties of biological tissues: II. Measurements in the frequency range 10 Hz to 20 GHz. *Phys. Med. Biol.* 41, 2251–2269. doi: 10.1088/0031-9155/41/11/002

Gardner, P. I., Ursell, P. C., Fenoglio, J. J., and Wit, A. L. (1985). Electrophysiologic and anatomic basis for fractionated electrograms recorded from healed myocardial infarcts. *Circulation* 72, 596–611. doi: 10.1161/01.CIR.72.3.596

Gepstein, L., Hayam, G., and Ben-Haim, S. A. (1997). A novel method for nonfluoroscopic catheter-based electroanatomical mapping of the heart : *in vitro* and *in vivo* accuracy results. *Circulation* 95, 1611–1622. doi: 10.1161/01.CIR.95.6.1611

Gerstenfeld, E. P. (2013). Recurrent ventricular tachycardia after catheter ablation in post-infarct cardiomyopathy. *J. Am. Coll. Cardiol.* 61, 74–76. doi: 10.1016/j.jacc.2012.07.057

Geselowitz, D. B., and Miller, W. T. (1983). A bidomain model for anisotropic cardiac muscle. *Ann. Biomed. Eng.* 11, 191–206. doi: 10.1007/BF02363286

Gillette, K., Prassl, A., Bayer, J., Vigmond, E., Neic, A., and Plank, G. (2018). Automatic generation of bi-ventricular models of cardiac electrophysiology for patient specific personalization using non-invasive recordings. *Comput. Cardiol.* 45, 2–5. doi: 10.22489/CinC.2018.265

Gomez, J. F., Cardona, K., Martinez, L., Saiz, J., and Trenor, B. (2014). Electrophysiological and structural remodeling in heart failure modulate arrhythmogenesis. 2D simulation study. *PLoS ONE* 9:e103273. doi: 10.1371/journal.pone.0103273

Greenbaum, R. A., Ho, S. Y., Gibson, D. G., Becker, A. E., and Anderson, R. H. (1981). Left ventricular fibre architecture in man. *Heart* 45, 248–263. doi: 10.1136/hrt.45.3.248

Heidenreich, E. A., Ferrero, J. M., Doblaré, M., and Rodríguez, J. F. (2010). Adaptive macro finite elements for the numerical solution of monodomain equations in cardiac electrophysiology. *Ann. Biomed. Eng.* 38, 2331–2345. doi: 10.1007/s10439-010-9997-2

Hein, S., and Schaper, J. (2001). The extracellular matrix in normal and diseased myocardium. *J. Nucl. Cardiol.* 8, 188–196. doi: 10.1067/mnc.2001.113331

Hill, Y. R., Child, N., Hanson, B., Wallman, M., Coronel, R., Plank, G., et al. (2016). Investigating a novel activation-repolarisation time metric to predict localised Vulnerability to reentry using computational modelling. *PLoS ONE* 11:e0149342. doi: 10.1371/journal.pone.0149342

Holmes, A. A., Scollan, D. F., and Winslow, R. L. (2000). Direct histological validation of diffusion tensor MRI in formaldehyde-fixed myocardium. *Magn. Reson. Med.* 44, 157–161. doi: 10.1002/1522-2594(200007)44:1<157::AID-MRM22>3.0.CO;2-F

Hooks, D. A (2007). Myocardial segment-specific model generation for simulating the electrical action of the heart. *Biomed. Eng. Online* 6:21. doi: 10.1186/1475-925X-6-21

Hsu, E. W., Muzikant, A. L., Matulevicius, S. A., Penland, R. C., and Henriquez, C. S. (1998). Magnetic resonance myocardial fiber-orientation mapping with direct histological correlation. *AJP Hear. Circ. Physiol.* 274, H1627–H1634.

Hsu, L.-Y., Natanzon, A., Kellman, P., Hirsch, G. A., Aletras, A. H., and Arai, A. E. (2006). Quantitative myocardial infarction on delayed enhancement MRI. Part I: animal validation of an automated feature analysis and combined thresholding infarct sizing algorithm. *J. Magn. Reson. Imaging* 23, 298–308. doi: 10.1002/jmri.20496

Jacquemet, V. (2006). Pacemaker activity resulting from the coupling with nonexcitable cells. *Phys. Rev. E* 74:011908. doi: 10.1103/PhysRevE.74.011908

Jamiel, A., Ebid, M., Ahmed, A. M., Ahmed, D., and Al-Mallah, M. H. (2017). The role of myocardial viability in contemporary cardiac practice. *Heart Fail. Rev.* 22, 401–413. doi: 10.1007/s10741-017-9626-3

Jiang, M., Cabo, C., Yao, J.-A., Boyden, P. A., and Tseng, G.-N. (2000). Delayed rectifier K currents have reduced amplitudes and altered kinetics in myocytes from infarcted canine ventricle. *Cardiovasc. Res.* 48, 34–43. doi: 10.1016/S0008-6363(00)00159-0

Johnston, B., Barnes, J., and Johnston, P. (2016). "The effect of conductivity values on activation times and defibrillation thresholds," in *2016 Computing in Cardiology Conference (CinC)* (Vancouver, BC), 10–13.

Johnston, B. M., Coveney, S., Chang, E. T. Y., Johnston, P. R., and Clayton, R. H. (2018). Quantifying the effect of uncertainty in input parameters in a simplified bidomain model of partial thickness ischaemia. *Med. Biol. Eng. Comput.* 56, 761–780. doi: 10.1007/s11517-017-1714-y

Karim, R., Bhagirath, P., Claus, P., James Housden, R., Chen, Z., Karimaghaloo, Z., et al. (2016). Evaluation of state-of-the-art segmentation algorithms for left ventricle infarct from late Gadolinium enhancement MR images. *Med. Image Anal.* 30, 95–107. doi: 10.1016/j.media.2016.01.004

Keller, D. U. J., Weber, F. M., Seemann, G., and Dössel, O. (2010). Ranking the influence of tissue conductivities on forward-calculated ECGs. *IEEE Trans. Biomed. Eng.* 57, 1568–1576. doi: 10.1109/TBME.2010.2046485

Kim, R. J., Fieno, D. S., Parrish, T. B., Harris, K., Chen, E. L., Simonetti, O., et al. (1999a). Relationship of MRI delayed contrast enhancement to irreversible injury, infarct age, and contractile function. *Circulation* 100, 1992–2002. doi: 10.1161/01.CIR.100.19.1992

Kim, Y.-H., Xie, F., Yashima, M., Wu, T.-J., Valderrabano, M., Lee, M.-H., et al. (1999b). Role of papillary muscle in the generation and maintenance of reentry during ventricular tachycardia and fibrillation in isolated swine right ventricle. *Circulation* 100, 1450–1459. doi: 10.1161/01.CIR.100.13.1450

Klepfer, R. N., Johnson, C. R., and Macleod, R. S. (1997). The effects of inhomogeneities and anisotropies on electrocardiographic fields: a 3-D finite-element study. *IEEE Trans. Biomed. Eng.* 44, 706–719. doi: 10.1109/10.605427

Kohl, P., and Gourdie, R. G. (2014). Fibroblast–myocyte electrotonic coupling: does it occur in native cardiac tissue? *J. Mol. Cell. Cardiol.* 70, 37–46. doi: 10.1016/j.yjmcc.2013.12.024

Kolipaka, A., Chatzimavroudis, G. P., White, R. D., O'Donnell, T. P., and Setser, R. M. (2005). Segmentation of non-viable myocardium in delayed enhancement magnetic resonance images. *Int. J. Cardiovasc. Imaging* 21, 303–311. doi: 10.1007/s10554-004-5806-z

Krueger, M. W., Schulze, W. H. W., Rhode, K. S., Razavi, R., Seemann, G., and Dössel, O. (2013). Towards personalized clinical *in-silico* modeling of atrial anatomy and electrophysiology. *Med. Biol. Eng. Comput.* 51, 1251–1260. doi: 10.1007/s11517-012-0970-0

Lazzara, R., and Scherlag, B. J. (1984). Electrophysiologic basis for arrhythmias in ischemic heart disease. *Am. J. Cardiol.* 53, B1–B7. doi: 10.1016/0002-9149(84)90493-4

Lopez-Perez, A., Sebastian, R., and Ferrero, J. M. (2015). Three-dimensional cardiac computational modelling: methods, features and applications. *Biomed. Eng. Online* 14:35. doi: 10.1186/s12938-015-0033-5

MacCannell, K. A., Bazzazi, H., Chilton, L., Shibukawa, Y., Clark, R. B., and Giles, W. R. (2007). A mathematical model of electrotonic interactions between ventricular myocytes and fibroblasts. *Biophys. J.* 92, 4121–4132. doi: 10.1529/biophysj.106.101410

MacLeod, R. S., Johnson, C. R., and Ershler, P. R. (1991). "Construction of an inhomogeneous model of the human torso for use in computational electrocardiography," in *Proceedings of the Annual Conference on Engineering in Medicine and Biology* (Publ by IEEE), 688–689. doi: 10.1109/IEMBS.1991.684145

Mahoney, V. M., Mezzano, V., and Morley, G. E. (2016). A review of the literature on cardiac electrical activity between fibroblasts and myocytes. *Prog. Biophys. Mol. Biol.* 120, 128–133. doi: 10.1016/j.pbiomolbio.2015.12.006

Mantziari, L., Butcher, C., Kontogeorgis, A., Panikker, S., Roy, K., Markides, V., et al. (2015). Utility of a novel rapid high-resolution mapping system in the catheter ablation of arrhythmias. *JACC Clin. Electrophysiol.* 1, 411–420. doi: 10.1016/j.jacep.2015.06.002

Marchlinski, F. E., Callans, D. J., Gottlieb, C. D., and Zado, E. (2000). Linear ablation lesions for control of unmappable ventricular tachycardia in patients with ischemic and nonischemic cardiomyopathy. *Circulation* 101, 1288–1296. doi: 10.1161/01.CIR.101.11.1288

Martinez-Mateu, L., Romero, L., Ferrer-Albero, A., Sebastian, R., Rodríguez Matas, J. F., Jalife, J., et al. (2018). Factors affecting basket catheter detection of real and phantom rotors in the atria: a computational study. *PLOS Comput. Biol.* 14:e1006017. doi: 10.1371/journal.pcbi.1006017

Matsushita, T., Oyamada, M., Fujimoto, K., Yasuda, Y., Masuda, S., Wada, Y., et al. (1999). Remodeling of cell-cell and cell-extracellular matrix interactions at the border zone of rat myocardial infarcts. *Circ. Res.* 85, 1046–1055. doi: 10.1161/01.RES.85.11.1046

McDowell, K. S., Arevalo, H. J., Maleckar, M. M., and Trayanova, N. A. (2011). Susceptibility to arrhythmia in the infarcted heart depends on myofibroblast density. *Biophys. J.* 101, 1307–1315. doi: 10.1016/j.bpj.2011.08.009

Mendonca Costa, C., Plank, G., Rinaldi, C. A., Niederer, S. A., and Bishop, M. J. (2018). Modeling the electrophysiological properties of the infarct border zone. *Front. Physiol.* 9:356. doi: 10.3389/fphys.2018.00356

Mewton, N., Liu, C. Y., Croisille, P., Bluemke, D., and Lima, J. A. C. (2011). Assessment of myocardial fibrosis with cardiovascular magnetic resonance. *J. Am. Coll. Cardiol.* 57, 891–903. doi: 10.1016/j.jacc.2010.11.013

Miragoli, M., Gaudesius, G., and Rohr, S. (2006). Electrotonic modulation of cardiac impulse conduction by myofibroblasts. *Circ. Res.* 98, 801–810. doi: 10.1161/01.RES.0000214537.44195.a3

Moon, J. C., Reed, E., Sheppard, M. N., Elkington, A. G., Ho, S., Burke, M., et al. (2004). The histologic basis of late gadolinium enhancement cardiovascular magnetic resonance in hypertrophic cardiomyopathy. *J. Am. Coll. Cardiol.* 43, 2260–2264. doi: 10.1016/j.jacc.2004.03.035

Nguyen, T. P., Qu, Z., and Weiss, J. N. (2014). Cardiac fibrosis and arrhythmogenesis: the road to repair is paved with perils. *J. Mol. Cell. Cardiol.* 70, 83–91. doi: 10.1016/j.yjmcc.2013.10.018

Nowbar, A. N., Howard, J. P., Finegold, J. A., Asaria, P., and Francis, D. P. (2014). 2014 Global geographic analysis of mortality from ischaemic heart disease by country, age and income: Statistics from World Health Organisation and United Nations. *Int. J. Cardiol.* 174, 293–298. doi: 10.1016/j.ijcard.2014.04.096

Okada, J., Washio, T., Maehara, A., Momomura, S., Sugiura, S., and Hisada, T. (2011). Transmural and apicobasal gradients in repolarization contribute to T-wave genesis in human surface ECG. *Am. J. Physiol. Circ. Physiol.* 301, H200–H208. doi: 10.1152/ajpheart.01241.2010

Ongstad, E., and Kohl, P. (2016). Fibroblast–myocyte coupling in the heart: potential relevance for therapeutic interventions. *J. Mol. Cell. Cardiol.* 91, 238–246. doi: 10.1016/j.yjmcc.2016.01.010

Ortiz-Pérez, J. T., Rodríguez, J., Meyers, S. N., Lee, D. C., Davidson, C., and Wu, E. (2008). Correspondence between the 17-segment model and coronary arterial anatomy using contrast-enhanced cardiac magnetic resonance imaging. *JACC Cardiovasc. Imaging* 1, 282–293. doi: 10.1016/j.jcmg.2008.01.014

Palamara, S., Vergara, C., Faggiano, E., and Nobile, F. (2015). An effective algorithm for the generation of patient-specific Purkinje networks in computational electrocardiology. *J. Comput. Phys.* 283, 495–517. doi: 10.1016/j.jcp.2014.11.043

Pashakhanloo, F., Herzka, D. A., Mori, S., Zviman, M., Halperin, H., Gai, N., et al. (2017). Submillimeter diffusion tensor imaging and late gadolinium enhancement cardiovascular magnetic resonance of chronic myocardial infarction. *J. Cardiovasc. Magn. Reson.* 19:9. doi: 10.1186/s12968-016-0317-3

Patel, H., Mazur, W., Williams, K. A., and Kalra, D. K. (2017). Myocardial viability–State of the art: is it still relevant and how to best assess it with imaging? *Trends Cardiovasc. Med.* 28, 24–37. doi: 10.1016/j.tcm.2017.07.001

Paul, T., Moak, J. P., Morris, C., and Garson, A. (1990). Epicardial mapping: how to measure local activation? *Pacing Clin. Electrophysiol.* 13, 285–292. doi: 10.1111/j.1540-8159.1990.tb02042.x

Pedersen, C. T., Kay, G. N., Kalman, J., Borggrefe, M., Della-Bella, P., Dickfeld, T., et al. (2014). EHRA/HRS/APHRS expert consensus on ventricular arrhythmias. *Hear. Rhythm* 11, e166–e196. doi: 10.1016/j.hrthm.2014.07.024

Perez-David, E., Arenal, Á., Rubio-Guivernau, J. L., del Castillo, R., Atea, L., Arbelo, E., et al. (2011). Noninvasive identification of ventricular tachycardia-related conducting channels using contrast-enhanced magnetic resonance imaging in patients with chronic myocardial infarction. *J. Am. Coll. Cardiol.* 57, 184–194. doi: 10.1016/j.jacc.2010.07.043

Perotti, L. E., Krishnamoorthi, S., Borgstrom, N. P., Ennis, D. B., and Klug, W. S. (2015). Regional segmentation of ventricular models to achieve repolarization dispersion in cardiac electrophysiology modeling. *Int. J. Numer. Method. Biomed. Eng.* 31:e02718. doi: 10.1002/cnm.2718

Pokorney, S. D., Friedman, D. J., Calkins, H., Callans, D. J., Daoud, E. G., Della-Bella, P., et al. (2016). Catheter ablation of ventricular tachycardia: lessons learned from past clinical trials and implications for future clinical trials. *Hear. Rhythm* 13, 1748–1754. doi: 10.1016/j.hrthm.2016.04.001

Prakosa, A., Arevalo, H. J., Deng, D., Boyle, P. M., Nikolov, P. P., Ashikaga, H., et al. (2018). Personalized virtual-heart technology for guiding the ablation of infarct-related ventricular tachycardia. *Nat. Biomed. Eng.* 2, 732–740. doi: 10.1038/s41551-018-0282-2

Prassl, A. J., Kickinger, F., Ahammer, H., Grau, V., Schneider, J. E., Hofer, E., et al. (2009). Automatically generated, anatomically accurate meshes for cardiac electrophysiology problems. *IEEE Trans. Biomed. Eng.* 56, 1318–1330. doi: 10.1109/TBME.2009.2014243

Priori, S. G., Blomström-Lundqvist, C., Mazzanti, A., Blom, N., Borggrefe, M., Camm, J., et al. (2015). 2015 ESC Guidelines for the management of patients with ventricular arrhythmias and the prevention of sudden cardiac death. *Eur. Heart J.* 36, 2793–2867. doi: 10.1093/eurheartj/ehv316

Pu, J., and Boyden, P. A. (1997). Alterations of Na+ currents in myocytes from epicardial border zone of the infarcted heart : a possible ionic mechanism for reduced excitability and postrepolarization refractoriness. *Circ. Res.* 81, 110–119. doi: 10.1161/01.RES.81.1.110

Quinn, T. A., Camelliti, P., Rog-Zielinska, E. A., Siedlecka, U., Poggioli, T., O'Toole, E. T., et al. (2016). Electrotonic coupling of excitable and nonexcitable cells in the heart revealed by optogenetics. *Proc. Natl. Acad. Sci. U S A.* 113, 14852–14857. doi: 10.1073/pnas.1611184114

Rantner, L. J., Arevalo, H. J., Constantino, J. L., Efimov, I. R., Plank, G., and Trayanova, N. A. (2012). Three-dimensional mechanisms of increased vulnerability to electric shocks in myocardial infarction: altered virtual electrode polarizations and conduction delay in the peri-infarct zone. *J. Physiol.* 590, 4537–4551. doi: 10.1113/jphysiol.2012.229088

Relan, J., Chinchapatnam, P., Sermesant, M., Rhode, K., Ginks, M., Delingette, H., et al. (2011). Coupled personalization of cardiac electrophysiology models for prediction of ischaemic ventricular tachycardia. *Interface Focus* 1, 396–407. doi: 10.1098/rsfs.2010.0041

Ringenberg, J., Deo, M., Filgueiras-Rama, D., Pizarro, G., Ibañez, B., Peinado, R., et al. (2014). Effects of fibrosis morphology on reentrant ventricular tachycardia inducibility and simulation fidelity in patient-derived models. *Clin. Med. Insights. Cardiol.* 8, 1–13. doi: 10.4137/CMC.S15712

Rog-Zielinska, E. A., Norris, R. A., Kohl, P., and Markwald, R. (2016). The living scar - cardiac fibroblasts and the injured heart. *Trends Mol. Med.* 22, 99–114. doi: 10.1016/j.molmed.2015.12.006

Rohr, S. (2012). Arrhythmogenic implications of fibroblast-myocyte interactions. *Circ. Arrhythmia Electrophysiol.* 5, 442–452. doi: 10.1161/CIRCEP.110.957647

Roney, C. H., Bayer, J. D., Zahid, S., Meo, M., Boyle, P. M. J., Trayanova, N. A., et al. (2016). Modelling methodology of atrial fibrosis affects rotor dynamics and electrograms. *Europace* 18, 146–155. doi: 10.1093/europace/euw365

Roth, B. J. (1988). The electrical potential produced by a strand of cardiac muscle: a bidomain analysis. *Ann. Biomed. Eng.* 16, 609–637. doi: 10.1007/BF02368018

Rutherford, S. L., Trew, M. L., Sands, G. B., LeGrice, I. J., and Smaill, B. H. (2012). High-resolution 3-dimensional reconstruction of the infarct border zone: impact of structural remodeling on electrical activation. *Circ. Res.* 111, 301–311. doi: 10.1161/CIRCRESAHA.111.260943

Schaper, W., Görge, G., Winkler, B., and Schaper, J. (1988). The collateral circulation of the heart. *Prog. Cardiovasc. Dis.* 31, 57–77. doi: 10.1016/0033-0620(88)90011-4

Schuleri, K. H., Centola, M., George, R. T., Amado, L. C., Evers, K. S., Kitagawa, K., et al. (2009). Characterization of peri-infarct zone heterogeneity by contrast-enhanced multidetector computed tomography. *J. Am. Coll. Cardiol.* 53, 1699–1707. doi: 10.1016/j.jacc.2009.01.056

Schwab, B. C., Seemann, G., Lasher, R. A., Torres, N. S., Wulfers, E. M., Arp, M., et al. (2013). Quantitative analysis of cardiac tissue including fibroblasts using three-dimensional confocal microscopy and image reconstruction: towards a basis for electrophysiological modeling. *IEEE Trans. Med. Imaging* 32, 862–872. doi: 10.1109/TMI.2013.2240693

Scollan, D. F., Holmes, A., Winslow, R., and Forder, J. (1998). Histological validation of myocardial microstructure obtained from diffusion tensor magnetic resonance imaging. *AJP Hear. Circ. Physiol.* 275, H2308–H2318.

Sebastian, R., Zimmerman, V., Sukno, F., Bijnens, B. B., and Frangi, A. F. (2009). "Cardiac modelling for pathophysiology research and clinical applications. the need for an automated pipeline," in *World Congress on Medical Physics and Biomedical Engineering 2009*, eds O. Dössel and W. C. Schlegel (Berlin; Heidelberg: Springer-Verlag), 2207–2210.

Seg3D, C. (2013). *Volumetric Image Segmentation and Visualization.* Scientific Computing and Imaging Institute.

Seidel, T., Edelmann, J.-C., and Sachse, F. B. (2016). Analyzing remodeling of cardiac tissue: a comprehensive approach based on confocal microscopy and 3D reconstructions. *Ann. Biomed. Eng.* 44, 1436–1448. doi: 10.1007/s10439-015-1465-6

Severs, N. J., Bruce, A. F., Dupont, E., and Rothery, S. (2008). Remodelling of gap junctions and connexin expression in diseased myocardium. *Cardiovasc. Res.* 80, 9–19. doi: 10.1093/cvr/cvn133

Si, H., and Gärtner, K. (2005). "Meshing piecewise linear complexes by constrained delaunay tetrahedralizations," in *Proceedings of the 14th International Meshing Roundtable*, ed B. W. Hanks (Berlin; Heidelberg: Springer-Verlag), 147–163.

Sicouri, S., and Antzelevitch, C. (1991). A subpopulation of cells with unique electrophysiological properties in the deep subepicardium of the canine ventricle. *The M Cell. Circ. Res.* 68, 1729–1741. doi: 10.1161/01.RES.68.6.1729

Sicouri, S., Fish, J., and Antzelevitch, C. (1994). Distribution of M cells in the canine ventricle. *J. Cardiovasc. Electrophysiol.* 5, 824–837. doi: 10.1111/j.1540-8167.1994.tb01121.x

Smith, J. H., Green, C. R., Peters, N. S., Rothery, S., and Severs, N. J. (1991). Altered patterns of gap junction distribution in ischemic heart disease. An immunohistochemical study of human myocardium using laser scanning confocal microscopy. *Am. J. Pathol.* 139, 801–21.

Smith, N., de Vecchi, A., McCormick, M., Nordsletten, D., Camara, O., Frangi, A. F., et al. (2011). euHeart: personalized and integrated cardiac care using patient-specific cardiovascular modelling. *Interface Focus* 1, 349–364. doi: 10.1098/rsfs.2010.0048

Soejima, K., Stevenson, W. G., Maisel, W. H., Sapp, J. L., and Epstein, L. M. (2002). Electrically unexcitable scar mapping based on pacing threshold for identification of the reentry circuit isthmus: feasibility for guiding ventricular tachycardia ablation. *Circulation* 106, 1678–1683. doi: 10.1161/01.CIR.0000030187.39852.A7

Sosa, E., and Scanavacca, M. (2005). Epicardial mapping and ablation techniques to control ventricular tachycardia. *J. Cardiovasc. Electrophysiol.* 16, 449–452. doi: 10.1046/j.1540-8167.2005.40710.x

Sosa, E., Scanavacca, M., D'Avila, A., Oliveira, F., and Ramires, J. A. F. (2000). Nonsurgical transthoracic epicardial catheter ablation to treat recurrent ventricular tachycardia occurring late after myocardial infarction. *J. Am. Coll. Cardiol.* 35, 1442–1449. doi: 10.1016/S0735-1097(00)00606-9

Sosa, E., Scanavacca, M., D'Avila, A., and Pilleggi, F. (1996). A new technique to perform epicardial mapping in the electrophysiology laboratory. *J. Cardiovasc. Electrophysiol.* 7, 531–536. doi: 10.1111/j.1540-8167.1996.tb00559.x

Soto-Iglesias, D., Butakoff, C., Andreu, D., Fernández-Armenta, J., Berruezo, A., and Camara, O. (2016). Integration of electro-anatomical and imaging data of the left ventricle: an evaluation framework. *Med. Image Anal.* 32, 131–144. doi: 10.1016/j.media.2016.03.010

Spach, M. S., and Boineau, J. P. (1997). Microfibrosis produces electrical load variations due to loss of side-to-side cell connections: a major mechanism of structural heart disease arrhythmias. *Pacing Clin. Electrophysiol.* 20, 397–413. doi: 10.1111/j.1540-8159.1997.tb06199.x

Spach, M. S., Miller, W. T., Miller-Jones, E., Warren, R. B., and Barr, R. C. (1979). Extracellular potentials related to intracellular action potentials during impulse conduction in anisotropic canine cardiac muscle. *Circ. Res.* 45, 188–204. doi: 10.1161/01.RES.45.2.188

Stevenson, W. G., Khan, H., Sager, P., Saxon, L. A., Middlekauff, H. R., Natterson, P. D., et al. (1993). Identification of reentry circuit sites during catheter mapping and radiofrequency ablation of ventricular tachycardia late after myocardial infarction. *Circulation* 88, 1647–1670. doi: 10.1161/01.CIR.88.4.1647

Stevenson, W. G., and Soejima, K. (2005). Recording techniques for clinical electrophysiology. *J. Cardiovasc. Electrophysiol.* 16, 1017–1022. doi: 10.1111/j.1540-8167.2005.50155.x

Streeter, D. D., Spotnitz, H. M., Patel, D. P., Ross, J., and Sonnenblick, E. H. (1969). Fiber orientation in the canine left ventricle during diastole and systole. *Circ. Res.* 24, 339–347. doi: 10.1161/01.RES.24.3.339

Sun, Y., Kiani, M. F., Postlethwaite, A. E., and Weber, K. T. (2002). Infarct scar as living tissue. *Basic Res. Cardiol.* 97, 343–347. doi: 10.1007/s00395-002-0365-8

Taggart, P., Sutton, P. M., Opthof, T., Coronel, R., Trimlett, R., Pugsley, W., et al. (2000). Inhomogeneous transmural conduction during early ischaemia in patients with coronary artery disease. *J. Mol. Cell. Cardiol.* 32, 621–630. doi: 10.1006/jmcc.2000.1105

Tedrow, U., and Stevenson, W. G. (2009). Strategies for epicardial mapping and ablation of ventricular tachycardia. *J. Cardiovasc. Electrophysiol.* 20, 710–713. doi: 10.1111/j.1540-8167.2008.01427.x

ten Tusscher, K., and Panfilov, A. (2006). Alternans and spiral breakup in a human ventricular tissue model. *AJP Hear. Circ. Physiol.* 291, H1088–H1100. doi: 10.1152/ajpheart.00109.2006

Trayanova, N. a., and Boyle, P. M. (2013). Advances in modeling ventricular arrhythmias: from mechanisms to the clinic. *Wiley Interdiscip. Rev. Syst. Biol. Med.* 6, 209–224. doi: 10.1002/wsbm.1256

Trayanova, N. A., Boyle, P. M., Arevalo, H. J., and Zahid, S. (2014). Exploring susceptibility to atrial and ventricular arrhythmias resulting from remodeling of the passive electrical properties in the heart: a simulation approach. *Front. Physiol.* 5, 1–12. doi: 10.3389/fphys.2014.00435.

Trayanova, N. A., O'Hara, T., Bayer, J. D., Boyle, P. M., McDowell, K. S., Constantino, J., et al. (2012). Computational cardiology: how computer simulations could be used to develop new therapies and advance existing ones. *Europace* 14, v82–v89. doi: 10.1093/europace/eus277

Trayanova, N. A., Pashakhanloo, F., Wu, K. C., and Halperin, H. R. (2017). Imaging-Based Simulations for Predicting Sudden Death and Guiding Ventricular Tachycardia Ablation. *Circ. Arrhythmia Electrophysiol.* 10:435. doi: 10.1161/CIRCEP.117.004743

Tschabrunn, C. M., Roujol, S., Nezafat, R., Faulkner-Jones, B., Buxton, A. E., Josephson, M. E., et al. (2016). A swine model of infarct-related reentrant ventricular tachycardia: electroanatomic, magnetic resonance, and histopathological characterization. *Hear. Rhythm* 13, 262–273. doi: 10.1016/j.hrthm.2015.07.030

Ukwatta, E., Arevalo, H., Li, K., Yuan, J., Qiu, W., Malamas, P., et al. (2016). Myocardial infarct segmentation from magnetic resonance images for personalized modeling of cardiac electrophysiology. *IEEE Trans. Med. Imaging* 35, 1408–1419. doi: 10.1109/TMI.2015.2512711

Ursell, P. C., Gardner, P. I., Albala, A., Fenoglio, J. J., and Wit, a L. (1985). Structural and electrophysiological changes in the epicardial border zone of canine myocardial infarcts during infarct healing. *Circ. Res.* 56, 436–451. doi: 10.1161/01.RES.56.3.436

van den Borne, S. W. M., Diez, J., Blankesteijn, W. M., Verjans, J., Hofstra, L., and Narula, J. (2010). Myocardial remodeling after infarction: the role of myofibroblasts. *Nat. Rev. Cardiol.* 7, 30–37. doi: 10.1038/nrcardio.2009.199

Varga-Szemes, A., van der Geest, R. J., Schoepf, U. J., De Cecco, C. N., Tesche, C., Fuller, S. R., et al. (2016). MRI post-processing methods for myocardial infarct quantification. *Curr. Radiol. Rep.* 4:30. doi: 10.1007/s40134-016-0159-7

Vergara, C., Palamara, S., Catanzariti, D., Nobile, F., Faggiano, E., Pangrazzi, C., et al. (2014). Patient-specific generation of the Purkinje network driven by clinical measurements of a normal propagation. *Med. Biol. Eng. Comput.* 52, 813–826. doi: 10.1007/s11517-014-1183-5

Vigmond, E., Vadakkumpadan, F., Gurev, V., Arevalo, H., Deo, M., Plank, G., et al. (2009). Towards predictive modelling of the electrophysiology of the heart. *Exp. Physiol.* 94, 563–577. doi: 10.1113/expphysiol.2008.044073

Wagner, A., Mahrholdt, H., Holly, T. A., Elliott, M. D., Regenfus, M., Parker, M., et al. (2003). Contrast-enhanced MRI and routine single photon emission computed tomography (SPECT) perfusion imaging for detection of subendocardial myocardial infarcts: an imaging study. *Lancet* 361, 374–379. doi: 10.1016/S0140-6736(03)12389-6

Walton, R. D., Pashaei, A., Martinez, M. E., Constantin, M., Duchateau, J., Bear, L., et al. (2018). Compartmentalized structure of the moderator band provides a unique substrate for macroreentrant ventricular tachycardia. *Circ. Arrhythmia Electrophysiol.* 11:e005913. doi: 10.1161/CIRCEP.117.005913

Wijnmaalen, A. P., van der Geest, R. J., van Huls van Taxis, C. F. B., Siebelink, H.-M. J., Kroft, L. J. M., Bax, J. J., et al. (2011). Head-to-head comparison of contrast-enhanced magnetic resonance imaging and electroanatomical voltage mapping to assess post-infarct scar characteristics in patients with ventricular tachycardias: real-time image integration and reversed registration. *Eur. Heart J.* 32, 104–114. doi: 10.1093/eurheartj/ehq345

Wilber, D. J. (2008). Catheter ablation of ventricular tachycardia: two decades of progress. *Hear. Rhythm* 5, S59–S63. doi: 10.1016/j.hrthm.2008.02.001

Winklhofer, S., Stoeck, C. T., Berger, N., Thali, M., Manka, R., Kozerke, S., et al. (2014). Post-mortem cardiac diffusion tensor imaging: detection of myocardial infarction and remodeling of myofiber architecture. *Eur. Radiol.* 24, 2810–2818. doi: 10.1007/s00330-014-3322-7

Wu, M.-T., Tseng, W.-Y. I., Su, M.-Y. M., Liu, C.-P., Chiou, K.-R., Wedeen, V. J., et al. (2006). Diffusion tensor magnetic resonance imaging mapping the fiber architecture remodeling in human myocardium after infarction: correlation with viability and wall motion. *Circulation* 114, 1036–1045. doi: 10.1161/CIRCULATIONAHA.105.545863

Xie, Y., Garfinkel, A., Camelliti, P., Kohl, P., Weiss, J. N., and Qu, Z. (2009). Effects of fibroblast-myocyte coupling on cardiac conduction and vulnerability to reentry: a computational study. *Hear. Rhythm* 6, 1641–1649. doi: 10.1016/j.hrthm.2009.08.003

Yamada, T. (2014). Catheter ablation of epicardial ventricular tachycardia. *J. Arrhythmia* 30, 262–271. doi: 10.1016/j.joa.2014.04.011

Yamashita, S., Sacher, F., Mahida, S., Berte, B., Lim, H. S., Komatsu, Y., et al. (2016). Image integration to guide catheter ablation in scar-related ventricular tachycardia. *J. Cardiovasc. Electrophysiol.* 27, 699–708. doi: 10.1111/jce.12963

Yan, A. T. (2006). Characterization of the peri-infarct zone by contrast-enhanced cardiac magnetic resonance imaging is a powerful predictor of post-myocardial infarction mortality. *Circulation* 114, 32–39. doi: 10.1161/CIRCULATIONAHA.106.613414

Yan, G.-X., Shimizu, W., and Antzelevitch, C. (1998). Characteristics and distribution of M cells in arterially perfused canine left ventricular wedge preparations. *Circulation* 98, 1921–1927. doi: 10.1161/01.CIR.98.18.1921

Yao, J.-A., Hussain, W., Patel, P., Peters, N. S., Boyden, P. A., and Wit, A. L. (2003). Remodeling of gap junctional channel function in epicardial border zone of healing canine infarcts. *Circ. Res.* 92, 437–443. doi: 10.1161/01.RES.0000059301.81035.06

Yokokawa, M., Desjardins, B., Crawford, T., Good, E., Morady, F., and Bogun, F. (2013). Reasons for recurrent ventricular tachycardia after catheter ablation of post-infarction ventricular tachycardia. *J. Am. Coll. Cardiol.* 61, 66–73. doi: 10.1016/j.jacc.2012.07.059

Zeigler, A. C., Richardson, W. J., Holmes, J. W., and Saucerman, J. J. (2016). Computational modeling of cardiac fibroblasts and fibrosis. *J. Mol. Cell. Cardiol.* 93, 73–83. doi: 10.1016/j.yjmcc.2015.11.020

NOMENCLATURE

2D	Two-dimensional
3D	Three-dimensional
AP	Action potential
APD	Action potential duration
BCL	Basic cycle length
SCC	Slow conducting channel
DE-MRI	Delayed enhancement-MRI
EAM	Electroanatomical map/mapping
ECG	Electrocardiogram
EGM	Electrogram
FEM	Finite-element method
LAT	Local activation time
LV	Left ventricle
MI	Myocardial infarction
RFA	Radiofrequency ablation
RV	Right ventricle
SD	Standard deviation
VT	Ventricular tachycardia
DTI	Diffusion tensor imaging
EP	Electrophysiology/electrophysiological

3

MRI-Based Computational Torso/Biventricular Multiscale Models to Investigate the Impact of Anatomical Variability on the ECG QRS Complex

Ana Mincholé[1†], Ernesto Zacur[2†], Rina Ariga[3], Vicente Grau[2‡] and Blanca Rodriguez[1‡]*

[1] *Department of Computer Science, University of Oxford, Oxford, United Kingdom,* [2] *Institute of Biomedical Engineering (IBME), University of Oxford, Oxford, United Kingdom,* [3] *Division of Cardiovascular Medicine, Radcliffe Department of Medicine, University of Oxford, Oxford, United Kingdom*

Correspondence:
Ana Mincholé
ana.minchole@gmail.com

† These authors have contributed equally to this work as first authors

‡ These authors have contributed equally to this work as senior authors

Aims: Patient-to-patient anatomical differences are an important source of variability in the electrocardiogram, and they may compromise the identification of pathological electrophysiological abnormalities. This study aims at quantifying the contribution of variability in ventricular and torso anatomies to differences in QRS complexes of the 12-lead ECG using computer simulations.

Methods: A computational pipeline is presented that enables computer simulations using human torso/biventricular anatomically based electrophysiological models from clinically standard magnetic resonance imaging (MRI). The ventricular model includes membrane kinetics represented by the biophysically detailed O'Hara Rudy model modified for tissue heterogeneity and includes fiber orientation based on the Streeter rule. A population of 265 torso/biventricular models was generated by combining ventricular and torso anatomies obtained from clinically standard MRIs, augmented with a statistical shape model of the body. 12-lead ECGs were simulated on the 265 human torso/biventricular electrophysiology models, and QRS morphology, duration and amplitude were quantified in each ECG lead for each of the human torso-biventricular models.

Results: QRS morphologies in limb leads are mainly determined by ventricular anatomy, while in the precordial leads, and especially V1 to V4, they are determined by heart position within the torso. Differences in ventricular orientation within the torso can explain morphological variability from monophasic to biphasic QRS complexes. QRS duration is mainly influenced by myocardial volume, while it is hardly affected by the torso anatomy or position. An average increase of 0.12 ± 0.05 ms in QRS duration is obtained for each cm^3 of myocardial volume across all the leads while it hardly changed due to changes in torso volume.

Conclusion: Computer simulations using populations of human torso/biventricular models based on clinical MRI enable quantification of anatomical causes of variability in the QRS complex of the 12-lead ECG. The human models presented also pave the way toward their use as testbeds *in silico* clinical trials.

Keywords: clinical MRI-based torso/ventricular anatomical models, computer simulations, electrocardiogram, computational modeling, cardiac magnetic resonance imaging

INTRODUCTION

The electrocardiogram (ECG) is the most widely used clinical tool for evaluation of cardiac function. It records the electrical activity of the heart from electrodes positioned on the patient's torso, and the duration, amplitude, and morphology of ECG waveforms in the different leads are used for patients' diagnosis (Macfarlane and Lawrie, 2010).

Electrocardiogram features, and specifically its QRS complex, are affected not only by microstructural and physiological factors such as fiber orientation, Purkinje, myocardial conduction pathways and ionic currents (Boineau and Spach, 1968), but also by anatomical characteristics such as heart size and orientation, ventricular wall thickness, and body mass index (Hoekema et al., 1999, 2001; van Oosterom et al., 2000; Corlan et al., 2005). Quantitative information on the latter is, however, scarce. An experimental study showed large changes in QRS with varying heart locations, using one isolated perfused dog heart suspended in an electrolytic torso tank (MacLeod et al., 2000). Computer simulation studies are ideally placed to provide insight on the underlying basis of the ECG. Most of the previous computational studies focused on simulating the ECG using a single heart anatomy as (Keller et al., 2010; Zemzemi et al., 2013; Zemzemi and Rodriguez, 2015; Neic et al., 2017; Potse, 2018). More recently, a computational study using torso-biventricular anatomical models for five patients with heart failure showed that heart position and orientation strongly altered QRS amplitude, but only slightly, QRS duration (Nguyên et al., 2015). Sánchez et al. (2018) also provided insights into the key factors determining the ECG characteristics based on data for six heart failure patients. These studies highlight the potential of computer simulation studies using image-based models to shed light into the anatomical basis governing ECG variability and the QRS complex.

Whereas the dense volumetric information and high resolution of current CT scans is a clear advantage in the construction of cardiac anatomical models (Nazarian and Halperin, 2018) for ECG simulations, the radiation involved limits their use, for example in healthy subjects. The alternative of using magnetic resonance imaging (MRI) scans is very attractive as they provide good quality cardiac images safely and non-invasively. Clinical protocols, however, focus on the heart and therefore information on the torso is scarce. This is why previous studies have used MRI scans obtained using dedicated imaging protocols, not suitable for routine clinical practice (Potse et al., 2014; Sánchez et al., 2018). Methodological advances are therefore needed to exploit clinically standard MRI databases in computer simulations studies using image-based human torso/biventricular anatomical models.

The goal of this study is to conduct a computer simulation study using a population of 265 torso-ventricular anatomical models based on clinically standard MRI to dissect and quantify the individual contribution of ventricular and torso anatomy on QRS biomarkers in the 12-lead ECG. We hypothesize that QRS complexes in each of the standard 12-lead ECGs are affected differently by geometrical factors such as ventricular anatomy, heart orientation and location, or torso anatomy. To test this hypothesis, we develop a computational pipeline to conduct high-performance computing (HPC) electrophysiological simulations using biophysically detailed computational human models with ventricular and torso anatomies obtained from clinically standard cardiac MRI acquisitions. In a clinical scenario, the new insights could facilitate an improved discrimination in clinical ECG recordings between the contributions of patient's anatomical features and those arising from a cardiac condition or disease.

MATERIALS AND METHODS

Reconstruction of Ventricular and Torso Anatomical Meshes From Clinical MRI

In this study, a total of 265 combined torso-ventricles anatomical models were considered to quantify the effect of ventricular and torso volumes, and heart position and orientation on the QRS complex. Initially, as described in **Figure 1**, twenty-five human heart-torso models were generated by combining the bi-ventricular geometries (H1–H5) and torsos (T1–T5) (including corresponding heart orientations and positions) extracted from clinical MRI acquisition from 5 healthy subjects. The MRI datasets were selected to include ventricular end diastolic myocardial volumes between 75 and 170 cm^3 and torso volumes between 23 and 54 dm^3. Then, either rotation or translation was applied to each bi-ventricular model within each torso. 5° steps up to (±40° were considered both around the long axis (LA) and around the left-to-right-ventricle axis (LR) (Nguyên et al., 2015). Translation was considered in 1 cm steps up to (±4 cm either along the lateral or along cranio-caudal directions.

The MRI scans were obtained in five healthy subjects (three females and two males) with a range of ventricular end-diastolic myocardial volumes between 75 and 170 cm^3 and torso volumes between 23 and 54 dm^3, recruited at John Radcliffe Hospital, Oxford, United Kingdom. Subjects were non-smokers without cardiovascular disease, hypertension or diabetes, and no family history of cardiomyopathy or sudden cardiac death (SCD).

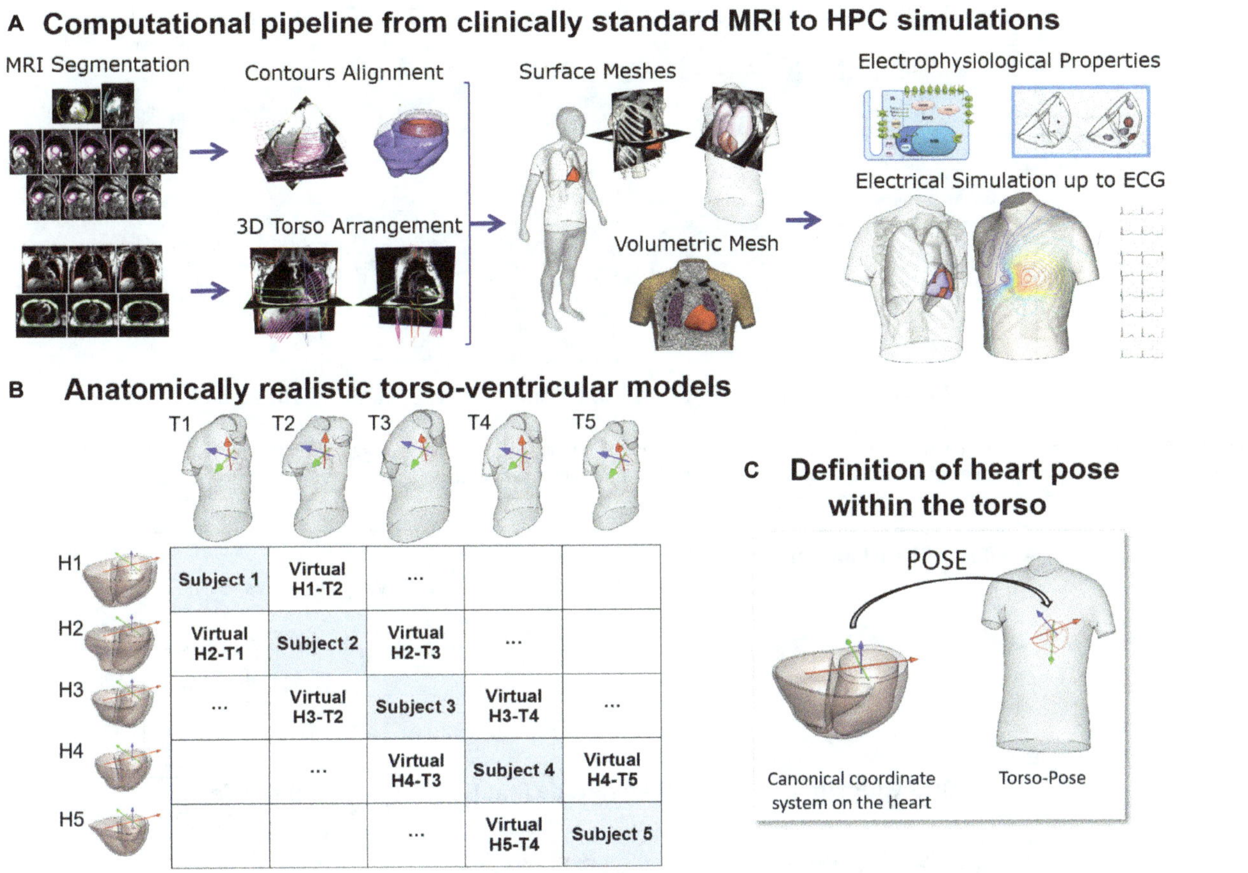

FIGURE 1 | (A) Computational pipeline from clinical MRI segmentations through construction of heart and torso geometries to the HPC simulation of electrophysiology from ionic to body surface potentials. Following MRI segmentations, heart surface is obtained by removing breath misalignment and torso surface by using the sparse information from the MRI contours together with a statistical body shape model. With the volumetric meshes, electrophysiological properties such as an action potential model and an activation model are used to simulate electrical activity from cell to torso and calculate the 12-lead ECG. **(B)** 25 torso-ventricular anatomical models combining five torsos (T1–T5) and five ventricles (H1–H5) of varying volumes. **(C)** Heart pose within the torso defined as the transformation from a canonical coordinate system of the ventricular geometry to the torso coordinate system.

Clinically standard cine cardiac MRI acquisition was performed for each subject, including long axis (LAX) and a stack of short axis (SAX) views. More specifically, for each subject, the data includes a 2 chamber LAX view, 4 chamber view, and a stack of SAX view from apex to base with 10 mm of separation between adjacent slices in the stack (8 mm slice thickness plus 2 mm gap). Image resolution ranges from 1.4 to 1.6 mm per pixel. An expert with several years of experience in cardiac MRI segmented the images at end-diastole including the following structures: left epicardium, left ventricle (LV) endocardium excluding the papillary muscles, and right ventricle (RV) endocardium (see **Figure 1A**, Segmentation). As the image resolution in standard MRI acquisitions does not allow to differentiate right ventricular epicardial and endocardial contours in the right ventricle, we synthesized right epicardial contours by a 3.5 mm offset from the endocardial contours (Prakash, 1978). Spatial misalignments in slice images and spatial discrepancies between the contours due to acquisitions at different breath holds were corrected by aligning intensity profiles of intersecting slices using a 3D rigid transformation for each image (Villard et al., 2017) (see **Figure 1A**, Contours alignment). Bi-ventricular geometries were built from the aligned contours using the end-diastole frames from the standard CINE acquisition as in Villard et al. (2018) and Zacur et al. (2017).

For the construction of the torso geometries, semi-automatic tools were developed and used to delineate the torso skin and lungs (Zacur et al., 2017). In brief, on each subject, the scout images (localizers), as well as, most of the MRI images (SAX and LAX images) with a large enough field of view were used and contoured. The sparse 3D geometrical information from the torso images is insufficient for the use of classical segmentation to surface methods such as isocontouring tools (**Figure 1A**, 3-Dimensional torso arrangement). Thus, we developed and applied a methodology to fit a statistical shape model of the human body to the skin contours (Zacur et al., 2017). The torso contours together with subject height, weight and gender information were used to reconstruct a body surface belonging to a learned class of plausible body shapes from the statistical shape model (Pishchulin et al., 2017; Zacur et al., 2017). The average discrepancy between MRI-based contours and model surface is

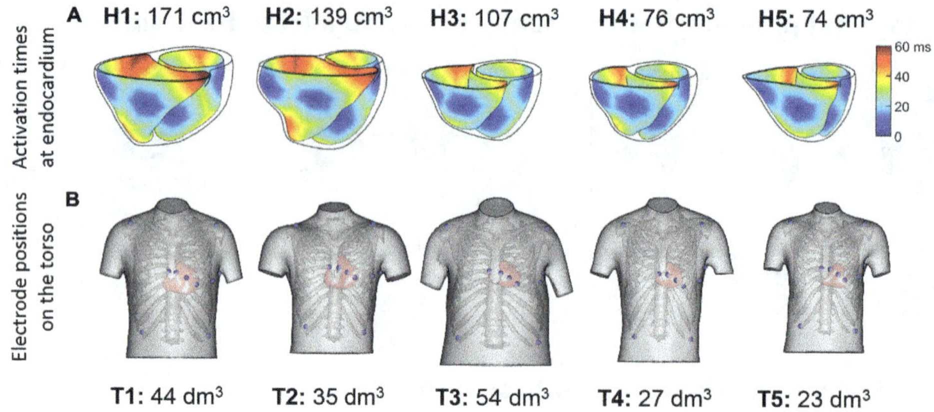

FIGURE 2 | (A) Endocardial activation maps for the five ventricular geometries. Information about ventricular volumes is also provided. **(B)** Homologous 12-lead electrode positions for the five virtualized subjects. Information about the torso volumes is provided.

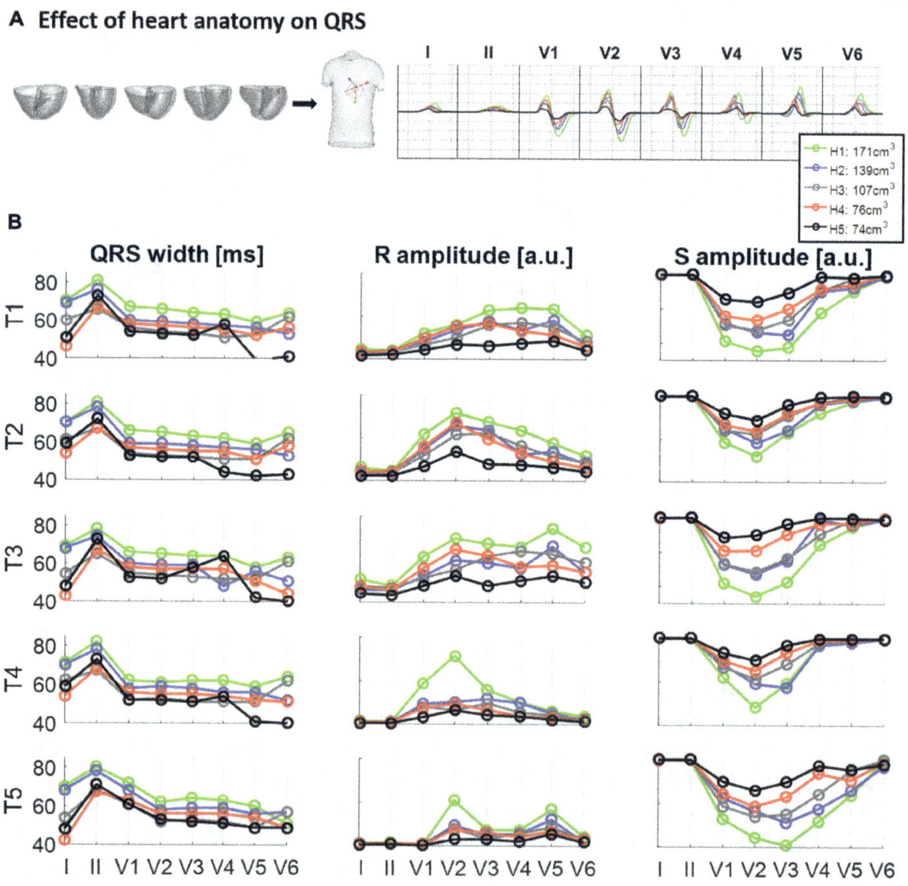

FIGURE 3 | Effect of ventricular geometry on QRS duration, and S and R wave amplitude. **(A)** Simulated QRS complexes obtained for five ventricular geometries placed in the torso-pose of Subject 3 (T3). **(B)** QRS duration (left), S and R amplitude (middle and right, respectively) obtained from simulations using the five ventricular geometries (H1 to H5) placed in each of the five torso-poses (T1 to T5). The term "a.u." stands for arbitrary units.

3 mm in terms of root mean square, being the 90th percentile 5 mm. A template-based approach was used to place other internal structures such as the lungs and the ribs (**Figure 1A**, Surface meshes). Full details about the procedure are provided in Zacur et al. (2017).

All surfaces were remeshed with different element sizes to ensure numerical convergence of the finite element software Chaste for electrophysiological simulations (Pitt-Francis et al., 2009; Dutta et al., 2016) as described in **Supplementary Material S1**. Finally, tetrahedral volumetric meshes were constructed from these surfaces (see **Supplementary Material S1**). The surface and volumetric meshes can be downloaded from http://www.cs.ox.ac.uk/ccs/home.

Figure 1B shows the reconstructed ventricular geometries and, the torso geometries including their corresponding heart orientations and positions, constrained by chest boundaries. The generation of a new virtual torso-ventricular geometry requires the transformation of the ventricular geometry from a canonical reference frame to the position defined by the torso (pose, see **Figure 1C**). Hereinafter, torso-pose is defined as the torso geometry including the heart pose, which represents the coordinate system and location of the heart. This torso-pose linking is supported by physical constraints such as chest boundaries, since one specific torso anatomy does not allow any heart position (Engblom et al., 2005). Further information is found in **Supplementary Material S1**.

Electrophysiological Simulations

The anatomical torso-ventricular model combinations described above were used to compute 265 QRS complexes from computer simulations as follows. The propagation of the electrical activity in the human ventricles and torso was modeled using the fully coupled heart-torso bidomain equations and solved with the Chaste software (Pitt-Francis et al., 2009). Human ventricular membrane kinetics were simulated with a modified version of the O'Hara-Rudy action potential model (O'Hara et al., 2011) published in Dutta et al. (2017). Myocardial and torso conductivities, and, myocardial fiber structure were set as described in **Supplementary Material S2**. An anisotropic myocardial fiber architecture was implemented using the Streeter rule (Streeter et al., 1969). The three orthotropic intracellular and extracellular myocardial conductivities were set as in Cardone-Noott et al. (2016). Transmural, apex-to-base and interventricular cell electrophysiological heterogeneities were introduced based on experimental and clinical data and as described in **Supplementary Material S2**. The QRS complex is hardly affected by the electrophysiological heterogeneities included in our models as they mainly affect the repolarization properties and the T wave. However, they provide our computational pipeline with all the state of the art capabilities to extend the work to investigate variability in T wave morphology, as well as under disease and drug action.

Sinus rhythm was simulated using a phenomenological activation model with early endocardial activation initiated by root nodes and a fast endocardial layer representing a tightly packed endocardial Purkinje network (Cardone-Noott et al., 2016). In short, 7 root nodes are positioned in the ventricles on the endocardium: four in the LV (LV mid septum, LV anterior paraseptal, and two LV mid-posterior) and three in the RV (RV mid septum, two RV free wall), as shown in **Supplementary Material S2**. Simulated ventricular activation times for these models show the LV endocardial surfaces are fully activated within a range of 39 to 51 ms, and the latest moments of activation occurs in a range from 57 to 76 ms. This is in agreement with the *ex vivo* microelectrode recordings by Durrer et al. (1970) reporting around 45 ms in endocardial LV activation, and from 60 to 80 ms the latest moments of whole ventricular activation.

The aim of this study is to investigate, analyze and quantify the effect of anatomical/geometrical variability on the QRS complexes in an electrophysiological computer simulation framework. It is not to construct personalized electrophysiology models to replicate each of the patients' data. In order to isolate the effect of ventricular anatomy from differences in activation patterns, the endocardial speed was set to 120 cm/s in all models, and the locations of the root nodes were mapped to anatomically homologous locations from the geometry used in a previous study (Cardone-Noott et al., 2016). The coupled epicardial, RV and LV endocardial surfaces and ventricular insertion points from the original geometry (Cardone-Noott et al., 2016) were diffeomorphically registered to each ventricular geometry using a composition of approximated Thin-Plate Splines (TPS) deformations (Rohr et al., 2001). The deformation method was guided by an iterated closest point between the corresponding source and target surfaces/structures (left and right endo- and epicardial surfaces, atrio-ventricular planes, and anterior and posterior interventricular grooves). The successive deformations were performed by following an annealing process in the smoothness parameter of approximated TPS (Amberg et al., 2007). The resulting registered deformation was applied to the early activation sites from the original geometry resulting in the anatomically homologous locations that lead to similar activation sequences (see **Figure 2A**). The resulting deformations and the mapped activation sites were visually evaluated and approved by an expert cardiologist. This technique was used given its broad acceptance and success in the medical imaging and shape analysis field but the universal ventricular coordinates could represent an alternative (Bayer et al., 2018).

QRS complexes from the 12-lead ECGs were simulated by placing virtual electrodes in the standard 12-lead ECG positions for each torso. Since the statistical shape model used for reconstructing the torsos is based on anatomical correspondences, the virtual electrodes are located in anatomically homologous locations for all the torsos (see **Figure 2B**). These electrode positions correspond to analogous intercostal spaces for all subjects. Electrode coordinates are given for each of the torso geometries, and can be downloaded from http://www.cs.ox.ac.uk/ccs/home.

To simulate the QRS complex for 265 combinations of ventricular/torso positions and orientations while minimizing the number of expensive HPC simulations, extracellular potentials were computed from the ventricular potentials following the integral of dipole source density formulation (Gima and Rudy, 2002; Plonsey and Barr, 2007) as:

$$\phi(e) = \int_{\Omega} \left(-D\nabla V_m \cdot \left(\nabla \frac{1}{||r-e||} \right) \right) dr,$$

where $e = (e_x, e_y, e_z)$ are the electrode position coordinates, D is the diffusion tensor, and V_m is the membrane potential. The integral is calculated over the whole myocardium volume, Ω. Bidomain simulations coupled with the Poisson equation to propagate the electrical activity to the body surface were compared to the integration of dipole source density formulation for the torso propagation. The resulting QRS complexes were very similar as shown in **Supplementary Figure S3** from

Supplementary Material S2. The propagation model based on the integration of dipole source density formulation was chosen in order to simplify the numerical complexity of the computations and to avoid re-meshing the torso volume for each scenario in which the ventricular geometry was rotated, translated or permuted. Although this method does not allow the inclusion of tissue inhomogeneities in the torso, several studies suggest minimal differences in the resulting body surface potentials and the QRS complex when assuming homogeneous or inhomogeneous torso models (Ramanathan and Rudy, 2001; Geneser et al., 2008).

Quantification of QRS-Based Features and Descriptors

Clinically used features from the QRS, such as duration and amplitude, were extracted for each of the simulated 12-lead ECGs. QRS duration is calculated by using a relative threshold on the absolute value of the slopes of the ECG signal to identify QRS onset and offset as in Martínez et al. (2004). We compared the simulation results with those reported in the literature and also clinical ECG recordings from healthy volunteers, as part of a prospective study approved by the National Research Ethics Committee (REC ref 12/LO/1979). Informed written consent was obtained from each participant (Lyon et al., 2018a).

Furthermore, in order to quantify the effect of anatomical variability in QRS morphology, we proposed a similarity measure to quantify QRS morphological differences, invariant to QRS amplitude and duration. The new metric (PC*) is based on a continuous generalization of the Pearson coefficient (PC), which in order to ensure independence from QRS duration, includes the invariance to a uniform warping (time scaling) in time of the QRS complex. Therefore, PC* between two QRS complexes is 1 when these have the same morphology regardless of the amplitude or the duration.

Let f and g be two functions defined on the domains $\mathrm{dom}(f) = \left[t_0^f, t_1^f\right]$ and $\mathrm{dom}(g) = \left[t_0^g, t_1^g\right]$, respectively. Let's assume that $\mathrm{dom}(f) \cap \mathrm{dom}(g) \neq \emptyset$ and let's consider the combined domain $[t_0, t_1] = \mathrm{dom}(f) \cup \mathrm{dom}(g)$, where $t_0 = \min\left(t_0^f, t_0^g\right)$ and $t_1 = \max\left(t_1^f, t_1^g\right)$. On this combined domain, let $\tilde{f}$ be the replicated extension of the original function f,

$$\tilde{f} = \begin{cases} f(t) & \text{if } t \in \left[t_0^f, t_1^f\right] \\ f(t_0^f) & \text{if } t < t_0^f \\ f(t_1^f) & \text{if } t < t_1^f \end{cases}$$

and equivalently for $\tilde{g}$.

Our proposed generalized PC is given by

$$\mathrm{PC}_{f,g} = \frac{1}{t_1 - t_0} \int_{t_0}^{t_1} \frac{\tilde{f}(t) - \mu_{\tilde{f}}}{\sigma_{\tilde{f}}} \cdot \frac{\tilde{g}(t) - \mu_{\tilde{g}}}{\sigma_{\tilde{g}}} dt \qquad (1)$$

where $\mu_{\tilde{f}}$ and $\mu_{\tilde{g}}$ are means, and $\sigma_{\tilde{f}}$ and $\sigma_{\tilde{g}}$ are the standard deviations of the functions $\tilde{f}(t)$ and $\tilde{g}(t)$, respectively,

$$\mu_{\tilde{f}} = \frac{1}{t_1 - t_0} \int_{t_0}^{t_1} \tilde{f}(t)dt, \qquad \sigma_{\tilde{f}} = \sqrt{\frac{1}{t_1 - t_0} \int_{t_0}^{t_1} \left(\tilde{f}(t) - \mu_{\tilde{f}}\right)^2 dt}$$

and equivalently for $\mu_{\tilde{g}}$ and $\sigma_{\tilde{g}}$. The subtraction of the means $\mu_{\tilde{f}}$ and $\mu_{\tilde{g}}$ in Eq. (1) ensures the invariance of PC under changes in the baseline levels. Likewise, normalizations by $\sigma_{\tilde{f}}$ and $\sigma_{\tilde{g}}$, endow PC with invariance to scaling. The normalization by $(t_1 - t_0)$ allows independence from time units. Thus, PC values are within the $[-1, 1]$ interval.

In order to ensure independence from QRS duration, we include the invariance to a uniform warping (time scaling) in time through the following similarity measurement PC*:

$$\mathrm{PC}^*_{f,g} = \max_{s \in \mathbb{R}^+} \mathrm{PC}_{f(\cdot), g(s\cdot)},$$

where $g(s\cdot)$ is a uniformly time-warped version of g. It is worth mentioning that since $\mathrm{dom}(g(s\cdot)) = 1/s \cdot \mathrm{dom}(g) = \left[t_0^g/s, t_1^g/s\right]$, the integral interval in Eq.(1) is updated accordingly, and the resulting PC* keeps having comparable values.

In the following, we will explain how to quantify a global similarity for a set of N functions $\{f_1(\cdot), f_2(\cdot), \cdots, f_N(\cdot)\}$. We propose to compute, the best time warping factors for the N functions simultaneously, in order to optimally align the set. Therefore, we search for

$$\{s_1, s_2, \ldots, s_N\} = \underset{s_1,\ldots,s_N \in \mathbb{R}^+}{\mathrm{argmax}} \min_{\substack{i=1\ldots N \\ j=i+1\ldots N}} \mathrm{PC}_{f_i(s_i\cdot), f_j(s_j\cdot)}$$

Once these optimal time warping factors have been computed, the global similarity for the functions $\{f_1(\cdot), f_2(\cdot), \cdots, f_N(\cdot)\}$ is given by

$$\mathrm{PC}^*_{f_1, f_2, \ldots f_N} = \max_{\substack{i=1\ldots N \\ j=i+1\ldots N}} \mathrm{PC}_{f_i(s_i\cdot), f_j(s_j\cdot)}$$

with this, the worst aligned pair defines the similarity of the whole set.

RESULTS

Effect of Ventricular Geometry on QRS Duration and Amplitude

Figure 3 illustrates the effect of different ventricular geometries within the same torso with corresponding heart position (hereinafter referred to as torso-pose) on QRS duration and amplitude. **Figure 3A** shows the QRS complexes obtained in leads I, II and V1–V6 for each of the five ventricles (H1–H5) placed in the torso-pose of Subject 3 (T3). **Figure 3B** shows QRS complex duration as well as S and R wave amplitude for all 25 torso-pose and ventricular combinations. For all torso-poses, QRS complexes decrease in amplitude and increase in duration with an increase in myocardial volume (green versus black traces corresponding to the largest versus the smallest ventricular volumes, respectively). An average increase of 0.12 ± 0.05 ms in QRS duration for each cm^3 of myocardial volume across all the leads was found. Relationships between QRS durations and ventricular myocardial volumes for each of the leads is shown in **Supplementary Material S4. Supplementary Figure S4** shows the 12 lead QRS complexes of different ventricular geometries within the same torso-pose for each of the five subjects.

Effect of Torso-Heart Position on QRS Duration and Amplitude

Figure 4 shows the effect of different torso-poses on QRS duration and amplitude. **Figure 4A** shows as an example, the QRS complexes obtained for the ventricular geometry H3 when placed in all the torso-poses, and **Figure 4B** provides quantification of QRS duration and R and S wave amplitudes for the five ventricular geometries. QRS duration does not change substantially for different torso-poses, and this suggests that QRS duration is mainly determined by the ventricular geometry. Indeed, a slight increase in QRS duration of 0.01 ± 0.03 ms for dm^3 of torso volume across all leads is observed (further information regarding the relationship between QRS duration and torso volume can be found in **Supplementary Material S4**). However, both S and R wave amplitudes are mainly determined by torso volumes, with larger QRS amplitudes corresponding to smaller torso volumes. Exceptionally, QRS complexes in T4 with a torso volume of 27 dm^3 exhibit larger amplitudes in V1 to V3 compared to T5 (23 dm^3) that exhibit larger amplitudes in V4 to V6. For these two torsos with similar volumes, heart position plays an important role in QRS amplitude. By comparing the ventricular positions for T4 and T5 (see **Figure 2**), we observe that for T5, V5 and V6 electrode positions are closer to the ventricles resulting in larger QRS amplitudes, whilst V2 and V3 electrodes are further away, resulting in smaller amplitudes.

Effect of Ventricular Geometry and Torso-Pose on QRS Morphology

Figure 5A displays the similarity measurement computed from the modified Pearson correlation PC*, which measures differences in QRS morphology due to differences in ventricular geometry and torso-pose.

Results show that for limb leads (I, II, aVR, aVL and aVF), and V5, QRS morphology is more similar (and PC* higher) for fixed ventricular geometry (with varying torso-pose) than for fixed torso-pose (with varying ventricular geometry). Therefore, in these leads, the ventricular geometry mainly determines the QRS morphology.

On the contrary, for leads V1 to V4 and V6, QRS morphology is more similar (as shown by the higher PC* values) for fixed torso-poses than for fixed ventricular geometry. Thus, in these leads, QRS morphology is mostly determined by torso-pose rather than by ventricular geometry.

These results are further illustrated in **Figures 5B,C** for two representative leads, aVL and V1. Simulated QRS morphology is mostly determined by the ventricular geometry and torso-pose in leads aVL and V1, respectively. Simulated QRS complexes obtained with the same ventricular geometry are shown in the same row while those obtained with the same torso-pose are shown in the same column. The warped QRS complexes from which PC* is computed are shown in **Supplementary Material S5**.

Effect of Heart Orientation and Position on the QRS Morphology

Figures 6, 7 illustrate the results obtained from the 265 simulations conducted to evaluate the effect of rotation around the long axis and left-to-right ventricle directions and translation along the lateral and cranio-caudal directions of the ventricles within the torso in the QRS complex. **Figure 6** displays simulated QRS complexes obtained for a representative anatomical model (H3 within T3), whereas **Figure 7** shows quantification of the QRS morphology similarity metric (PC*) for all subject specific torso-ventricular geometries.

As shown in **Figures 6A, 7A**, rotation along the long axis mainly affects the R and S amplitudes of leads V1 to V3. The amplitude of the R wave is larger when the LV faces the chest plane (orange traces) and decreases as the RV gets positioned between the LV and the chest (blue trace). The amplitude of the S wave also decreases in the precordial leads in ventricular positions where the RV faces the chest. Quantitative results regarding changes in QRS amplitudes with heart orientation and position can be found in **Supplementary Material S6**.

Figures 6B, 7B show that rotation around the left-to-right ventricle axis severely affects the QRS morphology in leads II, and V1 to V5. More horizontal hearts (orange traces) result in larger R wave amplitudes in leads I, V1, and V6 while more vertical ones (blue traces) result in larger R and S wave amplitudes in leads V2 to V5.

Figures 6C, 7C show that hearts located in more medial positions result in taller R and S waves in septal V1 to V3 leads while shorter R waves are observed in the precordial lateral leads V5 and V6. This is due to the closer ventricular location to V1 to V3 electrode positions and further from V5 and V6. On the other hand, hearts located in more lateral positions (toward the left-arm) displayed negatively deflected rS or even QS complexes in the septal V1 to V2 leads and larger R wave amplitudes in V5 to V6 (blue solid lines).

Figures 6D, 7D show the effect of shifting the ventricles up along the cranio-caudal (superior-inferior) direction leads to larger R wave amplitudes in lead I, and longer R and S waves in V1 to V5 (blue lines). However, shifting the heart down leads to shorter R waves in leads I, V1 and V6 (orange line). The changes would be equivalent to changing the electrode position with respect to the ventricles.

Comparison to Clinical Data

Simulated ECGs obtained from our population of models exhibit QRS axis (computed from QRS complexes in leads I and III) ranging from 50° to 75° [normal range –30° to 90° as shown in Engblom et al. (2005)], QRS durations per lead from 45 to 80 ms [normal range including all leads 78 ± 8 ms as shown in van Oosterom et al. (2000)], and amplitudes from 0.5 to 3.5 mV [healthy: 2 ± 0.6 mV as shown in van Oosterom et al. (2000)].

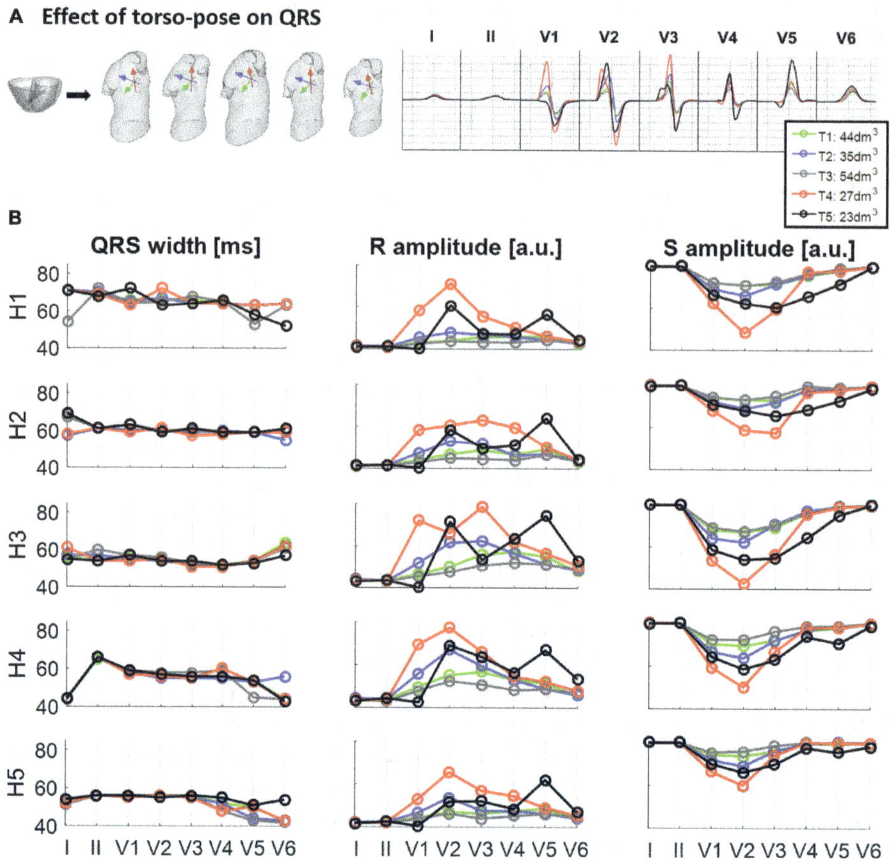

FIGURE 4 | Effect of torso-pose on QRS duration, and S and R wave amplitude. **(A)** Simulated QRS complexes obtained using the ventricular model from Subject 3 (H3) placed in the five different torsos-poses. **(B)** QRS duration (left), and S and R amplitudes (middle and right, respectively) from simulations using each of the five hearts (H1 to H5) placed in the different torso-poses (T1 to T5).

Thus, all these quantitative measurements are in agreement with clinical ECGs from healthy subjects (van Oosterom et al., 2000; Engblom et al., 2005; Stewart et al., 2011), supporting the credibility of the simulations.

Figure 8 shows a comparison of the variability exhibited in simulated and clinical 12 lead ECG QRS complexes. Simulated QRS complexes show variability in terms of morphology, especially in the precordial leads. The normal upright (positive) QRS complexes in both, lead I and lead aVF, result in a normal QRS axis. Furthermore, simulated QRS complexes show positive deflection with large, upright R wave in leads I, II, V4–V6 and a predominant negative deflection with a large, deep S wave in aVR, V1 and V2 (see **Figure 8A**). This is in agreement with the three clinical recordings shown in **Figure 8B**. Lead III in simulated ECGs shows biphasic QRS complexes with a negative deflection followed by a positive one as in the clinical recording of Subject 1 (**Figure 8B**). On the contrary, simulated lead aVL shows biphasic QRS complex with first a positive deflection followed by a negative one, as in clinical recordings of Subjects 1 and 3 (**Figure 8B**).

Precordial QRS complexes show R wave progression from V1 to V6, with an increasing R wave and a decreasing S wave when moving from V1 to V6. This progression is observed in both simulated (**Figure 8A**) and clinical ECGs (**Figure 8B**). QRS complexes in lead V1 show morphological variability from biphasic QRS complexes (positive-negative deflections) to downright QRS complexes (**Figure 8A**). This is in agreement with the variability in clinical recordings (**Figure 8B**).

DISCUSSION

The present study demonstrates the computational evaluation of the effect of heart-torso position and anatomy on the QRS complex using human torso/biventricular electrophysiology models derived from clinically standard MRI. The first contribution of the study is the computational pipeline to build the torso/biventricular anatomies initiating from standard clinical cardiac MRI augmented with a statistical shape model of the body (Zacur et al., 2017). This methodology enables exploiting clinical databases to evaluate the functional impact of MRI-extracted anatomical and structural features (Lyon et al., 2018b). Furthermore, human MRI-informed modeling and simulation based on this technology could accelerate the development of tailored pharmacological and electrical therapy

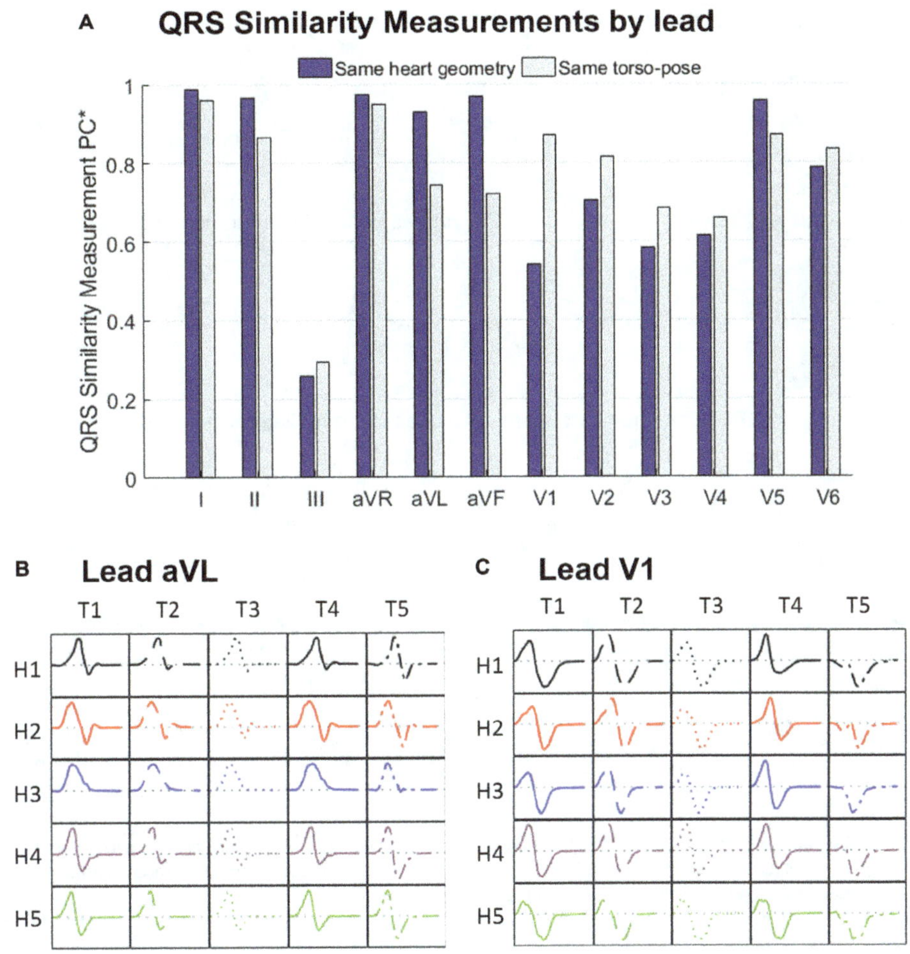

FIGURE 5 | (A) Similarity measurement (PC*) of the simulated QRS morphologies for fixed ventricular geometry (and varying torso-pose) (blue), and for fixed torso-pose (and varying ventricular geometry (gray). Panels **(B,C)** Simulated QRS morphologies obtained with the five ventricular geometries (H1 to H5) placed in the five torso-poses (T1 to T5) for leads aVL **(B)** and V1 **(C)**.

and the goal for precision care. Firstly, being able to reconstruct the patient's specific torso and ventricular model from standard cardiac MRI is a step forward to personalized computer modeling and simulation. The human models constructed have the biophysical detail required to enable future simulation studies into the response to disease and pharmacological treatment. Additionally, the simulation results demonstrate the influence of anatomical features on the QRS complex in healthy control conditions. This quantification of normal QRS complex variability is important to inform the evaluation of response to disease and treatment.

Analysis of the simulated QRSs yields the following findings: (i) QRS morphologies in limb leads I and II are mainly determined by the geometry of the ventricles whereas QRS morphologies in the precordial leads, and especially V1 to V4, are determined by the torso-pose. (ii) QRS duration is mainly influenced by myocardial volume while it is hardly affected by the torso geometry or heart position; (iii) QRS amplitude increases with large ventricular volumes and decreases with larger torso volumes. Quantification of the contribution of the individual heart structure, orientation and body habitus on the ECG is critical to aid the clinical interpretation of potential ECG abnormalities driven by disease or pharmacological treatment. In synergy with clinical databases, they could also drive the personalization of score metrics for risk stratification by discriminating in clinical recordings between the contribution of each patient's specific anatomy and those arising from their disease state.

Populations of Heart-Torso Electrophysiological Models From Standard Clinical MRI

In this paper, we present multiscale electrophysiological simulations using heart-torso anatomical models from standard cardiac MRI acquisitions (**Figure 1**). The generation of the subject-specific geometries is performed from standard cardiac MRI acquisitions allowing to be used directly on available clinical datasets. The scarce information of torso anatomy from standard cardiac MRI acquisitions makes the use of traditional

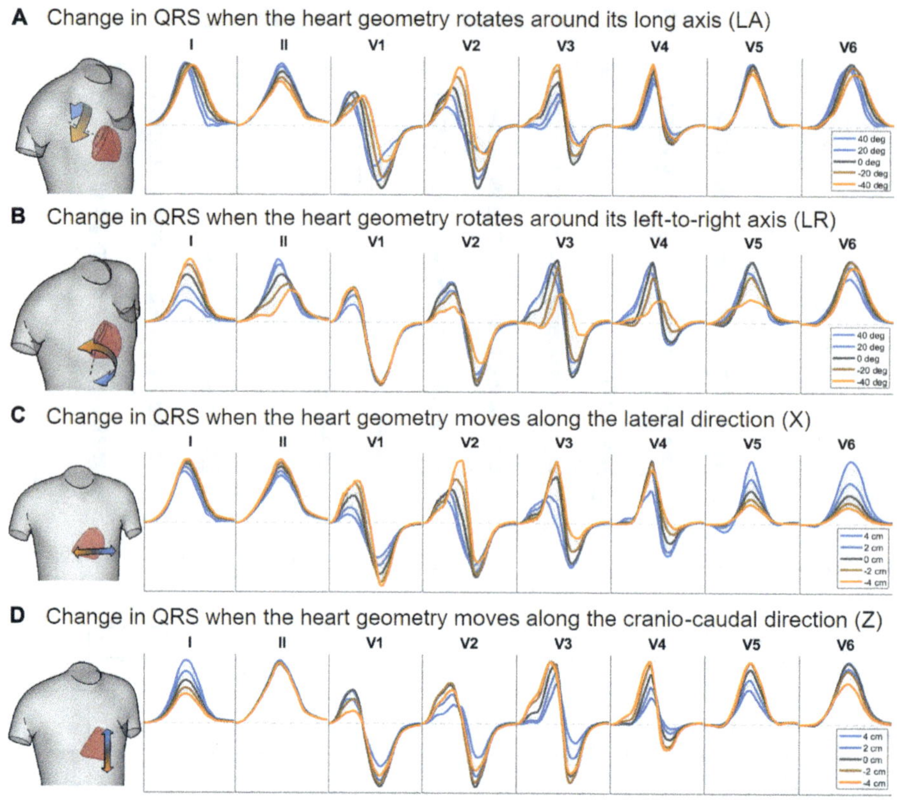

FIGURE 6 | Simulated QRS complex in leads I, II and V1 to V6 for different rotation angles around the long axis **(A)** and the left-to-right-ventricle direction **(B)**, and for different heart translations along the lateral **(C)** and cranio-caudal **(D)** directions. Gray lines correspond to intermediate results showing how the signals evolve from one colored state to another. The heart and torso geometries correspond to subject 3.

image-to-surface methods difficult and therefore, previous studies have required the use of dedicated imaging protocols (Potse et al., 2014). In the present pipeline, we make use of a statistical shape model together with the MRI information to accurately build the patient-specific torso geometry (Pishchulin et al., 2017; Zacur et al., 2017).

The comprehensive computational pipeline connects the outputs and inputs of different technologies, including the generation of torso-ventricular geometrical surfaces, the tetrahedralization into a multimaterial volumetric mesh, the generation of fiber orientations in the myocardium, the different input files to be used in the Chaste software to derive the fiber orientations and the endocardial layer for fast stimulation mimicking the Purkinje system, to assign different electrophysiological cell properties and finally to simulate the electrical activity and the 12-lead ECG. All files and torso-ventricular geometrical meshes are available for future studies.

In the evaluation of the role of anatomical features on the ECG, previous studies have typically performed perturbations to anatomical features (i.e., heart positioning and orientation) around a reference/original position to explore their individual effect (Corlan et al., 2005; Nguyên et al., 2015). In the present study, we sample the space of plausible anatomies and generate plausible instances by swapping ventricular anatomies together with torso-poses using their corresponding heart position and orientations (torso-poses) (see section "Reconstruction of Ventricular and Torso Anatomical Meshes From Clinical MRI"). This approach allows us to explore the role of ventricular anatomy on the QRS complex without the need to define a high dimensional parametrization of the ventricular shape. In particular, this population provides a generic open framework for further studies aimed to explore how anatomy and its variability influence the signature of the cardiac function in the ECG.

QRS Morphologies Are Determined by Ventricular Geometry in the Limb Leads and by Heart Orientation in Septal Leads

Ventricular geometry and not the torso-pose mainly determines the QRS morphology in the limb leads I and II, augmented leads, and V5 (see **Figure 5**). This finding may explain the weak correlation found in a number of studies between the anatomical heart orientation and the cardiac electrical axis (Dougherty, 1970; Horan, 1987; Engblom et al., 2005; Pellicori et al., 2015; Sathananthan et al., 2015). Cardiac electrical axis (Kashou and Kashou, 2018) is mainly estimated using the QRS complexes from leads I, II and aVF which, as shown in **Figures 5, 7**, are more influenced by ventricular geometry than by heart orientation. Therefore,

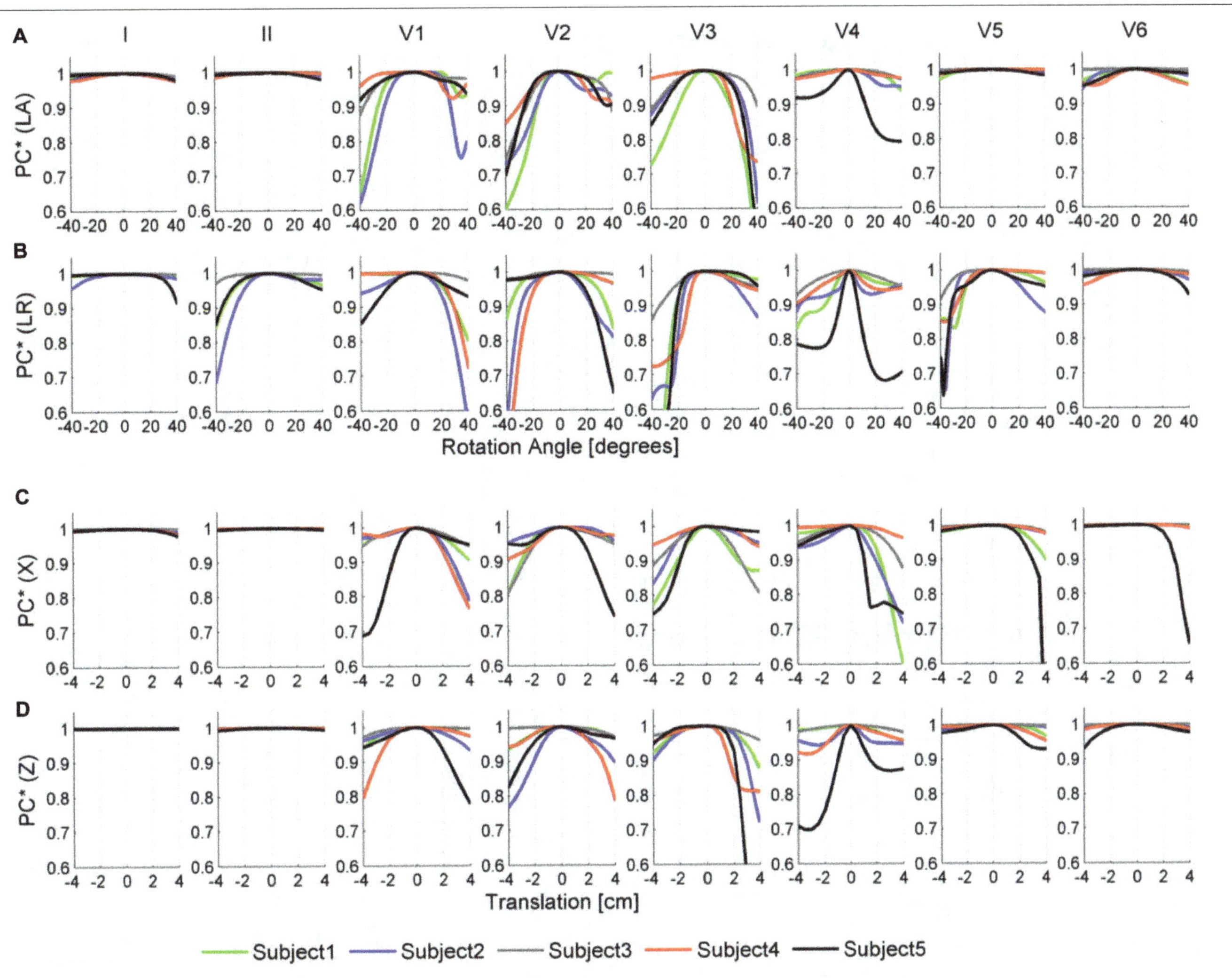

FIGURE 7 | Similarity measurement (PC*) for each lead (I, II, V1–V6) between the QRS at the original pose and the QRS when the heart is rotated along the long axis (LA) in panel **(A)**, the left-to-right-ventricles axis (LR) in panel **(B)**, and when translated in the lateral and cranio-caudal directions in panels **(C,D)**, respectively. Rotation angles range from –40° to 40° and translations range from –4 to 4 cm.

this results in a lower correlation between the electrical and anatomical axis.

On the other hand, QRS morphology in septal and anterior leads V1 to V4, III and V6 is mostly determined by the torso anatomy and its linked heart positioning. This could also result from changes in electrode position. The two different sources of variation, ventricular anatomy and torso-pose, affecting mainly limb/augmented leads and precordial leads, respectively, may have implications on the normal variability of QRS morphology in the different leads.

The proposed QRS similarity measurement is a global morphological measurement able to quantify differences in the QRS morphology due to the effect of anatomical variability. Unlike other studies proposing feature based differences as for example (Giffard-Roisin et al., 2017; Sánchez et al., 2018), we have measured differences in QRS morphology complementary and independent of QRS duration and amplitude. Our quantification allows a lead-wise evaluation of the influence of ventricular anatomy and torso-pose on the QRS morphology.

Importantly, the results on the contribution of the ventricular anatomy and the torso-pose on the QRS morphology of each of the leads do not depend on the endocardial and myocardial conduction (see **Supplementary Material S7**).

QRS Duration Depends Primarily on Ventricular Size and Is Hardly Affected by Heart Pose and Orientation

This study shows a positive correlation between ventricular volume and QRS duration (see **Figure 3**). Even if this finding is intuitive, little data exist on the influence of heart size and body weight on QRS duration. This correlation may have implications for the normal ranges of QRS duration and thus on the diagnosis of QRS prolongation. Most of the studies relating QRS duration and ventricular mass are in the context

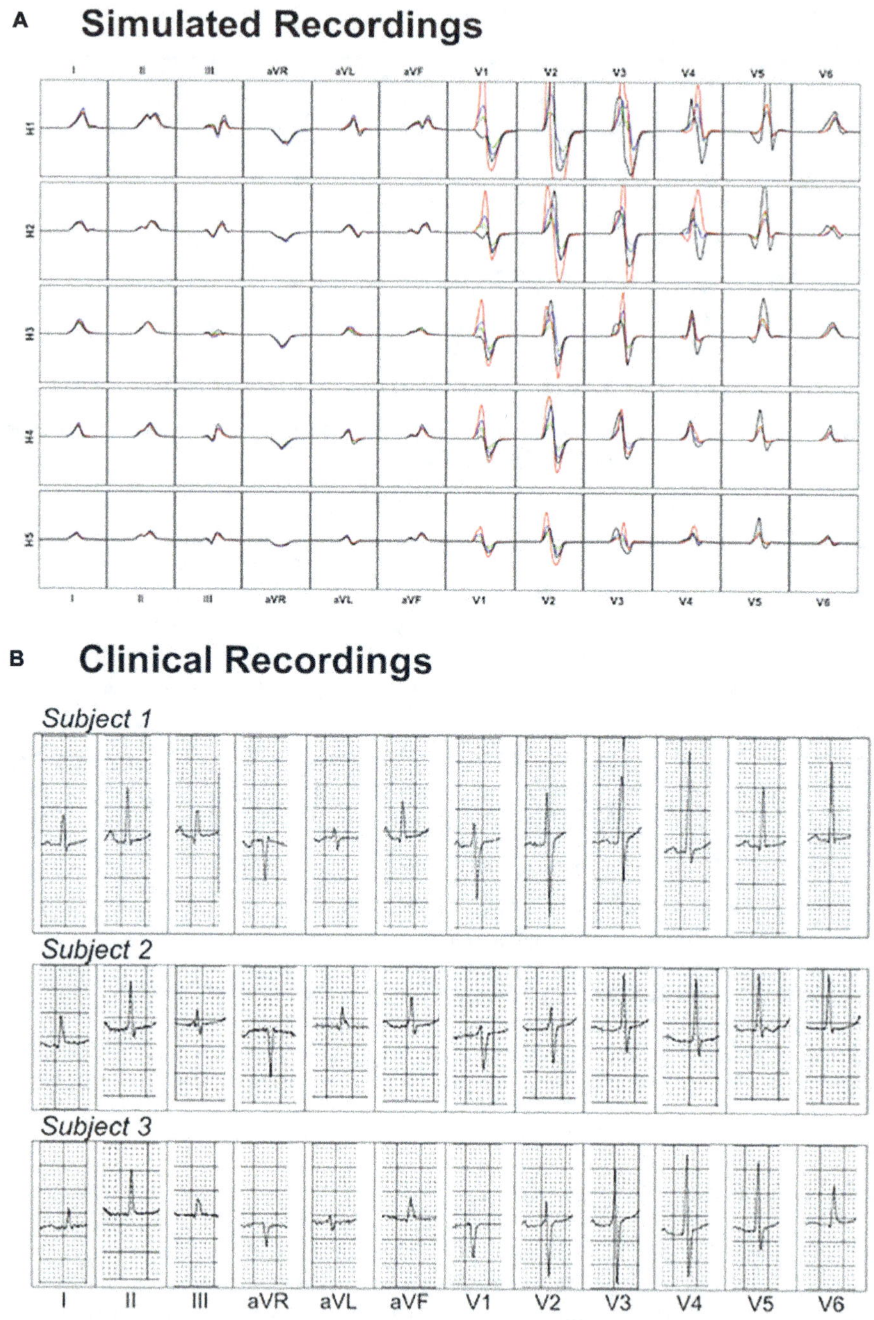

FIGURE 8 | Comparison between simulated and clinical 12-lead ECG recordings. Panel **(A)** shows the simulated 12-lead QRS complexes obtained using each of the ventricular models (H1–H5) placed in the five different torsos-poses. Panel **(B)** shows three exemplary clinical 12-lead ECG recordings from healthy subjects.

of patients at high cardiovascular risk (Stewart et al., 2011) and do not consider control subjects. Therefore, many factors may intervene for long QRS duration such as a reduced LV ejection fraction (Murkofsky et al., 1998) or ventricular dys-synchrony that are unrelated to LV hypertrophy (Oikarinen et al., 2004). On the contrary, we show that the torso-pose hardly modifies the QRS duration for any of the ventricular geometries (see **Figure 4**). This is in agreement with (Nguyên et al., 2015) that quantifies QRS duration differences from −6 to 10% in five heart failure patients.

Both Torso and Heart Geometrical Factors Have a Role in the QRS Amplitude

Ventricular and torso volumes are generally related since large body masses usually correspond to large hearts. Indeed, a recent paper in the large-scale population-based study UK-Biobank showed that higher LV mass was associated with increasing body mass index (BMI) (Petersen et al., 2017), explaining the BMI 72% of the global LV mass variability. However, myocardial and torso volumes affect the QRS amplitude in opposite ways. While larger ventricular geometries result in larger R and S wave amplitudes due to the increase of excitable myocardial tissue (see **Figure 3**), larger torso volumes result in lower R and S wave amplitudes due to the larger distance between the ventricles and the electrodes (see **Figure 4**). These two opposite effects coexist and lead to an ascending-descending behavior of the R wave amplitude with BMI as observed in clinical data (Kurisu et al., 2015). More specifically, precordial lateral leads display a slight increase in R wave from underweight to normal weight subjects followed by an abrupt decrease in the R amplitude for obese subjects (Kurisu et al., 2015). Despite the role of heart and body sizes, heart diseases and clinical conditions also affect QRS amplitude. Low QRS amplitude has been associated to different clinical conditions such as large infarct sizes (Katragadda et al., 2017), or to an increased risk of mortality in individuals free of apparent cardiovascular diseases (Usoro et al., 2014), while increased QRS amplitude has been associated to diseases such as left ventricular hypertrophy. Our study provides digital evidence in agreement with those findings and allows a systematic analysis of the effect of both ventricular and torso volumes in QRS amplitude.

Heart Rotation and Position Mainly Affect QRS Morphology in Leads V1 to V4

The independent effect of heart position and orientation on QRS complex has also been investigated in the different heart-torso geometries showing slight differences in QRS duration with rotation around LA and LR axis directions and translation in the lateral and cranio-caudal directions (**Figures 6, 7**). Large morphological and amplitude changes of QRS in V1 to V3 leads are observed with rotation around the LA direction, whereas V1 to V5 are mainly affected by rotation around LR direction. QRS morphologies in V1 to V4 are mainly affected by translation of the heart within the torso in the lateral and cranio-caudal directions. This is in agreement with studies reporting that variations in the magnitude of the electrocardiogram as observed through leads placed on the anterior thorax are dominated by the solid angle (van Oosterom et al., 2000). Small rotation angles in the range of $\pm 10^\circ$ could be considered as mimicking pose changes caused by respiration (McLeish et al., 2002; Shechter et al., 2004). These resulted in QRS morphological changes mainly in the anterior leads V3 and V4, with very minor scaling amplitudes in V1 to V4 (see **Supplementary Material S6**) in agreement with (Carey et al., 2016). Large changes in heart position and orientation lead to remarkable changes in QRS morphology and amplitude in agreement with body position changes that significantly affect the ECG (Mincholé et al., 2014).

LIMITATIONS AND FUTURE WORK

The QRS complex reflects the ventricular depolarization and its pattern is determined by the electrical activation sequence of the ventricles, as well as the geometric relationship between the heart and the body surface anatomy as shown in this study. The activation sequence is, in turn, related not only to ventricular geometry but also to Purkinje, myocardial conduction pathways, and, other tissue conductivities (Boineau and Spach, 1968; Keller et al., 2010). In this study, we focused on evaluating the role of anatomical ventricular/torso properties on the QRS complex. Further studies can evaluate the role of additional factors on the QRS complex such as for example variability in the Purkinje system (Wallman et al., 2014), myocardial conductivities, and disease conditions (Lyon et al., 2018b).

We have selected a wide range of ventricular and torso geometries with volumes from 75 to 170 cm^3, and from 23 to 54 dm^3, respectively. However, the total variability of control human geometries may not be represented by this dataset. The results showed in this study are not however, expected to change qualitatively with consideration of a larger dataset in healthy subjects. Considering disease conditions will include additional factors determining variability in QRS morphology (Lyon et al., 2018a,b).

We have tackled the reconstruction of the shape of the surface body by completing the sparse information obtained from the MRI with a statistical shape model of the body surface. The agreement of the reconstructed torso and the MRI contours is high (no more than few millimeters of discrepancy for all the cases). However, there are large areas where we have no information of the body shape and we rely on the shape plausibility provided by the statistical shape model. This may result in differences between the reconstructed torso and the real one, and, therefore, in differences in the simulated ECG. This is a limitation for the accuracy of the reconstruction pipeline, but does not invalidate the main message of the work, in which we evaluate scenarios with plausible anatomies without claiming personalization of the subjects.

The propagation of the electrical activity in the torso by means of the integration of dipole source density formulation is chosen in order to simplify the numerical complexity of the computations and to avoid re-meshing in each scenario. Although this method does not allow the inclusion of tissue inhomogeneities in the torso, previous studies (Ramanathan and Rudy, 2001; Geneser et al., 2008), and, our own evaluations (see **Supplementary Figure 3**) have suggested that differences in the QRS complex between homogeneous and heterogeneous torsos are minimal. The inclusion of vasculature close to the heart and all tissue inhomogeneities may result in differences in the QRS complex between homogeneous and heterogeneous torsos. For these inclusions, different numerical models should be chosen such as the coupled bidomain model by the finite element methods.

CONCLUSION

A population of 265 human torso-ventricular models is constructed based on clinical MRI using a computational pipeline for image analysis, construction of MRI-based anatomical models and HPC electrophysiological simulations. The technology demonstrated here can further exploit clinical databases to evaluate the functional implications of MRI-extracted features (Lyon et al., 2018b). Analysis of ECG simulations demonstrates that ventricular anatomy mostly determines QRS morphology in limb leads I and II, whereas heart position within the torso determines QRS morphology in the precordial leads, and especially V1 to V4. QRS duration is mainly influenced by myocardial volume, whereas QRS amplitude increases with large ventricular volumes and decreases with larger torso volumes. The new insights provided here are expected to aid in the discrimination in clinical recordings between the contribution of each patient's specific anatomy and those arising from their disease state, and to contribute to accelerating the development of individualized score metrics for risk stratification, and therefore an improved tailoring of their pharmacological and electrical therapy.

AUTHOR CONTRIBUTIONS

AM, EZ, VG, and BR contributed to the conception and design of the study. AM performed the electrophysiological simulations and ECG analysis. EZ performed the personalization of the geometrical models. RA acquired the MRI of the patients. AM and EZ worked on the analysis of the results and writing of the manuscript. All authors contributed to manuscript revision, and read and approved the submitted version.

ACKNOWLEDGMENTS

This work used the facilities of the UK National Supercomputing Service (Archer RAP and Archer Leadership Award e462), and the facilities of MareNostrum at Barcelona Supercomputing Center (BSC), Spain (PRACE project pr1efz00).

REFERENCES

Amberg, B., Romdhani, S., and Vetter, T. (2007). "Optimal step nonrigid ICP algorithms for surface registration," in *Proceedings of the 2007 IEEE Conference on Computer Vision and Pattern Recognition*, (Minneapolis, MN: IEEE), doi: 10.1109/CVPR.2007.383165

Bayer, J., Prassl, A. J., Pashaei, A., Gomez, J. F., Frontera, A., Neic, A., et al. (2018). Universal ventricular coordinates: a generic framework for describing position within the heart and transferring data. *Med. Image Anal.* 45, 83–93. doi: 10.1016/j.media.2018.01.005

Boineau, J. P., and Spach, M. S. (1968). The relationship between the electrocardiogram and the electrical activity of the heart. *J. Electrocardiol.* 1, 117–124. doi: 10.1016/S0022-0736(68)80014-7

Cardone-Noott, L., Bueno-Orovio, A., Mincholé, A., Zemzemi, N., and Rodriguez, B. (2016). Human ventricular activation sequence and the simulation of the electrocardiographic QRS complex and its variability in healthy and intraventricular block conditions. *Europace* 18, iv4–iv15. doi: 10.1093/europace/euw346

Carey, M. G., Al-Zaiti, S. S., Kozik, T. M., Schell-Chaple, H., and Pelter, M. M. (2016). QRS amplitude variation during monitoring. *Am. J. Crit. Care* 25, 97–98. doi: 10.4037/ajcc2016791

Corlan, A. D., Macleod, R. S., and De Ambroggi, L. (2005). The effect of intrathoracic heart position on electrocardiogram autocorrelation maps. *J. Electrocardiol.* 38, 87–94. doi: 10.1016/j.jelectrocard.2004.10.006

Dougherty, J. D. (1970). The relation of the frontal QRS axis to the anatomic position of the heart. *J. Electrocardiol.* 3, 267–284. doi: 10.1016/s0022-0736(70)80054-1

Durrer, D., van Dam, R. T., Freud, G. E., Janse, M. J., Meijler, F. L., and Arzbaecher, R. C. (1970). Total excitation of the isolated human heart. *Circulation* 41, 899–912. doi: 10.1161/01.CIR.41.6.899

Dutta, S., Mincholé, A., Quinn, T. A., and Rodriguez, B. (2017). Electrophysiological properties of computational human ventricular cell action potential models under acute ischemic conditions. *Prog. Biophys. Mol. Biol.* 129, 40–52. doi: 10.1016/j.pbiomolbio.2017.02.007

Dutta, S., Mincholé, A., Zacur, E., Quinn, T. A., Taggart, P., and Rodriguez, B. (2016). Early afterdepolarizations promote transmural reentry in ischemic human ventricles with reduced repolarization reserve. *Prog. Biophys. Mol. Biol.* 120, 236–248. doi: 10.1016/j.pbiomolbio.2016.01.008

Engblom, H., Foster, J. E., Martin, T. N., Groenning, B., Pahlm, O., Dargie, H. J., et al. (2005). The relationship between electrical axis by 12-lead electrocardiogram and anatomical axis of the heart by cardiac magnetic resonance in healthy subjects. *Am. Heart J.* 150, 507–512. doi: 10.1016/j.ahj.2004.10.041

Geneser, S. E., Kirby, R. M., and MacLeod, R. S. (2008). Application of stochastic finite element methods to study the sensitivity of ECG forward modeling to organ conductivity. *IEEE Trans. Biomed. Eng.* 55, 31–40. doi: 10.1109/TBME.2007.900563

Giffard-Roisin, S., Jackson, T., Fovargue, L., Lee, J., Delingette, H., Razavi, R., et al. (2017). Noninvasive personalization of a cardiac electrophysiology model from body surface potential mapping. *IEEE Trans. Biomed. Eng.* 64, 2206–2218. doi: 10.1109/TBME.2016.2629849

Gima, K., and Rudy, Y. (2002). Ionic current basis of electrocardiographic waveforms: a model study. *Circ. Res.* 90, 889–896. doi: 10.1161/01.res.0000016960.61087.86

Hoekema, R., Uijen, G. J., van Eming, L., and van Oosterom, A. (1999). Interindividual variability of multilead electrocardiographic recordings. Influence of heart position. *J. Electrocardiol.* 32, 137–148. doi: 10.1016/S0022-0736(99)90092-4

Hoekema, R., Uijen, G. J., and van Oosterom, A. (2001). Geometrical aspects of the interindividual variability of multilead ECG recordings. *IEEE Trans. Biomed. Eng.* 48, 551–559. doi: 10.1109/10.918594

Horan, L. G. (1987). Manifest orientation: the theoretical link between the anatomy of the heart and the clinical electrocardiogram. *J. Am. Coll. Cardiol.* 9, 1049–1056. doi: 10.1016/s0735-1097(87)80307-8

Kashou, A. H., and Kashou, H. E. (2018). *"Electrical axis (normal, right axis deviation, and left axis deviation)," in StatPearls, (Treasure Island (FL): StatPearls Publishing).* Available at: http://www.ncbi.nlm.nih.gov/books/NBK470532/ (accessed September 12, 2018).

Katragadda, S., Alagesan, M., Rathakrishnan, S., Kaliyaperumal, D., and Mambatta, A. K. (2017). Correlation of reciprocal changes and QRS amplitude in ECG to left ventricular dysfunction, wall motion score and clinical outcome in first time St elevation myocardial infarction. *J. Clin. Diagn. Res.* 11, OC04–OC08. doi: 10.7860/JCDR/2017/26021.10155

Keller, D. U. J., Weber, F. M., Seemann, G., and Dössel, O. (2010). Ranking the influence of tissue conductivities on forward-calculated ECGs. *IEEE Trans. Biomed. Eng.* 57, 1568–1576. doi: 10.1109/TBME.2010.2046485

Kurisu, S., Ikenaga, H., Watanabe, N., Higaki, T., Shimonaga, T., Ishibashi, K., et al. (2015). Electrocardiographic characteristics in the underweight and obese in accordance with the world health organization classification. *IJC Metab. Endocr.* 9, 61–65. doi: 10.1016/j.ijcme.2015.10.006

Lyon, A., Ariga, R., Mincholé, A., Mahmod, M., Ormondroyd, E., Laguna, P., et al. (2018a). Distinct ECG phenotypes identified in hypertrophic cardiomyopathy using machine learning associate with arrhythmic risk markers. *Front. Physiol.* 9:213. doi: 10.3389/fphys.2018.00213

Lyon, A., Bueno-Orovio, A., Zacur, E., Ariga, R., Grau, V., Neubauer, S., et al. (2018b). Electrocardiogram phenotypes in hypertrophic cardiomyopathy caused by distinct mechanisms: apico-basal repolarization gradients vs. Purkinje-myocardial coupling abnormalities. *Europace* 20, iii102–iii112. doi: 10.1093/europace/euy226

Macfarlane, P. W., and Lawrie, T. D. V. (2010). "The normal electrocardiogram and vectorcardiogram," in *Comprehensive Electrocardiology*, eds P. W. Macfarlane, A. van Oosterom, O. Pahlm, P. Kligfield, M. Janse, and J. Camm (London: Springer), doi: 10.1007/978-1-84882-046-3-13

MacLeod, R. S., Ni, Q., Punske, B., Ershler, P. R., Yilmaz, B., and Taccardi, B. (2000). Effects of heart position on the body-surface electrocardiogram. *J. Electrocardiol.* 33(Suppl.), 229–237. doi: 10.1054/jelc.2000.20357

Martínez, J. P., Almeida, R., Olmos, S., Rocha, A. P., and Laguna, P. (2004). A wavelet-based ECG delineator: evaluation on standard databases. *IEEE Trans. Biomed. Eng.* 51, 570–581. doi: 10.1109/TBME.2003.821031

McLeish, K., Hill, D. L. G., Atkinson, D., Blackall, J. M., and Razavi, R. (2002). A study of the motion and deformation of the heart due to respiration. *IEEE Trans. Med. Imaging* 21, 1142–1150. doi: 10.1109/TMI.2002.804427

Mincholé, A., Sörnmo, L., and Laguna, P. (2014). Detection of body position changes from the ECG using a laplacian noise model. *Biomed. Signal Process. Control* 14, 189–196. doi: 10.1016/j.bspc.2014.08.002

Murkofsky, R. L., Dangas, G., Diamond, J. A., Mehta, D., Schaffer, A., and Ambrose, J. A. (1998). A prolonged QRS duration on surface electrocardiogram is a specific indicator of left ventricular dysfunction [see comment]. *J. Am. Coll. Cardiol.* 32, 476–482. doi: 10.1016/s0735-1097(98)00242-3

Nazarian, S., and Halperin, H. R. (2018). "Computed tomography and magnetic resonance imaging for electrophysiology," in *Cardiac Electrophysiology: From Cell to Bedside*, (Amsterdam: Elsevier), 601–607. doi: 10.1016/B978-0-323-44733-1.00063-8

Neic, A., Campos, F. O., Prassl, A. J., Niederer, S. A., Bishop, M. J., Vigmond, E. J., et al. (2017). Efficient computation of electrograms and ECGs in human whole heart simulations using a reaction-eikonal model. *J. Comput. Phys.* 346, 191–211. doi: 10.1016/j.jcp.2017.06.020

Nguyên, U. C., Potse, M., Regoli, F., Caputo, M. L., Conte, G., Murzilli, R., et al. (2015). An in-silico analysis of the effect of heart position and orientation on the ECG morphology and vectorcardiogram parameters in patients with heart failure and intraventricular conduction defects. *J. Electrocardiol.* 48, 617–625. doi: 10.1016/j.jelectrocard.2015.05.004

O'Hara, T., Virág, L., Varró, A., and Rudy, Y. (2011). Simulation of the undiseased human cardiac ventricular action potential: model formulation and experimental validation. *PLoS Comput. Biol.* 7:e1002061. doi: 10.1371/journal.pcbi.1002061

Oikarinen, L., Nieminen, M. S., Viitasalo, M., Toivonen, L., Jern, S., Dahlöf, B., et al. (2004). QRS duration and QT interval predict mortality in hypertensive patients with left ventricular hypertrophy: the losartan intervention for endpoint reduction in hypertension study. *Hypertension* 43, 1029–1034. doi: 10.1161/01.HYP.0000125230.46080.c6

Pellicori, P., Joseph, A. C., Zhang, J., Lukaschuk, E., Sherwi, N., Bourantas, C. V., et al. (2015). The relationship of QRS morphology with cardiac structure and function in patients with heart failure. *Clin. Res. Cardiol.* 104, 935–945. doi: 10.1007/s00392-015-0861-0

Petersen, S. E., Sanghvi, M. M., Aung, N., Cooper, J. A., Paiva, J. M., Zemrak, F., et al. (2017). The impact of cardiovascular risk factors on cardiac structure and function: insights from the UK Biobank imaging enhancement study. *PLoS One* 12:e0185114. doi: 10.1371/journal.pone.0185114

Pishchulin, L., Wuhrer, S., Helten, T., Theobalt, C., and Schiele, B. (2017). Building statistical shape spaces for 3D human modeling. *Pattern Recogn.* 67, 276–286. doi: 10.1016/j.patcog.2017.02.018

Pitt-Francis, J., Pathmanathan, P., Bernabeu, M. O., Bordas, R., Cooper, J., Fletcher, A. G., et al. (2009). Chaste: a test-driven approach to software development for biological modelling. *Comput. Phys. Commun.* 180, 2452–2471. doi: 10.1016/j.cpc.2009.07.019

Plonsey, R., and Barr, R. C. (2007). *Bioelectricity: A Quantitative Approach*, 3rd Edn. Berlin: Springer.

Potse, M. (2018). Scalable and accurate ECG simulation for reaction-diffusion models of the human heart. *Front. Physiol.* 9:370. doi: 10.3389/fphys.2018.00370

Potse, M., Krause, D., Kroon, W., Murzilli, R., Muzzarelli, S., Regoli, F., et al. (2014). Patient-specific modelling of cardiac electrophysiology in heart-failure patients. *Europace* 16, iv56–iv61. doi: 10.1093/europace/euu257

Prakash, R. (1978). Determination of right ventricular wall thickness in systole and diastole. Echocardiographic and necropsy correlation in 32 patients. *Br. Heart J.* 40, 1257–1261. doi: 10.1136/hrt.40.11.1257

Ramanathan, C., and Rudy, Y. (2001). Electrocardiographic imaging: i. effect of torso inhomogeneities on body surface electrocardiographic potentials. *J. Cardiovasc. Electrophysiol.* 12, 229–240. doi: 10.1046/j.1540-8167.2001.00229.x

Rohr, K., Stiehl, H. S., Sprengel, R., Buzug, T. M., Weese, J., and Kuhn, M. H. (2001). Landmark-based elastic registration using approximating thin-plate splines. *IEEE Trans. Med. Imaging* 20, 526–534. doi: 10.1109/42.929618

Sánchez, C., D'Ambrosio, G., Maffessanti, F., Caiani, E. G., Prinzen, F. W., Krause, R., et al. (2018). Sensitivity analysis of ventricular activation and electrocardiogram in tailored models of heart-failure patients. *Med. Biol. Eng. Comput.* 56, 491–504. doi: 10.1007/s11517-017-1696-99

Sathananthan, G., Zahid, S., Aggarwal, G., Chik, W., Friedman, D., and Thiagalingam, A. (2015). Cardiac orientation: is there a correlation between the anatomical and the electrical axis of the heart? *Br. J. Cardiol.* 22, doi: 10.5837/bjc.2015.016

Shechter, G., Ozturk, C., Resar, J. R., and McVeigh, E. R. (2004). Respiratory motion of the heart from free breathing coronary angiograms. *IEEE Trans. Med. Imaging* 23, 1046–1056. doi: 10.1109/TMI.2004.828676

Stewart, R. A., Young, A. A., Anderson, C., Teo, K. K., Jennings, G., and Cowan, B. R. (2011). Relationship between QRS duration and left ventricular mass and volume in patients at high cardiovascular risk. *Heart* 97, 1766–1770. doi: 10.1136/heartjnl-2011-300297

Streeter, D. D., Spotnitz, H. M., Patel, D. P., Ross, J., and Sonnenblick, E. H. (1969). Fiber orientation in the canine left ventricle during diastole and systole. *Circ. Res.* 24, 339–347. doi: 10.1161/01.res.24.3.339

Usoro, A. O., Bradford, N., Shah, A. J., and Soliman, E. Z. (2014). Risk of mortality in individuals with low QRS voltage and free of cardiovascular disease. *Am. J. Cardiol.* 113, 1514–1517. doi: 10.1016/j.amjcard.2014.02.006

van Oosterom, A., Hoekema, R., and Uijen, G. J. (2000). Geometrical factors affecting the interindividual variability of the ECG and the VCG. *J. Electrocardiol.* 33(Suppl.), 219–227. doi: 10.1054/jelc.2000.20356

Villard, B., Grau, V., and Zacur, E. (2018). Surface mesh reconstruction from cardiac mri contours. *J. Imaging* 4:16. doi: 10.3390/jimaging4010016

Villard, B., Zacur, E., Dall'Armellina, E., and Grau, V. (2017). "Correction of slice misalignment in multi-breath-hold cardiac MRI scans," in *Proceedings of the STACOM 2016: Statistical Atlases and Computational Models of the Heart. Imaging and Modelling Challenges (Lecture Notes in Computer Science). International Workshop on Statistical Atlases and Computational Models of the Heart*, (Athens: Springer), doi: 10.1007/978-3-319-52718-5-4

Wallman, M., Smith, N. P., and Rodriguez, B. (2014). Computational methods to reduce uncertainty in the estimation of cardiac conduction properties from electroanatomical recordings. *Med. Image Anal.* 18, 228–240. doi: 10.1016/j.media.2013.10.006

Zacur, E., Minchole, A., Villard, B., Carapella, V., Ariga, R., Rodriguez, B., et al. (2017). "MRI-based heart and torso personalization for computer modeling and simulation of cardiac electrophysiology," in *Proceedings of the Imaging for Patient-Customized Simulations and Systems for Point-of-Care Ultrasound Lecture Notes in Computer Science*, (Cham: Springer), 61–70. doi: 10.1007/978-3-319-67552-7-8

Zemzemi, N., Bernabeu, M. O., Saiz, J., Cooper, J., Pathmanathan, P., Mirams, G. R., et al. (2013). Computational assessment of drug-induced effects on the electrocardiogram: from ion channel to body surface potentials. *Br. J. Pharmacol.* 168, 718–733. doi: 10.1111/j.1476-5381.2012.02200.x

Zemzemi, N., and Rodriguez, B. (2015). Effects of L-type calcium channel and human ether-a-go-go related gene blockers on the electrical activity of the human heart: a simulation study. *Europace* 17, 326–333. doi: 10.1093/europace/euu122

4

The Left and Right Ventricles Respond Differently to Variation of Pacing Delays in Cardiac Resynchronization Therapy: A Combined Experimental-Computational Approach

Erik Willemen[1], Rick Schreurs[1], Peter R. Huntjens[1,2], Marc Strik[3], Gernot Plank[4], Edward Vigmond[5], John Walmsley[1], Kevin Vernooy[3], Tammo Delhaas[1], Frits W. Prinzen[1] and Joost Lumens[1,2]*

[1] Cardiovascular Research Institute Maastricht (CARIM), Maastricht University, Maastricht, Netherlands, [2] IHU-LIRYC Electrophysiology and Heart Modeling Institute, Pessac, France, [3] Department of Cardiology, Maastricht University Medical Center, Maastricht, Netherlands, [4] Institute of Biophysics, Medical University of Graz, Graz, Austria, [5] Univeristy of Bordeaux, IMB UMR 5251, Talence, France

***Correspondence:**
Erik Willemen
e.willemen@maastrichtuniversity.nl

Introduction: Timing of atrial, right (RV), and left ventricular (LV) stimulation in cardiac resynchronization therapy (CRT) is known to affect electrical activation and pump function of the LV. In this study, we used computer simulations, with input from animal experiments, to investigate the effect of varying pacing delays on both LV and RV electrical dyssynchrony and contractile function.

Methods: A pacing protocol was performed in dogs with atrioventricular block (N = 6), using 100 different combinations of atrial (A)-LV and A-RV pacing delays. Regional LV and RV electrical activation times were measured using 112 electrodes and LV and RV pressures were measured with catheter-tip micromanometers. Contractile response to a pacing delay was defined as relative change of the maximum rate of LV and RV pressure rise (dP/dt_{max}) compared to RV pacing with an A-RV delay of 125 ms. The pacing protocol was simulated in the CircAdapt model of cardiovascular system dynamics, using the experimentally acquired electrical mapping data as input.

Results: Ventricular electrical activation changed with changes in the amount of LV or RV pre-excitation. The resulting changes in dP/dt_{max} differed markedly between the LV and RV. Pacing the LV 10–50 ms before the RV led to the largest increases in LV dP/dt_{max}. In contrast, RV dP/dt_{max} was highest with RV pre-excitation and decreased up to 33% with LV pre-excitation. These opposite patterns of changes in RV and LV dP/dt_{max} were reproduced by the simulations. The simulations extended these observations by showing that changes in steady-state biventricular cardiac output differed from changes in both LV and RV dP/dt_{max}. The model allowed to explain the discrepant changes in dP/dt_{max} and cardiac output by coupling between atria and ventricles as well as between the ventricles.

Conclusion: The LV and the RV respond in a opposite manner to variation in the amount of LV or RV pre-excitation. Computer simulations capture LV and RV behavior during pacing delay variation and may be used in the design of new CRT optimization studies.

Keywords: cardiac resynchronization therapy, right ventricle, optimization, computer simulation, therapy optimization studies, CircAdapt, hemodynamics, dyssynchrony

INTRODUCTION

Cardiac resynchronization therapy (CRT) is an established therapy for heart failure patients with a reduced left ventricular (LV) ejection fraction (EF), and left bundle branch block (LBBB) (Brignole et al., 2013). Through biventricular pacing, CRT aims to establish a more synchronous electrical activation of the ventricles and thereby improves cardiac pump function (Vernooy et al., 2007) and clinical outcome (Brignole et al., 2013). However, approximately one-third of the patients that receive CRT do not benefit from this therapy (Abraham et al., 2002; Cleland et al., 2005; Auricchio and Prinzen, 2011; Prinzen et al., 2013).

Programming of both atrioventricular (AV) and ventriculoventricular (VV) pacing delays strongly influences the contractile response to CRT, as determined by both ultrasound and maximum rate of LV pressure rise (LV dP/dt_{max}) (Bogaard et al., 2012; Auger et al., 2013; Strik et al., 2013b). However, meta-analyses of multiple optimization methods showed that pacing delay optimization fails to provide long-term improvement in clinical outcome (Auger et al., 2013). Suggested reasons for the absence of long-term benefits of such optimization are that the default "out-of-the-box" delays are already fairly good and that the optimization methods employed are not accurate or robust enough. An alternative explanation could be that most pacing delay optimization strategies that have been developed solely take LV function into account. Right ventricular (RV) function is often overlooked, although several studies show that RV failure is an independent predictor of mortality in patients with LV failure with and without CRT (Groote et al., 1998; Ricci et al., 2017). Two clinical studies indicated that there was a poor correlation between the pacing delay settings providing the highest LV dP/dt_{max} and RV dP/dt_{max} values (Sciaraffia et al., 2009; Hyde et al., 2016).

In recent years, computational models of cardiac electrophysiology, mechanics of the heart and cardiovascular system have increased our understanding of dyssynchronous heart failure and its treatment with CRT (Lee et al., 2018). Right ventricular function and its effect on CRT has, however, not been studied extensively using a computer modeling approach. Our group has been using the CircAdapt model of the heart and closed-loop circulatory system. While using a simplified cardiac anatomy, the advantages of this model are the inclusion of the entire (systemic and pulmonary) circulation and its high calculation speed (almost real time). In combination with experimental and clinical measurements, CircAdapt has shown to be able to identify and mechanistically understand the electromechanical substrates of the heart that are most responsive to CRT (Lumens et al., 2013, 2015; Huntjens et al., 2018).

A vast majority of the studies on the heart, also our aforementioned studies, are related largely to the LV. In the present study, we aim to study the changes in both LV and RV contractile response to variations of pacing delay settings in CRT, and to evaluate whether the CircAdapt computer model reliably simulates LV and RV pump function during these interventions. Subsequently we aim to use the computer modeling results to investigate how cardiac output is affected by differences between LV and RV contractile changes.

MATERIALS AND METHODS

Animal Experiments

Animal handling was performed according to the Dutch Law on Animal Experimentation and the European Directive for the Protection of Vertebrate Animals Used for Experimental and Other Scientific Purpose. The protocol was approved by the Animal Experimental Committee of Maastricht University. The animal experiments have been conducted in 2010–2011 and the methodology used has partially been described in a previous publication (Strik et al., 2013b), reporting on the LV pressure data. In the current study we analyzed both RV and LV pressure data and related them to the electrical conduction measurements. In short, 6 adult mongrel dogs were anesthetized using midazolam (0,25 mg/kg/h) and sufentanil (3 μg/kg/h) and a complete AV-block was induced by radiofrequency ablation. The dogs received pacing electrodes in the right atrium (A), RV apex and epicardially on the basal posterolateral wall via a left-sided thoracotomy.

Measurements were performed 12–21 weeks after inducing the AV-block using an external custom-built pacing system. RV-only pacing with an A to RV (A-RV) pacing delay of 125 ms was used as the baseline pacing setting, mimicking the activation pattern as seen in LBBB. The A-RV and A to LV (A-LV) delays were then programmed individually, ranging from 50 to 230 ms in steps of 20 ms, resulting in 100 possible combinations (**Figure 1A**). Pacing delay settings were assigned in a random order and baseline recordings were repeated after every 5th setting. During each setting, continuous, invasive hemodynamic and electrocardiographic measurements were performed (**Figure 1B**). 7F catheter-tip manometers were used for LV and RV pressure measurement. Epicardial electrograms of the LV free wall (LVFW) and RV free wall (RVFW) were recorded from 2 multielectrode custom-made bands holding 102 contact electrodes. Septal endocardial electrograms were recorded from

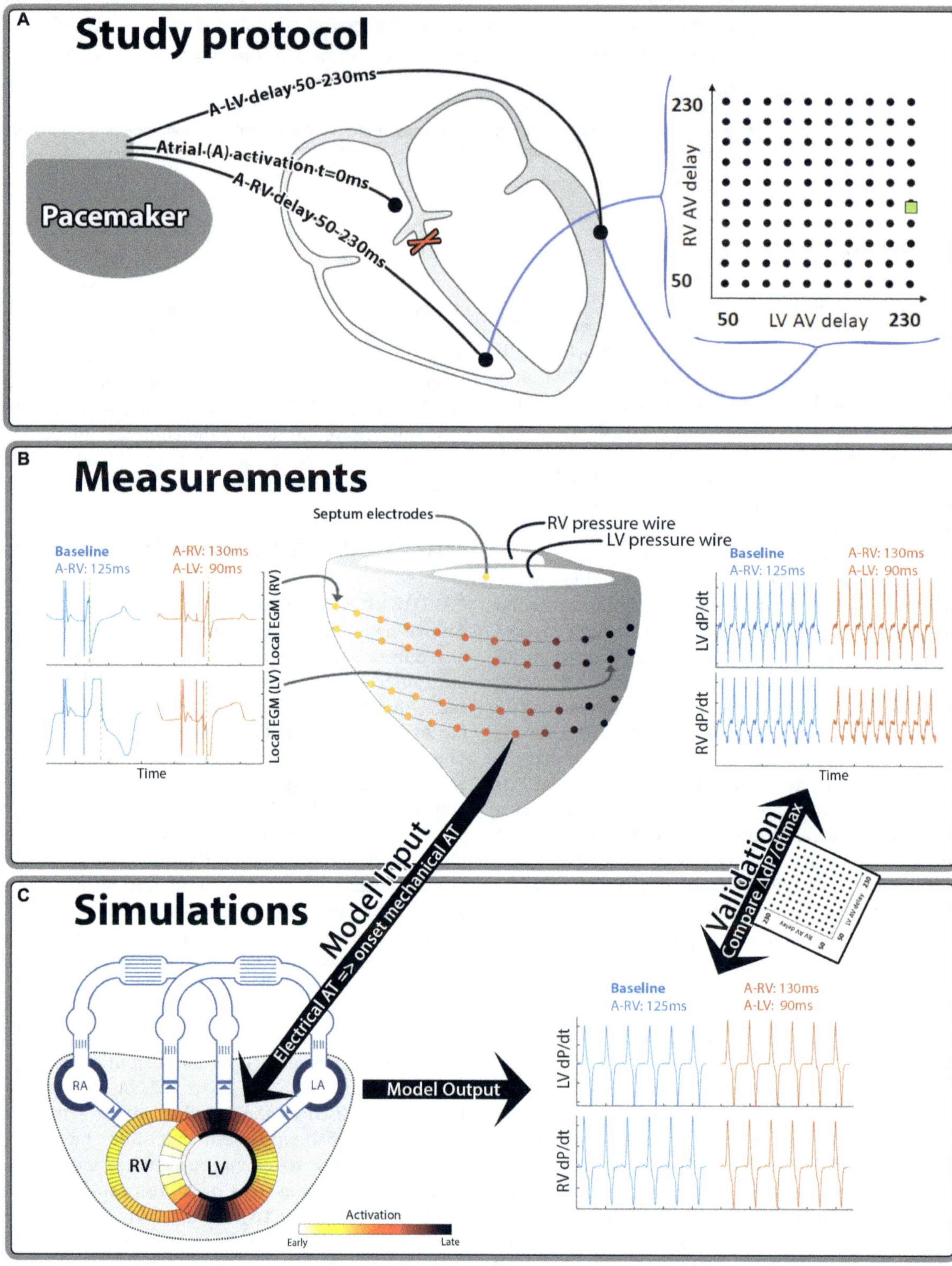

FIGURE 1 | Schematic representation of the methods used in this study. Hundred different A-LV/A-RV pacing delay combinations were programmed **(A)** while pressures and local electrical activation were measured **(B)**. Generic activation maps, derived from local electrograms, were used as onset of mechanical activation in the computer simulations **(C)**. The resulting output of the simulations and measurements was compared for validation purposes. The green square in the heat maps indicates the baseline pacing setting.

two multielectrode catheters with 7 contact electrodes on the RV septum and 3 on the LV septum. Measurements were recorded for a minimum of two respiratory cycles at each pacing delay setting.

Data Analysis

Local electrical activation times were determined as the duration between the atrial pace and the timepoint of steepest negative deflection of the electrogram using custom software (**Figure 1B**, green line in local EGM's). For quantification of intraventricular electrical dyssynchrony we calculated total activation time as the difference between earliest and latest activation time of the RVFW (RV TAT) and of the whole LV (LV TAT). The latter was calculated from the combination of epicardial LVFW and endocardial septal electrodes. To quantify electrical interventricular dyssynchrony we used the ventricular electrical uncoupling (VEU) index. VEU was defined as the difference between mean LVFW and mean RVFW activation times (Ploux et al., 2013).

For both the LV and the RV, response to pacing was defined as the relative change in dP/dt_{max} compared to the baseline setting. We applied quadratic LOESS fitting to account for measurement variability within each dog (Cleveland, 1979). Furthermore, in order to quantify a generic canine response to changes in pacing delay, we created a single representative canine dataset by taking the mean values of the dogs for each setting. We also applied linear 2D interpolation between the measurements in the heat map visualizations of all pacing delay settings. All these calculations were performed in Matlab 2016A (The Mathworks Inc., Natick, MA, United States).

Computer Simulations

The CircAdapt model of the entire heart and circulation (Arts et al., 2005; Lumens et al., 2009; Walmsley et al., 2015a), which can be downloaded from www.circadapt.org, was used to simulate cardiovascular mechanics and hemodynamics during pacing delay variations as applied in the animal experiments (**Figure 1C**). Previous experimental and clinical studies have shown that the CircAdapt model realistically relates local ventricular myofiber mechanics to global cardiovascular hemodynamics in dyssynchronous and paced hearts (Leenders et al., 2012; Huntjens et al., 2014; Lumens et al., 2015; Walmsley et al., 2015a,b).

The source code of the CircAdapt model used for all simulations as well as the Matlab® (The MathWorks, Natick, MA, United States) scripts to perform all simulations and analysis thereof are provided as an online supplement (**Supplementary Data Sheet S1**). In summary, the CircAdapt model is a reduced order model of the human four-chamber heart connected to a closed-loop cardiovascular system, with lumped pulmonary and systemic circulations. It uses a simplified ventricular geometry, where cardiac walls are represented by thick spherical shells consisting of contractile myocardium. The MultiPatch module enables cardiac walls to be subdivided into an arbitrary number of wall segments (patches). Tissue properties and activation time can differ between patches, but all patches within a wall share a common wall tension and curvature. Since wall tension is the same in all patches within a wall, spatial location within a wall is not required to calculate deformation in a patch.

In CircAdapt wall tension and curvature determine cavity pressure through Laplace's law (Lumens et al., 2009; Walmsley et al., 2015a) Fiber stress in a patch is the sum of an active component, representing myofiber contraction, and a passive component. The active stress component incorporates length-dependence of the force generated and the duration of contraction. The passive component provides a non-linear relationship between myofiber stress and strain. More details on the phenomenological model of myocardial contraction and the validation of the MultiPatch module are previously published by Walmsley et al. (2015a).

Simulating a Healthy Human Reference Heart and Circulation

Cardiac adaptation implemented in the CircAdapt model was used to obtain a reference parameterization that represents a healthy human cardiovascular system (Arts et al., 1994, 2005, 2012). The tissue volumes and areas in the cardiac walls and large blood vessels were adapted as described previously (Arts et al., 2005, 2012). A resting cardiac output of 5.1 l/min and heart rate of 70 bpm were assumed. Cardiac output was tripled and the heart rate was doubled during the stress-state of the adaptation process. Mean arterial pressure (MAP) was maintained at 92 mmHg during the adaptation process. The resulting reference simulation was used as the basis for subsequent pacing simulations.

Using Electrical Activation to Simulate the Pacing Delay Optimization Protocol

We divided the ventricular wall in the same amount of segments as the number of available electrodes (52 LV free wall, 50 RV free wall and 10 septal segments). Time of onset of activation was assigned based on the electrical activation times measured in the animal experiments. As previously stated, in the current MultiPatch module the segments were considered to be mechanically coupled in series, meaning that the order in which patches were placed was not significant (Walmsley et al., 2015a). This allowed sorting of the activation times per wall in each measurement, before taking the median of the dogs, to get a generic activation pattern. The benefit of this generic activation pattern is that it was less affected by differences in band placement, heart size and electrodes with insufficient contact in the dogs.

A representative baseline simulation was obtained by imposing the ventricular activation pattern measured during the experimental baseline condition, i.e., RV-only pacing with an A-RV delay of 125 ms. Systemic vascular resistance was adapted to obtain a MAP of 60 mmHg and heart rate was set to 80 bpm, both similar to the animal experiments. Furthermore, total circulating blood volume was adjusted so that cardiac output was maintained at 5.1 L/min. The resulting baseline simulation was used as the starting point for the pacing setting simulations. For each of the 100 pacing delay simulations, the pattern of ventricular activation was changed to the activation pattern measured in the canine experiments and the resulting beat-to-beat changes in ventricular mechanics and hemodynamics were stored until a new hemodynamic steady state was reached. During all pacing simulations, systemic vascular resistance and total circulating blood volume were kept constant in order to quantify the acute effect of pacing-induced changes of ventricular pump mechanics and cardiac hemodynamics. Simulated steady-state dP/dt_{max} values are compared with the experimental measurements. In addition, the simulations extended the animal experiments by providing quantitative insight in the beat-to-beat and steady-state changes of ventricular volumes and cardiac output.

RESULTS

Baseline characteristics for the AV-blocked dogs are described in **Table 1**.

Electrical Effects of Altering Pacing Delay Settings

Figure 2 shows the typical examples of electrical activation patterns acquired using contact mapping in a dog with AV block during LV pre-excitation, simultaneous RV and LV pacing and RV pre-excitation. In case of extreme pre-excitation, capture in the last paced ventricle was lost due to activation via the contralateral ventricle (indicated by the gray line). RV pre-excitation led to the largest LV TAT while LV pre-excitation resulted in an increase of RV TAT. During simultaneous pacing, two wave fronts originating from the RV and LV pacing electrodes fused and resynchronized the heart as indicated by a decrease in LV TAT.

Figure 3 shows the changes in electrical dyssynchrony indexes in dogs with variation of pacing delay settings. There was no change in LV and RV TAT and VEU when changing the AV delay during simultaneous activation of the LV and RV (left column). Both LV and RV TAT (first 2 rows of **Figure 3**) were lowest during simultaneous RV + LV pacing. The RV showed the largest TAT during LV pre-excitation or LV-only pacing (upper left corners in the heat maps). LV TAT showed a relatively large increase with large RV pre-excitation (right side of middle panels and lower right corners in heat maps), while RV TAT did not increase much. As indicated by the VEU (bottom row **Figure 3**), during LV-only pacing the LVFW was activated more than 40 ms before the RVFW. During RV-only pacing the LVFW was, on average, activated more than 20 ms later than the RVFW. The LVFW and RVFW were activated simultaneously with very slight LV pre-excitation (**Figure 3** bottom right, VEU = 0).

TABLE 1 | Baseline characteristics in median (range) of dogs during baseline (RV-only, A-RV 125 ms pacing).

	During baseline RV-only pacing
Weight (kg)	19.8 (19.4–21.4)
MAP (mmHg)	55 (42–71)
Systolic arterial pressure (mmHg)	70 (62–81)
Diastolic arterial pressure (mmHg)	45 (31–53)
LV dP/dt_{max} (mmHg/s)	1205 (1183–1646)
RV dP/dt_{max} (mmHg/s)	520 (345–700)
Weeks between AVB and Sacrifice (weeks)	13 (12–21)

Hemodynamic Effects of Altering Pacing Delay Settings

The changes in LV and RV dP/dt_{max} in response to changes in pacing delay settings are presented in **Figure 4** (top and bottom, respectively). Increasing AV delay during simultaneous RV and LV pacing (left column and identity line in the heat maps) hardly affected LV and RV dP/dt_{max} in both measurements and simulations. The relative effect of changing VV delay (green, second column from left) was largest in RV dP/dt_{max}. Changing pacing settings from RV to LV pre-excitation decreased RV dP/dt_{max} with more than 30% in the experiment. The decrease in RV dP/dt_{max} was less pronounced in the simulations but followed the same pattern. LV dP/dt_{max} was highest with LV pre-excitation and simultaneous pacing in both the experiment and simulations.

The heat maps of both the animal experiments and computer simulations (right side of **Figure 4**) show a qualitatively similar pattern where the largest changes in both LV and RV dP/dt_{max} are observed when changing the VV delay. The largest increase in LV dP/dt_{max} in the measurements was reached with a short A-LV (50 ms) and A-RV (90 ms). LV pre-excitation led to a larger increase in LV dP/dt_{max} than RV pre-excitation during all measurements and simulation, with an optimal LV pre-excitation range of 10–50 ms. For RV dP/dt_{max}, all LV pre-excitation pacing settings led to a decrease up to 33% in the experiment and 18% in the simulations, while RV pre-excitation caused little change compared to baseline (RV-only) pacing.

Changes in Simulated Cardiac Output at Different Pacing Delays

While dP/dt_{max} values are regarded as a measure of ventricular contractility, cardiac output may be more closely related to pump function of the entire heart. Note that due to the closed loop circulation, in a steady state situation cardiac output of the RV and LV are the same. Cardiac output was not determined in the experiments, but it was calculated in the model simulations. In these simulations the changes in cardiac output following a switch in pacing delay differed from the changes in both LV and RV dP/dt_{max} (**Figure 5**). Cardiac output was more sensitive to changes in AV-delay than to changes in VV-delay. AV-delays of 50 and 70ms led to the largest increases in cardiac output, amounting up to 9%.

In order to find an explanation for the differences in behavior between cardiac output and RV and LV dP/dt_{max} we compared the time course of these parameters as well as EDV during the first beats after start of a certain setting, in this case LV pre-excitation (**Figure 6**). In the first beat after the change in pacing setting and therefore also activation sequence (see above), both LV stroke volume and dP/dt_{max} increased while RV stroke volume and dP/dt_{max} decreased. In

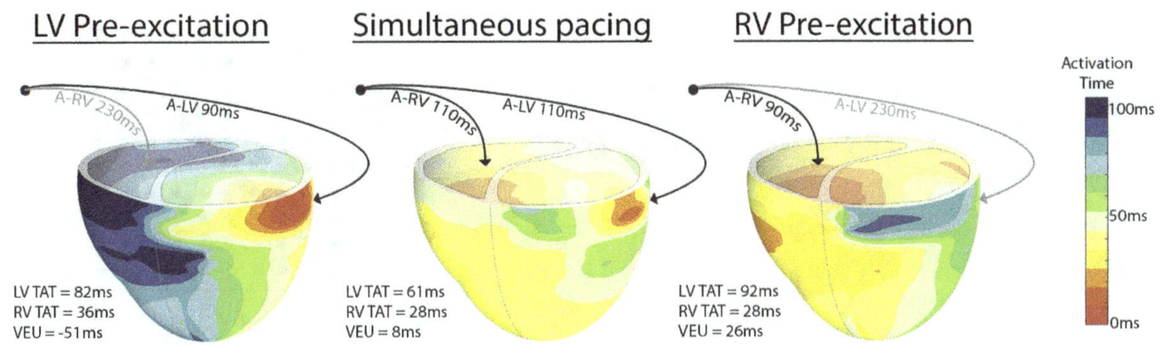

FIGURE 2 | Epicardial electric activation maps in a paced dog heart with complete AV block during LV pre-excitation **(left)**, simultaneous pacing **(middle)**, and RV pre-excitation **(right)**. Black arrows indicate capture, whereas gray arrows indicate loss of capture.

the subsequent beat RV EDV increased, due to the smaller SV of the previous beat, whereas LVEDV decreased. As a consequence of these EDV changes, RV SV recovered and LV SV decreased to some extent and in the third and subsequent beats an steady state (SS) was reached, with SV in both ventricles (and therefore cardiac output) increasing by about 3%. This example, representative for the other conditions, illustrates that dP/dt_{max} was largely independent of preload, whereas SV depended on it, most likely due to the length dependent activation, implemented in the CircAdapt model (see section "Materials and Methods").

Figure 7 shows the response of stroke volume of the LV and RV after simulated programming of nine different pacing settings. In the first beat RV SV remained either unchanged or decreased as compared to baseline, indicating little direct mechanical benefit of the change in pacing delay for the RV. However, similar to the example in **Figure 6**, copied into the left upper panel of **Figure 7**, RV stroke volume changed considerably in subsequent beats. While changes in LV SV initially differed from RV SV, a steady state was reached after several simulated beats. Note that the largest benefit in SV, and therefore cardiac output, was primarily dependent on AV-delay. For example, in the bottom row (A-RV 70 ms) the optimized RV filling improved stroke volume to such a degree that, through the serial coupling, LV preload increased, leading to a further increase in LV stroke volume after the second cycle. On the other hand, at longer AV-delays this atrial-ventricular coupling decreases, resulting in a lower steady-state cardiac output.

DISCUSSION

In this study we investigated the influence of LV and RV pacing delay settings on LV and RV electrical activation and contractility in animal studies and computer simulations. Both studies showed that LV TAT is smallest during synchronous RV and LV stimulation and increases when VV delays increase. RV TAT becomes larger in particular during LV pre-excitation. LV and RV contractility vary most, and in opposite direction, with changes in VV delay settings. After demonstrating the realistic simulations in the model, we used the model to calculate cardiac output changes and to explain why changes cardiac output differed from both RV and LV contractility. The latter findings demonstrate how a model like CircAdapt can extend mechanistic understanding of circulatory changes due to a device therapy.

LV and RV Contractility Respond in Opposite Manner to Variations in VV Pacing Delays

A key finding in the present study is that LV and RV dP/dt_{max} change in opposite direction when changing the VV pacing delay. Sciaraffia et al. (2009) previously demonstrated that RV and LV dP/dt_{max} identify different "optimal" VV delays in most of the patients included in their study. Furthermore, Houston et al. (2018) recently showed that in patients with dyssynchronous heart failure, RV-only pacing leads to higher RV dP/dt_{max} than LV-only or simultaneous LV + RV pacing. In an experimental study in pigs, different VV delays were tested at different pacing locations (Quinn et al., 2006). Similar to our study, these investigators found that RV pre-excitation led to a higher RV dP/dt_{max} than LV pre-excitation. The fact that findings were consistent in patients, animals and a computer model implies that the opposing changes in hemodynamics, caused by varying VV pacing delays, are caused by a universal mechanism.

Another key finding is that ventricular specific pre-excitation is required for a good contractile function in both the LV and RV. This is illustrated by LV pre-excitation increasing LV dP/dt_{max} and RV pre-excitation leading to the largest RV dP/dt_{max} values. In contrast, changes in AV delay have less effect on measured and simulated LV and RV dP/dt_{max}. In a previous study, in which we evaluated the relative importance of interventricular and intraventricular dyssynchrony for contractile response to CRT (change in LV dP/dt_{max}), it was demonstrated that interventricular dyssynchrony during intrinsic rhythm is the dominant electrical substrate driving response to CRT (Huntjens et al., 2018). In contrast, intraventricular dyssynchrony showed little effect on LV dP/dt_{max}, which is in line with experimental observations that reducing LV TAT by multipoint pacing does not improve LV dP/dt_{max} (Ploux et al., 2014). However, results

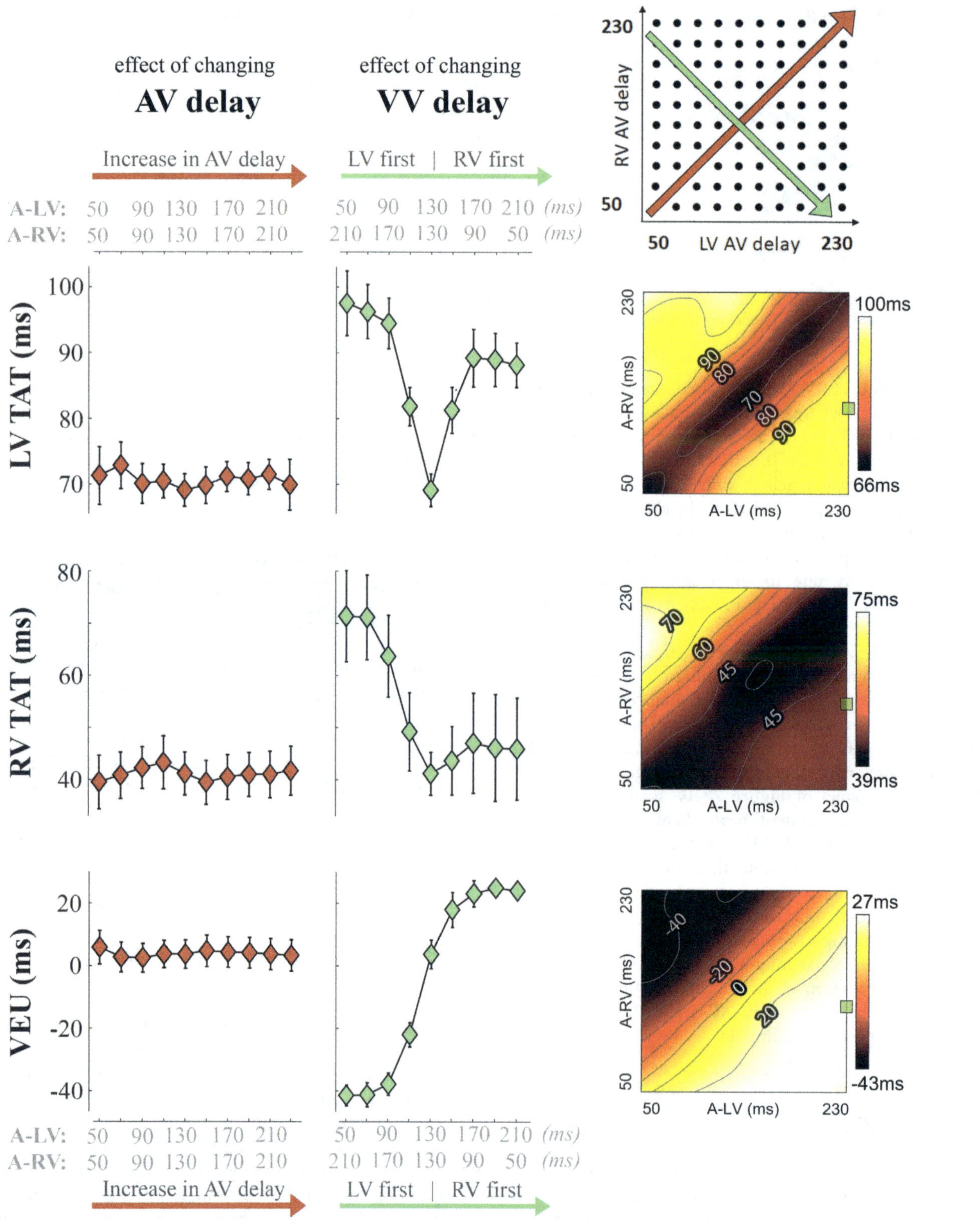

FIGURE 3 | Changes in electrical dyssynchrony indices during variation in pacing delay in the animal experiments. The left column shows the effect of increasing AV delay during simultaneous RV + LV pacing; the middle column shows changes in VV delay (green, from LV pre-excitation to RV pre-excitation) and the heat maps on the right are the results for all pacing setting (mean of six dogs, bars represent standard errors of the mean). From top to bottom: Total activation time (TAT) of the total LV (free wall and septum), RV free wall (RVFW), and VEU (Ventricular Electrical Uncoupling). The green square in each heat map indicate the baseline pacing setting.

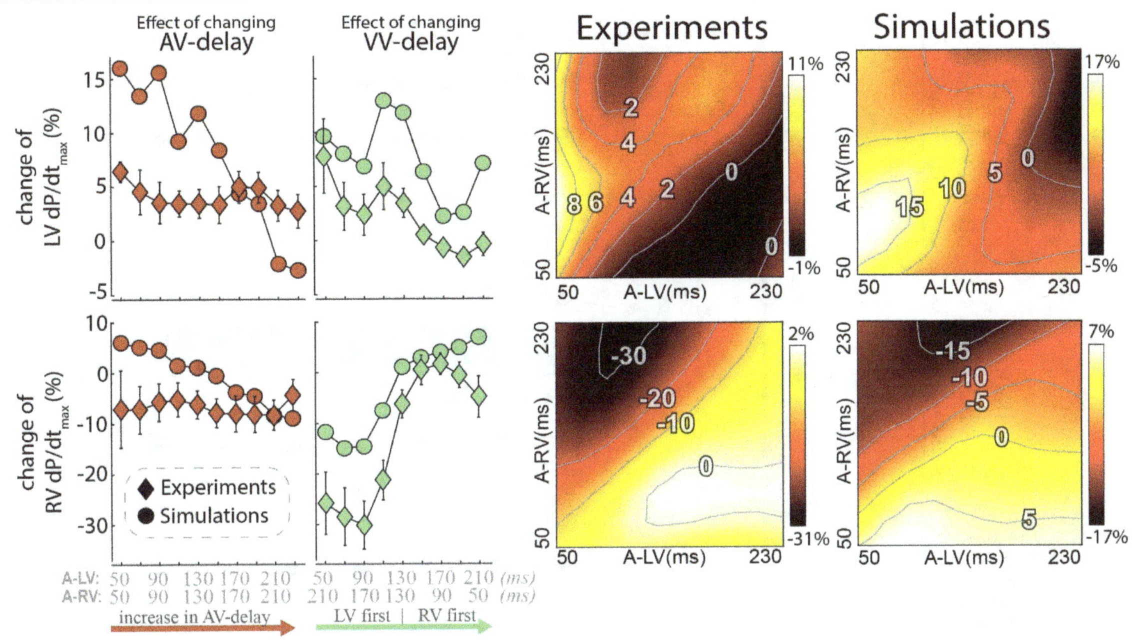

FIGURE 4 | Changes in contractile response as a result of changes in pacing delays in experiments and simulations. Percentile change from baseline of LV dP/dt_{max} (top) and RV dP/dt_{max} (bottom). The left rows depict the same AV and VV delay settings as in **Figure 3** are shown. Heat maps for both the experiment (3rd column) and simulations (4th column). Diamonds: Canine measurements (Mean (standard error of the mean) of six dogs; Circles: Simulation output.

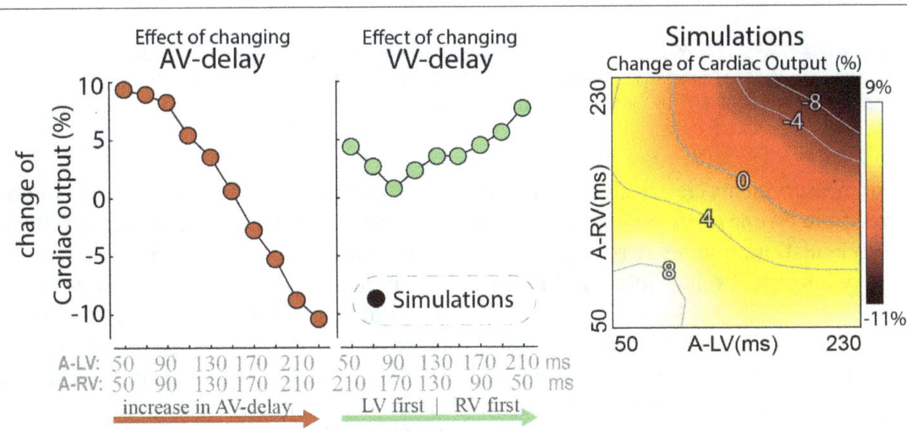

FIGURE 5 | Relative change in simulated steady-state cardiac output with a change in pacing delay settings. Depicted are the changes relative to baseline (see text).

in this study suggest that intraventricular dyssynchrony might still play a modulating role since increase in LV TAT, with large LV pre-excitation, led to a decrease in LV dP/dt_{max} compared to slight LV pre-excitation. Because RV TAT increases concurrently with decreases in VEU we cannot distinguish if either intra- or interventricular dyssynchrony has a larger effect on RV contractility.

In agreement with our observations, other studies in patients have shown that the lowest electrical dyssynchrony does not necessarily lead to the highest LV contractility or better clinical outcome (Thibault et al., 2011; Lumens et al., 2013). Optimization based on minimization of electrical dyssynchrony alone might therefore not be sufficient. Even if the optimal electrical activation for LV contractility is known, further clinical studies are required to investigate whether the gain in LV contractility outweighs the loss of RV contractility, especially since cardiac output might not match either or both but be a combination/compromise.

CircAdapt Simulations Capture Both LV and RV Contractile Response to Pacing Delay Changes

The present study demonstrates that the CircAdapt model can capture pacing-induced changes to both LV and RV contractile function. It is especially the response of the RV to pacing that has been less well studied, both by our group and by others.

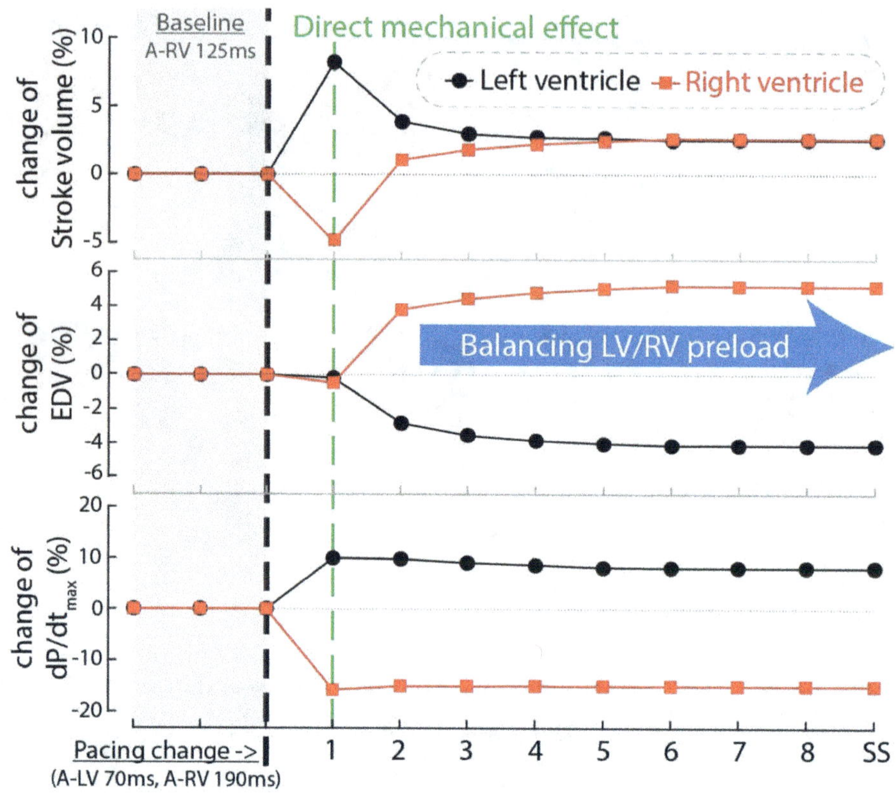

FIGURE 6 | Time courses of the relative change of stroke volume (top), end-diastolic volume (EDV, mid) and dP/dt_{max} of the LV (black circles) and RV (red squares) after changing pacing delay from baseline (A-RV 125 ms) to LV pre-excitation (A-LV 70 ms, A-RV 190 ms) in computer simulations. The black dashed line indicates the start of the change in pacing delay. The numbers in the blue bar indicate the number of simulated cardiac cycles. SS, steady state.

The use of experimental measurements electrical activation of the paced dog heart, derived from canine experiments, coupled to the simulation of the entire circulation, resulted in changes in RV and LV dP/dt_{max} that closely mimicked values measured in dog experiments.

Earlier studies have shown that CircAdapt enables realistic simulation of cardiac response to CRT, mostly focusing on LV function (Lumens et al., 2013, 2015; Huntjens et al., 2018). In one of those studies, it was demonstrated that the RV plays an important role in the improvement of LV function during LV-only pacing (Lumens et al., 2013). The present study extends the mechanistic insight in the working action of CRT in the context of pacing delay optimization, where the complex mechanical and hemodynamic interactions between the four cardiac cavities and the surrounding circulations are found to be important.

As demonstrated in this study, the CircAdapt model can capture the complexity of different LV and RV responses to CRT by incorporating several relevant components of cardiovascular interaction. Firstly, it realistically incorporates direct mechanical interaction between the three ventricular walls (Lumens et al., 2009). Secondly, it allows realistic simulation of regional myocardial mechanics in the ventricular walls of the asynchronously activated heart (Leenders et al., 2012; Walmsley et al., 2015a), thereby enabling experimentally measured activation times to be imposed and the related intraventricular heterogeneities in mechanical myofiber behavior to be simulated. Thirdly, it is a closed-loop system allowing for indirect (serial) hemodynamic interaction between the left and right side of the heart through the systemic and pulmonary circulations (Arts et al., 2005; Lumens et al., 2010). Fourthly, its four-chamber heart captures the dynamics of hemodynamic atrioventricular interactions (Jones et al., 2017). Lastly, it includes the mechanical interaction through pericardial constraint, with an increase in the volume of a chamber altering the pressure in the other chambers and, hence, diastolic filling and septal position (Palau-Caballero et al., 2017).

Simulation-Derived Mechanistic Insights

The ability of CircAdapt to realistically simulate both LV and RV hemodynamics during pacing allowed us to further study the impact of differences between both chambers on cardiac output. In particular, the model showed a difference in response between dP/dt_{max} and SV/CO. Similar differences have been observed in a clinical study where LV dP/dt_{max} responses differed from responses in stroke work (van Everdingen et al., 2018).

Our simulations provided a plausible explanation for this paradoxical observation. While LV and RV stroke volume

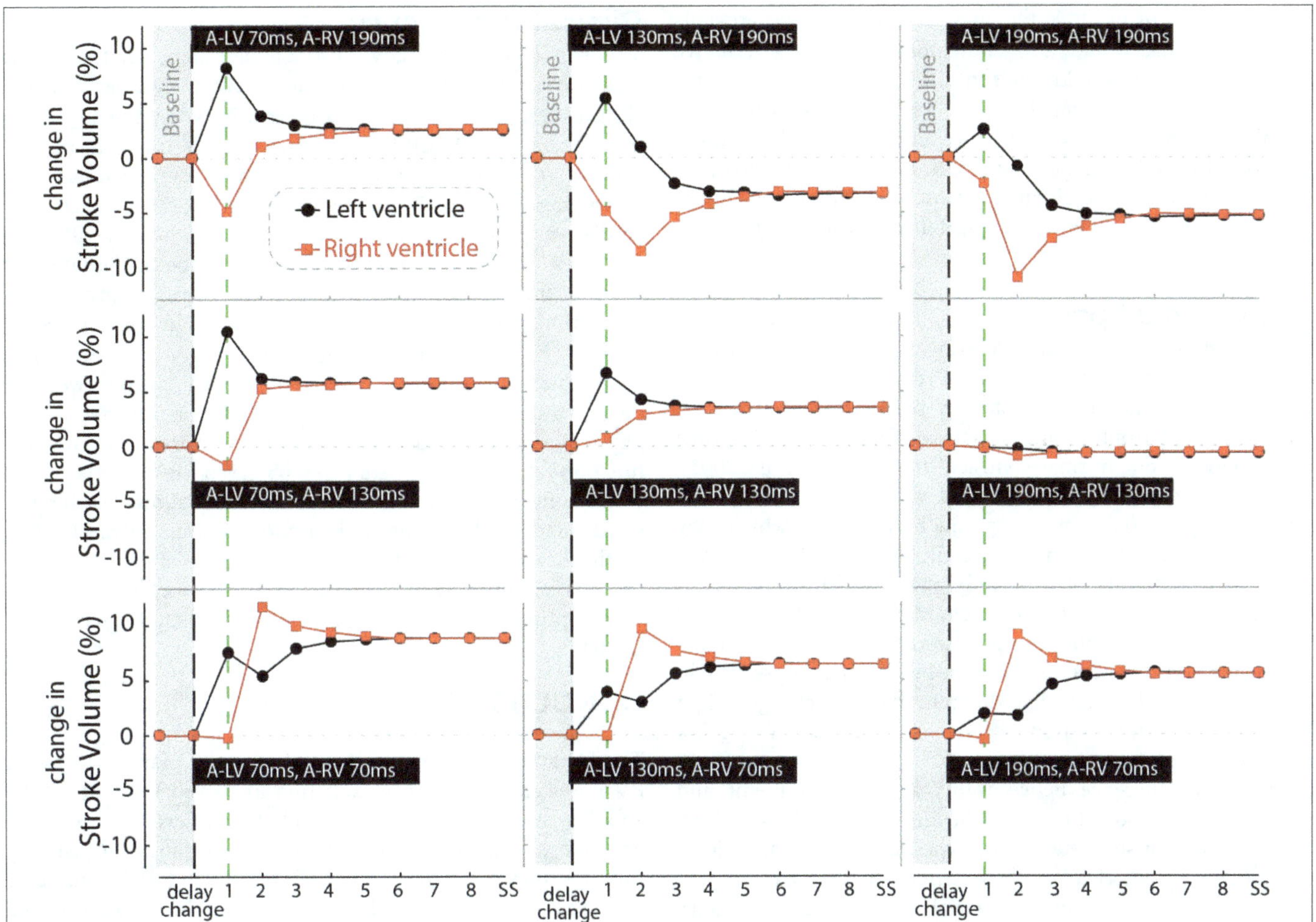

FIGURE 7 | Relative change in stroke volume of the left (black circles) and right (red squares) ventricle over a number of simulated cycles until steady-state (SS) after changing pacing delay (the nine settings shown in the black bars). Black dashed line indicates the moment of changing the pacing delays while the green line marks the first beat.

of the first beat after a change of pacing delay can differ substantially, a common steady-state stroke volume and thereby cardiac output is reached due to balancing ventricular preload conditions during the next few beats. There are three main determinants of the newly achieved steady-state preload condition. First, the changes in stroke volumes directly change the end-systolic volumes and thereby the end-diastolic volumes in the next beat. Second, the pacing-induced changes in effective left and right AV delays change the efficiency of atrial and ventricular diastolic filling and subsequent systolic contraction. Thirdly, changes in stroke volume affect the filling of the other ventricle through the systemic and pulmonary circulations.

While dP/dt_{max} changes congruently with first-beat stroke volume in the same ventricle, it is less affected by changes in preload. As a result, LV and RV dP/dt_{max} are much more sensitive to changes of VV-delay and, hence, asynchrony of electrical activation than to changes of AV-delay. On the other hand, changes of AV-delay affect cardiac output more than LV and RV dP/dt_{max}.

Computer Modeling in Therapy Optimization

Other cardiac computer modeling studies have been conducted to investigate other factors in the optimization of CRT therapy. For example, in a cohort of 648 virtual patients it was found that the location of the LV pacing site is an important factor in response to CRT (Crozier et al., 2016). Electrophysical cardiac computer modeling studies also demonstrated the importance of LV pacing site and the potential of simulations to predict the electrical optimal pacing location and setting (Reumann et al., 2007; Miri et al., 2009; Niederer et al., 2011). Our study shows, however, that an electrical optimum (lowest electrical dyssynchrony) might not necessarily be optimal for overall pump function.

The CircAdapt simulations performed for this study can run on a single core in real time. CircAdapt requires activation time as input and lacks the cardiac electrophysiological model necessary to extract this information from standard clinical data. This input could, however, potentially be generated by other models, for example the ones referred to in the previous paragraph. This would also allow for testing of alternative pacing sites, which would result in different activation patterns, which subsequently can be used as input for CircAdapt simulations. A workflow where fast and anatomically realistic cardiac electrophysiological simulations are combined with cardiac mechanical and circulatory CircAdapt simulations might further increase the clinical applicability of cardiac computer models.

Study Limitations

In this study the pacing experiments were performed in relatively healthy canine hearts. Previous work from our group showed that chronic total AV-block leads to structural changes (hypertrophy) and electrical remodeling (QT-time prolongation), but normal contractility (Peschar et al., 2003). On the other hand, patients treated with CRT have different levels of myocardial remodeling and heart failure, which may affect the response to pacing (Strik et al., 2013a, Nguyên et al., 2018). Results of this study might differ from patient data since long-term structural remodeling was not included in both the animal and computational experiments. On the other hand, differences in RV and LV response observed in this study could mean that different pacing settings might affect the positive and/or negative remodeling of the LV and RV.

A major difference between this animal experiment and patients in day-to-day life is that the animals were anesthetized. To allow comparison between the experiments and simulations, the model's LV afterload in the baseline situation was adapted to fit the measured mean arterial pressure in the dogs. After the change in activation delays regulation was disabled, which is likely similar to the anesthetic condition were regulation is slow. Caution should, however, be taken when translating results of this study toward the clinical setting considering that loading conditions potentially affect the effect of pacing delay changes (Quinn et al., 2009). Future studies are needed to investigate how load-dependent the observed effects of pacing delay optimization are and how homeostatic regulation interacts with changes in LV and RV contractility. A final limitation of the CircAdapt (and most other computer models in this field) is that changes in function of the autonomic nervous system are not taken into account.

Clinical Perspective

The results of this study raise the question what outcome measure is best to use for optimization of pacing delay. Current clinical practice focusses almost exclusively on the LV, using parameters like LV dP/dt_{max}, aortic outflow integral, and LV systolic (or aortic) pressure. This study demonstrates that improving LV function can reduce RV function. Furthermore, cardiac output is not necessarily increasing when LV dP/dt_{max} increases. Hence, An exclusive focus on the LV might not lead to the best overall outcome. Therefore, future studies on optimization of therapy should not exclusively focus on the LV but also include measures of RV and/or whole heart function. In our analysis of cardiac output we also demonstrated that the moment of measurement affects what physiological phenomenon is actually observed. Contractile function alone might better be observed in the first beats while longer lasting measurements, that allow reaching a steady state, will provide more information about the loading of the heart and its interaction with homeostatic regulation. Insights acquired in the present opens the way for designing better optimization protocols, possibly even including computer modeling.

CONCLUSION

The LV and the RV respond in an opposite manner to LV or RV pre-excitation. LV pre-excitation improved LV contractility and decreased RV contractility, while RV pre-excitation had the opposite effects. The CircAdapt computer model realistically captures these opposite responses of LV and RV contractile function. Computer simulations extend animal experimental findings by revealing that improving ventricular contractility does not necessarily lead to an improvement of cardiac output. This study demonstrates the potential of CircAdapt to provide a valuable and efficient *in silico* platform for further optimization studies for device therapy.

AUTHOR CONTRIBUTIONS

EW, PH, MS, JW, FP, and JL conceived and designed the experiments. EW, RS, and MS performed the experiments. EW, RS, PH, MS, GP, EV, FP, and JL analyzed and interpreted the data. MS, JW, FP, and JL contributed to materials and analysis tools. EW, RS, PH, MS, GP, EV, JW, KV, TD, FP, and JL wrote or provided the critical revision on the manuscript.

REFERENCES

Abraham, W. W. T., Fisher, W. G. W., Smith, A. L., Delurgio, D. B., Leon, A. R., Loh, E., et al. (2002). Cardiac resynchronization in chronic heart failure. *N. Engl. J. Med.* 346, 1845–1853. doi: 10.1056/NEJMoa013168

Arts, T., Delhaas, T., Bovendeerd, P., Verbeek, X., and Prinzen, F. (2005). Adaptation to mechanical load determines shape and properties of heart and circulation: the CircAdapt model. *Am. J. Physiol. Heart Circ. Physiol.* 288, 1943–1954. doi: 10.1152/ajpheart.00444.2004

Arts, T., Lumens, J., Kroon, W., and Delhaas, T. (2012). Control of whole heart geometry by intramyocardial mechano-feedback: a model study. *PLoS Comput. Biol.* 8:e1002369. doi: 10.1371/journal.pcbi.1002369

Arts, T., Prinzen, F. W., Snoeckx, L. H. E., Rijcken, J. M., and Reneman, R. S. (1994). Adaption of cardiac structure by mechanical feedback in the environment of the cell: a model study. *Biophys. J.* 66, 953–961. doi: 10.1016/S0006-3495(94)80876-8

Auger, D., Hoke, U., Bax, J. J., Boersma, E., and Delgado, V. (2013). Effect of atrioventricular and ventriculoventricular delay optimization on clinical and echocardiographic outcomes of patients treated with cardiac resynchronization therapy: a meta-analysis. *Am. Heart J.* 166, 20–29. doi: 10.1016/j.ahj.2013.03.021

Auricchio, A., and Prinzen, F. W. (2011). Non-responders to cardiac resynchronization therapy. *Circ. J.* 75, 521–527. doi: 10.1253/circj.CJ-10-1268

Bogaard, M. D., Meine, M., Tuinenburg, A. E., Maskara, B., Loh, P., and Doevendans, P. A. (2012). Cardiac resynchronization therapy beyond nominal settings: who needs individual programming of the atrioventricular and interventricular delay? *Europace* 14, 1746–1753. doi: 10.1093/europace/eus170

Brignole, M., Auricchio, A., Baron-Esquivias, G., Bordachar, P., Boriani, G., Breithardt, O.-A., et al. (2013). 2013 ESC guidelines on cardiac pacing and cardiac resynchronization therapy: the task force on cardiac pacing and resynchronization therapy of the European society of cardiology (ESC). Developed in collaboration with the European Heart Rhythm Association. *Eur. Heart J.* 34, 2281–2329. doi: 10.1093/eurheartj/eht150

Cleland, J. G., Daubert, J. C., Erdmann, E., Freemantle, N., Gras, D., Kappenberger, L., et al. (2005). The effect of cardiac resynchronization on morbidity and mortality in heart failure. *N. Engl. J. Med.* 352, 1539–1549.

Cleveland, W. S. (1979). Robust locally weighted regression and smoothing scatterplots. *J. Am. Stat. Assoc.* 74, 829–836. doi: 10.1080/01621459.1979.10481038

Crozier, A., Blazevic, B., Lamata, P., Plank, G., Ginks, M., Duckett, S., et al. (2016). The relative role of patient physiology and device optimisation in cardiac resynchronisation therapy: a computational modelling study. *J. Mol. Cell. Cardiol.* 96, 93–100. doi: 10.1016/j.yjmcc.2015.10.026

Groote, P. D. E., Millaire, A., Foucher-hossein, C., de Groote, P., Millaire, A., Foucher-hossein, C., et al. (1998). Right ventricular ejection fraction is an independent predictor of survival in patients with moderate heart failure. *J. Am. Coll. Cardiol.* 32, 948–954.

Houston, B. A., Sturdivant, J. L., Yu, Y., and Gold, M. R. (2018). Acute biventricular hemodynamic effects of cardiac resynchronization therapy in right bundle branch block. *Heart Rhythm* 15, 1525–1532. doi: 10.1016/j.hrthm.2018.05.017

Huntjens, P. R., Ploux, S., Strik, M., Walmsley, J., Ritter, P., Haissaguerre, M., et al. (2018). Electrical substrates driving response to cardiac resynchronization therapy. *Circ. Arrhythm. Electrophysiol.* 11:e005647. doi: 10.1161/CIRCEP.117.005647

Huntjens, P. R., Walmsley, J., Ploux, S., Bordachar, P., Prinzen, F. W., Delhaas, T., et al. (2014). Influence of left ventricular lead position relative to scar location on response to cardiac resynchronization therapy: a model study. *Europace* 16(Suppl. 4), iv62–iv68. doi: 10.1093/europace/euu231

Hyde, E. R., Behar, J. M., Crozier, A., Claridge, S., Jackson, T., Sohal, M., et al. (2016). Improvement of right ventricular hemodynamics with left ventricular endocardial pacing during cardiac resynchronization therapy. *Pacing Clin. Electrophysiol.* 39, 531–541. doi: 10.1111/pace.12854

Jones, S., Lumens, J., Sohaib, S. M. A., Finegold, J. A., Kanagaratnam, P., Tanner, M., et al. (2017). Cardiac resynchronization therapy: mechanisms of action and scope for further improvement in cardiac function. *Europace* 19, 1178–1186. doi: 10.1093/europace/euw136

Lee, A. W. C., Costa, C. M., Strocchi, M., Rinaldi, C. A., and Niederer, S. A. (2018). Computational modeling for cardiac resynchronization therapy. *J. Cardiovasc. Transl. Res.* 11, 92–108. doi: 10.1007/s12265-017-9779-4

Leenders, G. E., Lumens, J., Cramer, M. J., De Boeck, B. W. L., Doevendans, P. A., Delhaas, T., et al. (2012). Septal deformation patterns delineate mechanical dyssynchrony and regional differences in contractility: analysis of patient data using a computer model. *Circ. Heart Fail.* 5, 87–96. doi: 10.1161/CIRCHEARTFAILURE.111.962704

Lumens, J., Blanchard, D. G., Arts, T., Mahmud, E., and Delhaas, T. (2010). Left ventricular underfilling and not septal bulging dominates abnormal left ventricular filling hemodynamics in chronic thromboembolic pulmonary hypertension. *AJP Heart Circ. Physiol.* 299, H1083–H1091. doi: 10.1152/ajpheart.00607.2010

Lumens, J., Delhaas, T., Kirn, B., and Arts, T. (2009). Three-wall segment (TriSeg) model describing mechanics and hemodynamics of ventricular interaction. *Ann. Biomed. Eng.* 37, 2234–2255. doi: 10.1007/s10439-009-9774-2

Lumens, J., Ploux, S., Strik, M., Gorcsan, J., Cochet, H., Derval, N., et al. (2013). Comparative electromechanical and hemodynamic effects of left ventricular and biventricular pacing in dyssynchronous heart failure: electrical resynchronization versus left-right ventricular interaction. *J. Am. Coll. Cardiol.* 62, 2395–2403. doi: 10.1016/j.jacc.2013.08.715

Lumens, J., Tayal, B., Walmsley, J., Delgado-Montero, A., Huntjens, P. R., Schwartzman, D., et al. (2015). Differentiating electromechanical from non-electrical substrates of mechanical discoordination to identify responders to cardiac resynchronization therapy. *Circ. Cardiovasc. Imaging* 8:e003744. doi: 10.1161/CIRCIMAGING.115.003744

Miri, R., Graf, I. M., and DÖssel, O. (2009). Efficiency of timing delays and electrode positions in optimization of biventricular pacing: a simulation study. *IEEE Trans. Biomed. Eng.* 56, 2573–2582. doi: 10.1109/TBME.2009.2027692

Nguyên, U. C., Verzaal, N. J., van Nieuwenhoven, F. A., Vernooy, K., and Prinzen, F. W. (2018). Pathobiology of cardiac dyssynchrony and resynchronization therapy. *Europace* 6, 1660–1665. doi: 10.1093/europace/euy035

Niederer, S., Mitchell, L., Smith, N., and Plank, G. (2011). Simulating human cardiac electrophysiology on clinical time-scales. *Front. Physiol.* 2:14. doi: 10.3389/fphys.2011.00014

Palau-Caballero, G., Walmsley, J., Van Empel, V., Lumens, J., and Delhaas, T. (2017). Why septal motion is a marker of right ventricular failure in pulmonary arterial hypertension: mechanistic analysis using a computer model. *Am. J. Physiol. Heart Circ. Physiol.* 312, H691–H700. doi: 10.1152/ajpheart.00596.2016

Peschar, M., Vernooy, K., Vanagt, W. Y. R., Reneman, R. S., Vos, M. A., and Prinzen, F. W. (2003). Absence of reverse electrical remodeling during regression of volume overload hypertrophy in canine ventricles. *Cardiovasc. Res.* 58, 510–517. doi: 10.1016/S0008-6363(03)00331-6

Ploux, S., Lumens, J., Whinnett, Z., Montaudon, M., Strom, M., Ramanathan, C., et al. (2013). Noninvasive electrocardiographic mapping to improve patient selection for cardiac resynchronization therapy: beyond QRS duration and left bundle branch block morphology. *J. Am. Coll. Cardiol.* 61, 2435–2443. doi: 10.1016/j.jacc.2013.01.093

Ploux, S., Strik, M., Van Hunnik, A., Van Middendorp, L., Kuiper, M., and Prinzen, F. W. (2014). Acute electrical and hemodynamic effects of multisite left ventricular pacing for cardiac resynchronization therapy in the dyssynchronous canine heart. *Heart Rhythm* 11, 119–125. doi: 10.1016/j.hrthm.2013.10.018

Prinzen, F. W., Vernooy, K., and Auricchio, A. (2013). Cardiac resynchronization therapy: state-of-the-art of current applications, guidelines, ongoing trials, and areas of controversy. *Circulation* 128, 2407–2418. doi: 10.1161/CIRCULATIONAHA.112.000112

Quinn, T. A., Berberian, G., Cabreriza, S. E., Maskin, L. J., Weinberg, A. D., Holmes, J. W., et al. (2006). Effects of sequential biventricular pacing during acute right ventricular pressure overload. *Am. J. Physiol. Heart Circ. Physiol.* 291, H2380–H2387. doi: 10.1152/ajpheart.00446.2006

Quinn, T. A., Cabreriza, S. E., Richmond, M. E., Weinberg, A. D., Holmes, J. W., and Spotnitz, H. M. (2009). Simultaneous variation of ventricular pacing site and timing with biventricular pacing in acute ventricular failure improves function by interventricular assist. *Am. J. Physiol. Heart Circ. Physiol.* 297, H2220–H2226. doi: 10.1152/ajpheart.00802.2009

Reumann, M., Farina, D., Miri, R., Lurz, S., Osswald, B., and Dössel, O. (2007). Computer model for the optimization of AV and VV delay in cardiac resynchronization therapy. *Med. Biol. Eng. Comput.* 45, 845–854. doi: 10.1007/s11517-007-0230-x

Ricci, F., Mele, D., Bianco, F., Bucciarelli, V., De Caterina, R., and Gallina, S. (2017). Right heart-pulmonary circulation unit and cardiac resynchronization therapy. *Am. Heart J.* 185, 1–16. doi: 10.1016/j.ahj.2016.11.005

Sciaraffia, E., Malmborg, H., Lönnerholm, S., Blomström, P., and Blomström Lundqvist, C. (2009). Right ventricular contractility as a measure of optimal interventricular pacing setting in cardiac resynchronization therapy. *Europace* 11, 1496–1500. doi: 10.1093/europace/eup288

Strik, M., Van Deursen, C. J. M., Van Middendorp, L. B., Van Hunnik, A., Kuiper, M., Auricchio, A., et al. (2013a). Transseptal conduction as an important determinant for cardiac resynchronization therapy, as revealed by extensive electrical mapping in the dyssynchronous canine heart. *Circ. Arrhythm. Electrophysiol.* 6, 682–689. doi: 10.1161/CIRCEP.111.000028

Strik, M., Van Middendorp, L. B., Houthuizen, P., Ploux, S., Van Hunnik, A., Kuiper, M., et al. (2013b). Interplay of electrical wavefronts as determinant of the response to cardiac resynchronization therapy in dyssynchronous canine hearts. *Circ. Arrhythm. Electrophysiol.* 6, 924–931. doi: 10.1161/CIRCEP.113.000753

Thibault, B., Ducharme, A., Harel, F., White, M., Omeara, E., Guertin, M. C., et al. (2011). Left ventricular versus simultaneous biventricular pacing in patients with heart failure and a qrs complex =120 milliseconds. *Circulation* 124, 2874–2881. doi: 10.1161/CIRCULATIONAHA.111.032904

van Everdingen, W. M., Zweerink, A., Salden, O. A. E., Cramer, M. J., Doevendans, P. A., van Rossum, A. C., et al. (2018). Atrioventricular optimization in cardiac resynchronization therapy with quadripolar leads: should we optimize every pacing configuration including multi-point pacing? *Europace* 21, e11–e19. doi: 10.1093/europace/euy138

Vernooy, K., Cornelussen, R. N. M., Verbeek, X. A., Vanagt, W. Y., Van Hunnik, A., Kuiper, M., et al. (2007). Cardiac resynchronization therapy cures dyssynchronopathy in canine left bundle-branch block hearts. *Eur. Heart J.* 28, 2148–2155. doi: 10.1093/eurheartj/ehm207

Walmsley, J., Arts, T., Derval, N., Bordachar, P., Cochet, H., Ploux, S., et al. (2015a). Fast simulation of mechanical heterogeneity in the electrically asynchronous heart using the multipatch module. *PLoS Comput. Biol.* 11:e1004284. doi: 10.1371/journal.pcbi.1004284

Walmsley, J., Huntjens, P. R., Prinzen, F. W., Delhaas, T., and Lumens, J. (2015b). Septal flash and septal rebound stretch have different underlying mechanisms. *Am. J. Physiol. Heart Circ. Physiol.* 310, H394–H403. doi: 10.1152/ajpheart.00639.2015

5

Cellular Mechanisms of Sinus Node Dysfunction in Carriers of the *SCN5A*-E161K Mutation and Role of the H558R Polymorphism

Ronald Wilders*

Department of Medical Biology, Amsterdam University Medical Centers, Amsterdam, Netherlands

***Correspondence:**
Ronald Wilders
r.wilders@amc.uva.nl

Background: Carriers of the E161K mutation in the *SCN5A* gene, encoding the $Na_V1.5$ pore-forming α-subunit of the ion channel carrying the fast sodium current (I_{Na}), show sinus bradycardia and occasional exit block. Voltage clamp experiments in mammalian expression systems revealed a mutation-induced 2.5- to 4-fold reduction in I_{Na} peak current density as well as a +19 mV shift and reduced steepness of the steady-state activation curve. The highly common H558R polymorphism in $Na_V1.5$ limits this shift to +13 mV, but also introduces a −10 mV shift in steady-state inactivation.

Aim: We assessed the cellular mechanism by which the E161K mutation causes sinus node dysfunction in heterozygous mutation carriers as well as the potential role of the H558R polymorphism.

Methods: We incorporated the mutation-induced changes in I_{Na} into the Fabbri-Severi model of a single human sinoatrial node cell and the Maleckar et al. human atrial cell model, and carried out simulations under control conditions and over a wide range of acetylcholine levels.

Results: In absence of the H558R polymorphism, the E161K mutation increased the basic cycle length of the sinoatrial node cell from 813 to 866 ms. In the simulated presence of 10 and 25 nM acetylcholine, basic cycle length increased from 1027 to 1131 and from 1448 to 1795 ms, respectively. The increase in cycle length was the result of a significant slowing of diastolic depolarization. The mutation-induced reduction in I_{Na} window current had reduced the contribution of the mutant component of I_{Na} to the net membrane current during diastolic depolarization to effectively zero. Highly similar results were obtained in presence of the H558R polymorphism. Atrial excitability was reduced, both in absence and presence of the H558R polymorphism, as reflected by an increase in threshold stimulus current and a concomitant decrease in capacitive current of the atrial cell.

Conclusion: We conclude that the experimentally identified mutation-induced changes in I_{Na} can explain the clinically observed sinus bradycardia and potentially the occasional exit block. Furthermore, we conclude that the common H558R polymorphism does not significantly alter the effects of the E161K mutation and can thus not explain the reduced penetrance of the E161K mutation.

Keywords: computer simulations, electrophysiology, genetics, human, ion channel, sinus bradycardia, sinus node dysfunction, sodium current

INTRODUCTION

The"fast sodium current" (I_{Na}), which flows through $Na_V1.5$ sodium channels, is a key player in the electrical activity of the human heart (Zimmer et al., 2014), where it is responsible for the fast >150 V/s upstroke of individual atrial and ventricular cardio-myocytes (Workman et al., 2001; O'Hara et al., 2011). The cardiac-specific $Na_V1.5$ protein, encoded by the *SCN5A* gene, is the pore-forming α-subunit of the channel (Remme, 2013). I_{Na} has also been observed in patch-clamp recordings from isolated human sinoatrial (SA) node cells (Verkerk et al., 2009), in line with the observation by Chandler et al. (2009) that $Na_V1.5$ is expressed in human SA nodal tissue. Accordingly, I_{Na} was included in the comprehensive computational model of a single human SA nodal cell that was recently developed by Fabbri et al. (2017) and is known as the Fabbri-Severi model.

Mutations in genes encoding ion channel-related proteins may result in inherited arrhythmia disorders, in particular the long QT syndrome (LQTS) and the Brugada syndrome (BrS). Gain-of-function and loss-of-function mutations in *SCN5A* underlie LQTS type 3 (LQT3) and BrS type 1 (BrS1), respectively (Brugada et al., 2018; Giudicessi et al., 2018; Wilde and Amin, 2018). Mutations in *SCN5A* may also lead to overlapping phenotypes (*SCN5A* overlap syndromes), where clinical characteristics of LQTS, BrS, and other arrhythmia syndromes, e.g., conduction disease and sinus node dysfunction, coexist in a single family or even in a single patient (Remme et al., 2008; Giudicessi et al., 2018). Sinus node dysfunction is a relatively common observation in both LQT3 and BrS1 patients (Hayashi et al., 2018; Wilders and Verkerk, 2018). It should be noted that the "gain of function" in case of LQT3 refers to the persistent I_{Na} that prolongs the ventricular action potential and thus causes QT interval prolongation. If an LQT3 mutation is associated with sinus bradycardia, this mutation shows a concomitant "loss of function" in the voltage range of diastolic depolarization (Wilders and Verkerk, 2018).

In 2005, Smits et al. reported the clinical and biophysical features of a novel sodium channel mutation, E161K, i.e., the replacement of the highly conserved acidic residue glutamic acid (E) with the basic residue lysine (K) at position 161 of the $Na_V1.5$ protein (p.Glu161Lys; c.481G > A) (Smits et al., 2005). This loss-of-function mutation was identified in individuals of two non-related families. Affected patients had a complex clinical phenotype with symptoms of bradycardia, sinus node dysfunction, generalized conduction disease or BrS, or various combinations thereof. Sinus node dysfunction was observed in 8 out of 14 mutation carriers. Twenty-four-hour Holter recordings from 10 mutation carriers revealed that their absolute minimum heart rate, but not their maximum heart rate, was significantly lower compared to controls (39 ± 1 vs. 51 ± 0.6 beats/min, mean ± SEM). Furthermore, the incidence of signs of sinus node dysfunction in E161K mutation carriers was particularly high at night, when vagal tone is dominant.

Smits et al. (2005) assessed the biophysical effects of the E161K mutation by transfecting E161K or wild-type sodium channel α-subunit into tsA201 cells, together with wild-type β_1-subunit. Voltage clamp experiments on the transfected cells revealed a 2.5-fold reduction in peak I_{Na} at −20 mV for E161K sodium channels compared to wild-type channels. Furthermore, the steady-state activation curve of the mutant channels showed a +11.9 mV shift of its half-maximal activation potential ($V_{1/2}$) compared to wild-type (−30.7 ± 0.8 vs. −42.6 ± 1.4 mV, respectively). Also, the steepness of this curve was slightly reduced; its slope factor (k) amounted to 7.9 ± 0.3 vs. 6.7 ± 0.4 mV, respectively. Voltage dependence of steady-state inactivation, recovery from inactivation, and development of slow inactivation were not affected by the E161K mutation. Of note, these data were all obtained in H558 background, i.e., with histidine (H) at position 558 of the $Na_V1.5$ protein.

Iwasa et al. (2000) were the first to report on the c.1673A > G single nucleotide polymorphism ("SNP") in the *SCN5A* gene, which is responsible for the replacement of histidine (H) with arginine (R) at position 558 of the $Na_V1.5$ protein (p.His558Arg or H558R), in relation to familial LQTS. Ackerman et al. (2004) showed that H558R is the most common polymorphism in *SCN5A* and that this variant is present in all four ethnic groups, albeit at a significantly lower prevalence in Asians. In blacks, whites, and Hispanics, the prevalence of R558 instead of H558 amounts to 20–30%, whereas this prevalence is near 10% among Asians (Ackerman et al., 2004). Over the years, it has become clear that the H558R polymorphism can either mitigate or aggravate the effects of specific mutations in *SCN5A*. For example, this polymorphism has mitigating effects on the mutations M1766L (Ye et al., 2003) and P2006A (Shinlapawittayatorn et al., 2011), but aggravating effects on the mutations G400A (Hu et al., 2007) and A572D (Tester et al., 2010).

In 2010, Gui et al. (2010a,b) demonstrated that the H558R polymorphism also affects the E161K mutation. They carried out voltage clamp experiments on HEK-293 cells transfected with E161K mutant or wild-type sodium channel α-subunit. Like

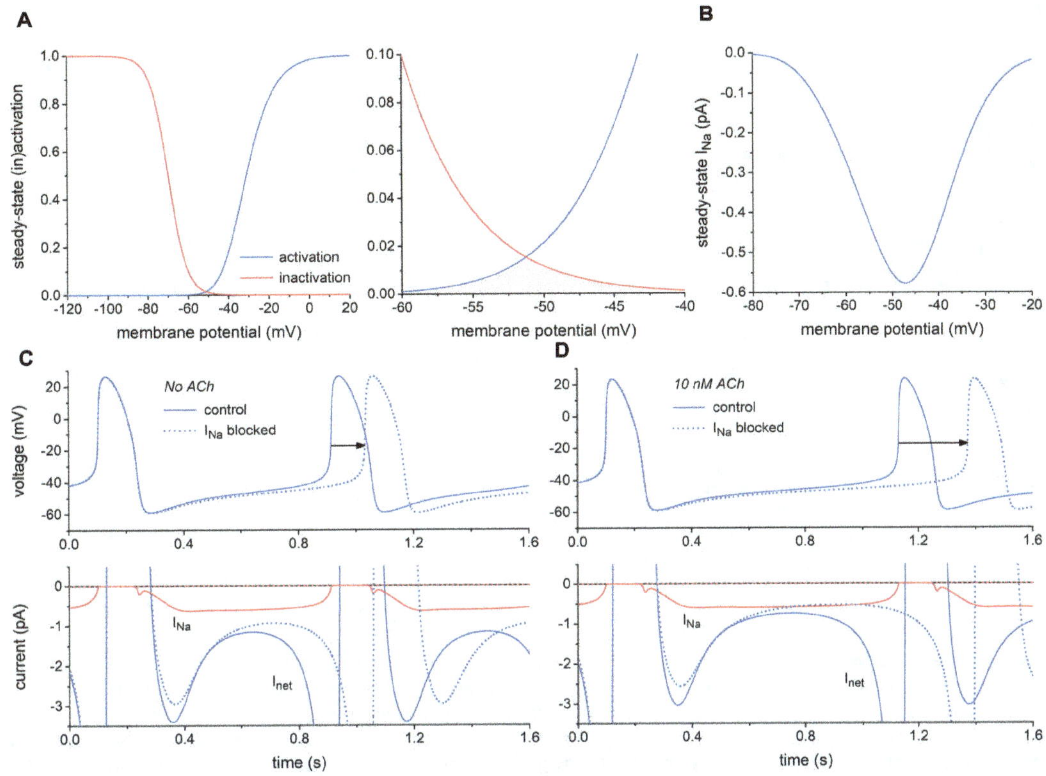

FIGURE 1 | Characteristics of the fast sodium current (I_{Na}) of the Fabbri-Severi model of a human SA nodal pacemaker cell. **(A)** Steady-state activation and inactivation curves (blue and red curves, respectively) of I_{Na} (left) and associated "window" of overlap (shaded area) in the voltage range between −60 and −40 mV (right). **(B)** Current–voltage relationship of steady-state I_{Na}. **(C)** Effect of full block of I_{Na} in the absence of acetylcholine (ACh). Spontaneous action potentials (top) and associated net membrane current (I_{net}) and I_{Na} (bottom). Horizontal arrow indicates increase in cycle length. **(D)** Effect of full block of I_{Na} during simulated administration of 10 nM ACh. Spontaneous action potentials (top) and associated I_{net} and I_{Na} (bottom). Horizontal arrow indicates increase in cycle length.

Smits et al. (2005), they observed a reduction in peak I_{Na} for E161K sodium channels compared to wild-type channels, both in H558 and R558 background. In either case, this reduction was approximately 4-fold, which is more pronounced than the 2.5-fold reduction in the study by Smits et al. (2005). With a value of ≈19 mV, the positive shift in $V_{1/2}$ of the steady-state activation curve in H558 background was also more pronounced. The steepness of this curve showed a reduction similar to that observed by Smits et al. (2005). In R558 background, the reduction in peak I_{Na} and steepness of the steady-state activation curve were both similar to those in H558 background (Gui et al., 2010b). However, the positive shift in $V_{1/2}$ of the steady-state activation curve was less pronounced, with a value of ≈13 mV rather than ≈19 mV. However, the potentially mitigating effects of this less pronounced shift in R558 background was counteracted by a −10 mV shift in $V_{1/2}$ of the steady-state inactivation curve, which was absent in H558 background.

To assess the mechanism by which the E161K mutation causes sinus node dysfunction as well as the potential role of the H558R polymorphism, we incorporated the mutation-induced changes in I_{Na} into the Fabbri-Severi model of a single human SA node cell (Fabbri et al., 2017). Furthermore, we incorporated these changes into the Maleckar et al. human atrial cell model (Maleckar et al., 2008, 2009) to assess the effects of the E161K mutation on atrial excitability, which may also play a role in sinus node dysfunction.

MATERIALS AND METHODS

Implementation of the E161K Mutation and H558R Polymorphism

Effects of the heterozygous E161K mutation in *SCN5A* were implemented in the CellML code (Cuellar et al., 2003) of the Fabbri-Severi human SA nodal cell model (Fabbri et al., 2017) by scaling the fully-activated conductance of I_{Na} (g_{Na}) and shifting the steady-state I_{Na} activation and/or inactivation curves, as detailed below, based on the experimental data from literature described in the Introduction and summarized in **Table 1**. The slight change in steepness of the steady-state activation curve was also included. These modifications were applied to half of the intrinsic I_{Na} channels, thus representing the heterozygous nature of the mutation, taking into account that a functional I_{Na} channel is built with a single $Na_V1.5$ protein.

Identical changes were applied to the Maleckar et al. (2009) human atrial cell model. The latter model, which is also known as the "human atrial myocyte with new repolarization"

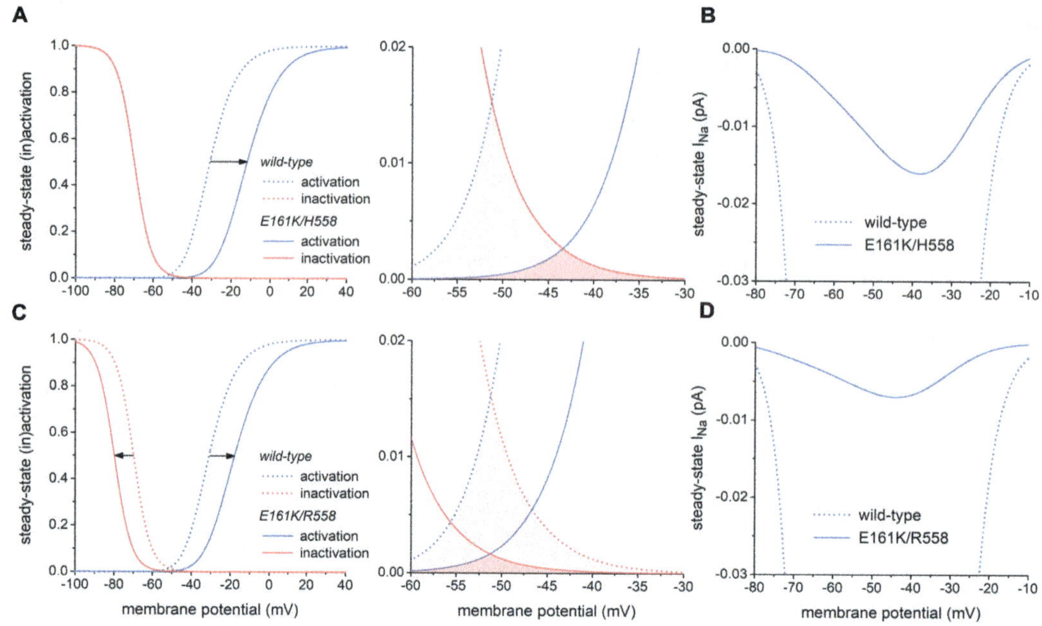

FIGURE 2 | Effects of the E161K mutation in *SCN5A*, either in H558 or R558 background, on biophysical properties of the fast sodium current (I_{Na}) of the Fabbri-Severi model of a human SA nodal pacemaker cell. **(A)** Shift and change in steepness of the steady-state activation curve (left) and effect on "window" (right) in H558 background. Horizontal arrow indicates the +19 mV shift. **(B)** Resulting effect on current–voltage relationship of steady-state I_{Na} in H558 background. **(C)** Shift and change in steepness of the steady-state activation curve and shift of steady-state inactivation curve (left) and effect on "window" (right) in R558 background. Horizontal arrows indicate the +13 and −10 mV shifts. **(D)** Resulting effect on current–voltage relationship of steady-state I_{Na} in R558 background.

(hAMr) model, was selected because it includes well-validated equations for the acetylcholine-activated potassium current $I_{K,ACh}$ (Maleckar et al., 2008), thus allowing simulations over a wide range of acetylcholine levels. Action potentials were elicited with a 1 ms, ≈50% suprathreshold stimulus current at a frequency of 1 Hz. The threshold stimulus current amplitude was determined by increasing the stimulus current amplitude in 0.1 pA/pF steps until a train of 200 action potentials

TABLE 1 | Experimental data on biophysical effects of the E161K mutation in *SCN5A*.

Study	Expression system	Background	Channel type	Peak current density (nA/pF)	Steady-state activation		*n*	Steady-state inactivation		*n*
					$V_{1/2}$ (mV)	k (mV)		$V_{1/2}$ (mV)	k (mV)	
Experimental Data										
Smits et al., 2005	tsA201 cells	H558	Wild-type	0.71 ± 0.11	−42.6 ± 1.4	6.7 ± 0.4	9	−89.4 ± 1.2	−4.9 ± 0.3	9
			E161K	0.28 ± 0.05*	−30.7 ± 0.8*	7.9 ± 0.3*	13	−88.5 ± 0.9	−4.4 ± 0.1	13
Gui et al., 2010a	HEK-293 cells	H558	Wild-type	0.87 ± 0.08	−34.7 ± 0.7	6.9 ± 0.2	23	−81.4 ± 0.7	−6.4 ± 0.1	24
			E161K	0.20 ± 0.03*	−14.9 ± 0.7*	9.0 ± 0.1*	19	−79.9 ± 0.9	−6.6 ± 0.1	21
Gui et al., 2010b	HEK-293 cells	H558	Wild-type	0.81 ± 0.08	−33.8 ± 0.7	6.7 ± 0.2	11	−80.3 ± 0.9	−6.2 ± 0.1	12
			E161K	0.19 ± 0.03*	−14.7 ± 0.6*	8.9 ± 0.1*	11	−78.4 ± 0.8	−6.5 ± 0.2	12
		R558	Wild-type	0.92 ± 0.17	−35.5 ± 1.3	6.8 ± 0.2	9	−81.8 ± 1.0	−6.5 ± 0.1	10
			E161K	0.15 ± 0.02*	−20.9 ± 1.2*	8.0 ± 0.1*	14	−88.8 ± 1.8*	−6.7 ± 0.2	10
Model Parameters										
Fabbri et al., 2017					−30.5	6.5		−69.8	−4.5	
Maleckar et al., 2009					−15.7	6.4		−63.6	−5.3	

*All experimental data obtained at room temperature and expressed as mean ± SEM. *P < 0.05 vs. wild-type.*

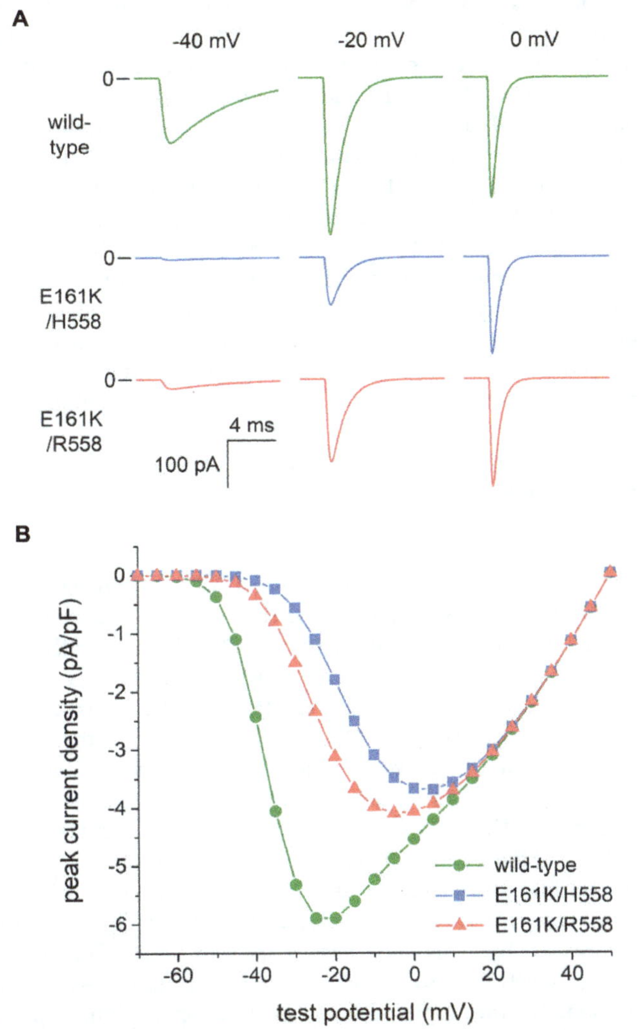

FIGURE 3 | Effects of the E161K mutation in *SCN5A*, either in H558 or R558 background, on the fast sodium current (I_{Na}) of the Fabbri-Severi model of a human SA nodal pacemaker cell during simulated voltage clamp experiments. **(A)** Control ("wild-type") and mutant I_{Na} during voltage clamp steps from a holding potential of −120 mV to test potentials of −40, −20, and 0 mV. **(B)** Current-voltage relationship of peak I_{Na}, as derived from these simulated voltage clamp experiments.

could successfully be elicited. To prevent slow drifts in ion concentrations, the intracellular Na^+ and K^+ concentrations were fixed, as were the cleft ion concentrations.

In H558 background, the E161K mutation was implemented by shifting the steady-state activation curve of the model I_{Na} by +19 mV. In R558 background, this curve was shifted by +13 mV, together with a −10 mV shift in the steady-state inactivation curve. In either background, a 50% decrease in g_{Na} was applied to arrive at an almost 4-fold decrease in peak current density of mutant I_{Na} during voltage clamp simulations. Furthermore, the slope factor of the steady-state activation curve of the model I_{Na} was increased by 20% to account for mutation-induced decrease in steepness of this curve.

Computer Simulations

The CellML code of both models, as available from the CellML Model Repository (Lloyd et al., 2008), was edited and run in version 0.9.31.1409 of the Windows based Cellular Open Resource (COR) environment (Garny et al., 2003b). All simulations were run for a sufficiently long time, i.e., for the duration of a train of 200 action potentials, to reach steady-state behavior. Data from the final ten action potentials were used for analysis.

RESULTS

Characteristics of the SA Nodal Fast Sodium Current

First, we characterized I_{Na} of the Fabbri-Severi model of a single human SA nodal pacemaker cell (Fabbri et al., 2017) and its effect on the spontaneous activity of this cell. **Figure 1A** shows the steady-state activation and inactivation curves of I_{Na} (left) and the associated "window" (area of overlap; right). The window is in the voltage range of diastolic depolarization, between −60 and −40 mV. Because of the relatively slow changes in membrane potential of the SA nodal cell and the relatively fast kinetics of I_{Na}, this window is the major determinant of the course of I_{Na} during the action potential, of course in combination with the fully-activated conductance of I_{Na} (g_{Na}), which amounts to 22.3 nS in the Fabbri-Severi model. The associated steady-state current-voltage relationship of I_{Na} is shown in **Figure 1B**.

With a value near 0.6 pA, the amplitude of I_{Na} during diastolic depolarization is small. However, this amplitude is relatively large in comparison to that of the net membrane current (I_{net}) (**Figure 1C**, solid lines). It is therefore not surprising that full block of I_{Na} results in a 117-ms increase in cycle length from 813 to 930 ms (**Figure 1C**, dotted lines), corresponding with a 13% decrease in beating rate from 74 to 64 beats/min. In the simulated presence of 10 nM acetylcholine (ACh), the amplitude of I_{net} during diastolic depolarization becomes considerably smaller, whereas that of I_{Na} does barely change. Accordingly, full block of I_{Na} now results in a more prominent increase in cycle length, by 245 ms from 1027 to 1272 ms (**Figure 1D**), corresponding with a 19% decrease in beating rate from 58 to 47 beats/min. Of note, I_{Na} hardly affects the cycle length through a change in action potential duration.

Now that the simulations of **Figure 1** had shown that changes in I_{Na} may modify the cycle length of the Fabbri-Severi model cell to a considerable extent, we first assessed the changes in peak and window I_{Na} caused by the E161K mutation in *SCN5A*, either in H558 or R558 background. Next, we tested the effects of these changes on the spontaneous pacemaker activity of the SA nodal model cell.

Effects of the E161K Mutation in SCN5A on Biophysical Properties of I_{Na}

The left panel of **Figure 2A** illustrates the changes in the steady-state I_{Na} activation and inactivation curves due to the E161K mutation in H558 background. These changes are limited to a +19 mV shift in the steady-state I_{Na} activation curve and a slight decrease in steepness of this curve, which is poorly discernible in **Figure 2A**. As a result, the window of overlap is significantly reduced and shifted to less negative values of membrane potential, now roughly ranging from −50 to −30 mV (**Figure 2A**, right) and thus limiting the contribution of I_{Na} to diastolic depolarization. This is reflected in the current–voltage relationship of steady-state I_{Na} (**Figure 2B**, solid line), which is strongly reduced in comparison with wild-type I_{Na}.

In R558 background, the shift in the steady-state I_{Na} activation curve is less pronounced (+13 vs. +19 mV), but accompanied by a −10 mV shift in the steady-state inactivation curve (**Figure 2C**, left). As a result, the window of overlap is smaller than in H558 background (**Figure 2C**, right). However, it better fits with the voltage range of diastolic depolarization. Yet, the steady-state I_{Na} in this voltage range is even more reduced in comparison with wild-type I_{Na} than in H558 background (**Figure 2D**, solid line).

Effects of the E161K Mutation in SCN5A on I_{Na} in Voltage Clamp Experiments

As set out in the Introduction, voltage clamp experiments on *SCN5A* channels expressed in tsA201 and HEK-293 cells (Smits et al., 2005; Gui et al., 2010a,b) had revealed that the E161K mutation induces a 2.5- to 4-fold decrease in I_{Na} peak current density, both in H558 and R558 background. To assess the extent to which this reduction is due to the changes in the I_{Na} steady-state activation and inactivation curves *per se*, we reconstructed current traces in response to voltage clamp steps from a holding potential of −120 mV to test potentials ranging from −100 to +50 mV. **Figure 3A** shows examples of wild-type and mutant current traces at test potentials of −40, −20, and 0 mV. These already demonstrate that the peak current density of the wild-type channels is higher than that of mutant channels, despite the identical value of g_{Na} used in the voltage clamp simulations. **Figure 3B** summarizes the simulation data. The changes in the steady-state activation and inactivation curves *per se* reduce the peak current density by ≈35%. To arrive at an almost 4-fold decrease in I_{Na} peak current density, in line with the experimental observations, we reduced the mutant g_{Na} by a factor of 2 in our further simulations. Thus we split the original g_{Na} of 22.3 nS of the Fabbri-Severi model cell into 11.15 nS for the wild-type I_{Na} channels and 5.575 nS for the E161K mutant I_{Na} channels, in either background.

Effects of the E161K Mutation on SA Nodal Pacemaker Activity

We applied the mutation-induced changes in I_{Na}, i.e., the shifts in steady-state activation and inactivation curves, the reduction in steepness of the steady-state activation curve, and the reduction in fully-activated conductance, to half of the I_{Na} channels in the Fabbri-Severi model to assess the effects of the heterozygous E161K mutation on the spontaneous pacemaker activity of a human SA nodal cell. **Figures 4A–G**, shows the effects on the action potential (**Figure 4A**), intracellular calcium concentration (**Figure 4B**) and underlying membrane currents (**Figures 4C–G**) under control conditions (no ACh), whereas the corresponding simulation data in the presence of 10 nM ACh are shown in **Figures 4H–N**. The simulated administration of ACh to the Fabbri-Severi model cell does not only activate the acetylcholine-activated potassium current $I_{K,ACh}$, which is zero under control conditions, but also reduces the hyperpolarization-activated "funny current" I_f (through a −4.95 mV shift in its voltage dependence of activation), the L-type calcium current I_{CaL} (through a 3.1% decrease in its maximal conductance), and the rate of Ca^{2+} uptake into the sarcoplasmic reticulum (SR) by the SERCA pump (through a 7.0% decrease in its maximum activity). Of note, the changes in I_{CaL} and Ca^{2+} uptake rate have only marginal effects at this level of ACh (Fabbri et al., 2017).

The main effect of the application of ACh is a prolongation of the basic cycle length from 813 to 1027 ms (**Figures 4A,H**, wild-type traces), which is associated with a decrease in the intracellular calcium concentration $[Ca^{2+}]_i$ (**Figures 4B,I**, wild-type traces), and sodium-calcium exchange current I_{NCX} during diastolic depolarization (**Figures 4E,L**, wild-type traces). I_f is also reduced (**Figures 4F,M**), as a result of the direct effect of ACh on its voltage dependence of activation. The remaining inward currents, i.e., the L-type calcium current I_{CaL} (**Figures 4D,K**), T-type calcium current I_{CaT} (**Figures 4E,L**) and I_{Na} (**Figures 4G,N**), are not largely affected. The total repolarizing current I_{repol} is also hardly affected, with an almost constant value of ≈9 pA during diastolic depolarization (**Figures 4D,K**). This is because it includes the ACh-activated $I_{K,ACh}$, which is also shown separately (**Figures 4F,M**), in addition to the rapid delayed rectifier potassium current I_{Kr}, the slow delayed rectifier potassium current I_{Ks}, the ultrarapid delayed rectifier potassium current I_{Kur}, the transient outward potassium current I_{to}, and the sodium-potassium pump current I_{NaK}, which are not shown separately in **Figure 4**. The reduction in the "pacemaker currents" I_f and I_{NCX} (Lakatta and DiFrancesco, 2009), in combination with the minor changes in other inward currents as well as I_{repol}, result in the reduction in the net membrane current I_{net} (**Figures 4C,J**) that underlies the observed increase in cycle length.

In absence of ACh, the mutation-induced reduction in I_{Na} (**Figure 4G**) causes a reduction in I_{net}, which becomes most prominent during the second half of diastolic depolarization (**Figure 4C**) and in turn results in a prolongation of the cycle length by 53 and 54 ms in H558 and R558 background, respectively (**Figure 4A**, horizontal arrow), from the basic cycle length of 813 ms, corresponding with a 6% decrease in beating rate from 74 to 69 beats/min in either background. Simulations with the wild-type model in which g_{Na} is reduced by 50% (labeled "50% g_{Na}"), thus simply blocking 50% of the channels, result in a cycle length prolongation of 55 ms and traces that are barely distinguishable from the mutant ones, thus demonstrating that the contribution

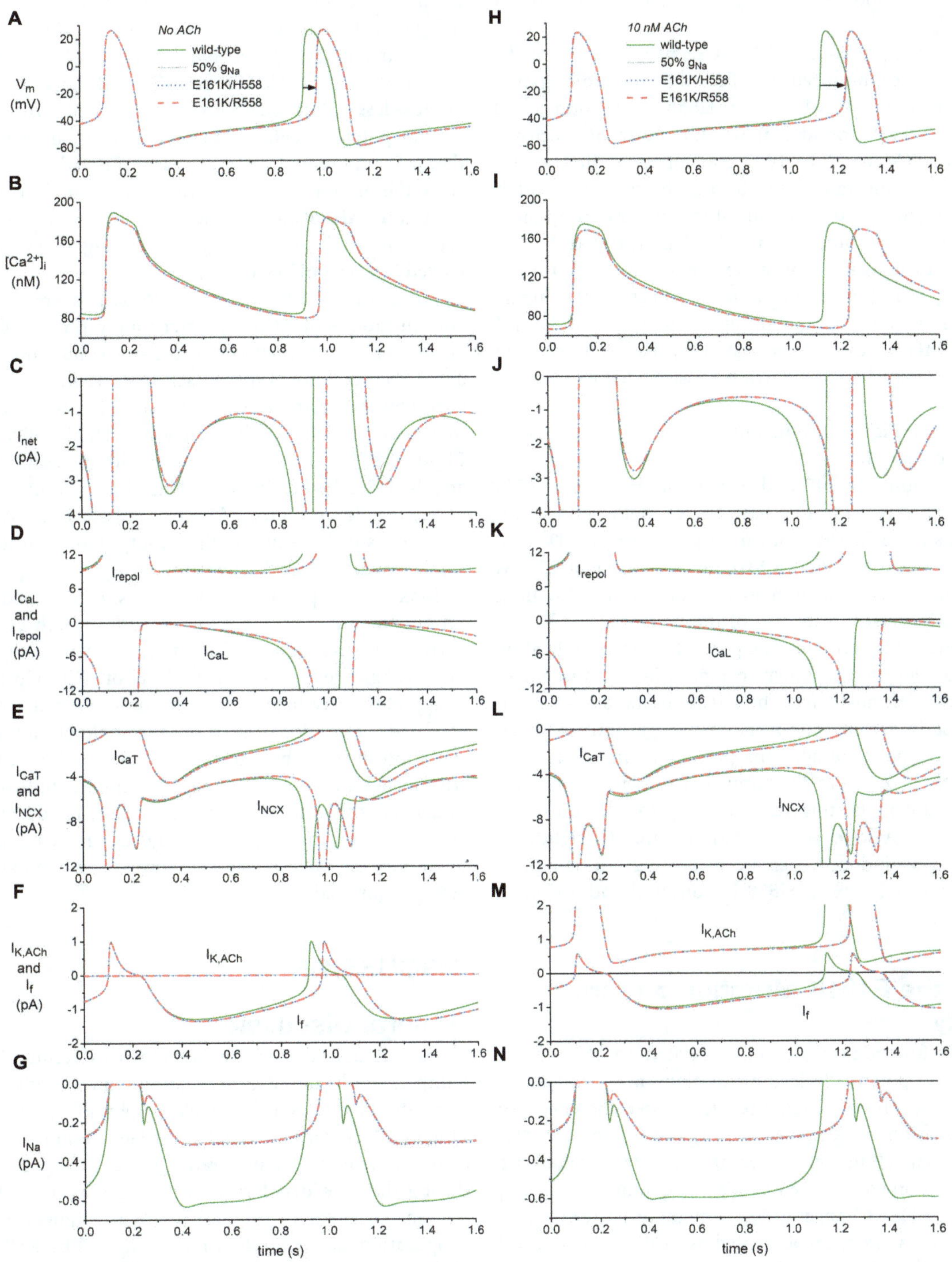

FIGURE 4 | Effects of the E161K mutation in *SCN5A*, either in H558 or R558 background, on the spontaneous activity of the Fabbri-Severi model of a human SA nodal pacemaker cell. **(A)** Membrane potential (V_m), and associated **(B)** intracellular calcium concentration ($[Ca^{2+}]_i$), **(C)** net membrane current (I_{net}), **(D)** L-type calcium current (I_{CaL}) and total repolarizing current (I_{repol}), **(E)** T-type calcium current (I_{CaT}) and sodium-calcium exchange current (I_{NCX}), **(F)** ACh-activated potassium current ($I_{K,ACh}$) and hyperpolarization-activated "funny current" (I_f), and **(G)** fast sodium current (I_{Na}) in the absence of ACh. **(H)** V_m, **(I)** $[Ca^{2+}]_i$, **(J)** I_{net}, **(K)** I_{CaL} and I_{repol}, **(L)** I_{CaT} and I_{NCX}, **(M)** $I_{K,ACh}$, and I_f, and **(N)** I_{Na} during simulated administration of 10 nM ACh. Solid gray lines show the effect of a 50% reduction in fully-activated conductance of I_{Na} (g_{Na}). Horizontal arrows indicate increase in cycle length. I_{repol} consists of $I_{K,ACh}$, the rapid delayed rectifier potassium current I_{Kr}, the slow delayed rectifier potassium current I_{Ks}, the ultrarapid delayed rectifier potassium current I_{Kur}, the transient outward potassium current I_{to}, and the sodium-potassium pump current I_{NaK}.

of the mutant component of I_{Na} to total I_{Na} is almost zero.

In the simulated presence of 10 nM ACh, the effects of the mutation are more pronounced, as reflected by the prolongation of the cycle length by 104 ms in H558 background and 105 ms in R558 background (**Figure 4H**, horizontal arrow), from the basic cycle length of 1027 ms, corresponding with a 9% decrease in beating rate from 58 to 53 beats/min in either background. Again, the contribution of the mutant component of I_{Na} to total I_{Na} is almost zero, as demonstrated by the highly similar prolongation of cycle length, by 107 ms, in case of 50% g_{Na}. The more pronounced effect of the highly similar reduction in I_{Na} in the simulated presence of 10 nM ACh (**Figures 4G,N**) can be explained by its occurrence in the setting of a smaller I_{net} during diastolic depolarization (**Figures 4C,J**).

As illustrated in **Figure 5A**, the mutation-induced increase in cycle length increases with increasing levels of ACh. At 25 nM, this increase amounts to 347 and 355 ms in H558 and R558 background, respectively, from a basic cycle length of 1448 ms, slightly less than the increase of 361 ms in case of 50% g_{Na}. In terms of beating rate (**Figure 5B**), an ACh level of 25 nM results in a rate of 41 beats/min in case of wild-type sodium channels and 33 beats/min in case of the heterozygous E161K mutation, in either background. The percent decrease in beating rate relative to wild type is shown in **Figure 5C**. In absence of ACh (**Figure 5C**, leftmost bars), the E161K mutation results in a 6.1% decrease in beating rate in H558 background and 6.2% decrease in R558 background. This percentage increases with increasing levels of ACh. In the simulated presence of 10 nM ACh, the decrease in beating rate amounts to 9.2 and 9.3%, respectively. At an ACh level of 25 nM (**Figure 5C**, rightmost bars), the mutation-induced decrease in beating rate is almost 20%, with values of 19.3% in H558 background and 19.7% in R558 background.

Effects of the E161K Mutation on Atrial Excitability

Sinus node dysfunction may also be related to changes in atrial excitability, potentially leading to sinus node exit block or atrial conduction block. Therefore, we assessed the effects of the E161K mutation on atrial excitability using the Maleckar et al. human atrial cell model (Maleckar et al., 2009), which we used in combination with its well-validated equations for $I_{K,ACh}$ (Maleckar et al., 2008). Changes in I_{Na}, simulating a heterozygous mutation in *SCN5A*, were implemented as in the Fabbri-Severi model. Of note, the effect of ACh on the Maleckar et al. model cell is limited to the activation of $I_{K,ACh}$.

Figure 6A shows atrial action potentials elicited at 1 Hz with a stimulus current of 1 ms duration under control conditions (no ACh). Both variants of the E161K mutation result in a reduction in the action potential overshoot and a less rapid activation, indicative of a decrease in capacitive current of the atrial cell (**Figure 6A**, inset). The associated I_{Na}, which is shown in **Figure 6B**, is approximately halved or – because the slower activation allows a larger fraction of the channels to inactivate during the activation process – even more than halved. In the simulated presence of 10 nM ACh, the resting membrane potential becomes more negative with a value of −79 mV vs. −74 mV (**Figure 6C**), which results in a larger I_{Na} because less sodium channels are inactivated at this more negative resting potential (**Figure 6D**). This does, however, not imply that action potential generation is facilitated in presence of ACh since the distance to action potential threshold is increased and an additional outward current, i.e., $I_{K,ACh}$, is activated. Again, activation is slowed and the underlying I_{Na} is approximately halved (**Figures 6C,D**, insets).

Atrial excitability was characterized, over a wide range of concentrations of ACh, by determining the threshold stimulus current of the atrial cell as well as its maximum upstroke velocity, as a direct measure of the capacitive current. Threshold stimulus current was determined with 1 ms stimuli of increasing amplitude that were applied at a frequency of 1 Hz. Results are shown in **Figure 7A**. The threshold increases with increasing levels of ACh and is 5–8% higher in case of the E161K mutation. Although barely visible in **Figure 7A**, the threshold in R558 background, with the smaller shift of the steady-state activation curve, is smaller than in H558 background.

Maximum upstroke velocity was determined by eliciting action potentials with a 1 ms, ≈50% suprathreshold stimulus current at a frequency of 1 Hz. As shown in **Figure 7B**, it is not strongly dependent on the level of ACh. Upstroke velocity is approximately halved, or even more than halved, in case of the E161K mutation. As for the threshold stimulus current, the mutation in R558 background is associated with (slightly) less strong effects than in H558 background. In contrast with the SA nodal cell, the mutant component of I_{Na} is not effectively zero, as revealed by the larger I_{Na} (**Figures 6B,D**, insets) and larger maximum upstroke velocity (**Figure 7B**) in comparison with the 50% g_{Na} simulations.

DISCUSSION

General Discussion

Our simulations demonstrate that the E161K mutation in *SCN5A* hampers both impulse generation and impulse propagation through its effects on the electrophysiological properties of human SA nodal and atrial cells. Generation of the SA nodal action potential is hampered by the strong decrease in I_{Na} during diastolic depolarization and the associated decrease in I_{net}, in particular in presence of ACh (**Figures 4, 5**). Impulse propagation, as comprehensively reviewed by Kléber and Rudy (2004), is hampered by the current-to-load mismatch that results from, on the one hand, the increase in threshold stimulus current and, on the other hand, the decrease in capacitive current of the atrial cell (**Figures 6, 7**). The highly common H558R polymorphism in *SCN5A* does not have a major effect on the outcome of the simulations, despite its effects on the biophysical properties of the E161K mutant channels (**Figures 2, 3**).

The E161K mutation has been subject of simulations since its discovery in 2005 (Smits et al., 2005). Smits et al. (2005)

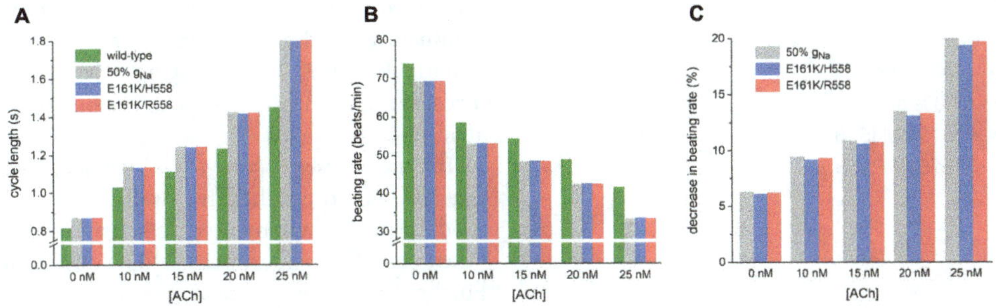

FIGURE 5 | Bradycardic effects of the E161K mutation in *SCN5A*, either in H558 or R558 background, on the Fabbri-Severi model of a human SA nodal pacemaker cell at different levels of ACh (0–25 nM). **(A)** Cycle length. **(B)** Associated beating rate. **(C)** Percent decrease in beating rate relative to wild-type. Solid gray bars show the effect of a 50% reduction in fully-activated conductance of I_{Na} (g_{Na}). Note the breaks in the vertical axes of **(A,B)**.

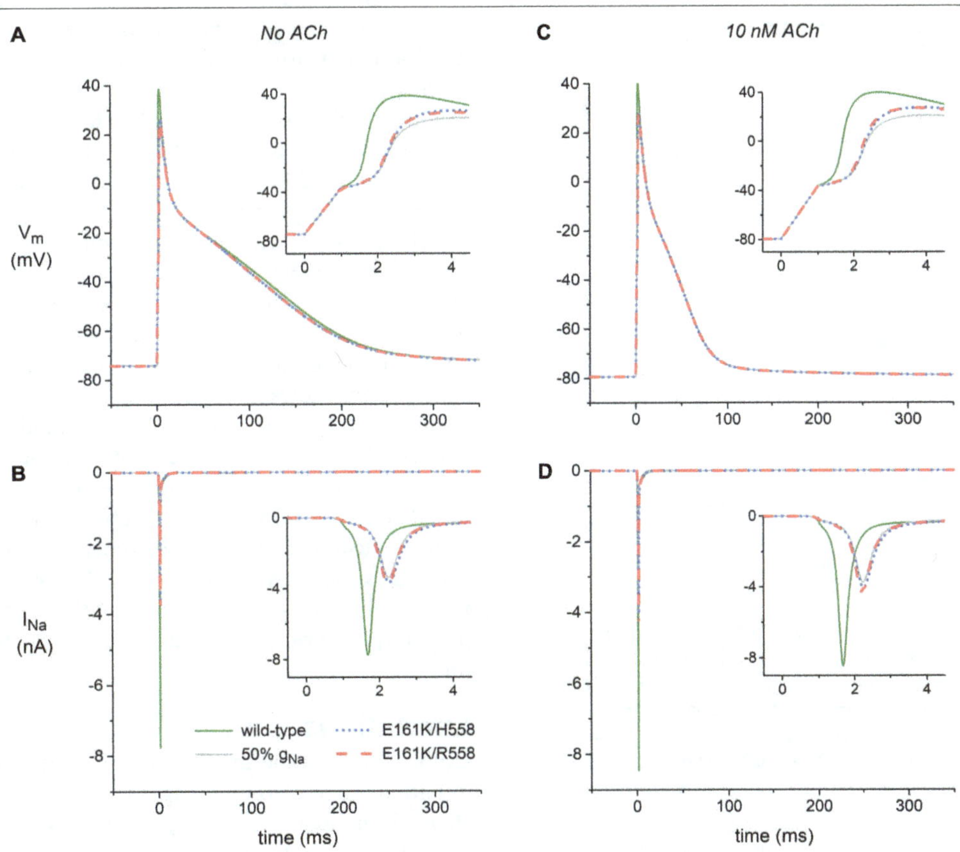

FIGURE 6 | Effects of the E161K mutation in *SCN5A*, either in H558 or R558 background, on the action potential and fast sodium current (I_{Na}) of the Maleckar et al. model of a human atrial myocyte. **(A)** Action potentials elicited at 1 Hz and **(B)** associated fast sodium current (I_{Na}) in the absence of ACh. **(C)** Action potentials elicited at 1 Hz and **(D)** associated I_{Na} during simulated administration of 10 nM ACh. Insets show membrane potential (V_m) and I_{Na} on an expanded time scale. Solid gray lines show the effect of a 50% reduction in fully-activated conductance of I_{Na} (g_{Na}).

showed that the E161K mutation impairs conduction in linear strands of atrial and ventricular cells, using the human atrial and ventricular cell models by Courtemanche et al. (1998) and Priebe and Beuckelmann (1998), respectively. Simulations were based on the observations by Smits et al. (2005) on E161K channels expressed in tsA201 cells. Mutation effects were relatively mild in comparison to later observations by Gui et al. (2010a,b) and obtained in H558 background. Smits et al. (2005) also carried out simulations on SA nodal cells, using the model of a peripheral rabbit SA nodal cell by Zhang et al. (2000), including equations for $I_{K,ACh}$ (Zhang et al., 2002). Despite the largely different time course of the human SA nodal action potential, with a much smaller I_{Na}, a much longer diastolic phase, and a significantly less negative maximum diastolic potential, the main findings of the present study are similar to those of Smits et al. (2005) regarding the SA

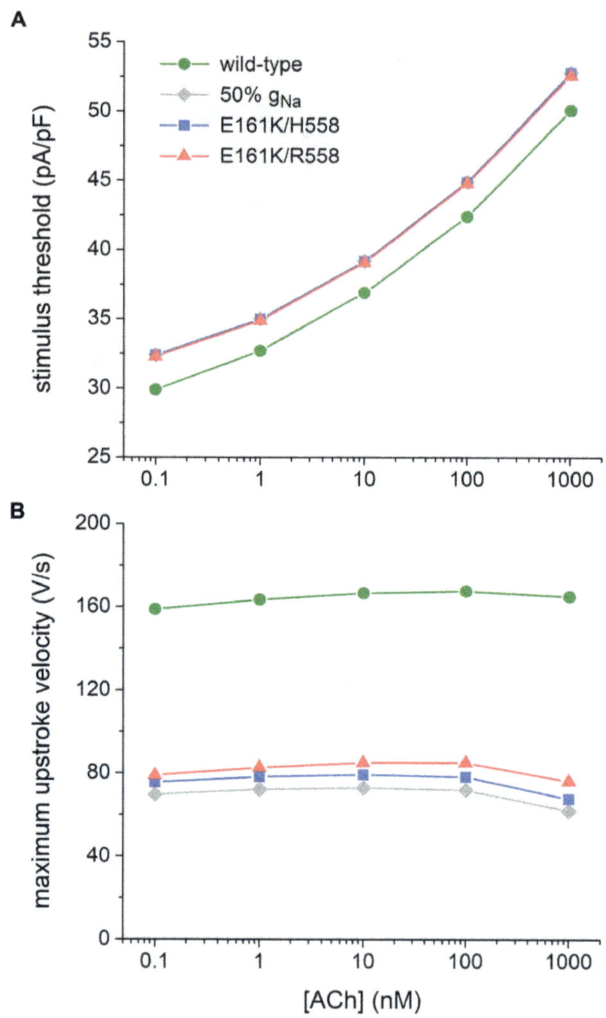

FIGURE 7 | Effects of the E161K mutation in *SCN5A*, either in H558 or R558 background, on the excitability of the Maleckar et al. model of a human atrial myocyte. **(A)** Threshold stimulus current amplitude for a stimulus of 1 ms duration and **(B)** maximum upstroke velocity at ACh concentrations ranging from 0.1 nM to 1 μM. Gray diamonds show the effect of a 50% reduction in fully-activated conductance of I_{Na} (g_{Na}). Note the logarithmic abscissa scale.

nodal action potential: the E161K mutation causes a decrease in diastolic depolarization rate that results in an increase in cycle length, which is much more pronounced in presence of ACh.

Butters et al. (2010) studied the effects of several mutations in *SCN5A*, including E161K, on cardiac pacemaking in a two-dimensional model of sino-atrial tissue based on a reconstruction of a single slice of the rabbit right atrium, using modified versions of the single cell models of rabbit SA nodal and atrial cells by Zhang et al. (2000, 2002) and Lindblad et al. (1996), respectively. Their simulations of the E161K mutation were again based on the observations by Smits et al. (2005). The mutation slowed down pacemaking and this effect was more pronounced in the presence of ACh. Furthermore, a conduction block in the direction toward the atrial septum occurred in the absence of ACh, while conduction in the direction toward the crista terminalis was sustained. With 15 nM ACh, exit block occurred in both directions and the SA node was unable to drive the surrounding atrium.

In the present study, we carried out simulations with the use of comprehensive well-validated human single cell models and implemented effects of the E161K mutation based on the experimental data by Gui et al. (2010a,b). Furthermore, we assessed the role of the highly common H558R polymorphism, also based on the experimental data by Gui et al. (2010a,b). We focused on cellular mechanisms and refrained from using two- or even three-dimensional models of sino-atrial interaction, with their coupling interactions between heterogeneous cells, because results of such simulations are critically dependent on the exact geometry and cell distribution (Garny et al., 2003a), which have not been fully elucidated.

Our simulations show that the effects of the E161K mutation are so large, both in H558 and R558 background, that the contribution of mutant I_{Na} to total I_{Na} of the SA nodal cell is effectively zero. Accordingly, it is not surprising that E161K mutation carriers show sinus node dysfunction as do carriers of several mutations in *SCN5A* that are associated with a complete or almost complete loss of function of the mutant channels, as reviewed by Lei et al. (2007, 2008) and Remme et al. (2008). In many cases, the sinus node dysfunction shows a reduced penetrance, as for the E161K mutation, where 8 out of 14 mutation carriers show the disease. Reduced penetrance is a common finding in primary electrical diseases, including those associated with mutations in *SCN5A* (Remme, 2013; Robyns et al., 2014). Several factors, including co-inherited genetic variants and alternative splicing sites, may play a role. However, our simulations suggest that it is highly unlikely that the common H558R polymorphism can explain the reduced penetrance of the E161K mutation.

Limitations

Unfortunately, experimental data on the effects of the E161K mutation are limited to voltage clamp data from mutant *SCN5A* channels in mammalian expression systems, viz. tsA201 and HEK-293 cells, obtained at room temperature and in the presence (Smits et al., 2005) or absence (Gui et al., 2010a,b) of a wild-type β-subunit. There are some quantitative differences in the experimental data, potentially due to differences in cell type or presence of β-subunit, with a more severe pattern in the data of Gui et al. (2010a,b), with a +19 mV shift of the steady-state activation curve in H558 background vs. the +11.9 mV shift reported by Smits et al. (2005) and a 4-fold vs. 2.5-fold reduction in peak current density. However, the latter difference may partly be explained by the larger shift in the steady-state activation curve. In our simulations, we have assumed that the experimentally observed effects of the mutation in mammalian expression systems at room temperature also hold for cardiac cells at the physiological temperature of 37°C. We cannot rule out that recordings at a more close-to-physiological temperature would have revealed additional effects of the E161K mutation, as has been the case for several other BrS-related mutations in *SCN5A* expressed in mammalian cell lines, like T1620M and Y1795H (Dumaine et al., 1999; Rivolta et al., 2001). Furthermore, we have to keep in mind that the cardiac sodium channel is part of a macromolecular complex that does not only comprise the α- and β-subunits, but also several other proteins that may regulate channel activity, such as ankyrin, caveolin and syntrophin, and may act differently in case of mutant channels (Ruan et al., 2009). Thus, it is uncertain to which extent the experimental data on the effects of the E161K mutation acquired in mammalian expression systems represent the mutant-induced changes that occur in human cardiac cells.

In our simulations, it is assumed that the Fabbri-Severi model of a human SA nodal cell (Fabbri et al., 2017) and the Maleckar et al. model of a human atrial cell (Maleckar et al., 2009) are fully representative of the biophysical properties of the corresponding real cells. However, experimental data on the biophysical properties of cardiac cells, and human cells in particular, are often incomplete or obtained under non-physiological conditions. Functional data on I_{Na} in human SA nodal cells, for example, are limited to accidental observations by Verkerk et al. (2009) when performing voltage clamp experiments on single human SA nodal pacemaker cells to record I_f. Accordingly, I_{Na} was included in the Fabbri-Severi model, but simply adopted from its parent model, i.e., the model of a rabbit SA nodal cell by Severi et al. (2012), who, in turn, used the equations of the SA nodal cell model by Noble et al. (1989). The latter equations were adopted from the model of SA nodal cell electrical activity by Noble and Noble (1984), who based their equations on the model of cardiac electrical activity by DiFrancesco and Noble (1985). The description of I_{Na} in the latter model is essentially that of Hodgkin and Huxley (1952), but with modifications based on data from experiments on rabbit cardiac Purkinje fibers at 10–26°C (Colatsky, 1980) and from isolated rat ventricular myocytes at 20–22°C (Brown et al., 1981). Activation and inactivation curves were shifted along the voltage axis to account for their observed temperature dependence, whereas rate constants were scaled to arrive at time constant values near the experimentally observed ones. The I_{Na} equations in the Maleckar et al. (2009) model are adopted from the model of an adult human atrial cell by Nygren et al. (1998), who used the voltage clamp data of Sakakibara et al. (1992) on I_{Na} in isolated human atrial myocytes at 17 ± 1°C to construct their model equations. Activation and inactivation curves were shifted in the positive direction along the voltage axis to reach a realistic activation threshold and stable resting potential. The time constants of activation and inactivation are very similar to those of the rabbit atrial cell model of Lindblad et al. (1996), who based their mathematical description of I_{Na} on the voltage clamp data of Wendt et al. (1992), acquired from cultured rabbit atrial myocytes at 17°C, and I_{Na} of the DiFrancesco-Noble model (DiFrancesco and Noble, 1985). Activation kinetics of I_{Na} were modified from those of the DiFrancesco-Noble model with the use of a Q_{10} of 1.7.

In our simulations, it is also assumed that mutation effects are limited to half of the intrinsic I_{Na} channels, thus representing the heterozygous nature of the mutation, taking into account that a functional I_{Na} channel is built with a single $Na_V1.5$ protein. This assumption is challenged by recent experimental findings of Clatot et al. (2018), who demonstrated that wild-type and mutant $Na_V1.5$ proteins can form dimers, enabling coupled gating of wild-type and mutant $Na_V1.5$ sodium channels that can be responsible for a dominant negative effect of the mutation. Thus, the cellular effects of the E161K mutation could be more severe than anticipated.

The action of ACh in the Fabbri-Severi model is, apart from the activation of $I_{K,ACh}$, limited to suppression of I_f, I_{CaL}, and Ca^{2+} uptake into the SR, thus simplifying the intracellular SR-based calcium clock signaling cascade through adenylyl cyclase, cyclic AMP and protein kinase A (Maltsev et al., 2014; Behar et al., 2016). This cascade is important for a detailed understanding of the action of ACh. Yet, in the present study, where the focus is on the effects of the E161K mutation in *SCN5A* and possible effects of the H558R polymorphism, it is sufficient that the suppression by ACh of I_f, I_{CaL}, and Ca^{2+} uptake into the SR, and that of I_{NCX} through the reduced intracellular calcium level, are included, in addition to the activation of $I_{K,ACh}$.

One should be careful in the interpretation of experimental data, not only because of the above considerations, but also because changes in biophysical parameters are not necessarily independent. This is nicely demonstrated by the decrease in peak current density shown in **Figure 3**. Such decrease is often interpreted as a reduction in the number of channels or a reduction in their single conductance. In this case, however, the E161K mutant-induced changes in steady-state activation and inactivation curves *per se* reduce the peak current density by ≈35%. This effect may, at least partly, explain the apparent discrepancy between the ≈30% decrease in cell surface expression of E161K/H558 channels in HEK-293 cells and the > 70% decrease in peak current density reported by Gui et al. (2010a). Similarly, an apparently slower inactivation of E161K/H558 channels at membrane potentials ranging from -40 to 0 mV can, at least partly, be explained by the +19 mV shift in their steady-state activation curve (Gui et al., 2010a). Because experimentally observed changes in time constants of (fast) inactivation or recovery from inactivation, if any, are already small, no attempts were made to include these changes in the simulations of the present study.

CONCLUSION

We conclude that the experimentally identified mutation-induced changes in I_{Na} can explain the clinically observed sinus bradycardia and potentially the occasional exit block. Furthermore, we conclude that the common H558R polymorphism does not significantly alter the effects of the E161K mutation and can thus not explain the reduced penetrance of the E161K mutation.

AUTHOR CONTRIBUTIONS

RW designed the experiments, acquired, analyzed and interpreted the data, and drafted, edited, and approved the manuscript.

ACKNOWLEDGMENTS

I thank the staff of the Departments of Medical Biology and Experimental Cardiology for their valuable contributions.

REFERENCES

Ackerman, M. J., Splawski, I., Makielski, J. C., Tester, D. J., Will, M. L., Timothy, K. W., et al. (2004). Spectrum and prevalence of cardiac sodium channel variants among black, white, Asian, and Hispanic individuals: implications for arrhythmogenic susceptibility and Brugada/long QT syndrome genetic testing. *Heart Rhythm* 1, 600–607. doi: 10.1016/j.hrthm.2004.07.013

Behar, J., Ganesan, A., Zhang, J., and Yaniv, Y. (2016). The autonomic nervous system regulates the heart rate through cAMP-PKA dependent and independent coupled-clock pacemaker cell mechanisms. *Front. Physiol.* 7:419. doi: 10.3389/fphys.2016.00419

Brown, A. M., Lee, K. S., and Powell, T. (1981). Sodium current in single rat heart muscle cells. *J. Physiol.* 318, 479–500. doi: 10.1113/jphysiol.1981.sp013879

Brugada, J., Campuzano, O., Arbelo, E., Sarquella-Brugada, G., and Brugada, R. (2018). Present status of Brugada syndrome: JACC State-of-the-art review. *J. Am. Coll. Cardiol.* 72, 1046–1059. doi: 10.1016/j.jacc.2018.06.037

Butters, T. D., Aslanidi, O. V., Inada, S., Boyett, M. R., Hancox, J. C., Lei, M., et al. (2010). Mechanistic links between Na^+ channel (SCN5A) mutations and impaired cardiac pacemaking in sick sinus syndrome. *Circ. Res.* 107, 126–137. doi: 10.1161/CIRCRESAHA.110.219949

Chandler, N. J., Greener, I. D., Tellez, J. O., Inada, S., Musa, H., Molenaar, P., et al. (2009). Molecular architecture of the human sinus node: insights into the function of the cardiac pacemaker. *Circulation* 119, 1562–1575. doi: 10.1161/CIRCULATIONAHA.108.804369

Clatot, J., Zheng, Y., Girardeau, A., Liu, H., Laurita, K. R., Marionneau, C., et al. (2018). Mutant voltage-gated Na^+ channels can exert a dominant negative effect through coupled gating. *Am. J. Physiol. Heart Circ. Physiol.* 315, H1250–H1257. doi: 10.1152/ajpheart.00721.2017

Colatsky, T. J. (1980). Voltage clamp measurements of sodium channel properties in rabbit cardiac Purkinje fibres. *J. Physiol.* 305, 215–234. doi: 10.1113/jphysiol.1980.sp013359

Courtemanche, M., Ramirez, R. J., and Nattel, S. (1998). Ionic mechanisms underlying human atrial action potential properties: insights from a mathematical model. *Am. J. Physiol.* 275, H301–H321. doi: 10.1152/ajpheart.1998.275.1.H301

Cuellar, A. A., Lloyd, C. M., Nielsen, P. F., Bullivant, D. P., Nickerson, D. P., and Hunter, P. J. (2003). An overview of CellML 1.1, a biological model description language. *Simulation* 79, 740–747. doi: 10.1177/0037549703040939

DiFrancesco, D., and Noble, D. (1985). A model of cardiac electrical activity incorporating ionic pumps and concentration changes. *Philos. Trans. R. Soc. Lond. B Biol. Sci.* 307, 353–398. doi: 10.1098/rstb.1985.0001

Dumaine, R., Towbin, J. A., Brugada, P., Vatta, M., Nesterenko, D. V., Nesterenko, V. V., et al. (1999). Ionic mechanisms responsible for the electrocardiographic phenotype of the Brugada syndrome are temperature dependent. *Circ. Res.* 85, 803–809. doi: 10.1161/01.RES.85.9.803

Fabbri, A., Fantini, M., Wilders, R., and Severi, S. (2017). Computational analysis of the human sinus node action potential: model development and effects of mutations. *J. Physiol.* 595, 2365–2396. doi: 10.1113/JP273259

Garny, A., Hunter, P. J., Noble, D., Boyett, M. R., and Kohl, P. (2003a). "Rabbit sino-atrial node modeling: from single cell to tissue structure," in *Proceedings of the 25th Annual International Conference of the IEEE Engineering in Medicine and Biology Society*, Piscataway, NJ: IEEE, 28–31. doi: 10.1109/IEMBS.2003.1279489

Garny, A., Kohl, P., and Noble, D. (2003b). Cellular Open Resource (COR): a public CellML based environment for modelling biological function. *Int. J. Bifurcat. Chaos* 13, 3579–3590. doi: 10.1142/S021812740300882X

Giudicessi, J. R., Wilde, A. A. M., and Ackerman, M. J. (2018). The genetic architecture of long QT syndrome: a critical reappraisal. *Trends Cardiovasc. Med.* 28, 453–464. doi: 10.1016/j.tcm.2018.03.003

Gui, J., Wang, T., Jones, R. P. O., Trump, D., Zimmer, T., and Lei, M. (2010a). Multiple loss-of-function mechanisms contribute to *SCN5A*-related familial sick sinus syndrome. *PLoS One* 5:e10985. doi: 10.1371/journal.pone.0010985

Gui, J., Wang, T., Trump, D., Zimmer, T., and Lei, M. (2010b). Mutation-specific effects of polymorphism H558R in *SCN5A*-related sick sinus syndrome. *J. Cardiovasc. Electrophysiol.* 21, 564–573. doi: 10.1111/j.1540-8167.2010.01762.x

Hayashi, H., Sumiyoshi, M., Nakazato, Y., and Daida, H. (2018). Brugada syndrome and sinus node dysfunction. *J. Arrhythm* 4, 216–221. doi: 10.1002/joa3.12046

Hodgkin, A. L., and Huxley, A. F. (1952). A quantitative description of membrane current and its application to conduction and excitation in nerve. *J. Physiol.* 117, 500–544. doi: 10.1113/jphysiol.1952.sp004764

Hu, D., Viskin, S., Oliva, A., Carrier, T., Cordeiro, J. M., Barajas-Martinez, H., et al. (2007). Novel mutation in the SCN5A gene associated with arrhythmic storm development during acute myocardial infarction. *Heart Rhythm* 4, 1072–1080. doi: 10.1016/j.hrthm.2007.03.040

Iwasa, H., Itoh, T., Nagai, R., Nakamura, Y., and Tanaka, T. (2000). Twenty single nucleotide polymorphisms (SNPs) and their allelic frequencies in four genes that are responsible for familial long QT syndrome in the Japanese population. *J. Hum. Genet.* 45, 182–183. doi: 10.1007/s100380050207

Kléber, A. G., and Rudy, Y. (2004). Basic mechanisms of cardiac impulse propagation and associated arrhythmias. *Physiol. Rev.* 84, 431–488. doi: 10.1152/physrev.00025.2003

Lakatta, E. G., and DiFrancesco, D. (2009). What keeps us ticking: a funny current, a calcium clock, or both? *J. Mol. Cell. Cardiol.* 47, 157–170. doi: 10.1016/j.yjmcc.2009.03.022

Lei, M., Huang, C. L.-H., and Zhang, Y. (2008). Genetic Na^+ channelopathies and sinus node dysfunction. *Prog. Biophys. Mol. Biol.* 98, 171–178. doi: 10.1016/j.pbiomolbio.2008.10.003

Lei, M., Zhang, H., Grace, A. A., and Huang, C. L.-H. (2007). *SCN5A* and sinoatrial node pacemaker function. *Cardiovasc. Res.* 74, 356–365. doi: 10.1016/j.cardiores.2007.01.009

Lindblad, D. S., Murphey, C. R., Clark, J. W., and Giles, W. R. (1996). A model of the action potential and underlying membrane currents in a rabbit atrial cell. *Am. J. Physiol.* 271, H1666–H1696. doi: 10.1152/ajpheart.1996.271.4.H1666

Lloyd, C. M., Lawson, J. R., Hunter, P. J., and Nielsen, P. F. (2008). The CellML model repository. *Bioinformatics* 24, 2122–2123. doi: 10.1093/bioinformatics/btn390

Maleckar, M. M., Greenstein, J. L., Giles, W. R., and Trayanova, N. A. (2009). K^+ current changes account for the rate dependence of the action potential in the human atrial myocyte. *Am. J. Physiol. Heart Circ. Physiol.* 297, H1398–H1410. doi: 10.1152/ajpheart.00411.2009

Maleckar, M. M., Greenstein, J. L., Trayanova, N. A., and Giles, W. R. (2008). Mathematical simulations of ligand-gated and cell-type specific effects on the action potential of human atrium. *Prog. Biophys. Mol. Biol.* 98, 161–170. doi: 10.1016/j.pbiomolbio.2009.01.010

Maltsev, V. A., Yaniv, Y., Maltsev, A. V., Stern, M. D., and Lakatta, E. G. (2014). Modern perspectives on numerical modeling of cardiac pacemaker cell. *J. Pharmacol. Sci.* 125, 6–38. doi: 10.1254/jphs.13R04CR

Noble, D., DiFrancesco, D., and Denyer, J. C. (1989). "Ionic mechanisms in normal and abnormal cardiac pacemaker activity," in *Neuronal and Cellular Oscillators*, ed. J. W. Jacklet (New York, NY: Marcel Dekker Inc.), 59–85.

Noble, D., and Noble, S. J. (1984). A model of sino-atrial node electrical activity based on a modification of the DiFrancesco-Noble (1984) equations. *Proc. R. Soc. Lond. B Biol. Sci.* 222, 295–304. doi: 10.1098/rspb.1984.0065

Nygren, A., Fiset, C., Firek, L., Clark, J. W., Lindblad, D. S., Clark, R. B., et al. (1998). Mathematical model of an adult human atrial cell: the role of K^+ currents in repolarization. *Circ. Res.* 82, 63–81. doi: 10.1161/01.RES.82.1.63

O'Hara, T., Virág, L., Varró, A., and Rudy, Y. (2011). Simulation of the undiseased human cardiac ventricular action potential: model formulation and experimental validation. *PLoS Comput. Biol.* 7:e1002061. doi: 10.1371/journal.pcbi.1002061

Priebe, L., and Beuckelmann, D. J. (1998). Simulation study of cellular electric properties in heart failure. *Circ. Res.* 82, 1206–1223. doi: 10.1161/01.RES.82.11.1206

Remme, C. A. (2013). Cardiac sodium channelopathy associated with *SCN5A* mutations: electrophysiological, molecular and genetic aspects. *J. Physiol.* 591, 4099–4116. doi: 10.1113/jphysiol.2013.256461

Remme, C. A., Wilde, A. A. M., and Bezzina, C. R. (2008). Cardiac sodium channel overlap syndromes: different faces of *SCN5A* mutations. *Trends Cardiovasc. Med.* 18, 78–87. doi: 10.1016/j.tcm.2008.01.002

Rivolta, I., Abriel, H., Tateyama, M., Liu, H., Memmi, M., Vardas, P., et al. (2001). Inherited Brugada and long QT-3 syndrome mutations of a single residue of the cardiac sodium channel confer distinct channel and clinical phenotypes. *J. Biol. Chem.* 276, 30623–30630. doi: 10.1074/jbc.M104471200

Robyns, T., Nuyens, D., Van Casteren, L., Corveleyn, A., De Ravel, T., Heidbuchel, H., et al. (2014). Reduced penetrance and variable expression of SCN5A mutations and the importance of co-inherited genetic variants: case report and review of the literature. *Indian Pacing Electrophysiol. J.* 14, 133–149. doi: 10.1016/S0972-6292(16)30754-9

Ruan, Y., Liu, N., and Priori, S. G. (2009). Sodium channel mutations and arrhythmias. *Nat. Rev. Cardiol.* 6, 337–348. doi: 10.1038/nrcardio.2009.44

Sakakibara, Y., Wasserstrom, J. A., Furukawa, T., Jia, H., Arentzen, C. E., Hartz, R. S., et al. (1992). Characterization of the sodium current in single human atrial myocytes. *Circ. Res.* 71, 535–546. doi: 10.1161/01.RES.71.3.535

Severi, S., Fantini, M., Charawi, L. A., and DiFrancesco, D. (2012). An updated computational model of rabbit sinoatrial action potential to investigate the mechanisms of heart rate modulation. *J. Physiol.* 590, 4483–4499. doi: 10.1113/jphysiol.2012.229435

Shinlapawittayatorn, K., Du, X. X., Liu, H., Ficker, E., Kaufman, E. S., and Deschênes, I. (2011). A common *SCN5A* polymorphism modulates the biophysical defects of *SCN5A* mutations. *Heart Rhythm* 8, 455–462. doi: 10.1016/j.hrthm.2010.11.034

Smits, J. P. P., Koopmann, T. T., Wilders, R., Veldkamp, M. W., Opthof, T., Bhuiyan, Z. A., et al. (2005). A mutation in the human cardiac sodium channel (E161K) contributes to sick sinus syndrome, conduction disease and Brugada syndrome in two families. *J. Mol. Cell. Cardiol.* 38, 969–981. doi: 10.1016/j.yjmcc.2005.02.024

Tester, D. J., Valdivia, C., Harris-Kerr, C., Alders, M., Salisbury, B. A., Wilde, A. A. M., et al. (2010). Epidemiologic, molecular, and functional evidence suggest A572D-SCN5A should not be considered an independent LQT3-susceptibility mutation. *Heart Rhythm* 7, 912–919. doi: 10.1016/j.hrthm.2010.04.014

Verkerk, A. O., Wilders, R., Van Borren, M. M. G. J., and Tan, H. L. (2009). Is sodium current present in human sinoatrial node cells? *Int. J. Biol. Sci.* 5, 201–204. doi: 10.7150/ijbs.5.201

Wendt, D. J., Starmer, C. F., and Grant, A. O. (1992). Na channel kinetics remain stable during perforated-patch recordings. *Am. J. Physiol.* 263, C1234–C1240. doi: 10.1152/ajpcell.1992.263.6.C1234

Wilde, A. A. M., and Amin, A. S. (2018). Clinical spectrum of *SCN5A* mutations: long QT syndrome, Brugada syndrome, and cardiomyopathy. *JACC Clin. Electrophysiol.* 4, 569–579. doi: 10.1016/j.jacep.2018.03.006

Wilders, R., and Verkerk, A. O. (2018). Long QT syndrome and sinus bradycardia—a mini review. *Front. Cardiovasc. Med.* 5:106. doi: 10.3389/fcvm.2018.00106

Workman, A. J., Kane, K. A., and Rankin, A. C. (2001). The contribution of ionic currents to changes in refractoriness of human atrial myocytes associated with chronic atrial fibrillation. *Cardiovasc. Res.* 52, 226–235. doi: 10.1016/S0008-6363(01)00380-7

Ye, B., Valdivia, C. R., Ackerman, M. J., and Makielski, J. C. (2003). A common human *SCN5A* polymorphism modifies expression of an arrhythmia causing mutation. *Physiol. Genomics* 12, 187–193. doi: 10.1152/physiolgenomics.00117.2002

Zhang, H., Holden, A. V., Kodama, I., Honjo, H., Lei, M., Varghese, T., et al. (2000). Mathematical models of action potentials in the periphery and center of the rabbit sinoatrial node. *Am. J. Physiol. Heart Circ. Physiol.* 279, H397–H421. doi: 10.1152/ajpheart.2000.279.1.H397

Zhang, H., Holden, A. V., Noble, D., and Boyett, M. R. (2002). Analysis of the chronotropic effect of acetylcholine on sinoatrial node cells. *J. Cardiovasc. Electrophysiol.* 13, 465–474. doi: 10.1046/j.1540-8167.2002.00465.x

Zimmer, T., Haufe, V., and Blechschmidt, S. (2014). Voltage-gated sodium channels in the mammalian heart. *Glob. Cardiol. Sci. Pract.* 2014, 449–463. doi: 10.5339/gcsp.2014.58

6

Extended Bidomain Modeling of Defibrillation: Quantifying Virtual Electrode Strengths in Fibrotic Myocardium

Jean Bragard[1*]*, Aparna C. Sankarankutty*[2,3] *and Frank B. Sachse*[2,3*]

[1] Department of Physics and Applied Mathematics, University of Navarra, Pamplona, Spain, [2] Nora Eccles Harrison Cardiovascular Research and Training Institute, University of Utah, Salt Lake City, UT, United States, [3] Department of Biomedical Engineering, University of Utah, Salt Lake City, UT, United States

Correspondence:
Jean Bragard
jbragard@unav.es
Frank B. Sachse
frank.sachse@utah.edu

Defibrillation is a well-established therapy for atrial and ventricular arrhythmia. Here, we shed light on defibrillation in the fibrotic heart. Using the extended bidomain model of electrical conduction in cardiac tissue, we assessed the influence of fibrosis on the strength of virtual electrodes caused by extracellular electrical current. We created one-dimensional models of rabbit ventricular tissue with a central patch of fibrosis. The fibrosis was incorporated by altering volume fractions for extracellular, myocyte and fibroblast domains. In our prior work, we calculated these volume fractions from microscopic images at the infarct border zone of rabbit hearts. An average and a large degree of fibrosis were modeled. We simulated defibrillation by application of an extracellular current for a short duration (5 ms). We explored the effects of myocyte-fibroblast coupling, intra-fibroblast conductivity and patch length on the strength of the virtual electrodes present at the borders of the normal and fibrotic tissue. We discriminated between effects on myocyte and fibroblast membranes at both borders of the patch. Similarly, we studied defibrillation in two-dimensional models of fibrotic tissue. Square and disk-like patches of fibrotic tissue were embedded in control tissue. We quantified the influence of the geometry and fibrosis composition on virtual electrode strength. We compared the results obtained with a square and disk shape of the fibrotic patch with results from the one-dimensional simulations. Both, one- and two-dimensional simulations indicate that extracellular current application causes virtual electrodes at boundaries of fibrotic patches. A higher degree of fibrosis and larger patch size were associated with an increased strength of the virtual electrodes. Also, patch geometry affected the strength of the virtual electrodes. Our simulations suggest that increased fibroblast-myocyte coupling and intra-fibroblast conductivity reduce virtual electrode strength. However, experimental data to constrain these modeling parameters are limited and thus pinpointing the magnitude of the reduction will require further understanding of electrical coupling of fibroblasts in native cardiac tissues. We propose that the findings from our computational studies are important for development of patient-specific protocols for internal defibrillators.

Keywords: defibrillation, cardiac tissue, fibrosis, computational modeling, multidomain modeling

INTRODUCTION

Several types of cardiac arrhythmias are treated with external or implanted defibrillators, which are devices for application of electrical current to a patient's thorax or heart (Al-Khatib et al., 2017). The electrical currents create an electrical field in the heart, which is determined by the location and geometry of the electrodes, the magnitude and waveform of the applied current, and the distribution, composition and electrical properties of tissues. Targets of defibrillation are constituents of cardiac muscle tissues, i.e., the myocytes. These cells respond to an extracellular electrical field caused by a defibrillator with changes of their transmembrane voltage. Modulated by the electrophysiological state of the myocytes, their transmembrane voltage will exhibit negative or positive shifts due to the electrical field. Thus, defibrillation might cause hyperpolarization and depolarization of myocytes. Also, defibrillation might trigger or modulate action potentials.

Several theories for mechanisms of defibrillation of the heart have been developed (Dosdall et al., 2010). The critical mass theory suggests that defibrillation success requires myocyte depolarization in a sufficient mass of tissue. The upper limit of vulnerability theory proposes the existence of a minimal electrical stimulus strength above which ventricular fibrillation cannot be induced even for stimuli occurring during the vulnerable period of the cardiac cycle. The sawtooth hypothesis and the syncytial heterogeneity hypothesis explains defibrillation effects on the transmembrane voltage of myocytes distally from the electrodes based on microscopic discontinuities of the intracellular space (Fishler, 1998). Similarly, the virtual electrode theory explains defibrillation effects based on structural heterogeneities such as endo- and epicardial surfaces as well as blood vessels. Virtual electrodes are thought to underlie local shifts of transmembrane voltages and thus trigger action potentials and elicit wave fronts that interfere with fibrillation. Recent work using computational modeling focused on understanding virtual electrodes caused by vessels (Connolly et al., 2017a,b) and related curvature of the surface of tissue heterogeneities to myocyte depolarization and initiation of wave fronts (Bittihn et al., 2012).

It is well-established that patients with myocardial fibrosis profit from defibrillator implantation (Iles et al., 2011), but it has also been reported that patients exhibit an increased mortality if they receive defibrillation shocks (Cevik et al., 2009). Several cardiac diseases including fibrosis are associated with discontinuity of the intracellular space and microstructural heterogeneity. For instance, myocardial infarction leads to scar regions with a decreased volume ratio of myocytes, but increased volume ratios of the extracellular space and fibroblasts. Also, our recent studies on a rabbit model of myocardial infarction revealed patches of fibrotic tissue interspersed within working myocardium distal from the scar (Seidel et al., 2017). Furthermore, several types of fibrosis of cardiac tissue are characterized by local increases of extracellular space and fibroblasts. Currently, our knowledge on defibrillation effects in fibrotic tissues is sparse and we do not even know if understanding these effects can help with parameterization of defibrillation protocols. Based on virtual electrode theory, it is conceivable that fibrotic tissue will exhibit substantial effects in response to defibrillation. However, experimental and computational studies on this subject have not been performed.

Here, we investigated the effects of defibrillation on transmembrane voltages in fibrotic tissues. We applied an extended bidomain model of electrical conduction in cardiac tissue. In contrast to the conventional bidomain model, which describes myocyte and extracellular domains only, the extended model comprises a description of a fibroblast domain. We performed simulations in one-dimensional (1D) and two-dimensional (2D) models of cardiac tissues with fibrotic patches of variable sizes, tissue composition and myocyte-fibroblast electrical coupling. We measured shifts of the myocyte membrane voltage caused by application of strong extracellular currents to assess the strength of virtual electrodes.

METHODS

Extended Bidomain Modeling of Cardiac Conduction

We utilized the extended bidomain model for computational simulations of defibrillation in 1D and 2D domains (Sachse et al., 2009). The model was developed based on the established bidomain model (Tung, 1978; Henriquez, 1993) and allows description of cardiac tissues comprising more than one cell species. The original extended bidomain model comprised two cell species, i.e., cardiac myocytes and fibroblasts. Intracellular domains for these two species together with the extracellular domain constitute three domains of interest.

The mathematical formulation of the extended bidomain model applies Kirchhoff's electrical current conservation law to myocardium (Plonsey and Barr, 2007). Here we followed the exposition in Sachse et al. (2009), which described the electrical dynamics of the myocardium in three "homogenized" continuous domains. In short, the expression of current conservation at any point in space mathematically translates into a Poisson equation for each of the three domains:

$$\nabla \cdot \left(\sigma_{myo} \nabla \phi_{myo}\right) = -f_{s,myo} + \beta_{myo,fib}\, I_{myo,fib} + \beta_{myo}\, I_{myo,e} \quad (1)$$

$$\nabla \cdot \left(\sigma_{fib} \nabla \phi_{fib}\right) = -f_{s,fib} - \beta_{myo,fib}\, I_{myo,fib} + \beta_{fib}\, I_{fib,e} \quad (2)$$

$$\nabla \cdot \left(\sigma_{e} \nabla \phi_{e}\right) = -f_{s,e} - \beta_{myo}\, I_{myo,e} - \beta_{fib}\, I_{fib,e} \quad (3)$$

where σ_{myo}, σ_{fib} and σ_e are the electrical conductivity tensors of the myocyte, fibroblast and extracellular domain, respectively, ϕ_{myo}, ϕ_{fib} , and ϕ_e are the intracellular potential of the myocyte, fibroblast and extracellular domain, respectively, and $f_{s,myo}$, $f_{s,fib}$, and $f_{s,e}$ (A/m^3), are the stimulus current source densities for the myocyte, fibroblast and extracellular domain, respectively. Membrane voltage of myocytes V_{myo} and fibroblasts V_{fib} was defined as the difference of their intracellular and extracellular potential. The number of myocytes per unit volume β_{myo} and fibroblasts per unit volume β_{fib} $(1/\mathrm{m}^3)$ were defined as:

$$\beta_{myo} = \frac{Vol_{myo}}{Vol_{myo,single}} \quad (4)$$

$$\beta_{fib} = \frac{Vol_{fib}}{Vol_{fib,single}} \quad (5)$$

with the volume fraction of myocytes Vol_{myo} and fibroblasts Vol_{fib} (dimensionless) as well as the individual volume for a myocyte $Vol_{myo,single}$ and fibroblast $Vol_{fib,single}$ (m^3). Currents between the myocyte and extracellular, fibroblast and extracellular, and myocyte and fibroblast domains are identified by $I_{myo,e}$, $I_{fib,e}$, and $I_{myo,fib}$ (A), respectively.

The current between the myocyte and fibroblast domain was defined as:

$$I_{myo,fib} = \frac{\phi_{myo} - \phi_{fib}}{R_{myo,fib}} \quad (6)$$

where $R_{myo,fib}$ is the resistance of gap junction channels (Ω). We defined the effective volume density $\beta_{myo,fib}$ ($1/m^3$) of electrical connections between fibroblasts and myocytes as:

$$\beta_{myo,fib} = \frac{Vol_{fib}}{Vol_{fib,single}} \quad (7)$$

We assumed that the conductivity tensors (S/m) for each domain have a linear relationship with their respective volume fractions:

$$\sigma_{myo} = Vol_{myo}\,\overline{\sigma}_{myo} \quad (8)$$

$$\sigma_{fib} = Vol_{fib}\,\overline{\sigma}_{fib} \quad (9)$$

$$\sigma_{e} = Vol_{e}\,\overline{\sigma}_{e} \quad (10)$$

where the tensors $\overline{\sigma}_{myo}$, $\overline{\sigma}_{fib}$ and $\overline{\sigma}_{e}$ described conductivity for volume ratios of 100%. In the subsequently described simulations, we vary $\overline{\sigma}_{fib}$ over a wide range of conductivities. We note that the range of σ_{fib} is smaller, due to scaling by the fibroblast volume fraction.

We applied a mathematical model of a rabbit ventricular myocyte (Mahajan et al., 2008) and a cardiac fibroblast (Sachse et al., 2008) to calculate the currents $I_{myo,e}$ and $I_{fib,e}$, respectively. Temperature of the fibroblast model was set to the same temperature as the myocyte model (308 K). We applied a temperature coefficient (Q10) of 2 to adjust rate coefficients of the time- and voltage dependent outward current of the fibroblast model.

Implementation of Extended Bidomain Model

The extended bidomain model was implemented using the finite volume method and the programming language Fortran. The Portable, Extensible Toolkit for Scientific Computation (PETSc) (Balay et al., 2018) was used for parallelization and solving the Poisson equation. The myocyte (Cellml, 2008b) and fibroblast (Cellml, 2008a) models were implemented from CellML (Garny et al., 2008).

A simple forward Euler scheme with a fixed time step of 0.5 or 1 μs was applied to solve the time evolution of the model. The Poisson equation for the cellular domain was solved at each time step with a relative tolerance of 10^{-12}. We applied the GMRES method, a member of the iterative Krylov methods that are implemented in PETSc. We used the additive Schwarz preconditioner in order to speed up the convergence for the iterative solver. The internal number of iterations for the Poisson solver for the 2D simulations was in the range of 50–100. This constituted the main burden of the numerical calculation. We checked for current conservation at each link of the discretized domain up to this precision (no numerical artifact of creation or annihilation of currents). In order to validate our numerical implementation, we also checked that the change in grid size discretization does not affect the results. We have compiled measured parameters in **Tables S1–S3** to show that variation of spatial resolution in the range of 25–100 μm has only minor effects. We further evaluated this new implementation of the extended bidomain model using our prior implementation (Sachse et al., 2009; Seemann et al., 2010). Modifications of the prior implementation were performed to account for discontinuity in the material properties of the cardiac tissue at the interface between the control and fibrotic regions.

Setup of 1D Simulations

We created 1D models of normal rabbit ventricular myocardium with an embedded central fibrotic patch (**Figure 1A**). The model was discretized with a spatial resolution of 50 or 100 μm. The patch exhibited differences in volume fractions of extracellular space, myocytes and fibroblasts measured in our previous work of fibrotic tissue (Greiner et al., 2018). Two different types of patches representing average and large fibrosis were configured (**Table 1**). We varied $R_{myo,fib}$ and $\overline{\sigma}_{fib}$ in simulations. The simulations started with applying 9 depolarizing myocyte membrane currents at the location 32.5–33 mm of the domain with an amplitude of 20 $\mu A/cm^2$ and a duration of 5 ms at a frequency of 4 Hz. At 250 ms after the last stimulus, extracellular currents were applied at 1–1.5 mm and 32.5–33 mm of the domain with an amplitude of 0.7×10^5 and -0.7×10^5 A/m^3, respectively. These injected currents created a nearly uniform electric field between the two sites of magnitude $E = 0.546$ V/cm (**Figure S1**). This electric field, in turn, was responsible for the generation of the virtual electrodes at the left (referred as point 1) and right (point 2) boundary of the fibrotic patch.

In order to measure virtual electrode strengths, we monitored the difference in the membrane voltage of the myocytes V_{myo} and fibroblasts V_{fib} at patch boundaries during the application of extracellular current with respect to the membrane voltages before current application. V_{myo} was not a monotonic function of time during the current application (**Figure S2**). Therefore, we reported the largest absolute value (maintaining its sign) of the monitored difference during the current application as a measure of the local virtual electrode strength. In addition, we quantified space constants λ_{myo} and λ_{fib} by fitting the spatial profile of V_{myo} and V_{fib}, respectively, at and proximal to the boundaries of the patch.

Setup of 2D Simulations

We generated 2D models of normal rabbit ventricular myocardium with an embedded fibrotic patch of square and disk-like shapes (**Figures 1B,C**). The square side length and

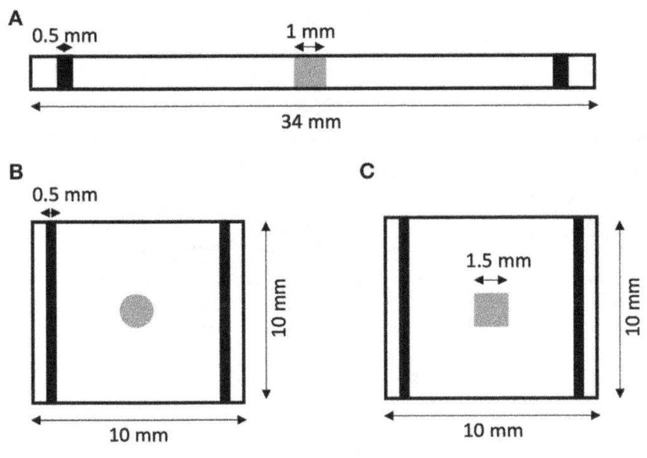

FIGURE 1 | Geometry of **(A)** 1D and **(B,C)** 2D models of rabbit ventricular tissue with central fibrotic patch. The sites of extracellular current application are marked in black. Fibrotic patches are shown in grey.

TABLE 1 | Parameters of extended bidomain model.

Parameter	Symbol	Region	Value
Extracellular volume fraction (%)	Vol_e	Control	32
		Average fibrosis	43
		Large fibrosis	60
Myocyte volume fraction (%)	Vol_{myo}	Control	65
		Average fibrosis	47
		Large fibrosis	20
Fibroblast volume fraction (%)	Vol_{fib}	Control	3
		Average fibrosis	10
		Large fibrosis	20
Extracellular conductivity (S/m)	$\overline{\sigma}_e$		1
Intra-myocyte conductivity (S/m)	$\overline{\sigma}_{myo}$		0.5
Intra-fibroblast conductivity (S/m)	$\overline{\sigma}_{fib}$		0, 0.1, 0.2, 0.5
Myocyte-fibroblast coupling resistance (MΩ)	$R_{myo,fib}$		$1–10^6$
Volume of single myocyte (pL)	$Vol_{myo,single}$		10.299
Volume of single fibroblast (pL)	$Vol_{fib,single}$		0.268
Membrane capacitance per unit area (μF/cm^2)			1
Myocyte surface to volume ratio (cm^{-1})			2,500
Fibroblast surface to volume ratio (cm^{-1})			16,800

the disk diameter were both set to 1.5 mm. We discretized the model with a spatial resolution of 50 μm in x and y direction. The computational domain was 1 cm x 1 cm in size. We applied four intracellular stimuli at 9–9.5 mm along the length and entire width with an amplitude of 20 μA/cm^2 for 5 ms at a frequency of 4 Hz. Two hundred and fifty milliseconds after the last stimulation, extracellular currents were applied at 0.5–1 mm and 9–9.5 mm along the length and throughout the width with an amplitude of 0.7×10^5 and -0.7×10^5 A/m^3, respectively. These injected currents created a nearly uniform electric field between the two electrodes of magnitude 0.530 V/cm.

Data Analysis

Effects of patch length W_p on ΔV_{myo} were analyzed using the fitting function:

$$\Delta V_{myo} = a\left(1 - e^{-\frac{W_p}{b}}\right) \tag{11}$$

with the parameters a and b. We used a different fitting function for ΔV_{fib}, because it was not always crossing the origin of axes:

$$\Delta V_{fib} = c - ae^{-\frac{W_p}{b}} \tag{12}$$

with the parameters a, b and c. We measured the fit quality using the adjusted R^2.

RESULTS

1D Simulations

We performed numerical simulations with the 1D extended bidomain model of control tissue with a central patch configured with parameters for average fibrosis (**Figure 1A**). The model was discretized with a spatial resolution of 100 μm. In **Figures 2A–C**, we present the results of a simulation of a propagating wave initiated by intracellular stimulation followed by application of extracellular current. The model parameters were $R_{myo,fib} = 4 \times 10^4$ MΩ and $\overline{\sigma}_{fib} = 0.1$ S/m. After scaling with the fibroblast volume fraction (Equation 9) in control tissue (3%) and patch (10%), σ_{fib} amounted to 0.003 and 0.01 S/m, respectively. In this case, the propagation of action potentials was only marginally affected by the fibrotic patch. Extracellular current altered ϕ_e as well as V_{myo} and V_{fib} at the application sites and the borders of the fibrotic patch.

We present the spatial distribution of ϕ_e, V_{myo}, and V_{fib} at the end ($t = 2.255$ s) of current application in **Figures 2D–F**, respectively. Due to current application, V_{myo} at the left border of the patch was increased from −84.95 mV before current application to −75.59 mV at the end of the current application. V_{fib} was reduced from −54.05 mV before current application to −58.97 mV at the end of the current application. At the right border of the patch V_{myo} was decreased from −85.00 to −93.44 mV. V_{fib} was increased from −54.21 to −51.18 mV. We determined the electric field for average and large fibrosis during the current application (**Figures S1A,B**, respectively). The spatial variation outside of the region for current application was small.

We applied the 1D model in a series of simulations varying $R_{myo,fib}$ and $\overline{\sigma}_{fib}$. Example simulated ϕ_e, V_{myo}, and V_{fib} are presented in **Figure S3**. Before current application, the biphasic relationship of V_{myo} with $R_{myo,fib}$ was nearly identical on both

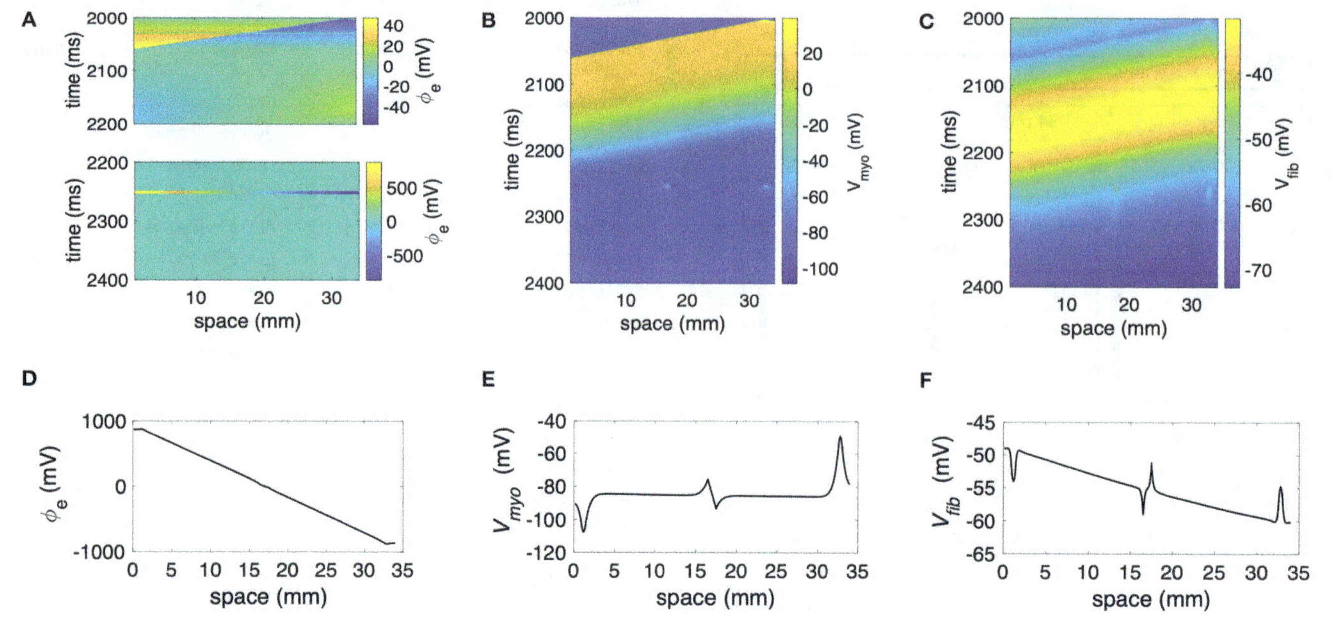

FIGURE 2 | Representative plots of **(A)** ϕ_e, **(B)** V_{myo}, and **(C)** V_{fib} for intracellular pacing and subsequent extracellular current application in the 1D model with the average fibrosis patch, $\overline{\sigma}_{fib}$ of 0.1 S/m and $R_{myo,fib}$ of 40 GΩ. Spatial distribution of **(D)** ϕ_e, **(E)** V_{myo}, and **(F)** V_{fib} at the end of application of extracellular currents. The extracellular current led to alterations of V_{myo} and V_{fib} not only at the application site, but also at the left and right border of the fibrotic patch.

boundaries of the patch (**Figures 3A,C**). Also, variation of $\overline{\sigma}_{fib}$ did not affect V_{myo}. After current application, the left border of the patch exhibited increased V_{myo}, measured as $\Delta V_{myo}^{(1)}$, dependent on $R_{myo,fib}$ and $\overline{\sigma}_{fib}$ (**Figure 3B**). At the right border of the patch, the reduction of V_{myo}, measured as $\Delta V_{myo}^{(2)}$, was dependent on $R_{myo,fib}$ and $\overline{\sigma}_{fib}$ (**Figure 3D**). At both borders of the patch, effects on V_{myo} were of similar magnitude for all $\overline{\sigma}_{fib}$ for large $R_{myo,fib}$.

We present corresponding measures on V_{fib} in **Figure 4**. The biphasic relationship of V_{fib} with $R_{myo,fib}$ before application of extracellular current (**Figures 4A,C**) was similar to the relationship of V_{myo} with $R_{myo,fib}$. For low $R_{myo,fib}$ (high myocyte-fibroblast coupling), V_{fib} was similar to the resting V_{myo} (**Figures 3A,C**). For high $R_{myo,fib}$ (low myocyte-fibroblast coupling), $V_{fib}$was close to the membrane voltage of isolated fibroblasts, i.e., ~58 mV (Shibukawa et al., 2005; Sachse et al., 2008). Similar as myocytes, fibroblasts at the borders of the patch exhibit alterations of their membrane voltage, $\Delta V_{fib}^{(1)}$ and $\Delta V_{fib}^{(2)}$, dependent on $R_{myo,fib}$ and $\overline{\sigma}_{fib}$ in response to current application (**Figures 4B,D**). For low $R_{myo,fib}$, ΔV_{fib} was roughly similar to the ΔV_{myo} at both borders. In contrast, for high $R_{myo,fib}$, ΔV_{fib} exhibited a reverse sign vs. the corresponding ΔV_{myo} at both borders. This results in the discontinuity in ΔV_{fib} for $R_{myo,fib}$ of 100–1,000 MΩ (**Figures 4B,D**).

Using the same geometrical model and experimental protocol, we also performed simulations using a patch with large fibrosis (**Figures 5, 6**). While the results were qualitatively similar as for the average case of fibrosis described above, we note important differences. In particular, the higher degree of fibrosis was associated with a higher magnitude of ΔV_{myo} and ΔV_{fib}. We observed conduction block for $R_{myo,fib}$ of 100–1,000 MΩ (**Figures 5A,C**). We confirmed that the magnitude ΔV_{myo} is a monotonously increasing function of the degree of fibrosis (**Figures 7A,B**). The parameter α described the variation between the low degree of fibrosis (α = 0) to the high degree of fibrosis (α = 1). In the range of settings that we have studied, the variation of ΔV_{myo} with α was roughly linear. Similarly, for low $R_{myo,fib}$ the magnitude ΔV_{fib} was a monotonously increasing function of α (**Figures 7C,D**). For high $R_{myo,fib}$, the magnitude ΔV_{fib} was approximately constant for α between 0 and 1.

We assessed the influence of patch length on virtual electrode strengths (**Figure 8**). The simulations were performed with a spatial resolution of 50 μm in order to explore smaller patch lengths. We present fit parameters of ΔV_{myo} and ΔV_{fib} in **Table 2**. The patch length was a major modulator of virtual electrode strengths. The larger the patch, the higher the effect on membrane voltages. However, there is a limit to this phenomenon, with the effect tapering off for longer patches. We assessed the length scale, which depends on the coupling between the myocyte and fibroblast domain through the coupling parameter $R_{myo,fib}$. For large $R_{myo,fib}$, the spatial length scales for the myocytes and fibroblasts correspond to their respective space constants λ_{myo} and λ_{fib}. In contrast, for low $R_{myo,fib}$ the spatial length scales were the same for the two species due to the coupling and settled at an intermediate value between λ_{myo} and λ_{fib}. Indeed, larger difference of the ΔV_{myo} and ΔV_{fib} were at the sub-millimeter scale (**Figure 8**), which is in agreement with the estimated values for of λ_{myo} and λ_{fib} (**Tables S1–S3**).

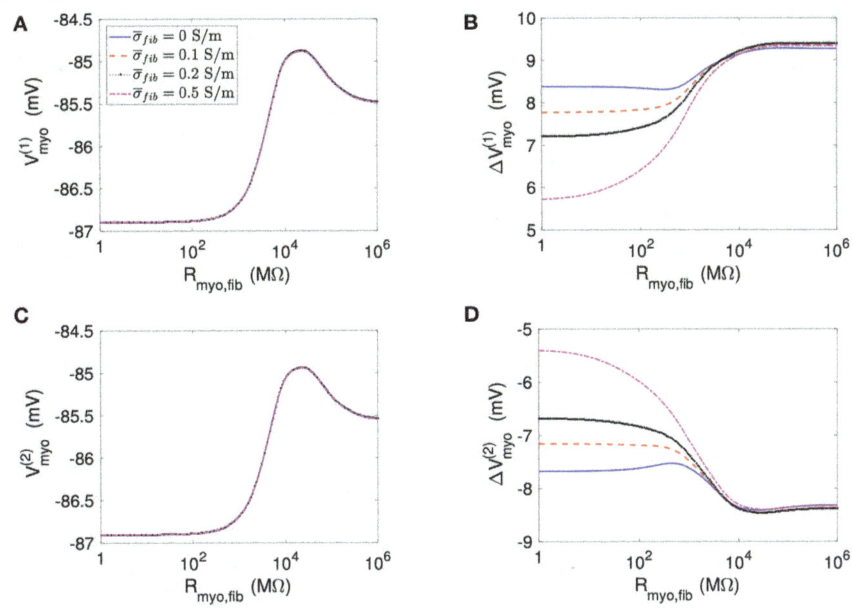

FIGURE 3 | Measurement of effects of extracellular current application on V_{myo} using the 1D model with the average fibrosis patch. Before application of extracellular currents, V_{myo} at the **(A)** left and **(C)** right border of the fibrotic patch was marginally affected by $R_{myo,fib}$ and $\bar{\sigma}_{fib}$. **(B)** At the end of current application, the left patch border exhibited a positive ΔV_{myo}. **(D)** In contrast, the right patch border exhibited a negative ΔV_{myo}.

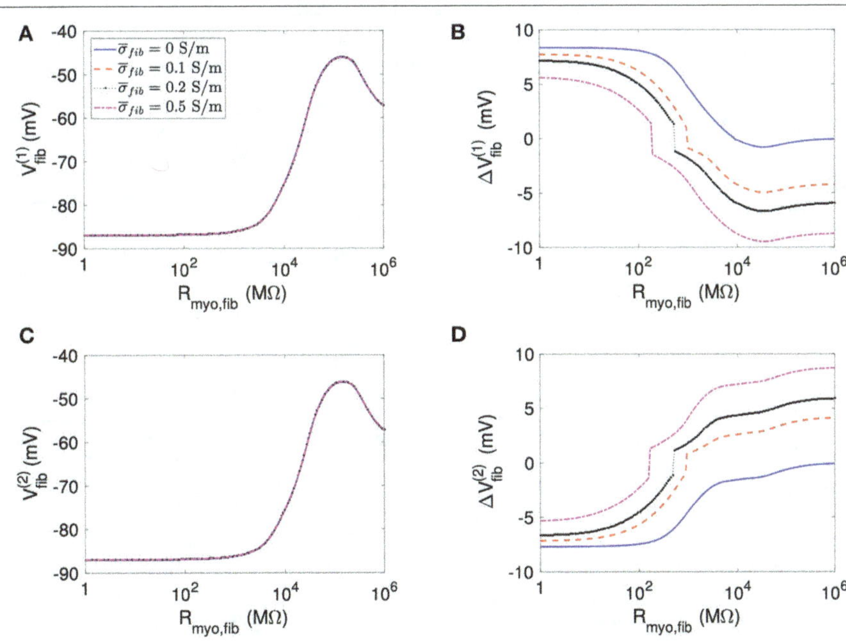

FIGURE 4 | Measurement of effects of extracellular current application on V_{fib} using the 1D model with the average fibrosis patch. Before application of extracellular currents, V_{fib} at the **(A)** left and **(C)** right border of the fibrotic patch was strongly affected by $R_{myo,fib}$ and $\bar{\sigma}_{fib}$. At the end of current application, the **(B)** left and **(D)** right border exhibited a ΔV_{fib} with magnitude and sign modulated by $R_{myo,fib}$ and $\bar{\sigma}_{fib}$.

2D Simulations

We investigated virtual electrodes in a 2D spatial domain of control tissue with central patches configured with parameters for average fibrosis (**Figures 1B,C**). Because we know from the 1D simulations that effects of the patch on ΔV_{myo} and ΔV_{fib} are larger at the millimeter than sub-millimeter scale, we set the patches (square and disk) to a size of 1.5 mm.

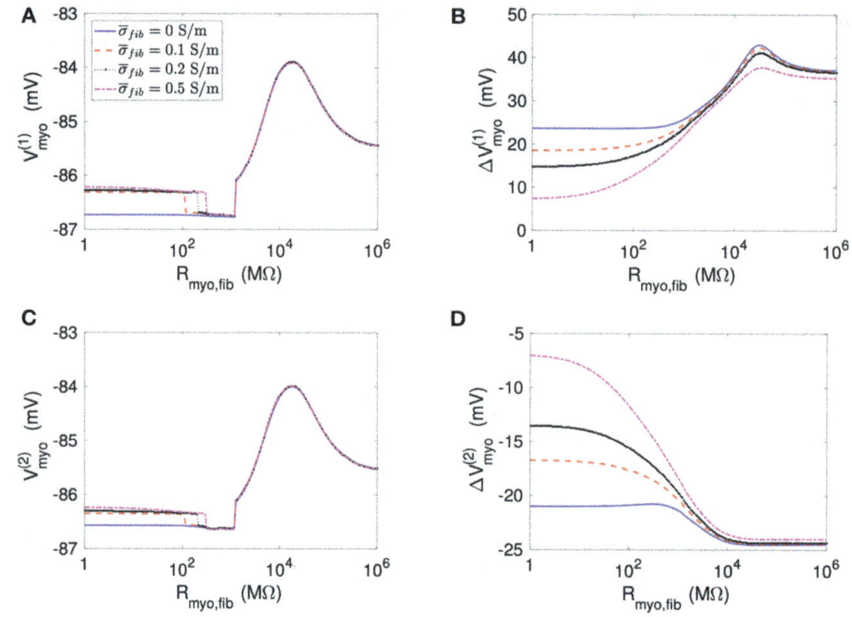

FIGURE 5 | Measurement of effects of extracellular current application on V_{myo} using the 1D model with the large fibrosis patch. Before application of extracellular currents, V_{myo} at the **(A)** left and **(C)** right border of the fibrotic patch was marginally affected by $R_{myo,fib}$ and $\overline{\sigma}_{fib}$. **(B)** At the end of current application, the left patch border exhibited a positive ΔV_{myo}. **(D)** In contrast, the right patch border exhibited a negative ΔV_{myo}.

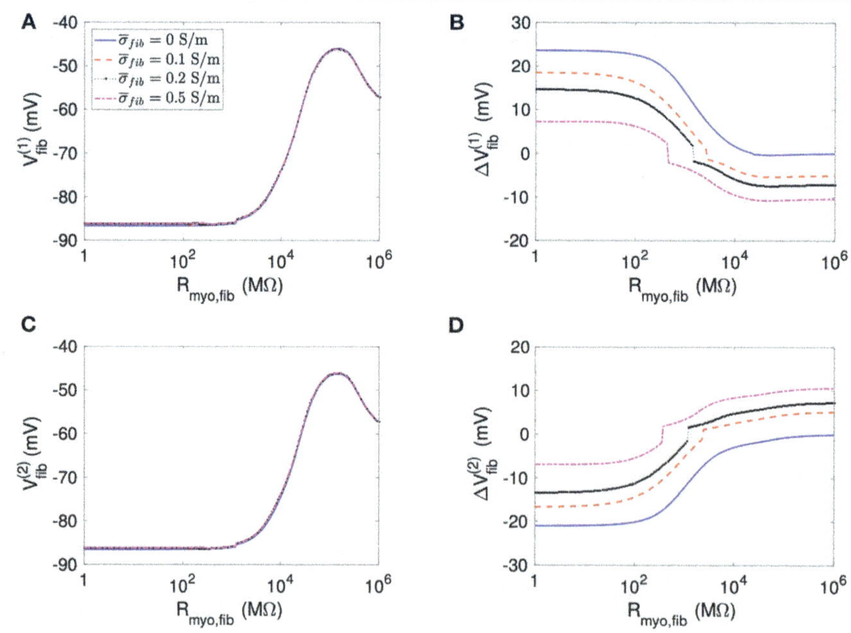

FIGURE 6 | Measurement of effects of extracellular current application on V_{fib} using the 1D model with the large fibrosis patch. Before application of extracellular currents, V_{fib} at the **(A)** left and **(C)** right border of the fibrotic patch was strongly affected by $R_{myo,fib}$ and $\overline{\sigma}_{fib}$. At the end of current application, the **(B)** left and **(D)** right border exhibited a ΔV_{fib} with magnitude and sign modulated by $R_{myo,fib}$ and $\overline{\sigma}_{fib}$.

Figure 9 displays the 3 main fields at the end of the extracellular current application in a model with a square-shaped patch, $\overline{\sigma}_{fib}$ of 0.1 S/m and $R_{myo,fib}$ of 1 GΩ. The injected currents at the electrode generated a fairly linear distribution for ϕ_e (**Figures 9A,D**), which implies a quasi-uniform electric field. Only close to the cathode (x≈9 mm) the field was distorted by a nascent wave initiated at the cathode location. Closer inspection revealed that the field is really uniform close to the patch

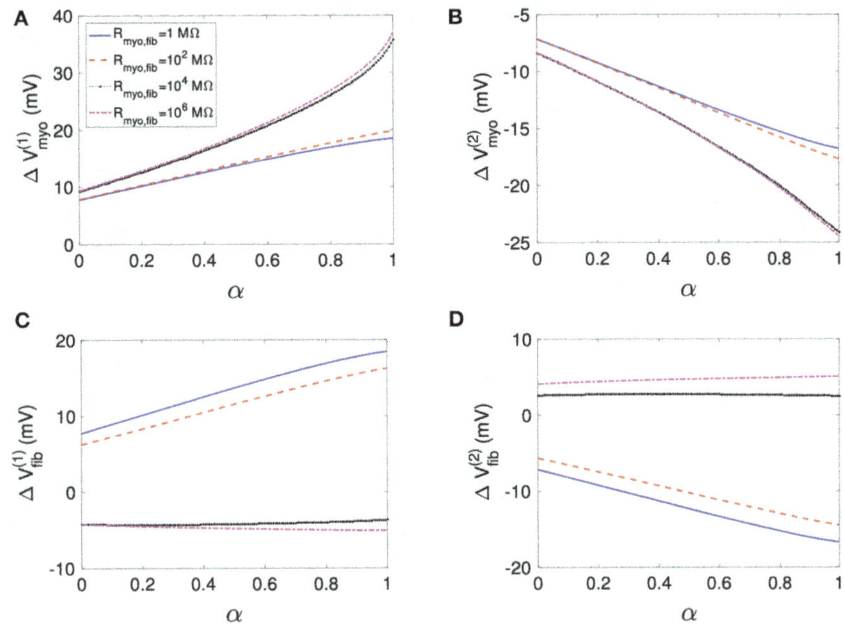

FIGURE 7 | Assessment of effects of extracellular current application on V_{myo} and V_{fib} simulated in 1D models with a patch of varying degrees of fibrosis. The degree of fibrosis ranged from average ($\alpha = 0$) to large ($\alpha = 1$). We also varied $R_{myo,fib}$. $\overline{\sigma}_{fib}$ was set to 0.1 S/m. The effects on the magnitude of ΔV_{myo} at the **(A)** left and **(B)** right boundary increased with the degree of fibrosis. Similarly, effects of ΔV_{fib} at the **(C)** left and **(D)** right boundary increased with the degree of fibrosis for small $R_{myo,fib}$. Marginal effects were present for larger $R_{myo,fib}$.

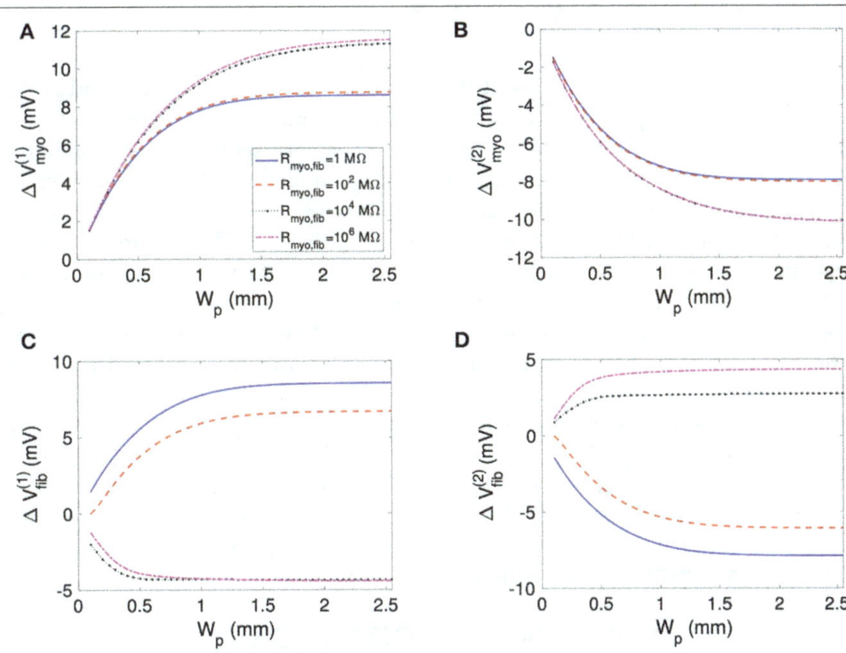

FIGURE 8 | Effects of patch length W_p on **(A,B)** V_{myo} and **(C,D)** V_{fib} at the boundary of the patch in response to application of the extracellular current. We varied $R_{myo,fib}$, but $\overline{\sigma}_{fib}$ was set on 0.1 S/m. For small W_p, V_{myo}, and V_{fib} were greatly reduced.

(**Figure 9D**). The corresponding spatial distribution of V_{myo} for the same time shows the virtual electrodes at the two edges of the square that are perpendicular to the applied field (**Figures 9B,E**). The edge corresponding to the small value of x exhibited a depolarization pattern (equivalent to point 1 in the 1D setting). On the contrary the other edge exhibited a hyperpolarization

TABLE 2 | Relationships of membrane voltage changes and W_p according to the fitting functions.

	$R_{myo,fib}$ (MΩ)	1	10^2	10^4	10^6
$\Delta V_{myo}^{(1)}$	a (mV)	8.778 (8.723, 8.833)	8.907 (8.862, 8.953)	11.65 (11.59, 11.71)	11.9 (11.84, 11.96)
	b (mm)	0.485 (0.473, 0.497)	0.4843 (0.4747, 0.494)	0.654 (0.6438,0.664)	0.6616 (0.651, 0.672)
	Adj. R^2	0.9965	0.9977	0.999	0.9989
$\Delta V_{myo}^{(2)}$	a (mV)	−8.049 (−8.087, −8.012)	−8.126 (−8.154, −8.097)	−10.24 (−10.25, −10.22)	−10.25 (−10.26, −10.23)
	b (mm)	0.4702 (0.4614, 0.479)	0.4671 (0.4606, 0.4737)	0.5756 (0.5725, 0.5787)	0.581 (0.578, 0.584)
	Adj. R^2	0.9979	0.9988	0.999	0.9999
$\Delta V_{fib}^{(1)}$	a (mV)	9.311 (9.171, 9.451)	8.965 (8.784, 9.146)	−4.682 (−4.902, −4.462)	−5.064 (−5.225, −4.903)
	b (mm)	0.447 (0.436, 0.4587)	0.455 (0.4396, 0.4709)	0.1521 (0.1454, 0.1588)	0.2181 (0.2103, 0.2259)
	c (mV)	8.677 (8.64, 8.714)	6.82 (6.771, 6.869)	−4.342 (−4.353, −4.33)	−4.374 (−4.389, −4.359)
	Adj. R^2	0.9985	0.9973	0.9944	0.9964
$\Delta V_{fib}^{(2)}$	a (mV)	−8.379 (−8.49, −8.26)	−8.106 (−8.265, −7.946)	3.136 (3.003, 3.269)	5.05 (4.887, 5.213)
	b (mm)	0.445 (0.435, 0.456)	0.454 (0.439, 0.4693)	0.1985 (0.1895, 0.2075)	0.2242 (0.216, 0.2324)
	c (mV)	−7.97 (−8.004, −7.94)	−6.17 (−6.213, −6.127)	2.728 (2.717, 2.738)	4.315 (4.299, 4.33)
	Adj. R^2	0.9988	0.9975	0.9941	0.9962

The values given in parentheses indicate a 95 % confidence interval for the parameter estimates.

pattern (equivalent to point 2 in the 1D setting). **Figures 9C,F** display the field for V_{fib}. In this example, $R_{myo,fib}$ was set to 1 GΩ, which is the value for which the coupling between the myocytes and the fibroblast cancels out the effect of the conductivity heterogeneities at the patch boundaries. According to the theory (see section Discussion), we expect to observe hyperpolarization for V_{fib} at point 1 and depolarization at point 2, which is the opposite of what happens to V_{myo}. However, the coupling term between the two domains caused that the V_{myo} is pulling the V_{fib} in the same direction. At the very edge of the patch (**Figure 9F**) the two effects cancel out.

We repeated the simulation using a disk-shaped patch with $R_{myo,fib} = 1$ TΩ, which represents negligible coupling between V_{fib} and V_{myo} (**Figure 10**). The simulation yielded a linear distribution for ϕ_e and the simulated electric field was almost identical as the field obtained with the square patch (**Figures 10A,D**). In **Figures 10B,E** we present the corresponding spatial distribution of V_{myo}. As before, we observed the two virtual electrodes at the edges of the patch. Due to the disk-shaped patch, the virtual electrodes were not so sharp and appeared diffuse also in the parallel direction of the electric field. **Figures 10C,F** confirmed that polarities of ΔV_{fib} are indeed opposite to the ΔV_{myo} at the patch boundary. Also, the spatial scale for the virtual electrode was much smaller than the virtual electrodes for the V_{myo} field, which agrees with the corresponding values for the space constants associated with the two fields.

Figure 11 and **Table S4** present quantitative measures for the virtual electrode strengths for the two patch geometries. We report the results for ΔV_{myo} and ΔV_{fib} at both locations of the patch boundaries as a function of $R_{myo,fib}$. We compared them with the corresponding values obtained for the 1D case. Using bidomain models it has been demonstrated that convex shape of boundaries leads to lower activation of the membrane (Entcheva et al., 1998, 1999; Pumir and Krinsky, 1999; Bittihn et al., 2012). This was confirmed in our simulation for ΔV_{myo} where the virtual electrode strengths were lower for the disk than for the square. However, the difference between the two geometries is rather minute. We measured an approximate 4% difference of ΔV_{myo} for low values of the $R_{myo,fib}$ and an approximate 5% difference for high values of the $R_{myo,fib}$. Also, ΔV_{myo} for the square-shaped were higher than for the disk-shaped patch, and close to the 1D patch geometry. ΔV_{fib} for the 1D and the two 2D geometries were similar (**Figures 11C,D**). For ΔV_{fib}, the influence of patch geometry was less pronounced.

DISCUSSION

Our computational study provided insights into the relationship between parameters of fibrotic patches and the strength of virtual electrodes caused by defibrillation. We applied the extended bidomain model to reflect that cardiac tissues comprise fibroblasts beyond myocytes. Our study showed that an increased degree of fibrosis and an increased size of the fibrotic patch cause an increased strength of virtual electrodes. Also, we found that the composition of tissue heterogeneities is a modulator

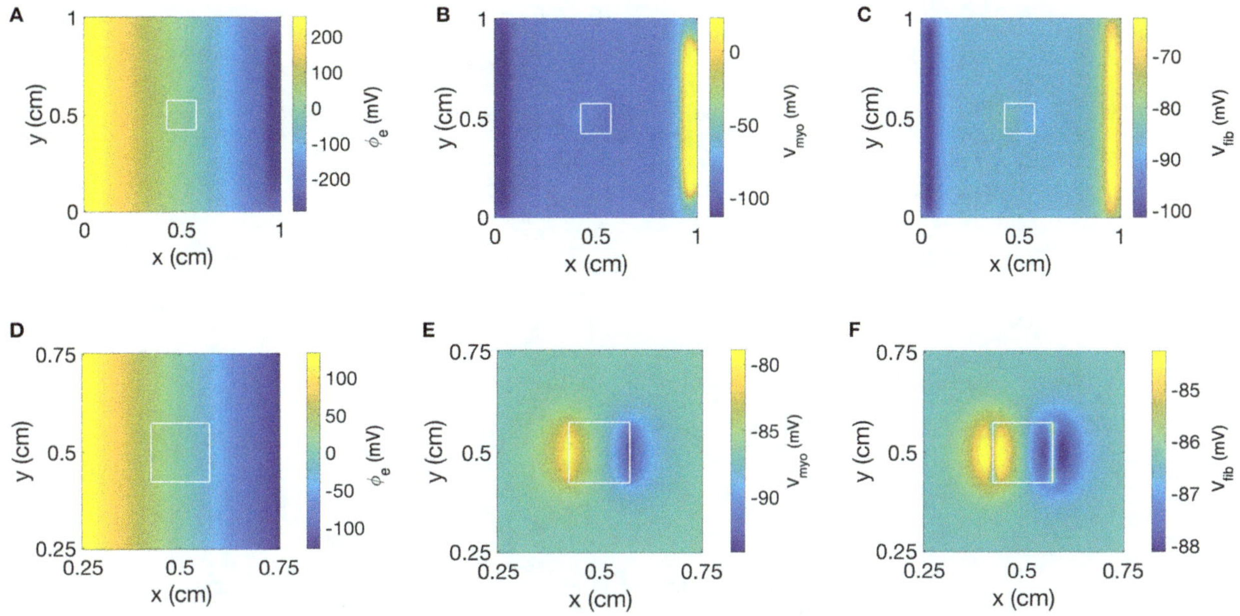

FIGURE 9 | Spatial distribution of **(A)** ϕ_e, **(B)** V_{myo}, and **(C)** V_{fib} at the end of extracellular current application in the 2D model with the square-shaped average fibrosis patch, $\overline{\sigma}_{fib}$ of 0.1 S/m and $R_{myo,fib}$ of 1 GΩ. Close-ups of the spatial distribution for **(D)** ϕ_e, **(E)** V_{myo}, and **(F)** V_{fib}. The extracellular current led to alterations of V_{myo} and V_{fib} not only at the application site, but also at the left and right border of the patch.

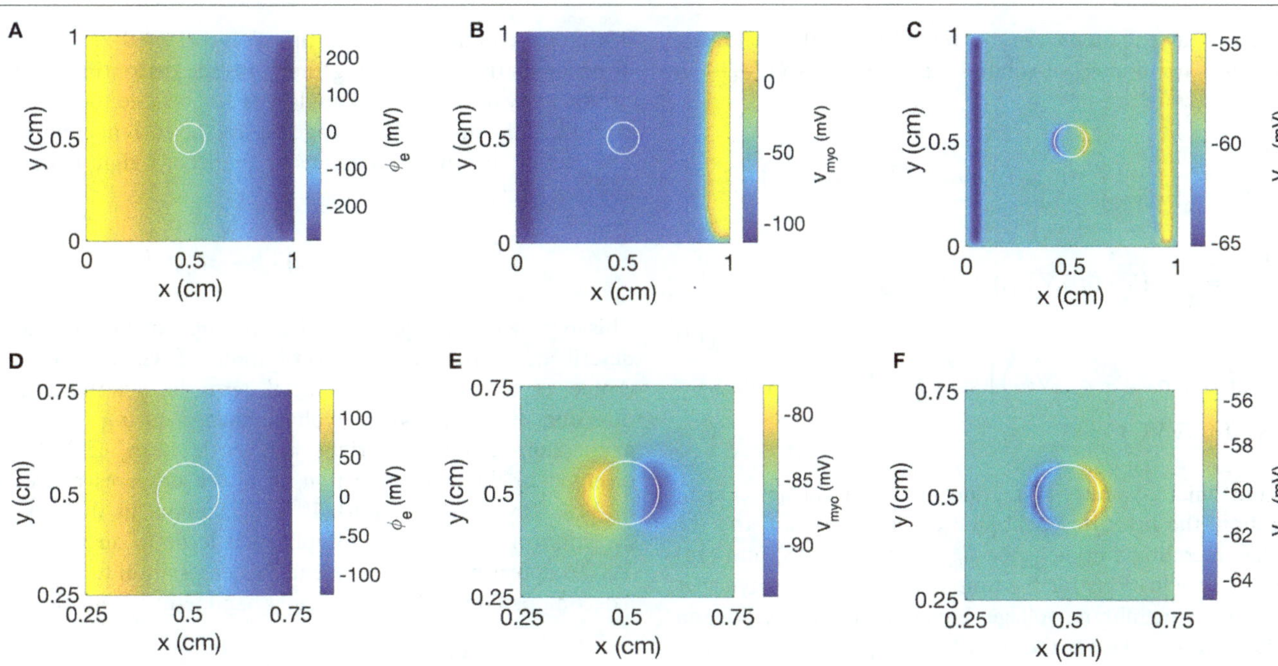

FIGURE 10 | Spatial distribution of **(A)** ϕ_e, **(B)** V_{myo}, and **(C)** V_{fib} at the end of extracellular current application in the 2D model with the disk-shaped average fibrosis patch, $\overline{\sigma}_{fib}$ of 0.1 S/m and $R_{myo,fib}$ of 1 TΩ. Close-ups of the spatial distribution for **(D)** ϕ_e, **(E)** V_{myo}, and **(F)** V_{fib} at the end of application of extracellular currents. The extracellular current led to alterations of V_{myo} and V_{fib} not only at the application site, but also at the left and right border of the patch.

of virtual electrode strength. Increased electrical coupling of myocytes with fibroblasts reduced the virtual electrode strength. Intra-fibroblast coupling reduced virtual electrodes in case of high myocyte-fibroblast coupling.

We explain our findings of depolarization and hyperpolarization of membranes during the application of the extracellular currents at the boundaries of the fibrotic patch based on reformulation of the equations for the extended

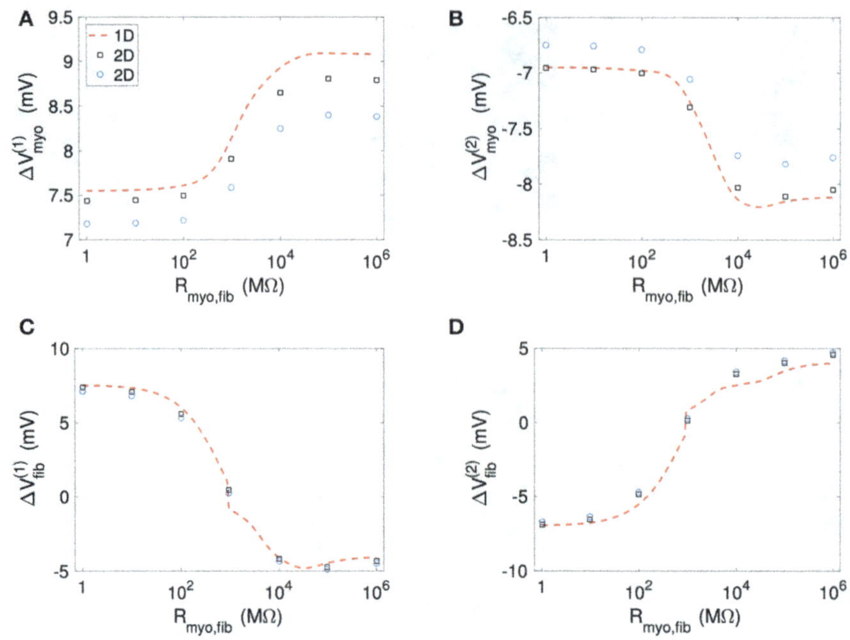

FIGURE 11 | Comparison of **(A,B)** V_{myo} and **(C,D)** V_{fib} from the 1D simulations and the 2D simulations with disk and square patch geometries. The square and circle symbols refer to the results for the respective square and disk patch geometry.

bidomain. The equations can be rewritten in the following simple form for numerical solution see Equations (17–20) in Sachse et al. (2009):

$$\frac{\partial V_{myo}}{\partial t} = \frac{1}{C_{myo}} \left(\nabla \cdot \left(\sigma_{myo} \nabla V_{myo} \right) + \nabla \cdot \left(\sigma_{myo} \nabla \phi_e \right) + \cdots \right) \tag{13}$$

$$\frac{\partial V_{fib}}{\partial t} = \frac{1}{C_{fib}} \left(\nabla \cdot \left(\sigma_{fib} \nabla V_{fib} \right) + \nabla \cdot \left(\sigma_{fib} \nabla \phi_e \right) + \cdots \right) \tag{14}$$

$$\nabla \cdot \left\{ \left(\sigma_e + \sigma_{myo} + \sigma_{fib} \nabla \phi_e \right) \right\} = -f_e - \nabla \cdot \left(\sigma_{myo} \nabla V_{myo} \right) - \nabla \cdot \left(\sigma_{fib} \nabla V_{fib} \right) \tag{15}$$

with the injected current f_e due to extracellular current application, the myocyte membrane capacitance C_{myo} and the fibroblast membrane capacitance C_{fib}. Equations (13) and (14) are parabolic equations for the time evolution of the myocytes and fibroblast membrane voltage. Equation (15) is the Poisson equation for calculating the extracellular potential. In these equations, $\cdots$ indicates terms that are not of interest for our initial discussion and hence omitted.

During the current application, we injected positive charge at the electrode located at 1–1.5 mm and negative charge of the same magnitude at the electrode located at 32.5–33 mm of the extracellular domain. This current injection produced a rather uniform gradient of ϕ_e (**Figure 2**). This corresponds to a quasi-uniform E in the system (**Figure S1**):

$$E = -\nabla \phi_e \tag{16}$$

With our computational set-up, E is oriented in the same direction as the x-axis. E together with the discontinuity of the conductivity at the patch boundary is responsible for the initial changes of the membrane voltage during the current application. This can be shown by decomposing the second right hand term of Equation (13) into:

$$\frac{\partial V_{myo}}{\partial t} \propto -\left(\nabla \sigma_{myo} \right) \cdot E + \sigma_{myo} \nabla^2 \phi_e \tag{17}$$

This represents the generalized activating function previously described to predict the distribution of virtual electrodes (Sobie et al., 1997). The crucial term in determining the direction of the membrane voltage change during the current application is the first right hand side term. If $\nabla \sigma_{myo}$ is oriented in the same direction as E one observes a decrease of V_{myo} (hyperpolarization). If $\nabla \sigma_{myo}$ points in the opposite direction of E, the current application leads to an increase of V_{myo} (depolarization). We extend this description for V_{fib} using a decomposition of the second right hand term of Equation (14):

$$\frac{\partial V_{fib}}{\partial t} \propto -\left(\nabla \sigma_{fib} \right) \cdot E + \sigma_{fib} \nabla^2 \phi_e \tag{18}$$

In our setup, due to the variations of the volume fraction of the myocytes and fibroblasts, $\nabla \sigma_{myo}$ is pointing in the opposite direction of E at point 1 of the domain, which results in a depolarization of V_{myo}. On the contrary, $\nabla \sigma_{fib}$ at point 1 is aligned with E, which results in a hyperpolarization of V_{fib} at point 1.

However, this simple mechanistic explanation ignores the coupling term between the fibroblast and the myocyte domain.

The current $I_{myo,fib}$, which is determined by the parameter $R_{myo,fib}$ and the voltage between the domains, explains why in some cases, V_{fib} follows V_{myo}. In particular, at high coupling between myocyte and fibroblast domain (i.e., low values of $R_{myo,fib}$), V_{myo} is very similar to V_{fib}. Interestingly, at intermediate values of $R_{myo,fib}$, the simulations revealed a competition of the two antagonistic effects for V_{fib} (**Figures 4, 6**). These two effects can even cancel each other out in a sort of tug of war situation, leaving V_{fib} at the patch boundary apparently unaffected by the application of the current (**Figure 9F**).

We note that the arguments presented here are valid in any spatial dimension. Based on the same arguments we also explain the mechanism behind the decrease of the virtual electrode strengths for large fibroblast-myocyte coupling. Our studies showed that due to heterogeneity of conductivity at the patch boundary, V_{fib} and V_{myo} tend to change in opposite directions. One membrane is depolarizing and the other one is hyperpolarizing, but the effect of the heterogeneities can be canceled out and even be inverted for V_{fib} because of current flow between the fibroblast and myocyte domain. This flow is lowering the effect of the conductivity heterogeneities and the virtual electrode strength. Theoretically, the current flow can go in either direction. If the fibroblast is the dominant constituent of the cardiac tissue at some heterogeneities, V_{fib} could pull V_{myo} to follow its electric depolarization or hyperpolarization. With the parameters applied in this study, myocytes were volume-wise dominant in the tissue. Thus, we did not observe such behavior.

For the 1D simulations, we reported extrema of the time evolution of ΔV_{fib} during the extracellular current application. In **Figures 4B,D**, the reported ΔV_{fib} is the largest absolute value (keeping its sign) of the monitored difference. These indicators exhibited a discontinuous behavior for intermediate values for the $R_{myo,fib}$ as exemplified in **Figures 4B,D**. The discontinuity is caused by the transition between dominant minima and maxima of V_{fib} as illustrated in **Figure S2B**. The transition occurred at decreased $R_{myo,fib}$, when increasing $\overline{\sigma}_{fib}$. This can be explained by the fact that the pull exerted by the myocytes on the fibroblasts diffuses faster when the diffusion is increased and is therefore less effective.

The 1D simulations for the large fibrosis revealed a complex behavior of V_{myo}. In **Figures 5A,C**, discontinuities occurred at intermediate values of $R_{myo,fib}$. This was caused by block of the propagating waves prior to the extracellular current application at the fibrotic patch, which modified the values of V_{myo}. Though this effect is important for the dynamics of the system, in the context of our study it did affect only marginally ΔV_{fib} and ΔV_{myo}.

In our 2D simulations, the influence of patch geometry on ΔV_{fib} was small (**Figures 11C,D**). This can be explained by the fact that the space constant for the fibroblast model is very small (computed previously around 0.15 mm) vs. the patch size of 1.5 mm. We refer the reader to Bittihn et al. (2012) for a more detailed description of the underlying mechanism.

A straightforward conclusion from our study is that fibrotic patches, similar as endo- and epicardial surfaces as well as blood vessels, constitute a potential site for wave initiation in response to defibrillation. This finding could help in parameterization of defibrillators. We suggest that further studies will lead to defibrillator protocols specifically for patients with known myocardial fibrosis to ensure defibrillation success. Also, based on our findings we propose that knowledge in the spatial distribution of fibrosis is valuable for optimization of positions for defibrillation electrodes. Potential clinical benefits of accounting for cardiac fibrosis are reduction in myocardial injury due to optimized defibrillation energy.

Prior studies on modeling of effects of fibrosis aimed at characterization of conduction and conduction defects as well as arrhythmogenesis and maintenance of arrhythmia in the atria and ventricles. Fibrosis was introduced in the models with various approaches including embedding of conduction barriers of various sizes and geometries, reduction of inter-myocyte coupling, regional replacement of myocytes with fibroblasts or myofibroblasts, and incorporation of myocyte-fibroblast coupling (Fishler, 1998; Fishler and Vepa, 1998; Mcdowell et al., 2012; Costa et al., 2014; Zeigler et al., 2016). Here, we applied the extended bidomain model to integrate various aspects of fibrotic remodeling.

A difficulty of applying the extended bidomain model is that we have only vague knowledge on parameters related to the fibroblast domain, in particular, the parameters $R_{myo,fib}$ and σ_{fib}. Quantitative measurements of these parameters have not been performed in normal and diseased myocardium (Kohl and Gourdie, 2014). However, a small number of *in vitro* measurements provided quantitative information to constrain these parameters. Beyond those, qualitative and indirect evidence suggests that etiologies and the progression of fibrotic remodeling affect the degree of myocyte-fibroblast and fibroblast-fibroblast electrical coupling in diseased myocardium. For these reasons, computational studies with the extended bidomain model and other computational modeling approaches commonly applied measurements from *in vitro* studies to justify parameter settings or varied parameters to reconstruct experimental findings. In this study, we chose to vary parameters within a wide range to go beyond the *in vitro* measurements and comprehensively explore potential effects of coupling.

We varied $R_{myo,fib}$ from 1 MΩ to 1 TΩ to describe strong and negligible electrical coupling, respectively, between fibroblasts and myocytes. The lower limit is close to the junctional resistance of a myocyte pair isolated from rabbit ventricular tissue (0.81 MΩ) (Kieval et al., 1992). The upper limit led to negligible currents between the fibroblast and myocyte domain, and effectively represents the case of electrical uncoupling of the domains. Experimental measurements on myocyte-fibroblast pairs in 24 h-old culture of neonatal rat hearts cells suggest that $R_{myo,fib}$ is variable and within a range of 125 MΩ and 3.23 GΩ (Rook et al., 1992). The variability was explained by the variable number of gap junction channels of the myocyte-fibroblast pairs. Prior modeling work applied measurements of gap junction channel conductances in the same preparation and assumed 10 to 30 gap junction channels per cell pair to vary $R_{myo,fib}$ from 1.11 to 3.33 GΩ for simulation of fibroblast effects in the sinoatrial node (Rook et al., 1989; Kohl et al., 1994). Assuming 0 to 75 gap junctions per cell pair, $R_{myo,fib}$ was varied from 0.44 to ∞ GΩ in a modeling study of fibroblast effects on conduction (Jacquemet and Henriquez, 2007). Based on the prior experimental and computational studies, the lower $R_{myo,fib}$ limit (1 MΩ) in our studies appears small. We note that effects of $R_{myo,fib}$ between 1 and 10 MΩ on virtual electrodes were in general similar. This range represents the extreme case of strong myocyte-fibroblast coupling. Increasing the lower limit of the parameter range to e.g., 1 GΩ does not change our conclusions on the relationship between $R_{myo,fib}$ and virtual electrodes.

We varied $\overline{\sigma}_{fib}$ from 0 to 0.5 S/m to describe absence of electrical coupling and strong coupling, respectively, within the fibroblast domain. The lower limit represents the case of electrical uncoupling of fibroblasts. The upper limit is identical to our setting of σ_{myo}. Dependent on Vol_{fib} (Equation 9), this led to a range of σ_{fib} of 0 and up to 0.1 S/m in the region with high fibrosis with Vol_{fib} of 20%. An experimental framework for estimating σ_{fib} comprises measurements of junctional conductance in pairs of cultured rat cardiac cells. Conductances of fibroblast-fibroblasts pairs were in the range of 175 pS and 6 nS (Rook et al., 1992). Measurements of conductance in myocyte-myocyte pairs were up to 42 nS (Rook et al., 1990). Estimates of conductance based on gap-junctional area in myocyte pairs range between 0.9 and 216.6 nS. These measurements and estimates of conductance between cell pairs are not sufficient to determine σ_{fib} in normal and diseased myocardium. Further information on fibroblast geometry, gap junction distribution and cytosolic conductivity would be required to estimate σ_{fib} using computational approaches introduced by us previously (Bauer et al., 2013; Greiner et al., 2018). Considering that conductances of freshly isolated ventricular myocyte-myocyte pairs from control rabbit hearts were much higher (1.24 ± 0.25 μS) (Kieval et al., 1992), it is also unclear how the *in vitro* measurements relate to conductance in native myocardium. However, based on this information and the explored volume fractions, we argue that σ_{fib} cannot be larger than σ_{myo} even in the region of high fibrosis with identical volume fractions for the fibroblast and myocyte domain. In this region, our calculations (Equations 8, 9) using the maximal $\overline{\sigma}_{fib}$ (0.5 S/m) led to identical σ_{fib} and σ_{myo} (0.1 S/m). Prior modeling studies of electrical conduction in human atrial tissues applied σ_{fib} in the range of 0.02–0.1 S/m (Greisas and Zlochiver, 2016). Also, σ_{fib} was set to 0.06 S/m in a study on rabbit heart (Corrias et al., 2012). Based on these arguments and the prior work, we limited the exploration of σ_{fib} to values up to 0.1 S/m in our simulations. We note that this value is the maximum in our simulations and it is likely that smaller values in the explored range are more realistic. For small Vol_{fib} and thus sparse inter-fibroblast coupling, we point the reader at our simulations with σ_{fib} equal to zero.

We note that, despite the large flexibility of the extended bidomain model to describe tissue remodeling, the computational demands of the model are similar as for conventional bidomain models. A minor increase of computational demands is caused by the integration of the fibroblast domain.

We suggest that the extended bidomain model provides a more comprehensive framework for modeling of conduction in control and diseased tissue than the conventional bidomain model. While the additional parameters enable already more detailed parameterization, various refinements can be envisioned. For instance, an alternative method to define the effective volume density (1/m^3) of electrical connections between fibroblasts and myocytes is:

$$\beta_{myo,fib} = \beta^{(r)} \frac{Vol_{fib}}{Vol_{fib,single}} \tag{19}$$

Because the electrical coupling between the fibroblasts and myocytes is mainly unknown and potentially varies from one situation to another we can define a parameter, $\beta^{(r)}$ (dimensionless), for characterizing this coupling. A value of $\beta^{(r)}$ = 1 corresponds to a situation where each of the fibroblasts has an electrical connection with the myocyte domain. A larger (smaller) value of $\beta^{(r)}$ allows changing this situation. For $\beta^{(r)} < 1$ not all the fibroblasts are coupled to a myocyte and conversely for $\beta^{(r)} > 1$ each fibroblast is coupled to more than one myocyte. Both, $R_{myo,fib}$ and $\beta^{(r)}$ are factors that contribute to the coupling between myocytes and fibroblasts and hence their effective influence can be combined in a single variable, $\beta^{(\mathrm{fract})}$ defined as:

$$\beta^{(fract)} = \frac{\beta^{(r)}}{R_{myo,fib}} \tag{20}$$

Limitations

We acknowledge several limitations related to the presented work. The studies were performed in 1D and 2D domains with isotropic conductivities. We did not consider unequal anisotropy ratios of conductivities. We applied simple descriptions of fibrotic remodeling derived from a rabbit model of cardiac infarction. While fibrotic remodeling is known to be a multi-faceted process comprising e.g., activation of fibroblasts, their differentiation into myofibroblasts, and subcellular remodeling of structural und electrophysiological properties, we primarily considered increased volume ratios of cells and the extracellular space in our study. Also, we applied mathematical models of normal myocytes and fibroblasts, and did not adjust these models to account for fibrosis and associated remodeling.

A limitation of our work is related to incomplete understanding of myocyte-fibroblast and fibroblast-fibroblast coupling in the heart. As discussed above, experimental measurements exist only for *in vitro* models and it is difficult to apply these measurements for parameterization of models of fibrotic remodeling in native myocardium. Also, we applied a simple linear model for scaling of σ_{fib} by Vol_{fib} (Equation 9). Non-linear models might be more realistic. In particular, for small Vol_{fib}, it is likely that fibroblasts are not electrically coupled with other fibroblasts, which can be reflected by a model using piece-wise defined functions. We note the controversy on myocyte-fibroblast coupling and the contribution of fibroblasts in physiological and pathophysiological conduction (Kohl and Gourdie, 2014). Based on our simulations, myocyte-fibroblast coupling is a major determinant of virtual electrode strength. However, for the entire simulated range of myocyte-fibroblast coupling, boundaries of fibrotic patches were associated with virtual electrodes.

In our comparison of software for extended bidomain modeling, we confirmed that the new and our prior implementation yielded very similar results when simulating a homogenous tissue. Peak V_{myo} and V_{fib} differed only by 5.08% (13.98 vs. 13.3 mV) and 5.23% (13.69 vs. 13.03 mV), respectively. However, we noticed that the approach for discretization of the patch boundary affects the magnitude of the altered membrane voltages. Conventional finite difference discretization (Sachse, 2004) led to significant differences vs. the finite volume discretization used in our studies. We reduced differences to the finite volume method by implementation of a finite difference approximation based on Kirchhoff's law (Witwer et al., 1972). However, the appropriate modeling approach should be dictated by the spatial distribution of the structural remodeling. While our finite volume approach described structural remodeling as an abrupt change from control tissue to the fibrotic patch, a gradual approach might be more appropriate (Seidel et al., 2017).

A related limitation of our study is the geometry and size of patches explored in the 2D simulations. We focused on disk and square shaped patches with a single size. Larger effects of geometry are expected for smaller sizes, i.e., below the millimeter scale, but we leave this for a future exploration. Also, we suggest that microscopic imaging can provide insights into the detailed distribution of remodeling.

AUTHOR CONTRIBUTIONS

JB and FS designed the study. All authors developed software for this project, analyzed, and interpreted the data, drafted and critically revised the manuscript, and approved the version to be published.

ACKNOWLEDGMENTS

We thank Mr. Marcus Blackburn, Mr. Joachim Greiner, and Dr. Gunnar Seemann for their help and discussions. We also thank Mr. Haonan Yang and Mrs. Nancy Allen for technical support.

REFERENCES

Al-Khatib, S. M., Stevenson, W. G., Ackerman, M. J., Bryant, W. J., Callans, D. J., Curtis, A. B., et al. (2017). 2017 AHA/ACC/HRS Guideline for Management of Patients With Ventricular Arrhythmias and the Prevention of Sudden Cardiac Death: A Report of the American College of Cardiology/American Heart Association Task Force on Clinical Practice Guidelines and the Heart Rhythm Society. *Circulation* 138:e272–e391. doi: 10.1161/CIR.0000000000000549

Balay, S., Abhyankar, S., Adams, M. F., Brown, J., Brune, P., Buschelman, K., et al. (2018). *PETSc Users Manual.* Argonne National Laboratory.

Bauer, S., Edelmann, J. C., Seemann, G., Sachse, F. B., and Dossel, O. (2013). Estimating intracellular conductivity tensors from confocal microscopy of rabbit ventricular tissue. *Biomed. Tech.* 58(Suppl. 1). doi: 10.1515/bmt-2013-4333. Available online at: https://www.degruyter.com/view/j/bmte.2013.58.issue-s1-N/bmt-2013-4333/bmt-2013-4333.xml

Bittihn, P., Horning, M., and Luther, S. (2012). Negative curvature boundaries as wave emitting sites for the control of biological excitable media. *Phys. Rev. Lett.* 109:118106. doi: 10.1103/PhysRevLett.109.118106

Cellml (2008a). *Electrophysiological Modeling of Fibroblasts and Their Interaction with Myocytes [Online].* Available online at: https://models.cellml.org/exposure/4e478093480e0d7e08a2f24177ec4906. (Accessed October 1, 2018).

Cellml (2008b). *A Rabbit Ventricular Action Potential Model Replicating Cardiac Dynamics at Rapid Heart Rates [Online].* Available online at: https://models.cellml.org/exposure/a5586b72d07ce03fc40fc98ee846d7a5 (Accessed October 1, 2018).

Cevik, C., Perez-Verdia, A., and Nugent, K. (2009). Implantable cardioverter defibrillators and their role in heart failure progression. *Europace* 11, 710–715. doi: 10.1093/europace/eup091

Connolly, A., Vigmond, E., and Bishop, M. (2017a). Virtual electrodes around anatomical structures and their roles in defibrillation. *PLoS ONE* 12:e0173324. doi: 10.1371/journal.pone.0173324

Connolly, A. J., Vigmond, E., and Bishop, M. J. (2017b). Bidomain predictions of virtual electrode-induced make and break excitations around blood vessels. *Front Bioeng Biotechnol.* 5:18. doi: 10.3389/fbioe.2017.00018

Corrias, A., Pathmanathan, P., Gavaghan, D. J., and Buist, M. L. (2012). Modelling tissue electrophysiology with multiple cell types: applications of the extended bidomain framework. *Integr. Biol.* 4, 192–201. doi: 10.1039/c2ib00100d

Costa, C. M., Campos, F. O., Prassl, A. J., Dos Santos, R. W., Sanchez-Quintana, D., Ahammer, H., et al. (2014). An efficient finite element approach for modeling fibrotic clefts in the heart. *IEEE Trans. Biomed. Eng.* 61, 900–910. doi: 10.1109/TBME.2013.2292320

Dosdall, D. J., Fast, V. G., and Ideker, R. E. (2010). Mechanisms of defibrillation. *Annu. Rev. Biomed. Eng.* 12, 233–258. doi: 10.1146/annurev-bioeng-070909-105305

Entcheva, E., Eason, J., Efimov, I. R., Cheng, Y., Malkin, R., and Claydon, F. (1998). Virtual electrode effects in transvenous defibrillation-modulation by structure and interface: evidence from bidomain simulations and optical mapping. *J. Cardiovasc. Electrophysiol.* 9, 949–961. doi: 10.1111/j.1540-8167.1998.tb00135.x

Entcheva, E., Trayanova, N. A., and Claydon, F. J. (1999). Patterns of and mechanisms for shock-induced polarization in the heart: a bidomain analysis. *IEEE Trans. Biomed. Eng.* 46, 260–270. doi: 10.1109/10.748979

Fishler, M. G. (1998). Syncytial heterogeneity as a mechanism underlying cardiac far-field stimulation during defibrillation-level shocks. *J. Cardiovasc. Electrophysiol.* 9, 384–394. doi: 10.1111/j.1540-8167.1998.tb00926.x

Fishler, M. G., and Vepa, K. (1998). Spatiotemporal effects of syncytial heterogeneities on cardiac far-field excitations during monophasic and biphasic shocks. *J. Cardiovasc. Electrophysiol.* 9, 1310–1324. doi: 10.1111/j.1540-8167.1998.tb00107.x

Garny, A., Nickerson, D. P., Cooper, J., Weber Dos Santos, R., Miller, A. K., Mckeever, S., et al. (2008). CellML and associated tools and techniques. *Philos. Trans. A Math. Phys. Eng. Sci.* 366, 3017–3043. doi: 10.1098/rsta.2008.0094

Greiner, J., Sankarankutty, A. C., Seemann, G., Seidel, T., and Sachse, F. B. (2018). Confocal microscopy-based estimation of parameters for computational modeling of electrical conduction in the normal and infarcted heart. *Front. Physiol.* 9:239. doi: 10.3389/fphys.2018.00239

Greisas, A., and Zlochiver, S. (2016). The multi-domain fibroblast/myocyte coupling in the cardiac tissue: a theoretical study. *Cardiovasc. Eng. Technol.* 7, 290–304. doi: 10.1007/s13239-016-0266-x

Henriquez, C. S. (1993). Simulating the electrical behavior of cardiac tissue using the bidomain model. *Crit. Rev. Biomed. Eng.* 21, 1–77.

Iles, L., Pfluger, H., Lefkovits, L., Butler, M. J., Kistler, P. M., Kaye, D. M., et al. (2011). Myocardial fibrosis predicts appropriate device therapy in patients with implantable cardioverter-defibrillators for primary prevention of sudden cardiac death. *J. Am. Coll. Cardiol.* 57, 821–828. doi: 10.1016/j.jacc.2010.06.062

Jacquemet, V., and Henriquez, C. S. (2007). Modelling cardiac fibroblasts: interactions with myocytes and their impact on impulse propagation. *Europace* 9(Suppl. 6), vi29–37. doi: 10.1093/europace/eum207

Kieval, R. S., Spear, J. F., and Moore, E. N. (1992). Gap junctional conductance in ventricular myocyte pairs isolated from postischemic rabbit myocardium. *Circ. Res.* 71, 127–136. doi: 10.1161/01.RES.71.1.127

Kohl, P., and Gourdie, R. G. (2014). Fibroblast-myocyte electrotonic coupling: does it occur in native cardiac tissue? *J. Mol. Cell. Cardiol.* 70, 37–46. doi: 10.1016/j.yjmcc.2013.12.024

Kohl, P., Kamkin, A. G., Kiseleva, I. S., and Noble, D. (1994). Mechanosensitive fibroblasts in the sino-atrial node region of rat heart: interaction with cardiomyocytes and possible role. *Exp. Physiol.* 79, 943–956. doi: 10.1113/expphysiol.1994.sp003819

Mahajan, A., Shiferaw, Y., Sato, D., Baher, A., Olcese, R., Xie, L. H., et al. (2008). A rabbit ventricular action potential model replicating cardiac dynamics at rapid heart rates. *Biophys. J.* 94, 392–410. doi: 10.1529/biophysj.106.98160

Mcdowell, K. S., Vadakkumpadan, F., Blake, R., Blauer, J., Plank, G., Macleod, R. S., et al. (2012). Methodology for patient-specific modeling of atrial fibrosis as a substrate for atrial fibrillation. *J. Electrocardiol.* 45, 640–645. doi: 10.1016/j.jelectrocard.2012.08.005

Plonsey, R., and Barr, R. C. (2007). *Bioelectricity: A Quantitative Approach.* New York, NY: Springer.

Pumir, A., and Krinsky, V. (1999). Unpinning of a rotating wave in cardiac muscle by an electric field. *J. Theor. Biol.* 199, 311–319. doi: 10.1006/jtbi.1999.0957

Rook, M. B., De Jonge, B., Jongsma, H. J., and Masson-Pevet, M. A. (1990). Gap junction formation and functional interaction between neonatal rat cardiocytes in culture: a correlative physiological and ultrastructural study. *J. Membr. Biol.* 118, 179–192. doi: 10.1007/BF01868475

Rook, M. B., Jongsma, H. J., and De Jonge, B. (1989). Single channel currents of homo- and heterologous gap junctions between cardiac fibroblasts and myocytes. *Pflugers Arch.* 414, 95–98. doi: 10.1007/BF00585633

Rook, M. B., Van Ginneken, A. C., De Jonge, B., El Aoumari, A., Gros, D., and Jongsma, H. J. (1992). Differences in gap junction channels between cardiac myocytes, fibroblasts, and heterologous pairs. *Am. J. Physiol.* 263, C959–977. doi: 10.1152/ajpcell.1992.263.5.C959

Sachse, F. B. (2004). *Computational Cardiology: Modeling of Anatomy, Electrophysiology, and Mechanics.* Berlin; New York, NY: Springer. doi: 10.1007/b96841

Sachse, F. B., Moreno, A. P., and Abildskov, J. A. (2008). Electrophysiological modeling of fibroblasts and their interaction with myocytes. *Ann. Biomed. Eng.* 36, 41–56. doi: 10.1007/s10439-007-9405-8

Sachse, F. B., Moreno, A. P., Seemann, G., and Abildskov, J. A. (2009). A model of electrical conduction in cardiac tissue including fibroblasts. *Ann. Biomed. Eng.* 37, 874–889. doi: 10.1007/s10439-009-9667-4

Seemann, G., Sachse, F. B., Karl, M., Weiss, D. L., Heuveline, V., and Dössel, O. (2010). "Framework for modular, flexible and efficient solving the cardiac bidomain equation using PETSc," in *Progress in Industrial Mathematics at ECMI 2008*, eds A. D. Fitt, J. Norbury, H. Ockendon, and E. Wilson (Berlin; Heidelberg: Springer), 363–369. doi: 10.1007/978-3-642-12110-4_55

Seidel, T., Sankarankutty, A. C., and Sachse, F. B. (2017). Remodeling of the transverse tubular system after myocardial infarction in rabbit correlates with local fibrosis: a potential role of biomechanics. *Prog. Biophys. Mol. Biol.* 130, 302–314. doi: 10.1016/j.pbiomolbio.2017.07.006

Shibukawa, Y., Chilton, E. L., Maccannell, K. A., Clark, R. B., and Giles, W. R. (2005). K+ currents activated by depolarization in cardiac fibroblasts. *Biophys. J.* 88, 3924–3935. doi: 10.1529/biophysj.104.054429

Sobie, E. A., Susil, R. C., and Tung, L. (1997). A generalized activating function for predicting virtual electrodes in cardiac tissue. *Biophys. J.* 73, 1410–1423. doi: 10.1016/S0006-3495(97)78173-6

Tung, L. (1978). *A Bi-Domain Model for Describing Ischemic Myocardial d-c Potentials.* Ph.D. Thesis, MIT, Cambridge, MA.

Witwer, J. G., Trezek, G. J., and Jewett, D. L. (1972). The effect of media inhomogeneities upon intracranial electrical fields. *IEEE Trans. Biomed. Eng.* 19, 352–362. doi: 10.1109/TBME.1972.324138

Zeigler, A. C., Richardson, W. J., Holmes, J. W., and Saucerman, J. J. (2016). Computational modeling of cardiac fibroblasts and fibrosis. *J. Mol. Cell. Cardiol.* 93, 73–83. doi: 10.1016/j.yjmcc.2015.11.020

7

Heterogeneous Effects of Fibroblast-Myocyte Coupling in Different Regions of the Human Atria Under Conditions of Atrial Fibrillation

*Jorge Sánchez, Juan F. Gomez, Laura Martinez-Mateu, Lucia Romero, Javier Saiz and Beatriz Trenor**

Centre for Research and Innovation in Bioengineering, Universitat Politècnica de València, Valencia, Spain

Correspondence:
Beatriz Trenor
btrenor@eln.upv.es

Background: Atrial fibrillation (AF), the most common cardiac arrhythmia, is characterized by alteration of the action potential (AP) propagation. Under persistent AF, myocytes undergo electrophysiological and structural remodeling, which involves fibroblast proliferation and differentiation, modifying the substrate for AP propagation. The aim of this study was to analyze the effects on the AP of fibroblast-myocyte coupling during AF and its propagation in different regions of the atria.

Methods: Isolated myocytes were coupled to different numbers of fibroblasts using the established AP models and tissue simulations were performed by randomly distributing fibroblasts. Fibroblast formulations were updated to match recent experimental data. Major ion current conductances of the myocyte model were modified to simulate AP heterogeneity in four different atrial regions (right atrium posterior wall, crista terminalis, left atrium posterior wall, and pulmonary vein) according to experimental and computational studies.

Results: The results of the coupled myocyte-fibroblast simulations suggest that a more depolarized membrane potential and higher fibroblast membrane capacitance have a greater impact on AP duration and myocyte maximum depolarization velocity. The number of coupled fibroblasts and the stimulation frequency are determining factors in altering myocyte AP. Strand simulations show that conduction velocity tends to homogenize in all regions, while the left atrium is more likely to be affected by fibroblast and AP propagation block is more likely to occur. The pulmonary vein is the most affected region, even at low fibroblast densities. In 2D sheets with randomly placed fibroblasts, wavebreaks are observed in the low density (10%) central fibrotic zone and when fibroblast density increases (40%) propagation in the fibrotic region is practically blocked. At densities of 10 and 20% the width of the vulnerable window increases with respect to control but is decreased at 40%.

Conclusion: Myocyte-fibroblast coupling characteristics heterogeneously affect AP propagation and features in the different atrial zones, and myocytes from the left atria are more sensitive to fibroblast coupling.

Keywords: atrial fibrillation, computer simulation, structural remodeling, myofibroblast, vulnerability

INTRODUCTION

Atrial fibrillation (AF) is the most common cardiac arrhythmia and is becoming more prevalent with population aging (Iwasaki et al., 2011). In persistent atrial fibrillation (PeAF), lasting longer than 7 days (Kirchhof et al., 2016), spontaneous, pharmacological, or ablative resumption of sinus rhythm is infrequent with prompt recurrences or commonly failed cardioversions (Jalife and Kaur, 2015).

In PeAF, cardiac tissue experiences structural and electrical remodeling driven by changes of the extracellular matrix, fibroblast differentiation, fatty and inflammatory infiltration, and ion channel remodeling, among other alterations (Kirchhof et al., 2016). The heterogeneities in the atrial substrate cause fiber discontinuities and local conduction disturbances favoring re-entries (Nattel and Dobrev, 2017).

The atria have a complex anatomical structure, differences between the right and left atrium, and complex structures like the pulmonary vein or left and right appendages (Sanchez-Quintana et al., 2012; Ferrer et al., 2015). They all have their own electrophysiological characteristics, which determine specific action potential (AP) waveforms and conduction velocities (CV), which are crucial to AF pathophysiology.

Approximately 75% of the adult myocardium tissue volume is occupied by myocytes, accounting for only 30–40% of the total number of cells (Biernacka and Frangogiannis, 2011). Fibroblasts are considered as the predominant non-myocyte cell. They become active under inflammatory response and then differentiate into myofibroblasts (Chacar et al., 2017) by different pathways (e.g., oxidative stress, atrial dilatation, calcium overload, and inflammation), although the precise mechanisms have not yet been established (Jalife and Kaur, 2015). Myofibroblasts differ from fibroblasts in that they develop contractile proteins and exhibit a more depolarized resting membrane potential (Salvarani et al., 2017) and greater membrane capacitance (Sridhar et al., 2017). The differences in resting membrane potential and membrane capacitance between fibroblasts and myofibroblasts might have an important repercussion on the electrophysiology of coupled myocytes.

Recent experimental studies have shown that fibroblasts express voltage-dependent sodium channels allowing an inward current (I_{Na}) (Chatelier et al., 2012; Koivumäki et al., 2014a; Poulet et al., 2016). Although they are not electrically excitable they may affect the myocytes' electrophysiological properties (Gaudesius et al., 2003; Kohl et al., 2005; Miragoli et al., 2006). Several animal experimental models have shown that fibroblasts electrically couple to myocytes and alter their AP (Rook et al., 1992; Gaudesius et al., 2003; Burstein et al., 2007; Rohr, 2011; Jalife and Kaur, 2015; Jousset et al., 2016; Quinn et al., 2016). Kohl et al. (1994) found that fibroblasts reacted electrically with myocytes through gap junctions and this was later corroborated *in vitro* in several animal species (Gaudesius et al., 2003; Camelliti et al., 2004; Kohl et al., 2005). However, the extent of (*in vivo*) fibroblast-myocyte electrotonic coupling in native myocardium remains controversial (Kohl and Gourdie, 2014). Recently, a study by Quinn et al. (2016) showed the existence of tunneling nanotube connections between excitable and non-excitable cells (e.g., myofibroblasts) in cardiac scar border tissue at the border zone of the scar in mice hearts. Similarly, Burstein et al. (2007) observed fibroblasts proliferation and differentiation into myofibroblasts during AF *in vivo* canine hearts. Fibroblast proliferation has also been observed in human hearts (Krul et al., 2015; Fukumoto et al., 2016), in regions with altered conduction velocity, although electrical coupling has not been demonstrated.

Computational simulations of the cellular electrophysiology have become a powerful tool for studying the role that fibroblasts play in the atrial substrate (MacCannell et al., 2007; Maleckar et al., 2009; Koivumäki et al., 2014a). Their flexibility permits modifying the cellular electrophysiology and varying different characteristics to analyze the impact of electrotonic coupling with electrically remodeled myocytes in PeAF (McDowell et al., 2013; Morgan et al., 2014; Sridhar et al., 2017). MacCannell et al. (2007) formulated an active and a passive model for fibroblasts electrophysiology, considering a capacitance and an ohmic resistance in the first case and a capacitance and four ionic currents in the second case. The active model is more realistic and has a major impact on myocytes, this is why in the present study the active model is implemented. Simulations also offer the possibility of studying how fibroblasts can change arrhythmia dynamics by reducing CV and introducing heterogeneities in the atrial substrate (Tanaka et al., 2007; Saha et al., 2018).

The present simulation study analyzes the effects of fibroblast-myocyte coupling in PeAF in specific structurally and electrophysiologically remodeled atrial tissues and compares the effect of fibroblasts and myofibroblasts on myocyte AP features, tissue conduction velocity and vulnerability to re-entries.

MATERIALS AND METHODS

Myocyte Electrophysiological Models

The human atrial AP model proposed by Koivumäki et al. (2011) was used to simulate atrial APs. To reproduce the tissue electrophysiology of different anatomical atrial regions, we modified the conductance of five ionic currents: transient outward K^+ current (I_{to}), potassium rapid current (I_{Kr}), potassium slow current (I_{Ks}), time independent K^+ current (I_{K1}), and L-type Ca^{2+} current (I_{CaL}) as proposed in previous simulation studies (Krueger et al., 2012; Ferrer et al., 2015). The conductance values, shown in **Table 1**, were modified according to the experimental values to reproduce the AP waveform in all four regions: right atrium posterior wall (RA), crista terminalis (CT), left atrium posterior wall (LA), and the pulmonary vein (PV) areas.

Ionic Remodeling

Table 2 shows the values used to introduce AF electrical remodeling in all atrial regions by modifying ion channel conductances for I_{CaL}, I_{to}, I_{K1}, sustained outward K^+ current

TABLE 1 | Ionic conductance modifications.

Channel conductance	RA	LA	PV	CT
g_{to}	1.0	1.0	0.25	0.55
g_{Kr}	1.0	1.6	4.8	0.55
g_{CaL}	1.0	0.67	0.3	1.0
g_{K1}	1.0	1.0	0.7425	1.0
g_{Ks}	1.0	1.0	5.12	1.0

Relative values for each atrial region (right atrium -RA-, left atrium -LA-, pulmonary veins -PV- and crista terminalis -CT-) with respect to the maximum conductance of the potassium transient outward current (g_{to}), potassium rapid current (g_{Kr}), calcium L-type current (g_{CaL}), and potassium slow current (g_{Ks}) in the Koivumäki et al. (2011) model.

(I_{sus}), Na^+/Ca^{2+} exchanger (NCX), sarcoplasmic reticulum Ca^{2+} ATPase (SERCA) pump, and ryanodine receptors (RyR), and specific calcium handling parameters, such as phospholamban (PLB), sarcolipin (SLN), and the baseline phosphorylation (phos). Dilation was also modeled by increasing the length of the cell by a factor of 1.1 (see **Table 2**) as described in Koivumäki et al. (2014b).

Fibroblast Electrophysiological Model

Fibroblast electrophysiology was represented according to the Koivumäki et al. (2014a) model. Membrane sodium current was updated to match recent experimental results (Poulet et al., 2016) (see **Supplementary Table S1**). The uncoupled fibroblast resting membrane potential (RMP_f) was set to −45 or −26 mV, as suggested by experimental data (Poulet et al., 2016; Salvarani et al., 2017). These values were obtained by shifting the gating variable for the time dependent potassium current as in previous simulation studies (Maleckar et al., 2009; Morgan et al., 2016), and shown in **Supplementary Table S2**. The fibroblast membrane capacitance (C_{mf}) values were varied within experimental ranges (6.3 and 50.4 pF) (MacCannell et al., 2007; Xie et al., 2009; McArthur et al., 2015; Poulet et al., 2016; Sridhar et al., 2017). Following previous experimental and simulation studies, we set RMP_f to −45 mV and C_{mf} to 6.3 pF for atrial fibroblasts (MacCannell et al., 2007; Maleckar et al., 2009), and a more depolarized RMP_f of −26 mV and a C_{mf} of 50.4 pF for atrial myofibroblasts (Morgan et al., 2016; Poulet et al., 2016; Salvarani et al., 2017; Sridhar et al., 2017). The code is available and can be found at http://hdl.handle.net/10251/120395.

TABLE 2 | Atrial fibrillation electrical remodeling.

L_{cell}	g_{CaL}	g_{to}	g_{sus}	g_{K1}	K_{NaCa}	cpumps	PLB	SLN	phos	RyR
1.1	0.41	0.38	0.62	1.62	1.5	0.84	1.18	0.6	2	2

Based on experimental observations/prior computational works (Koivumäki et al., 2014b), to account for persistent atrial fibrillation remodeling the ionic and cellular parameters modified were: cell length (L_{cell}), conductance of calcium L-type current (g_{CaL}), conductance of potassium transient outward current (g_{to}), conductance of potassium sustained current (g_{sus}), conductance of potassium inward rectifier (g_{K1}), maximum conductance of Na+/Ca2+ exchanger (K_{NaCa}), conductance of sarcoplasmic reticulum Ca2+ ATPase (SERCA) pump (cpumps), phospholamban (PLB), sarcolipin (SLN), baseline phosphorylation (phos), and ryanodine receptors (RyR). The values indicate the factor by which the original values are multiplied.

Cellular Simulations (0D)

To compute the membrane potential in a cell, Equations (1, 2, and 3) were used:

$$C_{myo}\frac{dV_{myo}}{dt} + I_{ion-myo} + I_{gap} = 0 \quad (1)$$

$$C_{fib}\frac{dV_{fib}}{dt} + I_{ion-fib} - I_{gap} = 0 \quad (2)$$

$$I_{gap} = \sum_{i=0}^{n} G_{gap}\left(V_{myo} - V_{fib_i}\right) \quad (3)$$

where C_{myo} is the membrane capacitance of the myocyte, $I_{ion-myo}$ is the total ionic current flowing through ionic channels of the myocyte, V_{myo} is the membrane potential in the myocyte, C_{fib} is the membrane capacitance of the fibroblast, $I_{ion-fib}$ is the total ionic current flowing through ionic channels of the fibroblast, V_{fib} the membrane potential in the fibroblast, I_{gap} is the total ionic current flowing through the gap junction, n is the number of coupled fibroblasts to one myocyte and G_{gap} is the coupling conductance between myocyte and fibroblast. G_{gap} was set to 0.5 nS (Morgan et al., 2016), a value within the range of 0.3–8 nS measured in cultured myocyte-fibroblast experiments as used in previous simulation studies (MacCannell et al., 2007; Rook et al., 1992). The number of fibroblasts coupled to a single myocyte varied from 0 to 9 (Koivumäki et al., 2014a), as shown in **Supplementary Figure S1**.

Stabilization of the cellular model of each region was achieved after 1000 stimuli of 2 ms duration and an amplitude of twice the threshold value. After this number of stimuli, APD_{90} values and ion concentration ranges reached steady state. The basic cycle length (BCL) was 1 s, 250 ms, or 2 s.

The following features of the myocyte AP were measured: AP duration at 90% repolarization (APD_{90}), depolarization upstroke velocity measured as the maximum variation of the depolarization phase (dV/dt_{max}), and the RMP.

Strand and Tissue Simulations

The diffusion-reaction Eq. (4) of the monodomain formalism was used to simulate AP electrical propagation:

$$\nabla \cdot (D\nabla V) = C_m\frac{dV}{dt} + I_{ion} \quad (4)$$

where D is the diffusion tensor, C_m is the membrane capacitance, and I_{ion} stands for ionic currents through the membrane. Diffusion coefficients were adjusted for the different atrial regions to achieve physiological CVs along a strand of myocytes in this particular tissue.

Diffusion coefficients for myocytes (Dm) were calculated and adjusted to achieve physiological CVs, yielding a Dm of 3.84 cm^2/s in RA and LA (CV = 70 cm/s), a Dm of 6.384 cm^2/s in CT (CV = 100 cm/s), and a Dm of 4.081 cm^2/s in PV (CV = 80 cm/s). In PeAF, the diffusion coefficient was reduced by 50% to reproduce gap junction remodeling (Harrild and Hen, 2000; Ten Tusscher et al., 2004; Krogh-madsen et al., 2012; McDowell et al., 2012).

For one-dimensional simulations (1D), a strand with a space discretization of 100 μm was used for myocytes (Satoh et al., 1996; Courtemanche et al., 1998; Nygren et al., 1998; Sachse et al., 2008) and 10 μm for fibroblasts-myofibroblasts (Sachse et al., 2008; Xie et al., 2009; Brown et al., 2015). Fibroblasts-myofibroblasts were randomly distributed along the strand at different densities (10, 20, and 40%) using a uniform random probabilistic function. One hundred random distributions were generated for each density value (see **Supplementary Figure S3**). The strand was paced with a BCL of 1 s for 50 s. The first element of the strand was stimulated with an amplitude of twice its threshold. CV was measured in the 50th pulse. The diffusion coefficient for elements with fibroblasts was halved with respect to the myocyte elements (Vasquez et al., 2004; Gomez et al., 2014b; Morgan et al., 2016).

Two-dimensional (2D) meshes representing cardiac tissues for RA and LA were built with a central fibrotic region of 2 cm diameter with different randomly distributed myofibroblast densities. Ten random distributions were implemented for each density (see **Supplementary Figures S1, S3**). The tissue grid had 524 × 524 elements with a spatial resolution of 100 μm. An anisotropic ratio of 2.86:1 was considered in RA and LA (Ferrer et al., 2015).

To study the effect of myofibroblasts on vulnerability to reentry, reentrant activity was generated using cross-field stimulation protocol S1-S2. S1 stimuli consisted of 10 pulses applied to the left border of the computational mesh to stabilize the tissue and S2 was applied to the bottom left corner of the tissue.

In order to obtain the instantaneous location of the rotors, we used phase singularity (PS) detections (Sabir et al., 1974; Gray et al., 1998; Gomez et al., 2014a; Martinez-Mateu et al., 2018) first building phase maps based on the Hilbert transform (HT) of the APs (Warren et al., 2003; Yamazaki et al., 2012) (5) by computing the instantaneous phase θ (6), whose values ranged from -π to π radians:

$$\mathrm{HT}\,[V\,(t)] = \frac{1}{\pi} \cdot \int_{-\infty}^{\infty} \frac{V\,(\tau)}{t - \tau} \cdot d\tau \quad (5)$$

$$\theta = \tan^{-1}\left(\frac{\mathrm{HT}\,[V\,(t)]}{V\,(t)}\right) \quad (6)$$

where V is the membrane potential. Then PSs, where all phases converge (7), were computed to track the rotor trajectory:

$$\oint \nabla\theta dr = \pm 2\pi \quad (7)$$

Phase singularity detections were also used to assess heterogeneity degree in the tissue due to the inclusion of fibrotic regions.

Implementation

The differential equations of the cellular models were solved using the Rush-Larsen method for the gating variables and the forward Euler method for all other ordinary differential equations with a time step of 10 μs. The monodomain Eq. (4) was solved using the finite elements method with "no flux" boundary condition.

Simulations were implemented in C++ and CUDA languages. Computations were performed on an Intel(R) Xeon(R) CPU E5-2603v3 processor with an NVIDIA Tesla K40c graphic card (see **Supplementary Figure S2**).

RESULTS

Cellular Simulations

Figure 1 shows the APs obtained in cellular simulations with a BCL of 1000 ms under normal sinus rhythm (Panel A) and PeAF (Panel B) conditions, highlighting the differences in APD_{90} for each atrial region. Under physiological conditions, the APD_{90} was 236.4 ms for RA, 214 ms for LA, 176.1 ms for PV, and 292.8 ms for CT. However, under PeAF conditions APD_{90} was 165.5 ms, 139.8 ms, 120.8 ms, and 180.2 ms for the RA, LA, PV, and CT, respectively. APD_{90} decreased by 40% for RA, LA, and CT and by approximately 30% for PV with respect to normal conditions (see Panel C). In PaAF, in addition to APD shortening, RMP dropped from −75 to −79 mV, and dV/dt_{max} increased from 163 V/s to 168 V/s for RA, CT, and LA. RMP fell from −68 to −78 mV, and dV/dt_{max} rose from 157 V/s to 165 V/s for PV (see Panels E and D).

When fibroblasts were coupled to a single myocyte, we analyzed the effect of their electrophysiological characteristics (RMP_f and C_{mf}) on myocyte electrical behavior (see **Figure 2**). When the number of coupled fibroblasts increased, the myocyte RMP became more depolarized and moved closer to the value of RMP_f. A higher C_{mf} value seemed to further reduce myocyte APD when RMP_f was −45 mV.

Figure 3 shows the effect of myocyte fibroblast coupling at different BCLs. As can be seen in Panel A, at a BCL of 300 ms myocyte AP was barely affected by coupling 1 fibroblast. APD_{90} was very slightly reduced at both RMP_f values (purple and green traces in panel A), for all BCLs.

In panel B at higher C_{mf} the effect on APD_{90}s was similar to Panel A, except for the fact that an RMP_f of −26 mV, APD_{90} was slightly higher than for an RMP_f of −45 mV, for all BCLs. As the number of fibroblasts increased (Panels C–F), the effects changed with the electrical characteristics of the fibroblasts and the BCL. Panels C and D show that for a different RMP_f, APD_{90} changed with BCL. Longer APD_{90}s were obtained for BCLs of 500 ms and 1000 ms for a RMPf of −26 mV. In Panel D, for a BCL of 300 ms, APD alternans arose, and APD_{90} increased with higher BCL at an RMPf of −26 mV. When the number of coupled fibroblasts increased (Panels E and F), APD_{90} was reduced to 50 ms for −45 mV and all BCLs and to less than 40 ms for an RMP_f of −26 mV.

We also analyzed myocyte RMP and dV/dt_{max} (see **Figure 4**). Myocyte RMP (Panel B) changed similarly when C_{mf} increased for both RMP_f values (−26 mV and −45 mV). Increasing the number of fibroblasts moved the myocyte RMP closer to RMP_f. The most significant change was in the dV/dt_{max} (Panel A), which was much lower at an RMP_f of −26 mV than the reduction obtained at an RMPf of −45 mV. When fibroblasts couple to myocytes their RMP_f move closer to each other and more Na^+ channels are available,

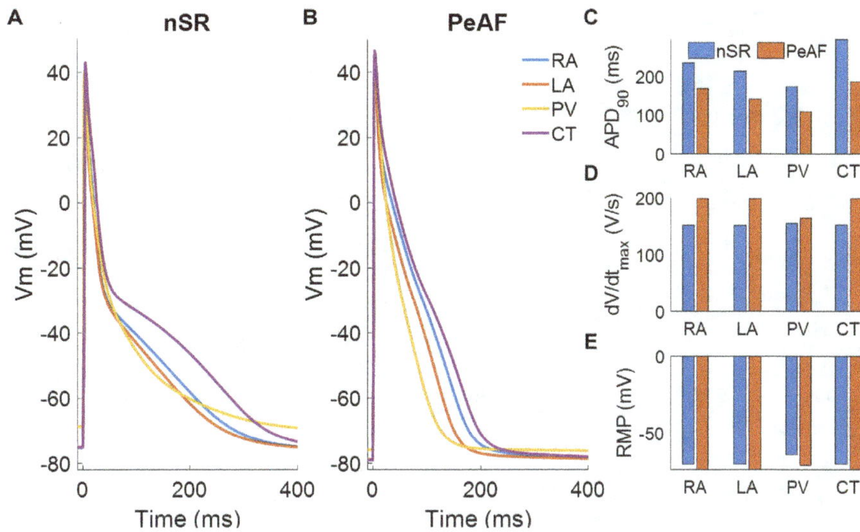

FIGURE 1 | Myocyte action potentials from four different regions of the atria: right atria (RA), left atria (LA), pulmonary vein (PV), and crista terminalis (CT). **(A)** Myocyte action potentials under normal sinus rhythm (nSR). **(B)** Myocyte action potentials under the effect of electrical remodeling during persistent atrial fibrillation (PeAF). **(C)** Myocyte action potential duration (APD_{90}) under nSR and PeAF. **(D)** Myocyte action potential maximum upstroke velocity (dV/dt_{max}) under nSR and PeAF. **(E)** Myocyte action potential resting membrane potential (RMP) under nSR and PeAF.

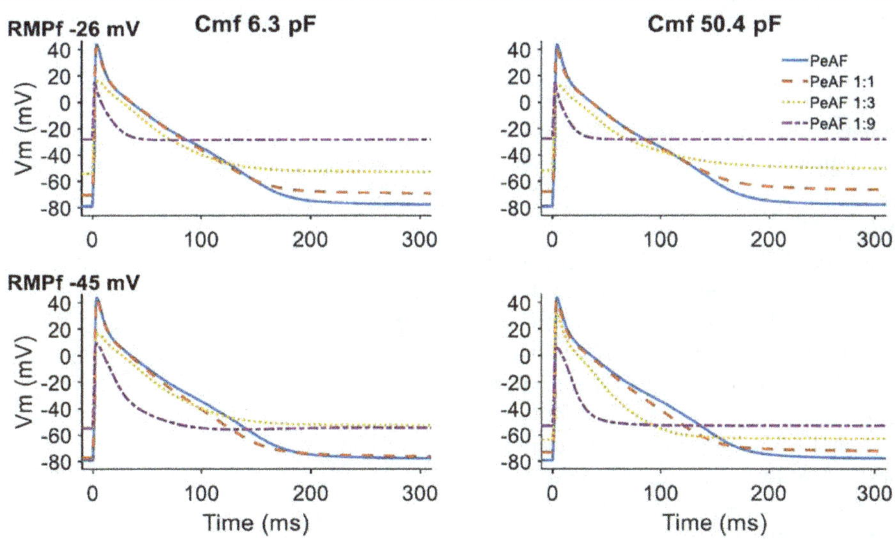

FIGURE 2 | Effect of fibroblast and myocyte coupling under persistent atrial fibrillation (PeAF) electrical remodeling in RA (baseline model). First and second rows show fibroblasts resting membrane potential (RMPf) of -26 and -45 mV, respectively, for a fibroblast membrane capacitance (Cmf) of 6.3 pF (first column) and 50.4 pF (second column). The different traces are action potentials of isolated myocytes under PeAF (blue), one myocyte under PeAF coupled to 1 fibroblast (1:1) (dashed orange), one myocyte under PeAF coupled to three fibroblasts (1:3) (dotted yellow), and one myocyte under PeAF coupled to nine fibroblasts (1:9) (dotted-dashed purple).

although myocyte Na^+ channel availability can be reduced due to a more depolarized RMP according to the number of coupled fibroblasts.

The experimental data agree with previous simulation studies in which fibroblasts presented an RMP of around −45 mV and a C_{mf} of 6.3 pF, while myofibroblasts have a more depolarized RMPf of −26 mV and a C_{mf} of 50.4 pF (Sridhar et al., 2017). In all the different atrial zones we analyzed the effects of coupling three fibroblasts or three myofibroblasts to a single myocyte (see **Figure 5**).

Panel A in **Figure 5** shows how APD_{90} was reduced when fibroblasts were coupled for all BCLs. When myofibroblasts were coupled, for a BCL of 300 ms APD alternans arose and for a BCL of 1000 ms APD_{90} increased. Panel B shows APD_{90s} in LA for different BCLs and similar fibroblast and myofibroblasts effects. The reduced APD_{90} in the PV case (Panel C) seems to be more

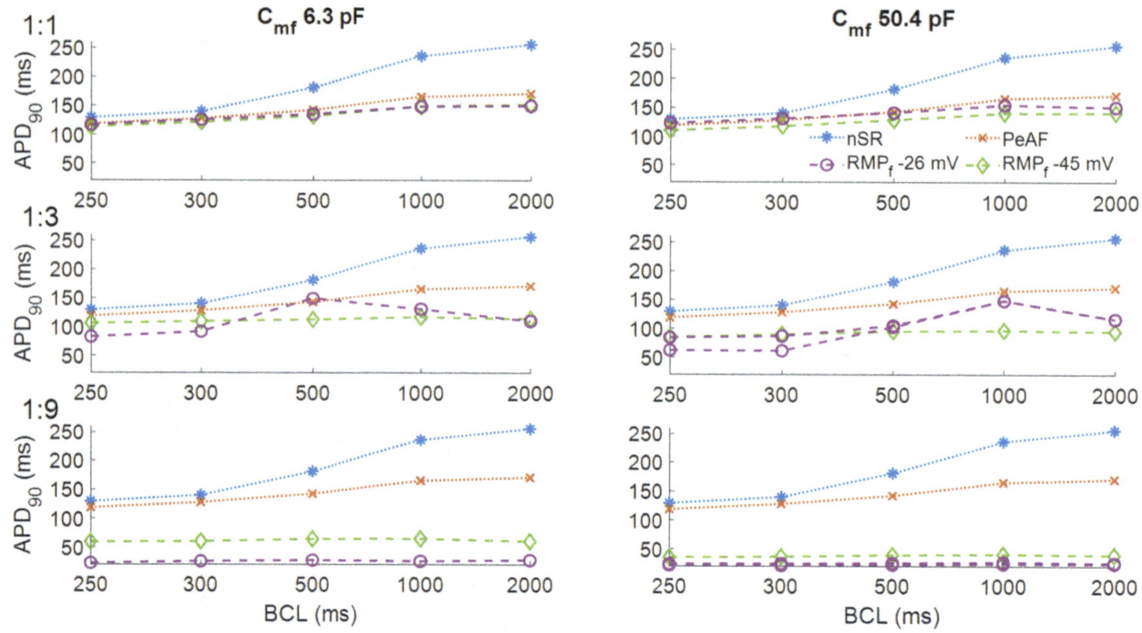

FIGURE 3 | Action potential durations of myocytes in normal sinus rhythm (nSR), under persistent atrial fibrillation electrical remodeling (PeAF) and after being coupled to fibroblasts with a resting membrane potential (RMPf) of −26 or −45 mV in RA (baseline model). In the first column the membrane capacitance of fibroblasts is 6.3 pF and in the second column 50.4 pF. One myocyte was coupled to one fibroblast (1:1) (first row), three fibroblasts (1:3) (second row), and nine fibroblasts (1:9) (third row).

pronounced in myofibroblast coupling. CT alternans also arose when myofibroblasts were coupled.

1D Strand Simulations

Conduction velocity in the atria changes locally according to the region's characteristics, as shown in **Figure 6**. During nSR and without fibroblasts, the RA has a CV of 70 cm/s, CT has a CV of 100 cm/s, LA has a CV of 70 cm/s, and PV has a CV of 80 cm/s (blue discontinuous lines) (Ferrer et al., 2015). AP propagation along the strand was affected by PeAF electrical remodeling (red discontinuous lines) and CVs dropped significantly. At higher fibroblast (yellow) or myofibroblasts (green) densities in the strand, CV dropped. Boxplot measurements of the CV are represented for the 100 random distributions of fibroblasts for each density (10, 20, and 40%). The region with the greatest differential effect on CV was the PV, depending on whether the distribution was with fibroblasts or myofibroblasts. PV also experienced conduction blocks in some of the random distributions (indicated by yellow asterisks). Conduction block was also seen in LA at a density of 40% in some distributions.

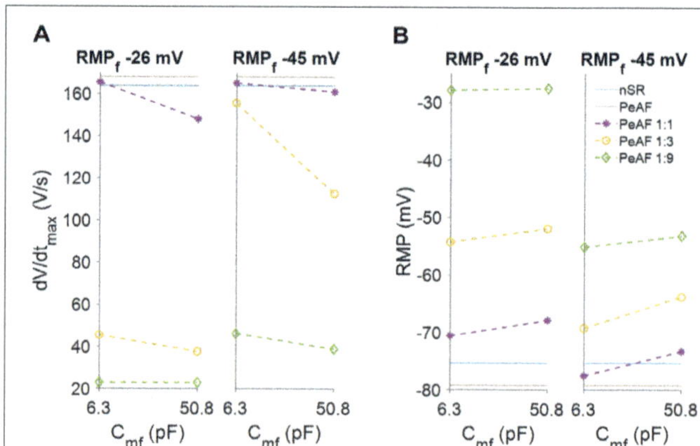

FIGURE 4 | Fibroblasts coupling effect on myocyte electrophysiology. **(A)** Myocyte maximum upstroke velocity (dV/dt_{max}). **(B)** Myocyte resting membrane potential (RMP). The levels for myocytes in normal sinus rhythm (nSR) and persistent atrial fibrillation (PeAF) conditions are given in blue and red, respectively. Discontinuous lines are myocytes in PeAF coupled to one fibroblast (1:1), 3 (1:3), or 9 (1:9).

2D Tissue Simulations

The 2D atrial tissue electrical activity in PeAF with different myofibroblast densities was analyzed to assess vulnerability to reentry. **Figure 7** shows snapshots of phase maps (taken at the same time). Re-entrant circuits can be seen in the RA (top panels) and in the LA (bottom panels) in PeAF remodeling and increasing levels of myofibroblast density from left to right (membrane potential snapshots can be seen in **Supplementary Figure S4**). In the absence of myofibroblasts a functional reentry was obtained in RA and LA. The tip of these rotors (**Figure 7**, first column), corresponding to the PS superimposed in white on the phase maps, describes a regular circular path, which agrees with the results obtained in previous simulation studies (Wilhelms et al., 2013). In LA, the rotor tip describes a smaller path due to the shorter wavelength caused by shorter

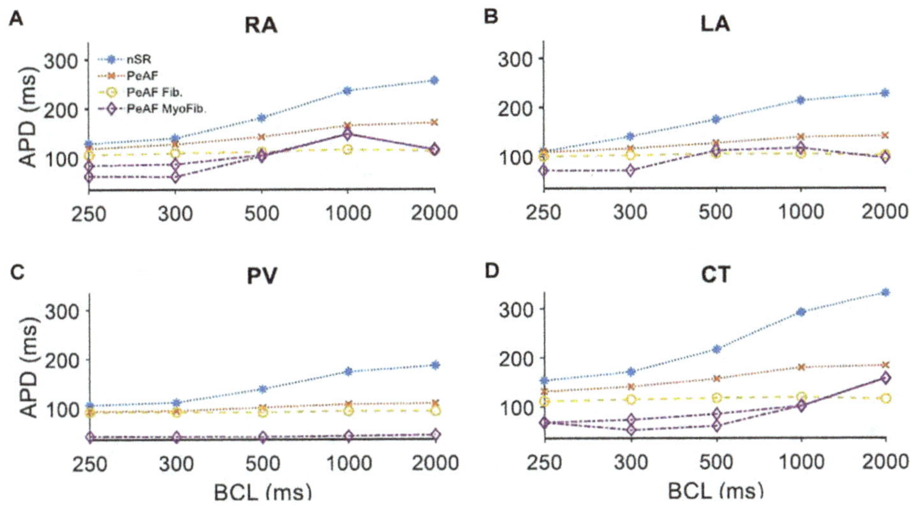

FIGURE 5 | Myocyte action potential duration (APD) of four different regions of the atria under persistent atrial fibrillation electrical remodeling (PeAF) coupled to three fibroblasts (Fib) or myofibroblasts (MyoFib) stimulated at different basic cycle lengths (BCLs). **(A)** Right atria (RA), **(B)** Left atria (LA), **(C)** Pulmonary vein (PV), and **(D)** Crista terminalis (CT).

LA ERP (Fernandez-Lozano et al., 2006; Krueger et al., 2012; Ferrer et al., 2015).

When myofibroblasts were present in the center of the tissue (see section "Materials and Methods"), the obstacle altered the reentrant activity. Small percentages of myofibroblasts (10–20%) allowed the wavefront to propagate through the fibrotic region, but the electrophysiological heterogeneities of myofibroblasts and myocytes caused wavebreaks, which were detected as PSs (quantified in **Supplementary Table S3**). However, propagation in the fibrotic region was practically blocked when myofibroblast density was raised to 40%, which produced an anatomical reentry surrounding the fibrotic obstacle. Since the wavefront did not propagate through the fibrotic region the number of wavebreaks was significantly reduced, as were the number of PSs detected (see **Supplementary Table S3**).

The myofibroblasts in the tissue increased reentry vulnerability, measured as the vulnerable window (VW), a time interval for which premature S2 stimulation generates a reentry (**Figure 8**). In the RA the vulnerable window in the absence of myofibroblasts was 37 ms. When myofibroblasts density was raised to 10%, the VW increased to 38 ± 0.0 ms. VW also increased (39 ± 0.63 ms) when density was raised to 20%, but at 40% VW dropped below the control value (35 ± 0.82 ms). Interestingly, LA was more sensitive to myofibroblasts with a larger VW than the RA. The LA VW in the absence of myofibroblasts was 40 ms. When myofibroblast density was raised to 10%, VW rose to 40 ± 0.0 ms, at 20% it increased to 40.5 ± 0.53 ms and at 40% it dropped to 38 ± 0.88 ms.

DISCUSSION

Computational modeling was used to investigate the effect of coupling fibroblasts and myofibroblasts to myocytes in four different regions of the atria during persistent AF. The study's major findings can be summarized as follows: (i) myocyte-fibroblast coupling heterogeneously shortens myocyte APD and depolarizes the myocyte resting membrane potential in the 4 different atrial regions These effects strongly depend on the fibroblast electrophysiology. (ii) Fibroblasts, and specially myofibroblasts, introduce heterogeneities in the atrial substrate which alter the propagation of the AP, slowing conduction velocity. (iii) Fibroblasts-myofibroblasts change the atrial substrate during PeAF, which alters the vulnerability to re-entries and the vulnerable window presents a biphasic behavior related to myofibroblast density. These results suggest that the heterogeneity of the atrial tissue in the presence of fibroblasts/myofibroblats promotes reentrant events and alters the dynamics of arrhythmogenic propagation.

Heterogeneous Effects of PeAF Remodeling and Electrical Coupling of Fibroblasts in Atrial Tissues

Atrial substrate is differently affected by PeAF remodeling and by the presence of fibroblasts, due to the electrophysiological heterogeneity of the different atrial regions. Our results from isolated single cells show differences in the RMP, dV/dt_{max}, and APD for the four different atrial regions (RA, LA, CT, and PV) in nSR and in PeAF. These differences are in agreement with the simulations carried out by Krueger et al. (2013), who reported the differential effects of AF remodeling in the different atrial regions. It has to be noted that in contrast to the Krueger study, our model presents a long-term stability in all regions in single-cell and tissue simulations and also considers the effect of fibroblast coupling. To our knowledge, this is the first simulation study including the three components (atrial heterogeneity, AF remodeling, and fibroblasts) using a detailed electrophysiological AP model for fibroblasts and focusing on the analysis of the different effects exerted by

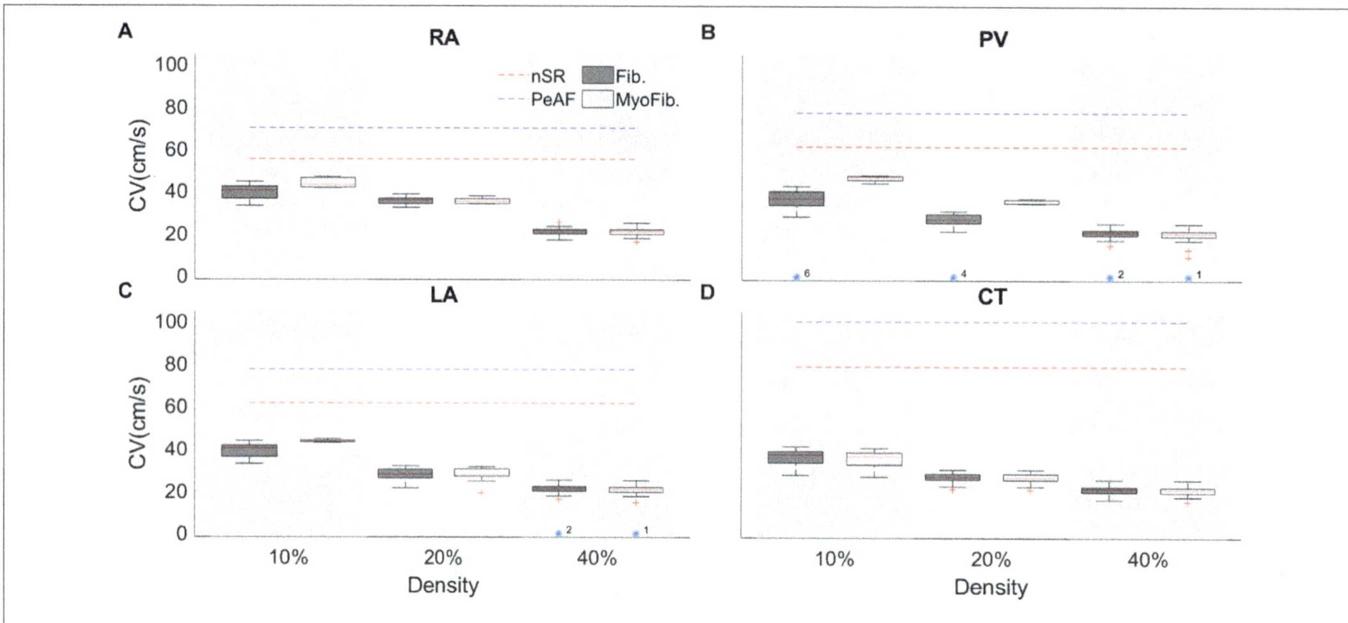

FIGURE 6 | Conduction velocity (CV) of a tissue strand in four different regions of the atria with random fibroblasts (Fib) or myofibroblast (MyoFib) distribution and different fibroblast densities. For each density 100 random configurations were simulated. CV measurements are represented in boxplots. **(A)** Right atria (RA). **(B)** Pulmonary vein (PV), **(C)** Left atria (LA), and **(D)** Crista terminalis (CT).

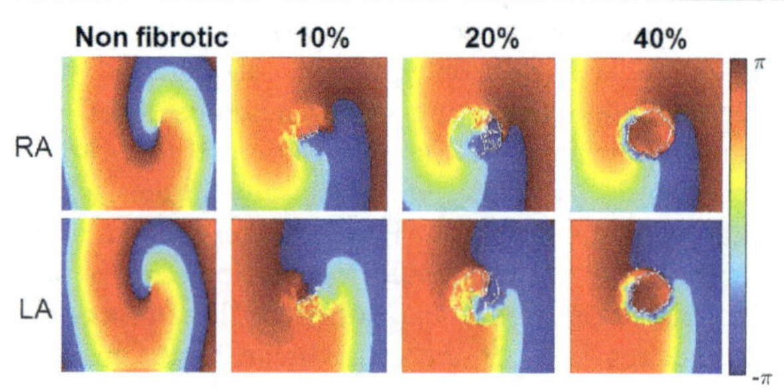

FIGURE 7 | Instantaneous phase maps and phase singularities (in white) for different densities of myofibroblasts (non-fibrotic, 10, 20, and 40%) in the right atria (RA) and left atria (LA) under conditions of persistent AF remodeling.

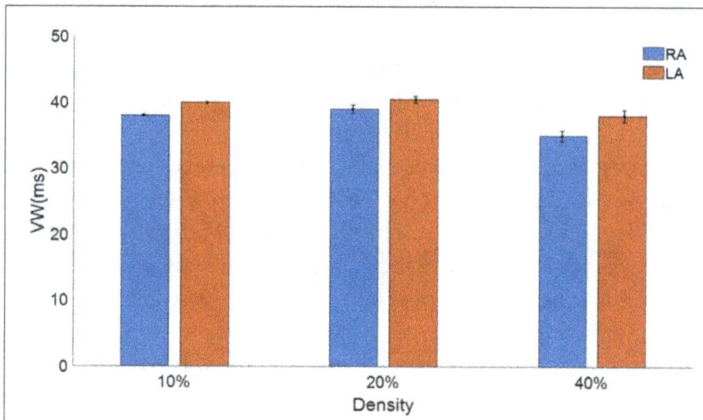

FIGURE 8 | Vulnerable window to reentry in atrial tissue with different densities of myofibroblasts indicated in percentage for the right atrial (RA) in blue and the left atrial (LA) in red subject to persistent atrial fibrillation remodeling.

fibrosis in the different atrial regions. A recent study by Roney et al. (2018) showed that high PS density in the PVs favored the effectiveness of PV isolation in ablation procedure. Their model also considered electrophysiological remodeling in AF, electrophysiological heterogeneities in different atrial regions, and fibrosis was simulated by changes in tissue conductivity. In a previous study (Roney et al., 2016), the same group modeled fibrosis by different methods and did not consider either electrophysiological heterogeneities in the atrial regions or AF remodeling to determine how different fibrosis models could affect rotor dynamics.

Different experimental studies show that atrial fibroblasts have a different electrophysiology from ventricular fibroblasts (MacCannell et al., 2007; Burstein and Nattel, 2008; Poulet et al., 2016; Salvarani et al., 2017). Morgan et al. (2016) found that fibroblast electrophysiology changes the dynamics of an arrhythmic process and provides relevant information on the effect of myocyte-fibroblast coupling in the atria. Our results indicate that RMPf, C_{mf}, and the number of coupled fibroblasts altered the behavior of myocytes AP, as was found in previous simulation studies (Maleckar et al., 2009; Koivumäki et al., 2014a; Sridhar et al., 2017). Furthermore, in the present study we found that introducing I_{Na} current into the fibroblast model had an interesting effect; due to the high RMP of isolated fibroblasts I_{Na} current was blocked but when fibroblasts were coupled with myocytes I_{Na} channels became available. Additionally, myocyte-fibroblast coupling led to a partial inactivation of the myocyte I_{Na} due to the higher RMP in the myocyte.

Fibroblast electrophysiology (RMPf and C_{mf}) changes myocyte AP characteristics (Jacquemet and Henriquez, 2008, 2009; Maleckar et al., 2009). Our simulation results also show that electrical coupling with myocytes increases atrial electrophysiological heterogeneity. Changes in the BCL altered the behavior of the coupled cells, with different responses in different regions. Interestingly, myofibroblast -myocyte coupling in regions with higher I_{K1} and I_{CaL} (RA and CT) exhibited more sensitivity to changes in frequency, while regions with smaller I_{K1} and I_{CaL} (PV) developed no AP for any of the BCLs. In contrast to McDowell et al. (2013), we defined different electric characteristics for the atrial myofibroblasts, which have a different effect on myocyte AP. Myofibroblasts act as the current source, raising the myocyte RMP (Jacquemet and Henriquez, 2007) according to the number of coupled myofibroblasts (Maleckar et al., 2009; Koivumäki et al., 2014a), thus leading to a partial inactivation of the myocyte I_{Na} current (see **Supplementary Figure S5**).

Heterogenous Effects of Fibrosis During PeAF in Atrial Tissues

Structural remodeling of the cardiac tissue contributes to reducing conduction velocity, delaying regional functional activations, and increasing structural heterogeneities, which are important factors for establishing a re-entrant driver or conduction block (Camelliti et al., 2005). Our results show that fibroblasts and myofibroblasts can alter the activation time in a 1D tissue strand, in agreement with different studies (Sachse et al., 2008; Xie et al., 2009). We implemented one hundred random configurations for different fibroblast/myofibroblast densities in the four atrial regions. Zhan et al. (2014) showed that fibroblasts can alter the CV and can lead to blocks in conduction with fibrosis densities of 40 and 45%, our results showed that a high density (40%) led to conduction blocks in the LA and that the PV was the most sensitive region to the presence of fibroblasts-myofibroblasts. Similarly, in an experimental study Miragoli et al. (2006) showed that myofibroblast proliferation changed the tissue conduction velocity and myocyte dV/dt_{max}. Our results showed a reduction in CV, in agreement with several other experimental and simulation studies that found that fibroblasts-myofibroblasts can establish an electric coupling with myocytes, reducing their dV/dt_{max} and activation time, reflected in reduced CV (Miragoli et al., 2006; Rohr, 2009; Xie et al., 2009; Yue et al., 2011). We also found a monotonic reduction in all four atrial regions.

Tanaka et al. (2007) have shown that local fibrosis distribution reduces CV in the different atrial regions, in agreement with our results, which showed a reduced CV with a tendency to homogenize in all four atrial regions. CV heterogeneity is responsible for giving the atria the characteristic activation times (Nguyen et al., 2012); if all the regions were to have a homogenous CV, this might induce the appropriate conditions for reentrant rhythms and conductions blocks (Gaspo et al., 1997). As the fast conduction systems' (CT) conduction velocity was significantly reduced, this may be an interesting mechanism for AF in the right atrium.

Vulnerability to Reentry During PeAF in Fibrotic Tissue

Structural remodeling and endo-epicardial dissociation alter the atrial substrate and could produce macroreentries and focal activity (Everett and Olgin, 2007; Verheule et al., 2014). When, we analyzed the propagation in different regions of the atria and at different myofibroblast densities, we found that a low myofibroblasts percentage increased the number of PSs due to the wavebreaks. However, at higher percentages, propagation through the fibrotic zone was blocked, the number of wavebreaks and PSs decreased, and an anatomical reentry was anchored around the fibrotic zone, in agreement with previous studies (McDowell et al., 2013; Roney et al., 2016). Several simulation studies have also shown that reentry dynamics is altered by heterogeneities of the AP in the cardiac tissue (Colman et al., 2014; Varela et al., 2016), the presence of fibroblasts (Ashihara et al., 2012; Gomez et al., 2014a; Morgan et al., 2016), and that PSs increase in the zones with fibroblasts (Saha et al., 2018).

Waks and Josephson (2014) demonstrated that the rotation dynamics depends on the atrial tissue (RA or LA) and its electrophysiological characteristics, as did we in the present study, in which vulnerability to reentries and the dynamics of the rotation depended on the atrial region. LA presented slightly higher VWs, due to its shorter APD.

Gomez et al. (2014b) showed that the density of fibroblasts had a biphasic impact on the ventricular vulnerable window for reentry, while our results showed the same VW biphasic behavior for the first time in atrial tissue. Krul et al. (2015) found that local fibrosis is associated with reentrant activity, comparable to our results at low fibroblast density (10%), which can be considered as a region of local diffuse fibrosis, presented higher tissue vulnerability and resulted in multiple wavebreaks. When myofibroblast density was raised (20%), tissue vulnerability to reentry rose and conduction blocks occurred. However, at higher densities (40%) the conduction blocks also occurred but VW dropped, as was found by Campos et al. (2018). This suggests that myocyte-fibroblast coupling in PeAF plays an important role in AF (Morgan et al., 2014), with different effects in different atrial regions.

Limitations

Several limitations must be considered when drawing conclusions from the present study. Firstly, we did not consider the effect of electrical remodeling due to cytokines like TGF-B, which have been reported during structural remodeling and are known to affect myocyte AP (Burstein and Nattel, 2008; Nattel et al., 2008; Zahid et al., 2016).

Secondly, as fibroblast electrophysiology and differentiation into myofibroblasts still remain unclear, the models we used should be considered as an approximation (Nattel, 2018). Myofibroblast electrophysiological characteristics are still not well understood. Furthermore, it is important to highlight that although animal models and *in vitro* experiments prove the existence of electrotonic coupling between myocytes and fibroblasts (Kohl et al., 2005; Miragoli et al., 2006; Grand et al., 2014; Salvarani et al., 2017), this has not been reported in humans *in vivo*. However, human cardiac tissue with fibrosis presents altered electrical behavior (Krul et al., 2015; Fukumoto et al., 2016).

Thirdly, the pulmonary vein AP model was built on the basis of the reported experimental data for dogs and sheep APD_{90} and RMP. Electrophysiological data from human isolated myocytes from PV are still unavailable (Ehrlich et al., 2003).

Fourthly, while AF mechanisms are still unclear, there are different pathways by which reentrant drivers can be generated and maintained. Several studies have shown how non-myocyte cells like fibroblasts, macrophages (Hulsmans et al., 2017) and adipocytes (De Coster et al., 2018) alter the atrial substrate and promote arrhythmias. The effects of non-myocytes or endo-epicardial dissociation have not been considered in the present study, although these are factors which might alter the reentry dynamics and would be interesting to analyze in future studies (Verheule et al., 2014).

Fifthly, we are aware that fibrosis is a complex structure involving different actors such as collagen deposition, inflammatory cytokines and proteins which may alter the myocyte electrophysiology. There are different approaches to simulating the fibrotic regions such as non-conductive elements (Ten Tusscher et al., 2004), the paracrine effect changing the myocyte ion channel conductance (Zahid et al., 2016) and coupling to elements with a static RMP (Majumder et al., 2011) and using ionic models to describe the electrophysiology of fibroblasts (McDowell et al., 2013; Morgan et al., 2016; Saha et al., 2018).

Finally, we did not include the effect of different sizes or locations of fibrotic regions in the tissue. The fibrotic regions can in fact attract rotors (Roy et al., 2018), and future studies in this line would shed light into the mechanisms of chaotic rhythms when fibroblasts proliferate. Additionally, 3D simulations have shown how fibroblasts and non-conductive areas can modify the dynamics of the reentry (McDowell et al., 2013; Morgan et al., 2014). Zahid et al. (2016) introduced the paracrine effect, modifying myocyte electrophysiology in the fibrotic region in 3D simulations reducing the AP duration and the conductivity of the fibrotic region. We are also aware that 3D simulations include further structural details. The work by Ferrer et al. (2015), among others, presents a highly detailed atrial model. However, these simulations have a high computational cost while 2D simulations are computationally more efficient and provide a detailed insight into arrhythmia dynamics. Despite these limitations, we consider that our simulations represent a realistic heterogeneous PeAF remodeling (electrophysiological and structural) scenario in the different atrial regions and contribute a great deal to the understanding of AF mechanisms.

CONCLUSION

The results of the present simulation study show that fibroblast electrophysiology alters myocyte AP characteristics and leads to slower conduction velocity in atrial tissues affected by PeAF. These changes are heterogeneous within the different atrial regions.

Myocyte-fibroblast coupling creates a substrate in which the dynamics of arrhythmic reentries changes with the fibroblast density. By increasing the density of fibroblasts, reentries evolve from functional to anatomical around the obstacle formed by the fibrotic region. We also observed biphasic behavior of tissue vulnerability to reentries. Low myofibroblast densities (10 and 20%) increase the vulnerability to reentry, while a higher density (40%) reduces tissue vulnerability.

AUTHOR CONTRIBUTIONS

JoS, JaS, and BT contributed to the conception and design of the study. JG, LR, and LM-M contributed to the development of the model. JoS performed the computational simulations and JoS, JaS, and BT performed the analysis and interpretation of the results. All authors contributed to drafting of the manuscript and all revised, and approved the submitted version.

REFERENCES

Ashihara, T., Haraguchi, R., Nakazawa, K., Namba, T., Ikeda, T., Nakazawa, Y., et al. (2012). The role of fibroblasts in complex fractionated electrograms during persistent/permanent atrial fibrillation: implications for electrogram-based catheter ablation. *Circ. Res.* 110, 275–284. doi: 10.1161/CIRCRESAHA.111.255026

Biernacka, A., and Frangogiannis, N. G. (2011). Aging and cardiac fibrosis. *Aging Dis.* 2, 158–173. doi: 10.1016/j.bbi.2008.05.010

Brown, T. R., Krogh-Madsen, T., and Christini, D. J. (2015). Computational approaches to understanding the role of fibroblast-myocyte interactions in cardiac arrhythmogenesis. *Biomed. Res. Int.* 2015:465714. doi: 10.1155/2015/465714

Burstein, B., and Nattel, S. (2008). Atrial fibrosis: mechanisms and clinical relevance in atrial fibrillation. *J. Am. Coll. Cardiol.* 51, 802–809. doi: 10.1016/j.jacc.2007.09.064

Burstein, B., Qi, X. Y., Yeh, Y. H., Calderone, A., and Nattel, S. (2007). Atrial cardiomyocyte tachycardia alters cardiac fibroblast function: a novel consideration in atrial remodeling. *Cardiovasc. Res.* 76, 442–452. doi: 10.1016/j.cardiores.2007.07.013

Camelliti, P., Borg, T. K., and Kohl, P. (2005). Structural and functional characterisation of cardiac fibroblasts. *Cardiovasc. Res.* 65, 40–51. doi: 10.1016/j.cardiores.2004.08.020

Camelliti, P., Devlin, G. P., Matthews, K. G., Kohl, P., and Green, C. R. (2004). Spatially and temporally distinct expression of fibroblast connexins after sheep ventricular infarction. *Cardiovasc. Res.* 62, 415–425. doi: 10.1016/j.cardiores.2004.01.027

Campos, F. O., Shiferaw, Y., Weber dos Santos, R., Plank, G., and Bishop, M. J. (2018). Microscopic isthmuses and fibrosis within the border zone of infarcted hearts promote calcium-mediated ectopy and conduction block. *Front. Phys.* 6:57. doi: 10.3389/fphy.2018.00057

Chacar, S., Farès, N., Bois, P., and Faivre, J.-F. (2017). Basic signaling in cardiac fibroblasts. *J. Cell. Physiol.* 232, 725–730. doi: 10.1002/jcp.25624

Chatelier, A., Mercier, A., Tremblier, B., Thériault, O., Moubarak, M., Benamer, N., et al. (2012). A distinct de novo expression of Na v 1.5 sodium channels in human atrial fibroblasts differentiated into myofibroblasts. *J. Physiol.* 590, 4307–4319. doi: 10.1113/jphysiol.2012.233593

Colman, M. A., Varela, M., Hancox, J. C., Zhang, H., and Aslanidi, O. V. (2014). Evolution and pharmacological modulation of the arrhythmogenic wave dynamics in canine pulmonary vein model. *Europace* 16, 416–423. doi: 10.1093/europace/eut349

Courtemanche, M., Ramirez, R. J., and Nattel, S. (1998). Ionic mechanisms underlying human atrial action potential properties: insights from a mathematical model. *Am. J. Physiol.* 275, H301–H321. doi: 10.1152/ajpheart.1998.275.1.H301

De Coster, T., Claus, P., Kazbanov, I. V., Haemers, P., Willems, R., Sipido, K. R., et al. (2018). Arrhythmogenicity of fibro-fatty infiltrations. *Sci. Rep.* 8, 2050. doi: 10.1038/s41598-018-20450-w

Ehrlich, J. R., Cha, T.-J., Zhang, L., Chartier, D., Melnyk, P., Hohnloser, S. H., et al. (2003). Cellular electrophysiology of canine pulmonary vein cardiomyocytes: action potential and ionic current properties. *J. Physiol.* 551, 801–813. doi: 10.1113/jphysiol.2003.046417

Everett, T. H., and Olgin, J. E. (2007). Atrial fibrosis and the mechanisms of atrial fibrillation. *Hear. Rhythm* 4, S24–S27. doi: 10.1016/j.hrthm.2006.12.040

Fernandez-Lozano, I., Toquero-Ramos, J., Escudero-Vela, C., Castedo-Mejuto, E., Escudier-Villa, J. M., and Alonso-Pulpon, L. (2006). [Left atrial posterior wall and pulmonary vein refractory periods are associated with atrial fibrillation inducibility in a swine model]. *Rev. Esp. Cardiol.* 59, 653–661.

Ferrer, A., Sebastián, R., Sánchez-Quintana, D., Rodríguez, J. F., Godoy, E. J., Martínez, L., et al. (2015). Detailed anatomical and electrophysiological models of human atria and torso for the simulation of atrial activation. *PLoS One* 10:e0141573. doi: 10.1371/journal.pone.0141573

Fukumoto, K., Habibi, M., Ipek, E. G., Zahid, S., Khurram, I. M., Zimmerman, S. L., et al. (2016). Association of left atrial local conduction velocity with late gadolinium enhancement on cardiac magnetic resonance in patients with atrial fibrillation. *Circ. Arrhythm. Electrophysiol.* 9:e002897. doi: 10.1161/CIRCEP.115.002897

Gaspo, R., Bosch, R. F., Talajic, M., and Nattel, S. (1997). Functional mechanisms underlying tachycardia-induced sustained atrial fibrillation in a chronic dog model. *Circulation* 96, 4027–4035. doi: 10.1161/01.CIR.96.11.4027

Gaudesius, G., Miragoli, M., Thomas, S. P., and Rohr, S. (2003). Coupling of cardiac electrical activity over extended distances by fibroblasts of cardiac origin. *Circ. Res.* 93, 421–428. doi: 10.1161/01.RES.0000089258.40661.0C

Gomez, J. F., Cardona, K., Martinez, L., Saiz, J., and Trenor, B. (2014a). Electrophysiological and structural remodeling in heart failure modulate arrhythmogenesis. 2D simulation study. *PLoS One* 10:e0117883. doi: 10.1371/journal.pone.0103273

Gomez, J. F., Cardona, K., Romero, L., Ferrero, J. M., and Trenor, B. (2014b). Electrophysiological and structural remodeling in heart failure modulate arrhythmogenesis. 1D simulation study. *PLoS One* 9:e106602. doi: 10.1371/journal.pone.0106602

Grand, T., Salvarani, N., Jousset, F., and Rohr, S. (2014). Aggravation of cardiac myofibroblast arrhythmogeneicity by mechanical stress. *Cardiovasc. Res.* 104, 489–500. doi: 10.1093/cvr/cvu227

Gray, R. A., Pertsov, A. M., and Jalife, J. (1998). Spatial and temporal organization during cardiac fibrillation. *Nature* 392, 75–78. doi: 10.1038/32164

Harrild, D. M., and Hen, C. S. (2000). A computer model of normal conduction in the human atria. *Circ. Res.* 87, e25–e36. doi: 10.1161/01.RES.87.7.e25

Hulsmans, M., Clauss, S., Xiao, L., Aguirre, A. D., King, K. R., Hanley, A., et al. (2017). Macrophages facilitate electrical conduction in the heart. *Cell* 169, 510.e20–522.e20. doi: 10.1016/j.cell.2017.03.050

Iwasaki, Y. K., Nishida, K., Kato, T., and Nattel, S. (2011). Atrial fibrillation pathophysiology: implications for management. *Circulation* 124, 2264–2274. doi: 10.1161/CIRCULATIONAHA.111.019893

Jacquemet, V., and Henriquez, C. S. (2007). Modelling cardiac fibroblasts: interactions with myocytes and their impact on impulse propagation. *Europace* 9(Suppl.6), vi29-vi37. doi: 10.1093/europace/eum207

Jacquemet, V., and Henriquez, C. S. (2008). Loading effect of fibroblast-myocyte coupling on resting potential, impulse propagation, and repolarization: insights from a microstructure model. *AJP Hear. Circ. Physiol.* 294, H2040–H2052. doi: 10.1152/ajpheart.01298.2007

Jacquemet, V., and Henriquez, C. S. (2009). Modulation of conduction velocity by nonmyocytes in the low coupling regime. *IEEE Trans. Biomed. Eng.* 56, 893–896. doi: 10.1109/TBME.2008.2006028

Jalife, J., and Kaur, K. (2015). Atrial remodeling, fibrosis, and atrial fibrillation. *Trends Cardiovasc. Med.* 25, 475–484. doi: 10.1016/j.tcm.2014.12.015

Jousset, F., Maguy, A., Rohr, S., and Kucera, J. P. (2016). Myofibroblasts electrotonically coupled to cardiomyocytes alter conduction: insights at the cellular level from a detailed in silico tissue structure model. *Front. Physiol.* 7:496. doi: 10.3389/fphys.2016.00496

Kirchhof, P., Benussi, S., Kotecha, D., Ahlsson, A., Atar, D., Casadei, B., et al. (2016). 2016 ESC guidelines for the management of atrial fibrillation developed in collaboration with EACTS. *Europace* 18, 1609–1678. doi: 10.1093/europace/euw295

Kohl, P., Camelliti, P., Burton, F. L., and Smith, G. L. (2005). Electrical coupling of fibroblasts and myocytes: relevance for cardiac propagation. *J. Electrocardiol.* 38, 45–50. doi: 10.1016/j.jelectrocard.2005.06.096

Kohl, P., and Gourdie, R. G. (2014). Fibroblast - myocyte electrotonic coupling: does it occur in native cardiac tissue? *J. Mol. Cell. Cardiol.* 70, 37–46. doi: 10.1016/j.yjmcc.2013.12.024

Kohl, P., Kamkin, A. G., Kiseleva, I. S., and Noble, D. (1994). Mechanosensitive fibroblasts in the sino-atrial node region of rat heart: interaction with cardiomyocytes and possible role. *Exp. Physiol.* 79, 943–956. doi: 10.1113/expphysiol.1994.sp003819

Koivumäki, J., Clark, R. B., Belke, D., Kondo, C., Fedak, P., Maleckar, M. M., et al. (2014a). Na+ current expression in human atrial myofibroblasts: identity and functional roles. *Front. Physiol.* 5:275. doi: 10.3389/fphys.2014.00275

Koivumäki, J. T., Seemann, G., Maleckar, M. M., and Tavi, P. (2014b). In silico screening of the key cellular remodeling targets in chronic atrial fibrillation. *PLoS Comput. Biol.* 10:e1003620. doi: 10.1371/journal.pcbi.1003620

Koivumäki, J. T., Korhonen, T., and Tavi, P. (2011). Impact of sarcoplasmic reticulum calcium release on calcium dynamics and action potential morphology in human atrial myocytes: a computational study. *PLoS Comput. Biol.* 7:e1001067. doi: 10.1371/journal.pcbi.1001067

Krogh-madsen, T., Abbott, G. W., and Christini, D. J. (2012). Effects of electrical and structural remodeling on atrial fibrillation maintenance?: a simulation study. *PLoS Comput. Biol.* 8:e1002390. doi: 10.1371/journal.pcbi.1002390

Krueger, M., Seemann, G., Rhode, K., Keller, D. U. J., Schilling, C., Arujuna, A., et al. (2012). Personalization of atrial anatomy and elelectophysiology as a basis for clinical modeling of radio-frequency-ablation of atrial fibrillation. *Med. Imaging IEEE Trans.* 32, 1–12. doi: 10.1109/TMI.2012.2201948

Krueger, M. W., Dorn, A., Keller, D. U. J., Holmqvist, F., Carlson, J., Platonov, P. G., et al. (2013). In-silico modeling of atrial repolarization in normal and atrial fibrillation remodeled state. *Med. Biol. Eng. Comput.* 51, 1105–1119. doi: 10.1007/s11517-013-1090-1

Krul, S. P. J., Berger, W. R., Smit, N. W., Van Amersfoorth, S. C. M., Driessen, A. H. G., Van Boven, W. J., et al. (2015). Atrial fibrosis and conduction slowing in the left atrial appendage of patients undergoing thoracoscopic surgical pulmonary vein isolation for atrial fibrillation. *Circ. Arrhythm. Electrophysiol.* 8, 288–295. doi: 10.1161/CIRCEP.114.001752

MacCannell, K. A., Bazzazi, H., Chilton, L., Shibukawa, Y., Clark, R. B., and Giles, W. R. (2007). A mathematical model of electrotonic interactions between ventricular myocytes and fibroblasts. *Biophys. J.* 92, 4121–4132. doi: 10.1529/biophysj.106.101410

Majumder, R., Nayak, A. R., and Pandit, R. (2011). Scroll-wave dynamics in human cardiac tissue: lessons from a mathematical model with inhomogeneities and fiber architecture. *PLoS One* 6:e18052. doi: 10.1371/journal.pone.0018052

Maleckar, M. M., Greenstein, J. L., Giles, W. R., and Trayanova, N. A. (2009). Electrotonic coupling between human atrial myocytes and fibroblasts alters myocyte excitability and repolarization. *Biophys. J.* 97, 2179–2190. doi: 10.1016/j.bpj.2009.07.054

Martinez-Mateu, L., Romero, L., Ferrer-Albero, A., Sebastian, R., Rodríguez Matas, J. F., Jalife, J., et al. (2018). Factors affecting basket catheter detection of real and phantom rotors in the atria: a computational study. *PLoS Comput. Biol.* 14:e1006017. doi: 10.1371/journal.pcbi.1006017

McArthur, L., Chilton, L., Smith, G. L., and Nicklin, S. A. (2015). Electrical consequences of cardiac myocyte: fibroblast coupling. *Biochem. Soc. Trans.* 43, 513–518. doi: 10.1042/BST20150035

McDowell, K. S., Vadakkumpadan, F., Blake, R., Blauer, J., Plank, G., MacLeod, R. S., et al. (2012). Methodology for patient-specific modeling of atrial fibrosis as a substrate for atrial fibrillation. *J. Electrocardiol.* 45, 640–645. doi: 10.1016/j.jelectrocard.2012.08.005

McDowell, K. S., Vadakkumpadan, F., Blake, R., Blauer, J., Plank, G., Macleod, R. S., et al. (2013). Mechanistic inquiry into the role of tissue remodeling in fibrotic lesions in human atrial fibrillation. *Biophys. J.* 104, 2764–2773. doi: 10.1016/j.bpj.2013.05.025

Miragoli, M., Gaudesius, G., and Rohr, S. (2006). Electrotonic modulation of cardiac impulse conduction by myofibroblasts. *Circ. Res.* 98, 801–810. doi: 10.1161/01.RES.0000214537.44195.a3

Morgan, R., Colman, M., Kruger, M., Seemann, G., Rhode, K., and Aslanidi, O. (2014). "Evaluating effects of fibrosis in atrial arrhythmogenesis using 3D computational modelling," in *Proceedings of the international conference on Computing in Cardiology 2014*, (Cambridge, MA), 765–768.

Morgan, R., Colman, M. A., Chubb, H., Seemann, G., and Aslanidi, O. V. (2016). Slow conduction in the border zones of patchy fibrosis stabilizes the drivers for atrial fibrillation: insights from multi-scale human atrial modeling. *Front. Physiol.* 7:474. doi: 10.3389/fphys.2016.00474

Nattel, S. (2018). Molecular and cellular mechanisms of atrial fibrosis in atrial fibrillation. *JACC Clin. Electrophysiol.* 3, 425–435. doi: 10.1016/j.jacep.2017.03.002

Nattel, S., Burstein, B., and Dobrev, D. (2008). Atrial remodeling and atrial fibrillation: mechanisms and implications. *Circ. Arrhythm. Electrophysiol.* 1, 62–73. doi: 10.1161/CIRCEP.107.754564

Nattel, S., and Dobrev, D. (2017). Controversies about atrial fibrillation mechanisms: aiming for order in chaos and whether it matters. *Circ. Res.* 120, 1396–1398. doi: 10.1161/CIRCRESAHA.116.310489

Nguyen, T. P., Xie, Y., Garfinkel, A., Qu, Z., and Weiss, J. N. (2012). Arrhythmogenic consequences of myofibroblastmyocyte coupling. *Cardiovasc. Res.* 93, 242–251. doi: 10.1093/cvr/cvr292

Nygren, A., Fiset, C., Firek, L., Clark, J. W., Lindblad, D. S., Clark, R. B., et al. (1998). Mathematical model of an adult human atrial cell: the role of K+ currents in repolarization. *Circ. Res.* 82, 63–81. doi: 10.1161/01.RES.82.1.63

Poulet, C., Künzel, S., Büttner, E., Lindner, D., Westermann, D., and Ravens, U. (2016). Altered physiological functions and ion currents in atrial fibroblasts from patients with chronic atrial fibrillation. *Physiol. Rep.* 4:e12681. doi: 10.14814/phy2.12681

Quinn, T. A., Camelliti, P., Rog-Zielinska, E. A., Siedlecka, U., Poggioli, T., O'Toole, E. T., et al. (2016). Electrotonic coupling of excitable and nonexcitable cells in the heart revealed by optogenetics. *Proc. Natl. Acad. Sci. U.S.A.* 113, 14852–14857. doi: 10.1073/pnas.1611184114

Rohr, S. (2009). Myofibroblasts in diseased hearts: new players in cardiac arrhythmias? *Hear. Rhythm* 6, 848–856. doi: 10.1016/j.hrthm.2009.02.038

Rohr, S. (2011). Cardiac fibroblasts in cell culture systems: myofibroblasts all along? *J. Cardiovasc. Pharmacol.* 57, 389–399. doi: 10.1097/FJC.0b013e3182137e17

Roney, C. H., Bayer, J. D., Cochet, H., Meo, M., Dubois, R., Jaïs, P., et al. (2018). Variability in pulmonary vein electrophysiology and fibrosis determines arrhythmia susceptibility and dynamics. *PLoS Comput. Biol.* 14:e1006166. doi: 10.1371/journal.pcbi.1006166

Roney, C. H., Bayer, J. D., Zahid, S., Meo, M., Boyle, P. M. J., Trayanova, N. A., et al. (2016). Modelling methodology of atrial fibrosis affects rotor dynamics and electrograms. *Europace* 18(Suppl. 4), iv146–iv155. doi: 10.1093/europace/euw365

Rook, M. B., Van Ginneken, A. C. G., de Jonge, B., el Aoumari, A., Gros, D., Jongsma, H. J., et al. (1992). Differences in gap junction channels between cardiac myocytes, fibroblasts, and heterologous pairs. *Am. J. Physiol.* 263, C959–C977. doi: 10.1152/ajpcell.1992.263.5.C959

Roy, A., Varela, M., and Aslanidi, O. (2018). Image-based computational evaluation of the effects of atrial wall thickness and fibrosis on re-entrant drivers for atrial fibrillation. *Front. Physiol.* 9:1352. doi: 10.3389/fphys.2018.01352

Sabir, M. A., Sosulski, F. W., and Finlayson, A. J. (1974). Chlorogenic acid-protein interactions in sunflower. *J. Agric. Food Chem.* 22, 575–578. doi: 10.1021/jf60194a052

Sachse, F. B., Moreno, A. P., and Abildskov, J. A. (2008). Electrophysiological modeling of fibroblasts and their interaction with myocytes. *Ann. Biomed. Eng.* 36, 41–56. doi: 10.1007/s10439-007-9405-8

Saha, M., Roney, C. H., Bayer, J. D., Meo, M., Cochet, H., Dubois, R., et al. (2018). Wavelength and fibrosis affect phase singularity locations during atrial fibrillation. *Front. Physiol.* 9:1207. doi: 10.3389/fphys.2018.01207

Salvarani, N., Maguy, A., De Simone, S. A., Miragoli, M., Jousset, F., and Rohr, S. (2017). TGF-β1(Transforming Growth Factor-β1) plays a pivotal role in cardiac myofibroblast arrhythmogenicity. *Circ. Arrhythm. Electrophysiol.* 10:e004567. doi: 10.1161/CIRCEP.116.004567

Sanchez-Quintana, D., Ramon Lopez-Mínguez, J., Pizarro, G., Murillo, M., and Angel Cabrera, J. (2012). Triggers and anatomical substrates in the genesis and perpetuation of atrial fibrillation. *Curr. Cardiol. Rev.* 8, 310–326. doi: 10.2174/157340312803760721

Satoh, H., Delbridge, L. M. D., Blatter, L. A., and Bers, D. M. (1996). Surface: volume relationship in cardiac myocytes studied with confocal microscopy and membrane capacitance measurements: species-dependence and developmental effects. *Biophys. J.* 70, 1494–1504. doi: 10.1016/S0006-3495(96)79711-4

Sridhar, S., Vandersickel, N., and Panfilov, A. V. (2017). Effect of myocyte-fibroblast coupling on the onset of pathological dynamics in a model of ventricular tissue. *Sci. Rep.* 7:40985. doi: 10.1038/srep40985

Tanaka, K., Zlochiver, S., Vikstrom, K. L., Yamazaki, M., Moreno, J., Klos, M., et al. (2007). Spatial distribution of fibrosis governs fibrillation wave dynamics in the posterior left atrium during heart failure. *Circ. Res.* 101, 839–847. doi: 10.1161/CIRCRESAHA.107.153858

Ten Tusscher, K., Noble, D., Noble, P. J., and Panfilov, A. V. (2004). A model for human ventricular tissue. *Am. J. Physiol. Circ. Physiol.* 286, H1573–H1589.

Varela, M., Colman, M. A., Hancox, J. C., and Aslanidi, O. V. (2016). Atrial heterogeneity generates re-entrant substrate during atrial fibrillation and anti-arrhythmic drug action: mechanistic insights from canine atrial models. *PLoS Comput. Biol.* 12:e1005245. doi: 10.1371/journal.pcbi.1005245

Vasquez, C., Moreno, A. P., and Berbari, E. J. (2004). Modeling fibroblast-mediated conduction in the ventricle. *Comput. Cardiol.* 2004, 349–352. doi: 10.1109/CIC.2004.1442944

Verheule, S., Eckstein, J., Linz, D., Maesen, B., Bidar, E., Gharaviri, A., et al. (2014). Role of endo-epicardial dissociation of electrical activity and transmural conduction in the development of persistent atrial fibrillation. *Prog. Biophys. Mol. Biol.* 115, 173–185. doi: 10.1016/j.pbiomolbio.2014.07.007

Waks, J. W., and Josephson, M. E. (2014). Mechanisms of atrial fibrillation – reentry, rotors and reality. *Arrhythm. Electrophysiol. Rev.* 3, 90–100. doi: 10.15420/aer.2014.3.2.90

Warren, M., Guha, P. K., Berenfeld, O., Zaitsev, A., Anumonwo, J. M. B., Dhamoon, A. S., et al. (2003). Blockade of the inward rectifying potassium current terminates ventricular fibrillation in the guinea pig heart. *J. Cardiovasc. Electrophysiol.* 14, 621–631. doi: 10.1046/j.1540-8167.2003.03006.x

Wilhelms, M., Hettmann, H., Maleckar, M. M., Koivumäki, J. T., Dössel, O., and Seemann, G. (2013). Benchmarking electrophysiological models of human atrial myocytes. *Front. Physiol.* 3:487. doi: 10.3389/fphys.2012.00487

Xie, Y., Garfinkel, A., Camelliti, P., Kohl, P., Weiss, J. N., and Qu, Z. (2009). Effects of fibroblast-myocyte coupling on cardiac conduction and vulnerability to reentry: a computational study. *Hear. Rhythm* 6, 1641–1649. doi: 10.1016/j.hrthm.2009.08.003

Yamazaki, M., Mironov, S., Taravant, C., Brec, J., Vaquero, L. M., Bandaru, K., et al. (2012). Heterogeneous atrial wall thickness and stretch promote scroll waves anchoring during atrial fibrillation. *Cardiovasc. Res.* 94, 48–57. doi: 10.1093/cvr/cvr357

Yue, L., Xie, J., and Nattel, S. (2011). Molecular determinants of cardiac fibroblast electrical function and therapeutic implications for atrial fibrillation. *Cardiovasc. Res.* 89, 744–753. doi: 10.1093/cvr/cvq329

Zahid, S., Cochet, H., Boyle, P. M., Schwarz, E. L., Whyte, K. N., Vigmond, E. J., et al. (2016). Patient-derived models link re-entrant driver localization in atrial fibrillation to fibrosis spatial pattern. *Cardiovasc. Res.* 110, 443–454. doi: 10.1093/cvr/cvw073

Zhan, H., Xia, L., Shou, G., Zang, Y., Liu, F., and Crozier, S. (2014). Fibroblast proliferation alters cardiac excitation conduction and contraction: a computational study. *J. Zhejiang Univ. Sci. B* 15, 225–242. doi: 10.1631/jzus.B1300156

8

In silico Assessment of Pharmacotherapy for Human Atrial Patho-Electrophysiology Associated with hERG-Linked Short QT Syndrome

***Dominic G. Whittaker*[1,2], *Jules C. Hancox*[2,3*] and *Henggui Zhang*[2,4,5,6*]**

[1] Faculty of Biological Sciences, School of Biomedical Sciences, University of Leeds, Leeds, United Kingdom, [2] Biological Physics Group, School of Physics and Astronomy, The University of Manchester, Manchester, United Kingdom, [3] Cardiovascular Research Laboratories, Department of Physiology, Pharmacology and Neuroscience, School of Medical Sciences, University of Bristol, Bristol, United Kingdom, [4] School of Computer Science and Technology, Harbin Institute of Technology, Harbin, China, [5] Space Institute of Southern China, Shenzhen, China, [6] Key Laboratory of Medical Electrophysiology of Ministry of Education and Medical Electrophysiological Key Laboratory of Sichuan Province, Institute of Cardiovascular Research, Southwest Medical University, Luzhou, China

***Correspondence:**
Jules C. Hancox
jules.hancox@bristol.ac.uk
Henggui Zhang
henggui.zhang@manchester.ac.uk

Short QT syndrome variant 1 (SQT1) arises due to gain-of-function mutations to the *human Ether-à-go-go-Related Gene* (*hERG*), which encodes the α subunit of channels carrying rapid delayed rectifier potassium current, I_{Kr}. In addition to QT interval shortening and ventricular arrhythmias, SQT1 is associated with increased risk of atrial fibrillation (AF), which is often the only clinical presentation. However, the underlying basis of AF and its pharmacological treatment remain incompletely understood in the context of SQT1. In this study, computational modeling was used to investigate mechanisms of human atrial arrhythmogenesis consequent to a SQT1 mutation, as well as pharmacotherapeutic effects of selected class I drugs–disopyramide, quinidine, and propafenone. A Markov chain formulation describing wild type (WT) and N588K-hERG mutant I_{Kr} was incorporated into a contemporary human atrial action potential (AP) model, which was integrated into one-dimensional (1D) tissue strands, idealized 2D sheets, and a 3D heterogeneous, anatomical human atria model. Multi-channel pharmacological effects of disopyramide, quinidine, and propafenone, including binding kinetics for I_{Kr}/hERG and sodium current, I_{Na}, were considered. Heterozygous and homozygous formulations of the N588K-hERG mutation shortened the AP duration (APD) by 53 and 86 ms, respectively, which abbreviated the effective refractory period (ERP) and excitation wavelength in tissue, increasing the lifespan and dominant frequency (DF) of scroll waves in the 3D anatomical human atria. At the concentrations tested in this study, quinidine most effectively prolonged the APD and ERP in the setting of SQT1, followed by disopyramide and propafenone. In 2D simulations, disopyramide and quinidine promoted re-entry termination by increasing the re-entry wavelength, whereas propafenone induced secondary waves which destabilized the re-entrant circuit. In 3D simulations, the DF of re-entry was reduced in a dose-dependent manner for disopyramide and quinidine, and propafenone to a lesser extent. All of the anti-arrhythmic agents promoted pharmacological conversion, most frequently terminating re-entry in the order quinidine > propafenone = disopyramide. Our findings provide further insight into mechanisms of SQT1-related AF and a rational basis for the pursuit of combined I_{Kr} and I_{Na} block based pharmacological strategies in the treatment of SQT1-linked AF.

Keywords: arrhythmia, short QT syndrome, atrial fibrillation, hERG, class I anti-arrhythmics, human atria, potassium channels

INTRODUCTION

The short QT syndrome (SQTS) is characterized primarily by a short QT interval on the ECG, which corresponds to abbreviated ventricular repolarisation. However, symptomatic atrial fibrillation (AF) has also been reported as a common first clinical presentation of the SQTS (Schimpf et al., 2005), suggesting that pathophysiological mechanisms leading to shortening of the QT interval also affect the atria, which can increase susceptibility to AF. The N588K mutation to the *human Ether-à-go-go-Related gene (hERG)*, which encodes the α subunit of channels carrying rapid delayed rectifier potassium current, I_{Kr}, underlies a form of SQTS variant 1 (SQT1) (Brugada et al., 2004), and has been associated with a high incidence of AF in affected probands—as high as 50% (Hu et al., 2017). Whilst ventricular arrhythmia substrates in SQT1 have received much attention (Zhang and Hancox, 2004; Patel and Antzelevitch, 2008; Adeniran et al., 2011), there have been comparatively fewer studies investigating mechanisms by which SQT1 mutations promote AF, which can be an important biomarker of the SQTS. Furthermore, effective management of AF remains a challenge, and is incompletely understood in the context of SQT1 (Enriquez et al., 2016; Hancox et al., 2018).

A previous simulation study (Loewe et al., 2014b) used the Courtemanche-Ramirez-Nattel (CRN) mathematical model of the human atrial action potential (AP) (Courtemanche et al., 1998) to demonstrate shortening of the atrial effective refractory period (ERP) and tissue excitation wavelength (WL) consequent to the N588K-hERG mutation. This was shown to facilitate initiation and sustenance of spiral waves in idealized two-dimensional (2D) sheets of human atrial tissue, which is a likely mechanism for increased susceptibility to AF. However, both the intrinsic electrical heterogeneities and complex anatomy of the human atria have also been suggested to influence arrhythmia vulnerability and dynamics in overall response to K^+ channel mutations (Colman et al., 2017; Whittaker et al., 2017b). Consequently, the first aim of the present study was to assess the arrhythmogenicity of the N588K-hERG mutation in anatomically-detailed models of the human atria with realistic structure and inclusion of regional differences in electrophysiology.

The class Ia anti-arrhythmic drug quinidine is typically used as the frontline therapy for QT interval normalization in SQT1 (Gaita et al., 2004; Giustetto, 2006; Hu et al., 2017), and disopyramide has been suggested as a possible alternative (Dumaine and Antzelevitch, 2006; Schimpf et al., 2007). Regarding management of atrial arrhythmias, the class Ic anti-arrhythmic drug propafenone has been reported to be effective at preventing recurrent episodes of (paroxysmal) AF mediated by the N588K mutation to hERG (Hong et al., 2005; Bjerregaard et al., 2006), maintaining 2 patients free of arrhythmia recurrence for >2 years (Hong et al., 2005). In an experimental setting in which a hERG activator was used to approximate SQT1, quinidine (a blocker of I_{Na} and I_{Kr}) was effective at extending atrial AP duration and ERP and preventing AF (Nof et al., 2010), more so than E-4031 (a selective I_{Kr} blocker) or lidocaine (an I_{Na} blocker) alone, suggesting that K^+ and Na^+ channel blocking effects combine synergistically for improved management of AF in SQT1. Similarly, in our previous study, a multi-scale computational modeling approach was used to investigate ventricular pharmacological effects of disopyramide and quinidine in SQT1 (Whittaker et al., 2017a), where combined I_{Na} and I_{Kr} block by both compounds was shown to prolong ERP to a greater extent than I_{Na} or I_{Kr} block alone. Mechanisms by which Na^+ and K^+-channel blocking agents may provide beneficial effects in the context of SQT1-mediated human atrial pro-arrhythmia remain unclear. A multi-scale cardiac modeling approach is being used increasingly for optimisation of therapy (Yuan et al., 2015). Consequently, the second aim of the present study was to assess the efficacy of the class I drugs disopyramide, quinidine, and propafenone on rate and rhythm control of human atrial arrhythmias mediated by SQT1, from cell to 3D tissue levels, using drug binding models (including reduced potency of drugs against SQT1 mutant I_{Kr}) with multi-channel pharmacology.

METHODS

Modeling Human Atrial Electrophysiology

Human atrial electrophysiology was simulated using the Colman et al. model (Colman et al., 2013), as updated recently (Ni et al., 2017), and is hereinafter referred to as the CNZ (Colman-Ni-Zhang) model. The equations for I_{Kr} in the CNZ model were replaced with previously developed and validated Markov chain formulations of wild type (WT) and N588K mutant I_{Kr}/hERG (Whittaker et al., 2017a). The maximal conductance of I_{Kr} was set to $g_{Kr} = 0.0111375 \cdot [K^+]_o^{0.59}$, where $[K^+]_o$ is the extracellular potassium concentration (Adeniran et al., 2011), resulting in an action potential duration (APD) at 90% repolarisation (APD_{90}) of 248.8 ms at 1 Hz in the baseline human atrial cell model, which is well within the experimentally-measured range of APDs in human atrial myocytes (Bosch et al., 1999; Kim et al., 2002; Dobrev and Ravens, 2003; Katoh et al., 2005; Redpath et al., 2006; Pau et al., 2007). A family of regional human atrial cell models was incorporated into the CNZ model, accounting for distinct differences in electrophysiology of the right and left atrium (RA and LA, respectively), right and left atrial appendages (RAA and LAA, respectively), crista terminalis (CT), pectinate muscles (PM), atrio-ventricular ring (AVR), atrial septum (AS), Bachmann's bundle (BB), and pulmonary veins (PV) (Colman et al., 2013). Changes to maximal ionic conductances relative to the RA model implemented in order to create a family of regional cell models are given in **Table S1**. The homozygous (N588K) form of SQT1 was modeled as consisting of 100% mutant subunits, whereas the heterozygous (WT-N588K) form was assumed to consist of a 1:1 WT:mutant subunit ratio (Whittaker et al., 2017a).

Modeling Pharmacological Actions of Disopyramide and Quinidine

In our previous study (Whittaker et al., 2017a), the actions of the class Ia anti-arrhythmic drugs disopyramide and quinidine on human ventricles were simulated in the setting of SQT1. State-dependent binding of disopyramide and quinidine to hERG channels was simulated through addition of drug-bound open and inactivated states to Markov chain formulations of I_{Kr}, and the guarded receptor model (Starmer et al., 1984) was used to describe use-dependent block of fast sodium current, I_{Na}, by both agents. Furthermore, the blocking actions of disopyramide and quinidine on slow delayed rectifier potassium current, I_{Ks}, L-type calcium current, I_{CaL}, transient outward potassium current, I_{to}, inward rectifier potassium current, I_{K1} (quinidine only), and late sodium current, I_{NaL} (quinidine only), were modeled using a simple "pore block" approach. In the present study, the actions of disopyramide and quinidine on human atrial electrophysiology were represented using the same formulations and IC_{50} (half maximal inhibitory concentration) values presented in Whittaker et al. (2017a). In addition, disopyramide and quinidine have both been reported to block the atrial-specific ultra-rapid delayed rectifier potassium current, I_{Kur}. For disopyramide, the IC_{50} for block of I_{Kur} was taken to be 25.0 μM (Aréchiga et al., 2008), and for quinidine the IC_{50} was taken to be 6.6 μM, as measured in human atrial myocytes (Nenov et al., 1998). As the CNZ model does not include late sodium current, quinidine block of I_{NaL} was not included in simulations. Full details of disopyramide and quinidine models can be found in Whittaker et al. (2017a).

Modeling Pharmacological Actions of Propafenone

Using the same approach as detailed for disopyramide and quinidine in Whittaker et al. (2017a), state-dependent models of drug block by propafenone were developed. Interactions between propafenone and I_{Kr}/hERG were developed based on experimental data obtained at 37°C (Paul et al., 2002; McPate et al., 2008), where estimation of parameters for drug-bound states of the Markov chain formulation of I_{Kr} was performed using the procedure outlined in Moreno et al. (2016). Binding and unbinding rates to activated and inactivated state channels were allowed to vary freely in order to minimize the difference between simulated and experimental dose-dependent steady state block (WT and N588K), mean fractional block of tail currents during a pulse protocol, and voltage-dependence of tail current block (Paul et al., 2002; McPate et al., 2008). The extended drug-free Markov chain model of I_{Kr}/hERG is shown in **Figure 1**, as well as the close concordance between simulated and experimental data regarding propafenone block of I_{hERG}. Parameters and state affinities are given in **Table S2**.

Propafenone is a class Ic sodium channel blocking anti-arrhythmic drug (Roden, 2014). Use-dependent block of sodium channels by propafenone was represented using the guarded receptor hypothesis (Starmer et al., 1984), as described for disopyramide and quinidine. Propafenone is predominantly an open state sodium channel blocker with little to no resting state block (Edrich et al., 2005; Burashnikov et al., 2012), and was thus assumed to bind only to activated and inactivated states. Binding and unbinding parameters were constrained based on the dose-dependent, use-dependent, and steady state block of I_{Na} by propafenone (Harmer et al., 2008), as shown in **Figure 2A**. Binding and unbinding parameters and state affinities are given in **Table S3**.

Whilst propafenone most potently blocks I_{Kr} and I_{Na}, it is a multi-channel blocker, and thus exerts secondary effects on other ion channels, which were modeled using a simple pore block based on IC_{50} values from the literature. Propafenone blocks I_{CaL} with an IC_{50} of 1.5–1.7 μM in mammalian cardiac myocytes (Fei et al., 1993; Hancox and Mitcheson, 1997). In human atrial myocytes, propafenone has been shown to block I_{to} with an IC_{50} of 4.8 μM (Gross and Castle, 1998; Seki et al., 1999) and I_{K1} with an IC_{50} of 16.8 μM (Amorós et al., 2013). Finally, I_{Kur} is blocked with an IC_{50} of 4.4 μM (Franqueza et al., 1998). The therapeutic range of propafenone has been estimated to be between 2 and 6 μM (Paul et al., 2002). Taking into account plasma protein binding, estimates of the most likely unbound concentrations have been given as 0.15–0.7 μM (Slawsky and Castle, 1994), 0.2–0.6 μM (Duan et al., 1993), and 0.33–1 μM (Seki et al., 1999). In this study, the effects of three equally-spaced concentrations which fell within this range were studied—0.2, 0.5, and 0.8 μM propafenone. It should be noted that these concentrations are not intended to be compared directly with those chosen for disopyramide and quinidine (1, 2, and 5 μM), which were taken from Whittaker et al. (2017a) and are not equally-spaced. A comparison of IC_{50} values used for disopyramide, quinidine, and propafenone is given in **Table S4**.

In order to assess whether the combined actions of propafenone in the model induced reasonable rate- and concentration- dependent effects on the AP under control conditions, alterations in the maximum upstroke velocity ($\dot{V}_{max}$) upon application of propafenone were compared with experimental data taken from canine atrial cells (Burashnikov et al., 2012). **Figure 2B** shows changes in $\dot{V}_{max}$ upon application of 0.3 and 1.5 μM propafenone at cycle lengths of 500 and 300 ms, where close concordance can be seen between simulation and experiment (**Figure 2C**). Although experimental data were taken from canine atrial myocytes, the human atrial simulation data nonetheless recapitulated the considerable reduction in $\dot{V}_{max}$ at both concentrations and cycle lengths, which is primarily due to the sodium channel blocking actions of propafenone.

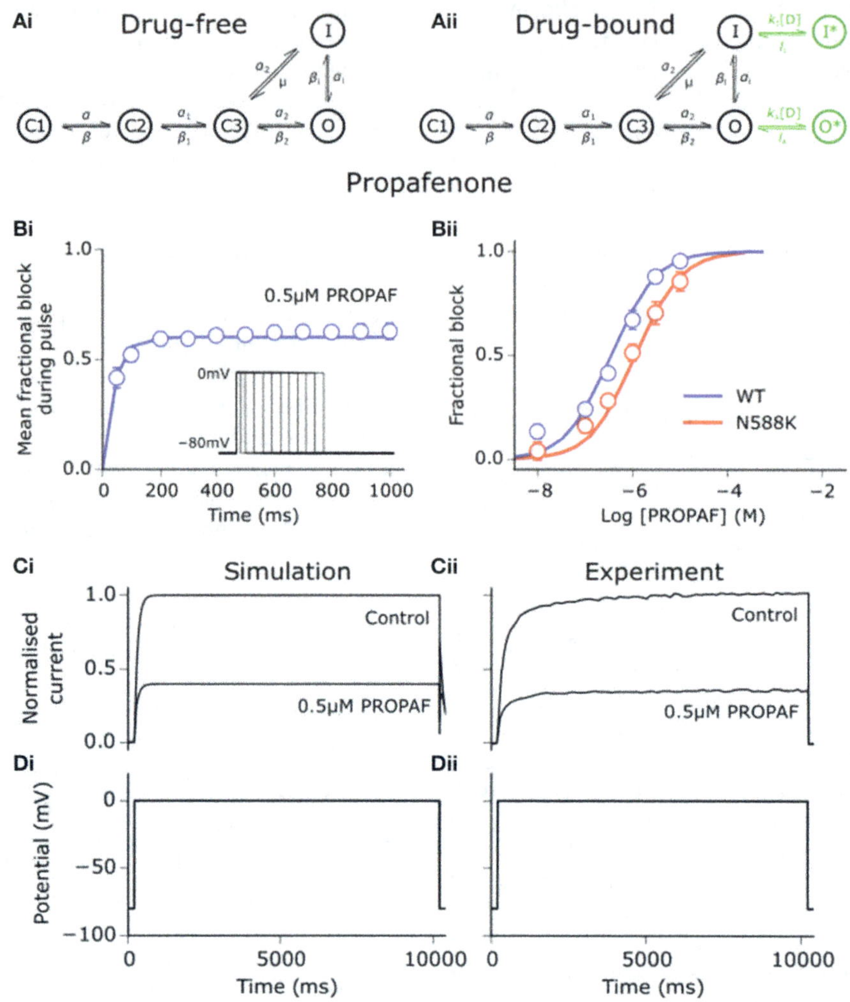

FIGURE 1 | Propafenone interactions with hERG channels. **(Ai)** Drug-free and **(Aii)** drug-bound (additional states shown in green) Markov chain models of I_{Kr}/hERG. Simulated (solid line) and experimental (points) mean fractional block by 0.5 μM propafenone (PROPAF) of I_{hERG} during pulse protocol (shown inset) **(Bi)**, and dose-response curve under WT (blue) and SQT1 mutant N588K (red) conditions **(Bii)**, where IC_{50} values are 390 nM and 936 nM (2.4-fold increase), respectively. **(Ci)** Simulated and **(Cii)** experimental current traces in response to a 10,000 ms depolarising voltage step to 0 mV from a holding potential of −80 mV **(Di,Dii)** under control conditions and with application of 0.5 μM PROPAF – these data were used to validate and not to further train the model. Experimental data at 37°C are taken from Paul et al. (2002) and McPate et al. (2008).

Tissue Simulations

Propagation of excitation waves in tissue was described using the monodomain equation,

$$\frac{\partial V}{\partial t} = \nabla(\mathbf{D}\nabla V) - \frac{I_{ion}}{C_m}, \tag{1}$$

where V is the transmembrane voltage, $\mathbf{D}$ is the global conductivity tensor, I_{ion} is the total ionic current, and C_m is the membrane capacitance. Equation (1) was solved using a finite difference PDE solver based on the explicit forward Euler method and Strang splitting scheme. Effects of the N588K-hERG mutation on ERP, WL, conduction velocity (CV), and spiral wave dynamics were determined using 1D and 2D models of RA tissue, as described previously (Whittaker et al., 2017b, 2018). Spiral waves were initiated in 2D models using an S1-S2 cross-shock protocol, and spiral wave core trajectories over a 5.0 s simulation period were traced by locating phase singularities (Bray and Wikswo, 2002). The behavior of re-entrant excitations in an anatomically-realistic setting was determined using a 3D human atrial structured grid geometry based on the Visible Female dataset (Seemann et al., 2006; Colman et al., 2013; Whittaker et al., 2017b) with rule-based fiber orientations (Krueger et al., 2011). The transverse value of the diffusion coefficient, $D_{\perp}$, was set to 0.1 mm^2 ms^{-1}, where an anisotropy ratio ($D_{||}$:$D_{\perp}$) of 3:1 in directions longitudinal and transverse to fibers was applied in the atrial working myocardium, and a ratio of 9:1 along the fast conducting bundles of the BB, CT, and PM (Colman et al., 2013; Whittaker et al., 2017b), which gave global and specific regional activation times in close agreement with experimental

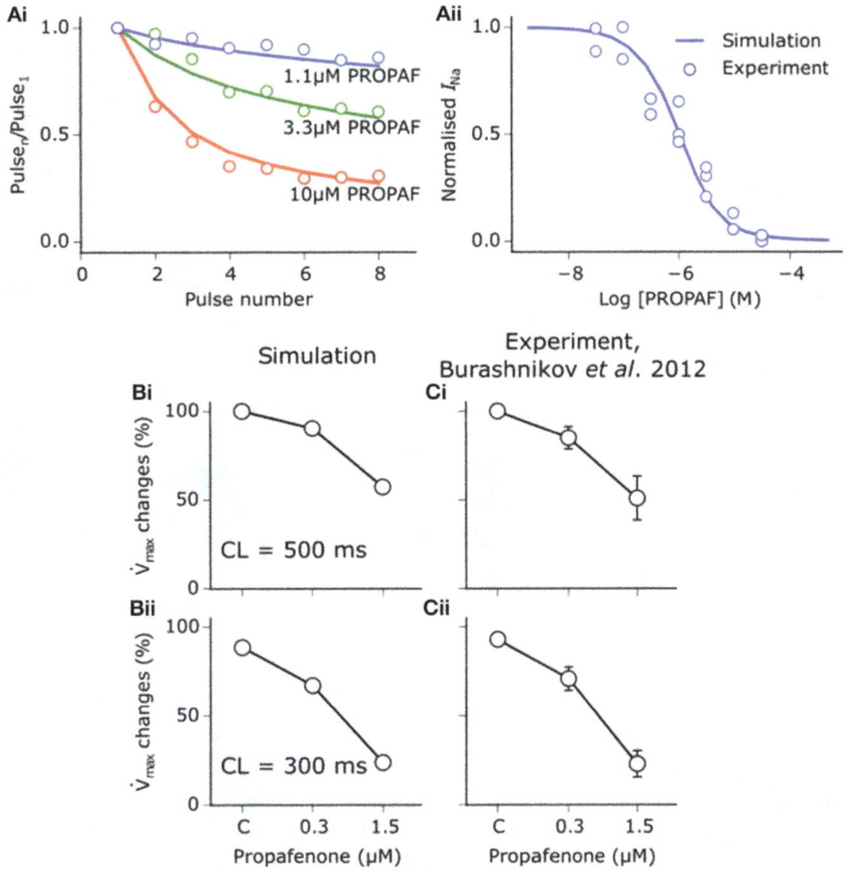

FIGURE 2 | Propafenone interactions with sodium channels. **(Ai)** Simulated (solid lines) and experimental (points) use-dependent block of sodium channels by propafenone (PROPAF) elicited using a series of 8 pulses from −90 mV to 0 mV at 3 Hz for three different test concentrations. **(Aii)** Steady state block of sodium channels using pulses from −90 mV to 0 mV at 3 Hz until a steady state was achieved. Experimental data are taken from Harmer et al. (2008), where the steady state block IC_{50} value is given as 1.4 μM. **(B)** Simulated and **(C)** experimentally-measured PROPAF-induced reduction in maximum upstroke velocity ($\dot{V}_{max}$) upon application of 0.3 and 1.5 μM PROPAF at a cycle length (CL) of (i) 500 ms and (ii) 300 ms. All $\dot{V}_{max}$ reductions are relative to the control (C) value at a CL of 500 ms. Experimental data, recorded from canine atrial myocytes, are taken from Burashnikov et al. (2012).

measurements (Lemery et al., 2007). The activation (ACT) time was defined as the time required for the membrane potential to reach −20 mV at each point in the geometry (Ni et al., 2017). Activation-recovery interval (ARI) was defined as the time interval between membrane potential depolarisation to −20 mV and repolarisation to −70 mV (adjusted to −65 mV in the PV region due to higher resting membrane potential) (Ni et al., 2017).

Re-entry was initiated using the phase distribution method (Biktashev and Holden, 1998; Whittaker et al., 2017a), by initiating either a clockwise or anti-clockwise scroll wave (as seen from a RA posterior wall view). Where sustained re-entrant activity was initiated, a power spectrum was obtained through fast Fourier transform analysis of pseudo ECG (pECG) time series (recorded from within the RA cavity). The dominant frequency (DF) was computed in Matlab from the largest peak in the power spectrum density. For simulating the effects of disopyramide, quinidine, and propafenone on re-entrant excitation, state variables for each node within the 3D anatomical model were saved after 2.5 s of a 10.0 s episode of sustained re-entrant activity in drug-free conditions. These were then used as initial conditions for new 3D simulations of duration 7.5 s (giving 10.0 s activity overall) in which varying concentrations of anti-arrhythmic drugs (1, 2, or 5 μM disopyramide and quinidine; 0.2, 0.5, or 0.8 μM propafenone) were applied immediately. This gave 18 simulations in total; 3 doses for each of the 3 anti-arrhythmic drugs, with 2 scroll wave initial conditions (both clockwise and anti-clockwise).

RESULTS

Effects of SQT1 Mutant I_{Kr} on Human Atrial Action Potentials

Both SQT1 mutant conditions shortened the human atrial APD at a pacing rate of 1 Hz (**Figure 3Ai**), from 248.8 ms in the WT condition to 195.4 and 163.3 ms in heterozygous (WT-N588K) and homozygous (N588K) mutation conditions, respectively. This was due to loss of inactivation associated with the N588K-hERG mutation, which increased I_{Kr} early

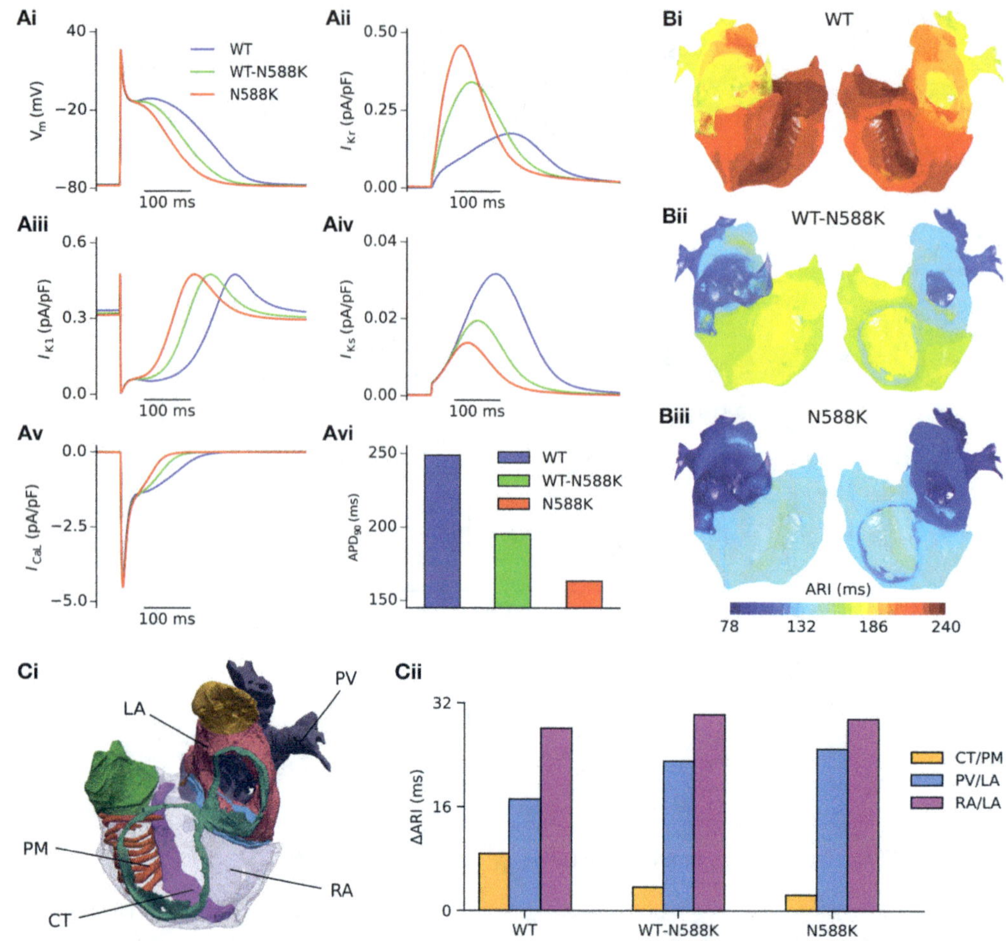

FIGURE 3 | Effects of the N588K-hERG mutation at the single cell and whole human atria level. **(Ai)** Single cell action potential profiles under WT (blue), WT-N588K (green), and N588K (red) conditions at a pacing frequency of 1 Hz, with corresponding current traces for **(Aii)** I_{Kr}, **(Aiii)** I_{K1}, **(Aiv)** I_{Ks}, and **(Av)** I_{CaL}, and **(Avi)** a summary of the measured APD_{90}. **(B)** Activation-recovery interval (ARI) maps under (i) WT, (ii) WT-N588K, and (iii) N588K conditions. **(Ci)** View looking into the cavities of the 3D anatomical human atria model, with the following regions highlighted: crista terminalis (CT), left atrium (LA), pectinate muscles (PM), pulmonary veins (PV), and right atrium (RA). **(Cii)** Measured dispersion of activation-recovery interval, ΔARI, between different atrial regions under WT and SQT1 mutation conditions.

during the AP and served to accelerate the repolarisation process (**Figure 3Aii**). Action potential abbreviation reduced considerably the duration of the plateau phase, causing I_{K1} to contribute to terminal repolarisation earlier during the AP (**Figure 3Aiii**), and lesser activation and reduced contribution of I_{Ks} (**Figure 3Aiv**). The SQT1 mutation also decreased net I_{CaL} due to the abbreviated plateau phase (**Figure 3Av**), shortening the APD_{90} under heterozygous and homozygous conditions (**Figure 3Avi**). In tissue, accelerated repolarisation under SQT1 conditions shortened the ERP and consequently the excitation WL. At the organ scale (in the 3D anatomical human atria model), both heterozygous and homozygous forms of the N588K-hERG mutation decreased global ARI (**Figure 3B**), whilst preserving the global dispersion of ARI. Furthermore, whereas ΔARI was decreased between CT/PM regions, it was increased between PV/LA and RA/LA regions under SQT1 conditions (**Figure 3C**). A summary of the effects of the N588K-hERG mutation on multi-scale human atrial AP biomarkers is given in **Table 1**.

Scroll Wave Dynamics in 3D Anatomical Human Atria Geometry

A summary of 3D scroll wave simulations in the anatomical human atria model under WT and SQT1 mutation conditions (in a clockwise configuration from a RA posterior wall aspect) is given in **Figure 4**. In the WT condition, scroll waves followed 2 transient, fragmented circuits around the RA, before self-terminating at ~0.7 s (**Video S1**), which precluded accurate measurement of the DF. In the WT-N588K condition, re-entrant wave activity sustained for the entire 10.0 s with a DF of 4.99 Hz, and was driven mostly by a macro re-entrant circuit around the right AVR, whilst also showing CT/isthmus driven activity in the RA (**Video S2**). Under homozygous N588K mutation conditions, scroll wave activity was also driven

TABLE 1 | A summary of multi-scale simulation results.

	Single cell		1D		3D	
	APD$_{90}$ (ms)	APD$_{50}$ (ms)	ERP (ms)	WL (ms)	ΔARI (ms)	DF (Hz)
WT	248.8	144.6	273	198.9	77	4.19*
WT-N588K	195.4	100.3	218	158.4	77	4.99
N588K	163.3	75.3	187	135.7	71	5.59

*Analysis biomarkers at the single cell, 1D, and 3D levels under WT, WT-N588K, and N588K conditions at a pacing rate of 1 Hz. ΔARI refers to global dispersion of ARI. DF was measured from the first 5.0 s of activity. APD$_{90}$ and APD$_{50}$, Action Potential Duration at 90% and 50% repolarisation respectively; ERP, Effective Refractory Period; WL, Excitation Wavelength; ARI, Activation-Recovery Interval; DF, Dominant Frequency. The DF is an average computed from two simulations with clockwise and anti-clockwise initial conditions, except in the case marked with *, in which only one value was used.*

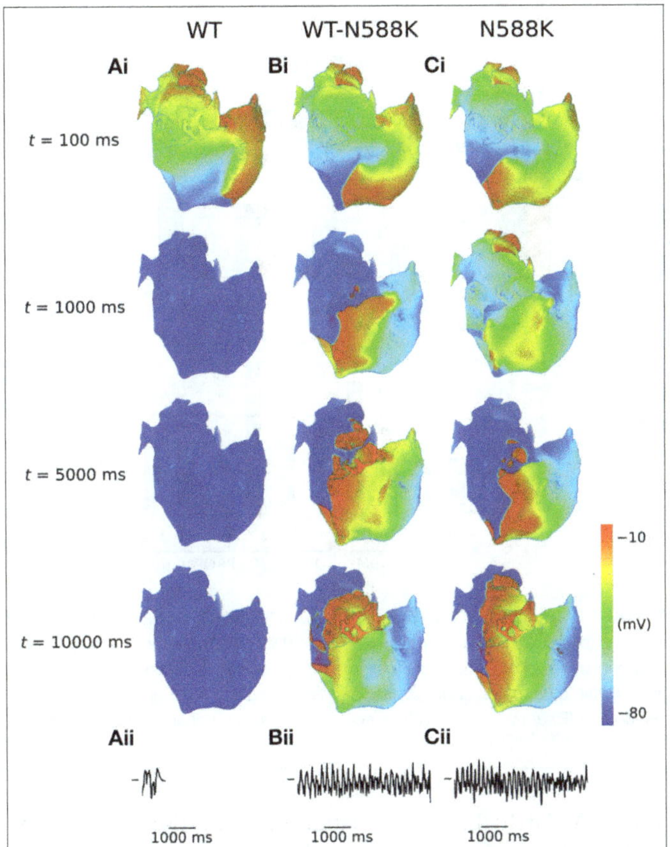

FIGURE 4 | Scroll waves under WT and SQT1 mutation conditions in the 3D anatomical human atria model. (i) Evolution of scroll waves following initiation of re-entry in a clockwise configuration (from a RA posterior wall aspect) at times $t = 100$ ms, $t = 1{,}000$ ms, $t = 5{,}000$ ms, and $t = 10{,}000$ ms under **(A)** WT, **(B)** WT-N588K, and **(C)** N588K conditions, with (ii) corresponding pseudo ECGs taken from the first 5.0 s of re-entry simulations.

predominantly by a re-entrant circuit around the AVR, with occasional existence of multiple waves on the RA free wall (**Video S3**), and a DF of 5.59 Hz. A summary of simulations using anti-clockwise scroll wave initial conditions is shown in **Figure S1**, and an average of the DF from both simulations (where applicable) measured from the first 5.0 s of activity is given in **Table 1**.

Effects of Class I Drugs on Human Atrial Action Potentials

In order to assess the actions of class I anti-arrhythmic drugs on the human atria at the cellular level, the effects of applying various concentrations of disopyramide, quinidine, and propafenone were investigated on the single cell AP under heterozygous WT-N588K (hereinafter referred to simply as SQT1) conditions. **Figure 5** shows AP profiles under drug-free SQT1 conditions and upon application of different concentrations of each drug at a pacing frequency of 1 Hz, with corresponding fractional block of I_{Kr} and I_{Na}. Application of all concentrations of disopyramide and propafenone produced only modest prolongation of the APD, failing to restore it to that of the WT condition. Quinidine, on the other hand, was more effective at prolonging the APD due to extensive I_{Kr} block, with the highest concentration (5 μM) prolonging the APD beyond that of the WT level. In contrast, all three agents prolonged the ERP effectively, restoring it to (or exceeding) that of the WT level at the highest respective concentrations tested, due to additional ERP-prolonging effects of I_{Na} block.

Conduction slowing due to sodium channel block by the three drugs caused an increase in activation time in the 3D anatomical human atria model (**Figure 5D**), which was most prominent for quinidine and least prominent for propafenone at the concentrations tested. A summary of the effects of pharmacological modulation across multiple scales is given in **Table 2**. In addition, in the 1D tissue model, the rate-dependent effects of disopyramide, quinidine, and propafenone on the ERP, CV, and WL are shown in **Figure S2**. Quinidine was shown to produce the most potent effects on CV and ERP at all pacing rates. Propafenone exerted the weakest effects on ERP at fast pacing rates, but had the greatest propensity to promote beat-to-beat alternans.

Pharmacological Effects of Class I Drugs on Re-entry Dynamics

In 2D simulations, under drug-free WT conditions the initiated spiral wave failed to re-enter the tissue (not shown). Under drug-free SQT1 conditions, the initiated spiral wave sustained for the 5.0 s duration of the simulation, eventually settling into a stationary, epicycloidal trajectory (**Figure 6Ai**). Application of 5 μM disopyramide was sufficient to terminate re-entry, as the re-entry wavelength was increased to such an extent that

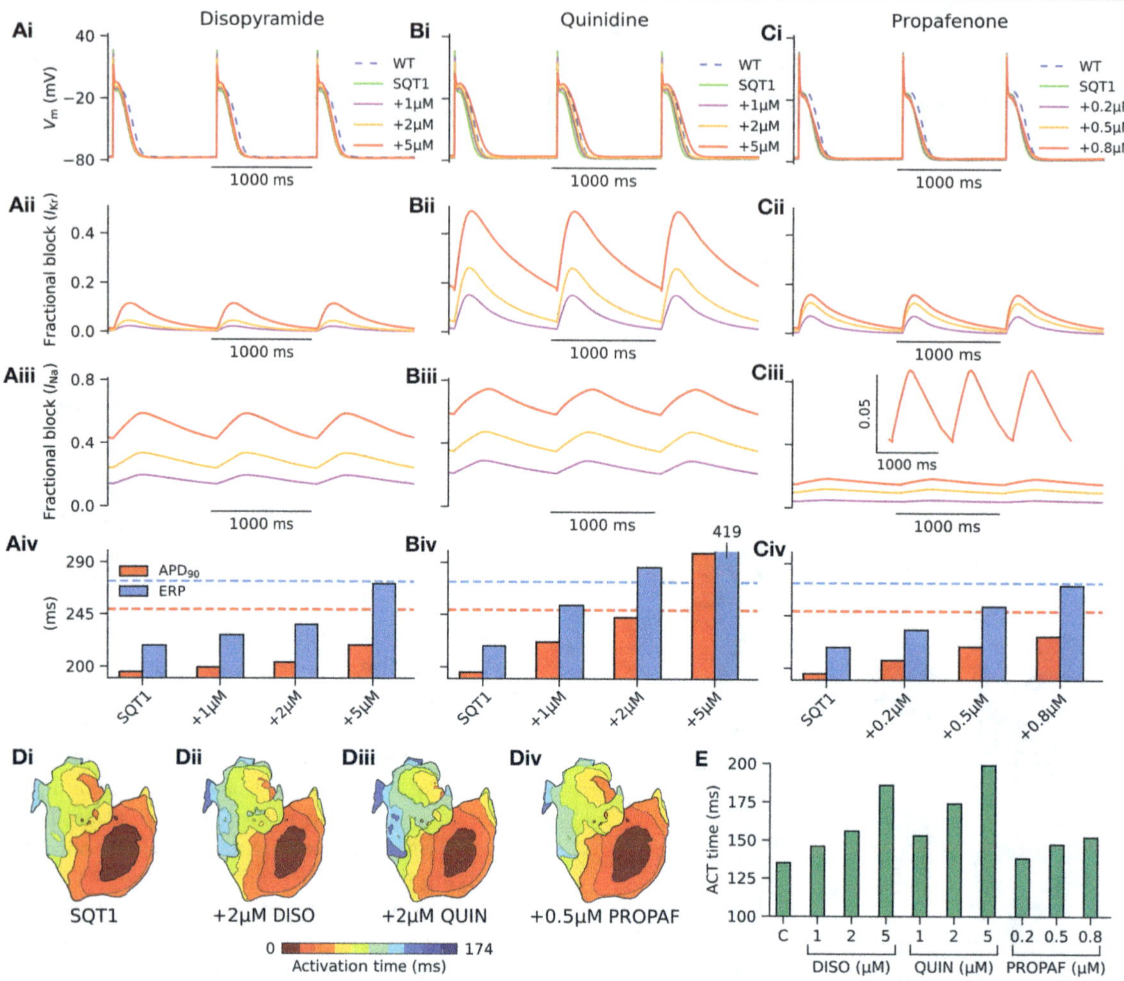

FIGURE 5 | Effects of class I drugs on human atrial electrophysiology in SQT1. Effects of **(A)** disopyramide (DISO), **(B)** quinidine (QUIN), and **(C)** propafenone (PROPAF) on (i) single human atrial cell action potentials (APs) under wild type (WT) conditions (blue, dashed line), drug-free WT-N588K (SQT1) conditions (green, solid line), and SQT1 + varying drug concentrations (purple, orange, and red solid lines). Corresponding fractional block of (ii) I_{Kr} and (iii) I_{Na}, and (iv) increase in APD_{90} (red) and effective refractory period (ERP; blue). **(D)** Activation sequences in the 3D anatomical human atria model under (i) drug-free SQT1 (control – C), (ii) SQT1 + 2 μM DISO, (iii) SQT1 + 2 μM QUIN, and (iv) SQT1 + 0.5 μM PROPAF conditions, with corresponding **(E)** activation (ACT) time summarized as a barchart. All simulations performed at a basic cycle length of 1,000 ms.

the spiral wave meandered out of the tissue (**Figure 6Aii**). On the other hand, both 1 and 2 μM disopyramide did not terminate re-entrant activity, but did increase the area over which spiral waves meandered (from 0.35 $mm^2\ ms^{-1}$ in the WT condition to 0.40 and 0.47 $mm^2\ ms^{-1}$, respectively '(**Figure 6B**). Similarly, 1 μM quinidine increased the area of meander to 0.44 $mm^2\ ms^{-1}$ without terminating re-entry, whereas 2 and 5 μM quinidine terminated re-entry without inducing wave break (**Figure 6C**). Application of 0.2 and 0.5 μM propafenone resulted in termination of re-entry by decreasing both the stationarity and stability of spiral waves (**Figure 6D**), whereas 0.8 μM propafenone did not terminate re-entry but did destabilize the re-entrant circuit and substantially increase the area of meander (to 0.75 $mm^2\ ms^{-1}$).

In 3D simulations using clockwise scroll wave initial conditions, quinidine terminated re-entry at all concentrations, and disopyramide terminated re-entry at concentrations of 1 and 5 μM (arrhythmia termination by 5 μM disopyramide and 2 μM quinidine are shown in **Videos S4, S5**, respectively). At a concentration of 2 μM disopyramide, the DF was reduced from 4.79 to 3.99 Hz (measured from the final 5.0 s of activity). Propafenone, on the other hand, was comparatively ineffective at reducing the DF at the concentrations tested, but terminated re-entry at a concentration of 0.5 μM (**Video S6**). Representative examples of arrhythmia termination by disopyramide, propafenone, and quinidine are shown in **Figure 7**. Disopyramide and quinidine produced a dose-dependent decrease in the DF which was greater than for propafenone (**Figure 7C**). In an anti-clockwise scroll wave configuration, the efficacy of anti-arrhythmic drugs was less favorable, with pharmacological conversion of re-entrant waves occurring only for 0.5 μM propafenone and 5 μM quinidine. A quantitative summary of all 2D and 3D re-entry simulations is given in **Table S5**.

TABLE 2 | A summary of multi-scale pharmacological simulation results.

		Single cell	1D			3D
		APD_{90} (ms)	ERP (ms)	CV (cm/s)	WL (mm)	ACT time (ms)
Drug-free	**SQT1**	195.4	218	72.7	158.4	135
DISO (μM)	**1**	199.3	227	68.7	155.9	146
	2	203.6	236	65.4	154.3	156
	5	218.4	271	57.8	156.5	186
QUIN (μM)	**1**	221.5	253	66.6	168.4	153
	2	242.6	286	61.6	176.1	174
	5	298.3	419	49.4	207.2	199
PROPAF (μM)	**0.2**	206.9	233	72.0	167.8	138
	0.5	218.6	253	70.6	178.7	147
	0.8	227.4	271	69.1	187.4	152

Analysis biomarkers at the single cell, 1D, and 3D levels at a pacing rate of 1 Hz under drug-free SQT1 conditions, and upon application of various concentrations of disopyramide (DISO), quinidine (QUIN), and propafenone (PROPAF). APD_{90}, Action Potential Duration at 90% repolarisation ; ERP, Effective Refractory Period; CV, Conduction Velocity; ACT time, Activation Time.

DISCUSSION

In this study, pathophysiological effects of the SQT1-related N588K-hERG mutation on human atrial electrophysiology were assessed, investigating mechanisms of increased susceptibility to the development of atrial arrhythmias in multi-scale cellular and tissue models incorporating electrical and anatomical heterogeneities. Furthermore, the actions of the class I anti-arrhythmic drugs disopyramide, quinidine, and propafenone were assessed in the context of sustained atrial arrhythmic excitations mediated by the SQT1 N588K mutation using drug simulations including binding kinetics, altered potency of I_{Kr}/hERG block in SQT1, and multiple ion channel block. Both quinidine and disopyramide have demonstrated efficacy in QT interval prolongation in the setting of SQT1 (Gaita et al., 2004; Schimpf et al., 2007; Mizobuchi et al., 2008; Giustetto et al., 2011; Hu et al., 2017), whereas propafenone has been used in 3 patients for management of episodes of paroxysmal AF mediated by SQT1, which prevented recurrence of arrhythmias but did not prolong the QT interval (Hong et al., 2005; Bjerregaard et al., 2006). This study provides clinically-relevant insights into pharmacology of SQT1 by evaluating and comparing the actions of all three drugs in the context of accelerated atrial repolarisation and arrhythmias mediated by SQT1, offering an important step toward *in silico* optimisation of pharmacological therapy in this context.

Main Findings

The major findings presented in this study are as follows. (1) Heterozygous and homozygous forms of the SQT1-linked N588K-hERG mutation shortened significantly the APD of human atrial cells, whilst preserving global dispersion of ARI, and increasing ΔARI between certain regions of the human atria. (2) The dominant frequency and lifespan of re-entry in 3D arrhythmia simulations was increased by heterozygous and homozygous forms of the N588K mutation. (3) Disopyramide, quinidine, and propafenone all produced ERP prolongation in the setting of SQT1, the extent of which was greatest for quinidine. (4) In 2D simulations, disopyramide and quinidine terminated re-entry at high concentrations due to increased re-entry wavelength, whereas propafenone terminated re-entry in a non-dose-dependent manner, by inducing secondary waves. (5) In 3D simulations, the DF of re-entry was reduced in a dose-dependent manner for clinically-relevant doses of disopyramide and quinidine, and propafenone to a lesser extent. (6) All three anti-arrhythmic agents demonstrated some efficacy in pharmacological rhythm control, most frequently terminating re-entry in the order quinidine > propafenone = disopyramide. A summary of findings regarding pro-arrhythmic mechanisms of the N588K-hERG mutation in human atria and anti-arrhythmic actions of selected class I drugs is given in **Figure 8**.

SQT1 Mutant I_{Kr} Promotes Human Atrial Arrhythmogenesis

The fact that the N588K-hERG mutation is associated with both a short QT interval and reports of AF (Hong et al., 2005) suggests that pathophysiological mechanisms leading to QT interval shortening in SQT1 also affect the atria and may promote AF. In an experimental model of SQT1, application of 20 μM of the I_{Kr} agonist PD-118057 shortened the APD in both CT and PM cell types of canine atrial tissue (Nof et al., 2010), as well as increasing APD dispersion between them. In the present study, at the cellular level heterozygous and homozygous forms of the N588K-hERG mutation produced a shortening of the human right atrial APD of 53.4 and 85.5 ms, respectively–values which are consistent with a previous simulation study (Loewe et al., 2014b). At the tissue level, global ΔARI was unaffected by the WT-N588K mutation condition, and was slightly decreased by the homozygous form. The model predicted an increase in ΔARI between PV/LA and RA/LA regions for both heterozygous and homozygous forms of the N588K mutation (**Figure 3C**), but not between CT/PM regions. This may be due to the fact that the effects of the hERG activator PD-118057 and of the N588K mutation on I_{Kr}/hERG are different: the former

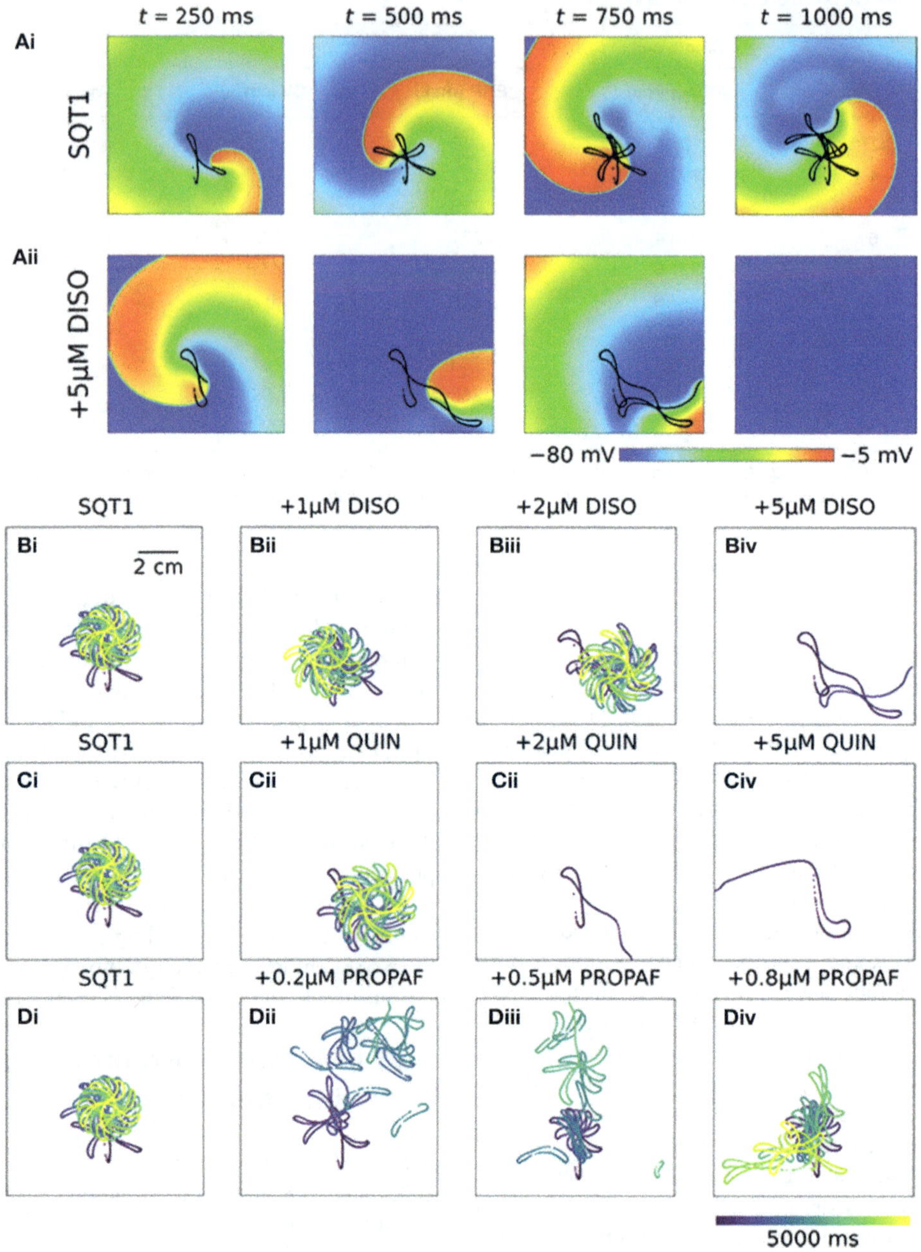

FIGURE 6 | Re-entry dynamics in homogeneous 2D sheets upon application of disopyramide, propafenone, and quinidine in SQT1 mutation conditions. **(A)** Representative snapshots of re-entrant spiral waves under (i) drug-free SQT1 and (ii) SQT1 + 5 μM disopyramide (DISO) conditions at times, $t = 250$, 500, 750, and 1,000 ms following re-entry initiation, with spiral wave core trajectories superimposed onto membrane potentials in black. Spiral wave core trajectories over a 5,000 ms period under **(Bi, Ci, Di)** drug-free SQT1 conditions, and upon application of **(Bii)** 1 μM, **(Biii)** 2 μM, and **(Biv)** 5 μM DISO, **(Cii)** 1 μM, **(Ciii)** 2 μM, and **(Civ)** 5 μM quinidine (QUIN), and **(Dii)** 0.2 μM, **(Diii)** 0.5 μM, and **(Div)** 0.8 μM propafenone (PROPAF).

increases I_{Kr}/hERG channel open probability without altering gating kinetics (Zhou et al., 2005), whereas the latter alters kinetics through profound attenuation of inactivation (Cordeiro et al., 2005; McPate et al., 2005).

Interestingly, there is clinical evidence of a LA-RA gradient in the DF in paroxysmal AF (Lazar et al., 2004), which may be underlain by APD differences between the RA and LA in pathological conditions which promote AF (Voigt et al., 2010). Furthermore, regional differences in APD between PV/LA regions have been identified previously as high frequency excitation or microreentrant sources underlying AF (Mandapati et al., 2000; Arora et al., 2003; Kumagai et al., 2004)–this suggests that localized increases in the spatial dispersion of repolarisation could be a mechanism by which atrial arrhythmogenesis is promoted in SQT1, as suggested in the previous experimental study (Nof et al., 2010).

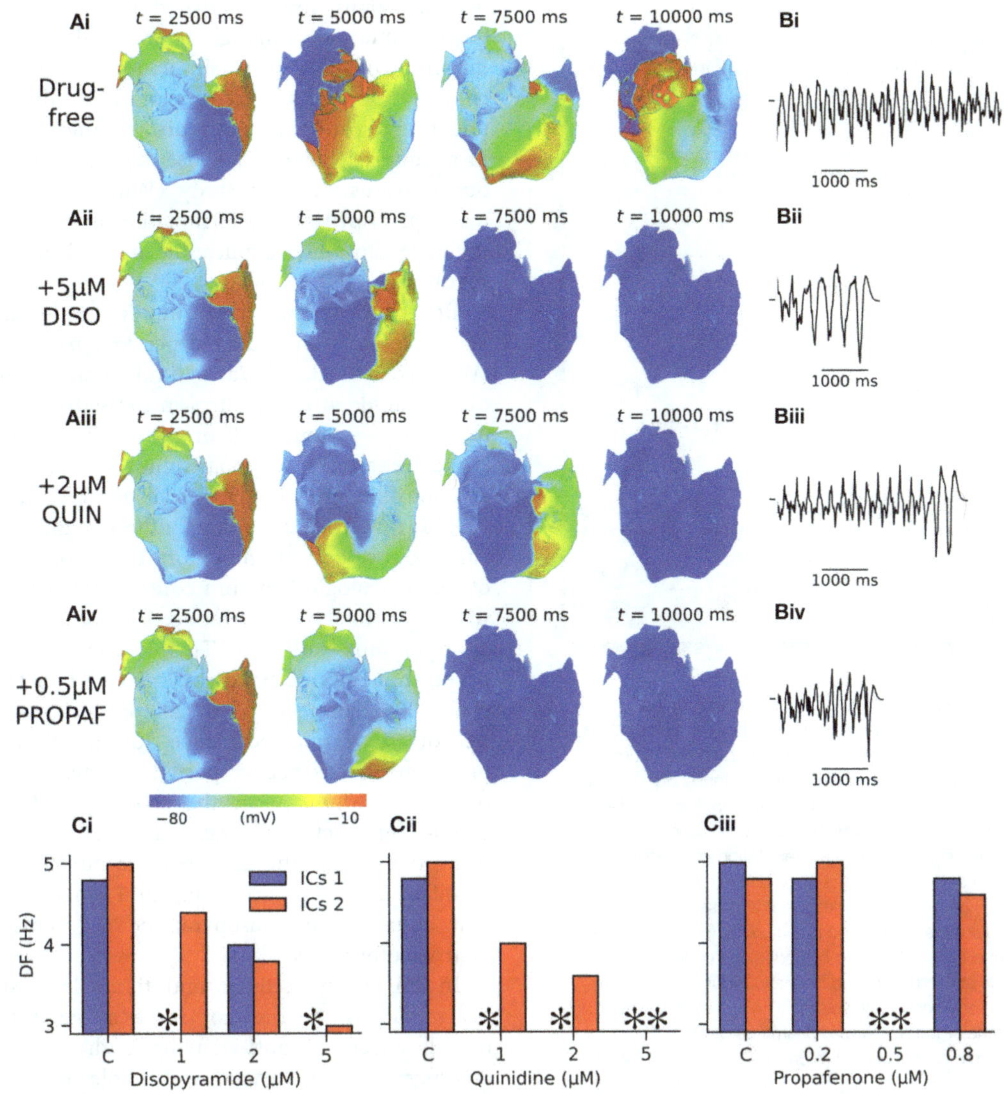

FIGURE 7 | Arrhythmia termination in 3D anatomical human atria by representative concentrations of disopyramide, propafenone, and quinidine under SQT1 mutation conditions. **(A)** Snapshots of re-entrant scroll waves in a clockwise configuration (viewed from RA posterior wall) at various time points after initiation of a scroll wave in the 3D anatomical human atrial model under (i) drug-free WT-N588K conditions, and upon application of (ii) 5 μM disopyramide (DISO), (iii) 0.5 μM propafenone (PROPAF), and (iv) 2 μM quinidine (QUIN) conditions, with **(B)** corresponding pseudo ECG recorded during the final 5.0 s. In pharmacological simulation drugs were applied at $t = 2{,}500$ ms. **(C)** Barcharts summarizing DF upon application of various concentrations of (i) DISO, (ii) PROPAF, and (iii) QUIN for clockwise and anti-clockwise initial conditions (ICs 1 and ICs 2, respectively). * denotes simulations in which DF was not calculated due to occurrence of re-entry termination.

In a previous simulation study (Loewe et al., 2014b), the N588K-hERG mutation in a 1:1 mutant to WT ratio was shown to increase inducibility and lifespan of rotors in idealized 2D sheets of human atrial tissue, but did not permit sustained re-entry. By contrast, in the present study, the heterozygous WT-N588K (SQT1) condition permitted the sustenance of spiral waves in 2D simulations. This may be due to several differences in the modeling, one of which is that the CRN model used in that study (Loewe et al., 2014b) produces an ERP restitution curve which is around 50 ms higher than available experimental data (Wilhelms et al., 2013), making re-entry more difficult to sustain, whereas the CNZ model ERP restitution curve lies mostly within the experimental range (**Figure S3**). In this study, the presence of realistic structure and heterogeneous electrophysiology, in addition to the cellular electrophysiological substrate induced by the N588K-hERG mutation, also favored the sustenance of re-entrant scroll waves in the 3D anatomical human atria model (using both clockwise and anti-clockwise scroll wave initial conditions), and could both prolong or shorten the lifespan of re-entrant excitations under pharmacological modulation conditions when compared directly to observations in 2D homogeneous sheets. This highlights the value of including both approaches in probing the arrhythmia substrate associated with genetic mutations in human atria, as behavior in heterogeneous

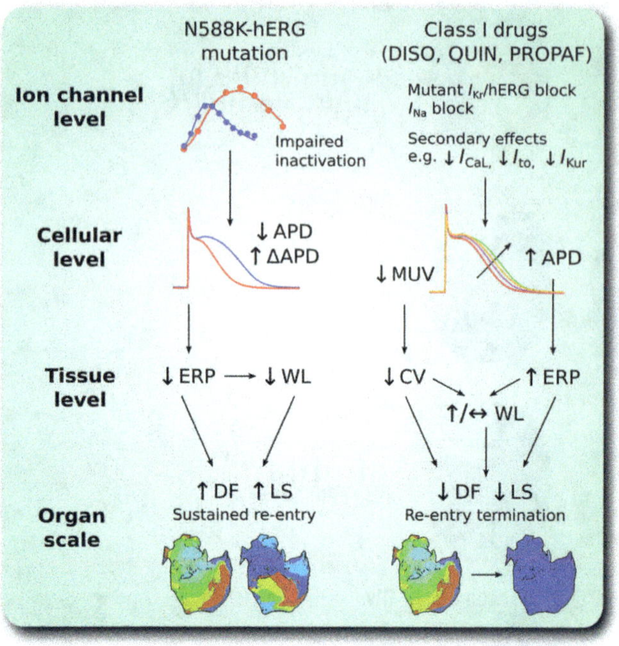

FIGURE 8 | A schematic summary of pro-arrhythmic effects of the N588K-hERG mutation in human atria and anti-arrhythmic effects of class I drugs. At the ion channel level, the N588K mutation impairs hERG channel inactivation, increasing I_{Kr} which shortens the action potential duration (APD) at the cellular level, and increases its dispersion, ΔAPD, between certain regions of the human atria. In tissue, shortened APD corresponds to shortened effective refractory period (ERP) and excitation wavelength (WL), promoting sustenance of arrhythmias at the organ scale through higher dominant frequency (DF) and lifespan (LS) of re-entry. Class I drugs disopyramide (DISO), quinidine (QUIN), and propafenone (PROPAF) exert effects at the ion channel level by blocking I_{Kr} and I_{Na}, in addition to secondary actions. This prolongs APD and ERP, and reduces maximum upstroke velocity (MUV) and conduction velocity (CV) at the cellular and tissue levels, respectively. At the organ scale these pharmacological actions promote arrhythmia rate and rhythm control through reduced DF and LS of re-entry.

3D anatomical models cannot necessarily be predicted from homogeneous 2D simulations, and vice versa. It should be noted nonetheless that electrical activity observed in 3D re-entry simulations in this study remained relatively organized and generally not driven by multiple wavelets. This lack of complex, chaotic behavior which is observed in persistent AF is consistent with reports of paroxysmal AF in some patients with the N588K-hERG mutation (Hong et al., 2005) - addition of electrical and intracellular gap junction remodeling or fibrosis in patients may be required to promote degeneration of paroxysmal AF into persistent AF.

Class I Drugs May Represent Useful SQT1-Specific Pharmacotherapy for AF

Despite the prevalence of AF and decades of research, anti-arrhythmic therapies for AF continue to have limited efficacy and safety (Workman et al., 2011). In this study, the class I anti-arrhythmic drugs disopyramide, quinidine, and propafenone were shown to be only moderately effective in the management of atrial arrhythmias mediated by the SQT1-linked N588K-hERG mutation, although it should be noted that the 7.5 s duration of 3D drug simulations is much shorter than clinical time scales. Pharmacological rhythm control occurred under application of both disopyramide and quinidine, but in an unpredictable, non-dose-dependent way, as observed in our previous *in silico* study (Whittaker et al., 2017a). One mechanism of re-entry termination involving reduction of the excitable gap under application of 5 μM quinidine is shown in **Figure S4**.

Both disopyramide and quinidine reduced consistently the DF of re-entry in a dose-dependent manner, although as in (Whittaker et al., 2017a) quinidine was more effective than disopyramide at rate control in the setting of SQT1, likely due to its more potent block of I_{Kr} (McPate et al., 2008) and I_{Na} (Koumi et al., 1992). Propafenone was comparatively ineffective at controlling the rate of atrial arrhythmias under the WT-N588K mutation condition, although did demonstrate some efficacy in re-entry termination. **Figure S5** shows a mechanism of pharmacological rhythm control by 0.5 μM propafenone, in which secondary waves induced by propafenone extinguished all re-entrant pathways. This is consistent with the use of propafenone to manage paroxysmal AF in SQT1 patients (Hong et al., 2005; Bjerregaard et al., 2006), which maintained 3 patients free of arrhythmia recurrence during follow up. However, as propafenone has been reported to have no prolonging effect on the QT interval in the setting of SQT1 (Hong et al., 2005)— an effect which was demonstrated with variable success using two leading human ventricle models (ten Tusscher and Panfilov, 2006; O'Hara et al., 2011) in **Figure S6**—it is likely that quinidine and disopyramide will remain more suitable pharmacotherapies.

In this study, cellular and tissue level simulations (in a 1D model) alone did not serve as good predictors of the overall effects of anti-arrhythmic drugs in the electrically-heterogeneous, 3D anatomical whole atria model, consistent with previous modeling studies (Varela et al., 2016; Whittaker et al., 2017b). For example, disopyramide was shown not to strongly affect the excitation WL in RA tissue (**Table 2**; **Figure S2**), and yet it decreased reliably the DF of re-entrant excitations under heterozygous N588K mutation conditions in 3D simulations. This is likely due to the fact that scroll waves were largely anatomically driven by a typical macro re-entrant atrial flutter/tachycardia circuit (Lee et al., 2012) which was larger than the functional WL; effects of disopyramide on CV were thus more important. In contrast, propafenone produced only modest changes to the CV and was thus less effective at rate control in the model, but did terminate re-entry under conditions in which the re-entrant circuit was abolished by interaction with secondary waves (**Figure S5**).

Insights Into the Efficacy of Class I Drugs in SQT1

Further support for quinidine as a useful pharmacotherapy for AF in the setting of SQT1 comes from the experimental use of the I_{Kr} agonist PD-118057 model (Nof et al., 2010). That study suggested that the combined blocking actions on I_{Kr} and I_{Na} are what made quinidine effective at preventing sustained AF in canine right atrial tissue preparations, as neither I_{Kr} nor I_{Na} block alone (by E-4031 or lidocaine, respectively) was effective at terminating AF. Similarly, in our previous simulation study of ventricular pharmacotherapy for SQT1 we showed that combined block of I_{Na} and I_{Kr} by disopyramide and quinidine prolonged the ERP to a greater extent than block of I_{Na} or I_{Kr} alone (Whittaker et al., 2017a). In this study, we sought to determine whether the greater ERP prolongation associated with the synergistic combination of I_{Na} and I_{Kr} block by class I drugs would also translate to greater efficacy in terminating re-entry in a 2D sheet of SQT1 mutant human atrial tissue. **Figure S7** shows that the actions of 5 μM of a hypothetical drug with disopyramide kinetics for I_{Na} and I_{Kr} block were able to terminate re-entry, whereas I_{Na} or I_{Kr} block alone did not, as combined block produced the greatest prolongation of the ERP. The spiral wave trajectories highlight the fact that I_{Na} block in particular destabilized the re-entrant circuit, which, when combined with I_{Kr} block, caused the spiral wave to meander out of the tissue boundaries (**Video S7**). The findings from *in silico* and *in vitro* experiments thus suggest that the combination of prolonged APD and refractoriness arising from K^+ and Na^+ channel inhibition is likely to be valuable in the setting of SQT1. Though selective blockers of I_{Ks} and I_{K1} are not yet clinically-available, this combination may also warrant investigation as a pharmacotherapeutic strategy for other forms of K^+-linked SQTS (SQT2 and SQT3).

LIMITATIONS

There are a number of limitations of the simulations presented in this study. The 3D anatomical human atria model which was employed for simulations in this study incorporated rule-based fiber orientations (Krueger et al., 2011), which may not capture sufficiently the complex cardiac microstructure of the human atria (Stephenson et al., 2017) which could contribute to the arrhythmia substrate. Whilst several hERG mutations have now been identified in SQT1 (Hancox et al., 2018), the present study focused only on the N588K-hERG mutation (which produces a more marked effect on hERG kinetics than some other mutations, Hancox et al., 2018), so the results here may not apply to all forms of SQT1. However, recently the S631A-hERG mutation (previously engineered for hERG structure-function studies), which produces a similar extent of attenuation of inactivation to N588K-hERG (McPate et al., 2008) has been reported in an SQT1 family (Akdis et al., 2018), and thus the findings of this study are likely also to be relevant to that form of SQT1. An additional potential limitation arises from the fact that mechanical contraction was not considered, which has been reported previously to be impaired in the setting of SQT1 in single human atrial cell simulations (Whittaker et al., 2015) as well as in organ-scale ventricle simulations (Adeniran et al., 2013), and based on clinical measurements (Frea et al., 2015).

The models of disopyramide and quinidine used in this study were adopted from (Whittaker et al., 2017a), in which the effects of anti-arrhythmic drugs were assessed in the setting of SQT1 in the human ventricles. However, both agents also exhibit modest anti-cholinergic effects in the atria (Nakajima et al., 1989) which were not accounted for, due to the absence of a formulation for acetylcholine-activated potassium current, $I_{K,ACh}$, in the CNZ model. Similarly, the β-adrenergic receptor blocking effects of propafenone were not considered (McLeod et al., 1984). Inclusion of these factors could give some insight into the response of the SQT1 phenotype to anti-arrhythmic drugs in the presence of autonomic modulation, and could give more favorable results in terms of arrhythmia prevention, especially for propafenone, which may be particularly effective against AF triggered by increased vagal tone. In addition, dynamic effects of agents due to the influence of circadian variations in drug concentration and heart rate on bioavailability were not investigated, which can give further insights into differing clinical efficacies of drugs (Loewe et al., 2014a). In relation to this, a further, more general limitation is that translation of drug concentrations from experiments and computer simulations to meaningful clinical concentrations is potentially problematic. Finally, whilst the 1:1 mutant to WT ratio, which was intended to represent the heterozygous state of the proband, may represent an oversimplification of the real hERG channel population in SQT1, the approach adopted in this and our previous studies (Adeniran et al., 2011, 2017; Whittaker et al., 2017a) reproduced quantitatively QT interval shortening and T wave morphology in SQTS conditions which was concordant with clinical observations.

CONCLUSIONS

The simulations performed in this study further substantiate a causative link between the SQTS-related N588K mutation and APD/ERP shortening in human atria, as well as increased spatial dispersion of repolarisation, which promotes development of AF. In 3D human atria simulations which included heterogeneous anatomy and electrophysiology, the N588K mutation was shown to increase the dominant frequency and lifespan of re-entrant excitation beyond that observed in WT conditions. Pharmacological simulations demonstrated that disopyramide and quinidine were more effective at rate control than propafenone in the setting of SQT1, and quinidine was most effective at rhythm control. Combined block of I_{Na} and I_{Kr} by a hypothetical drug was shown to be more beneficial in terms of re-entry termination in a 2D sheet of human atrial tissue than I_{Kr} or I_{Na} block alone in this context, suggesting useful targets for future pharmacotherapies. The multi-scale integrative cardiac modeling approach adopted in this study serves as a useful paradigm for optimisation of pharmacological therapy, allowing investigation of how genetic defects at the ion channel level influence organ scale propagation, arrhythmogenesis, and response to pharmacotherapies.

AUTHOR CONTRIBUTIONS

DW, JH, and HZ conceived the experiments and wrote the manuscript. DW developed and validated computer models and performed numerical experiments and analysis.

ACKNOWLEDGMENTS

JH gratefully acknowledges receipt of a University of Bristol research fellowship.

REFERENCES

Adeniran, I., Hancox, J. C., and Zhang, H. (2013). *In silico* investigation of the short QT syndrome, using human ventricle models incorporating electromechanical coupling. *Front. Physiol.* 4:166. doi: 10.3389/fphys.2013.00166

Adeniran, I., McPate, M. J., Witchel, H. J., Hancox, J. C., and Zhang, H. (2011). Increased vulnerability of human ventricle to re-entrant excitation in hERG-linked variant 1 short QT syndrome. *PLoS Comput. Biol.* 7:e1002313. doi: 10.1371/journal.pcbi.1002313

Adeniran, I., Whittaker, D. G., Harchi, A. E., Hancox, J. C., and Zhang, H. (2017). *In silico* investigation of a KCNQ1 mutation associated with short QT syndrome. *Sci. Rep.* 7:8469. doi: 10.1038/s41598-017-08367-2

Akdis, D., Saguner, A. M., Medeiros-Domingo, A., Schaller, A., Balmer, C., Steffel, J., et al. (2018). Multiple clinical profiles of families with the short QT syndrome. *EP Eur.* 20, f113–f121. doi: 10.1093/europace/eux186

Amorós, I., Dolz-Gaitón, P., Gómez, R., Matamoros, M., Barana, A., de la Fuente, M. G., et al. (2013). Propafenone blocks human cardiac Kir2.x channels by decreasing the negative electrostatic charge in the cytoplasmic pore. *Biochem. Pharmacol.* 86, 267–278. doi: 10.1016/j.bcp.2013.04.023

Aréchiga, I. A., Barrio-Echavarria, G. F., Rodríguez-Menchaca, A. A., Moreno-Galindo, E. G., Decher, N., Tristani-Firouzi, M., et al. (2008). Kv1.5 open channel block by the antiarrhythmic drug disopyramide: molecular determinants of block. *J. Pharmacol. Sci.* 108, 49–55. doi: 10.1254/jphs.08084FP

Arora, R., Verheule, S., Scott, L., Navarrete, A., Katari, V., Wilson, E., et al. (2003). Arrhythmogenic substrate of the pulmonary veins assessed by high-resolution optical mapping. *Circulation* 107, 1816–1821. doi: 10.1161/01.CIR.0000058461.86339.7E

Biktashev, V. N., and Holden, A. V. (1998). Reentrant waves and their elimination in a model of mammalian ventricular tissue. *Chaos. Interdiscip. J. Nonlinear Sci.* 8, 48–56. doi: 10.1063/1.166307

Bjerregaard, P., Jahangir, A., and Gussak, I. (2006). Targeted therapy for short QT syndrome. *Expert Opin. Ther. Targets* 10, 393–400. doi: 10.1517/14728222.10.3.393

Bosch, R. F., Zeng, X., Grammer, J. B., Popovic, K., Mewis, C., and Kühlkamp, V. (1999). Ionic mechanisms of electrical remodeling in human atrial fibrillation. *Cardiovasc. Res.* 44, 121–131. doi: 10.1016/S0008-6363(99)00178-9

Bray, M.-A., and Wikswo, J. P. (2002). Use of topological charge to determine filament location and dynamics in a numerical model of scroll wave activity. *IEEE Trans. Biomed. Eng.* 49, 1086–1093. doi: 10.1109/TBME.2002.803516

Brugada, R., Hong, K., Dumaine, R., Cordeiro, J., Gaita, F., Borggrefe, M., et al. (2004). Sudden death associated with Short-QT syndrome linked to mutations in HERG. *Circulation* 109, 30–35. doi: 10.1161/01.CIR.0000109482.92774.3A

Burashnikov, A., Belardinelli, L., and Antzelevitch, C. (2012). Atrial-selective sodium channel block strategy to suppress atrial fibrillation: ranolazine versus propafenone. *J. Pharmacol. Exp. Ther.* 340, 161–168. doi: 10.1124/jpet.111.186395

Colman, M. A., Aslanidi, O. V., Kharche, S., Boyett, M. R., Garratt, C., Hancox, J. C., et al. (2013). Pro-arrhythmogenic effects of atrial fibrillation-induced electrical remodelling: insights from the three-dimensional virtual human atria. *J. Physiol.* 591, 4249–4272. doi: 10.1113/jphysiol.2013.254987

Colman, M. A., Ni, H., Liang, B., Schmitt, N., and Zhang, H. (2017). *In silico* assessment of genetic variation in KCNA5 reveals multiple mechanisms of human atrial arrhythmogenesis. *PLOS. Comput. Biol.* 13:e1005587. doi: 10.1371/journal.pcbi.1005587

Cordeiro, J. M., Brugada, R., Wu, Y. S., Hong, K., and Dumaine, R. (2005). Modulation of IKr inactivation by mutation N588K in KCNH2: A link to arrhythmogenesis in short QT syndrome. *Cardiovasc. Res.* 67, 498–509. doi: 10.1016/j.cardiores.2005.02.018

Courtemanche, M., Ramirez, R. J., and Nattel, S. (1998). Ionic mechanisms underlying human atrial action potential properties: insights from a mathematical model. *Am. J. Physiol. Heart Circ. Physiol.* 275, H301–H321.

Dobrev, D., and Ravens, U. (2003). Remodeling of cardiomyocyte ion channels in human atrial fibrillation. *Basic Res. Cardiol.* 98, 137–148. doi: 10.1007/s00395-003-0409-8

Duan, D., Fermini, B., and Nattel, S. (1993). Potassium channel blocking properties of propafenone in rabbit atrial myocytes. *J. Pharmacol. Exp. Ther.* 264, 1113–1123.

Dumaine, R., and Antzelevitch, C. (2006). Disopyramide: although potentially life-threatening in the setting of long QT, could it be life-saving in short QT syndrome? *J. Mol. Cell. Cardiol.* 41, 421–423. doi: 10.1016/j.yjmcc.2006.06.070

Edrich, T., Wang, S.-Y., and Wang, G. K. (2005). State-dependent block of human cardiac hNav1.5 sodium channels by propafenone. *J. Membr. Biol.* 207, 35–43. doi: 10.1007/s00232-005-0801-4

Enriquez, A., Antzelevitch, C., Bismah, V., and Baranchuk, A. (2016). Atrial fibrillation in inherited cardiac channelopathies: from mechanisms to management. *Heart Rhythm.* 13, 1878–1884. doi: 10.1016/j.hrthm.2016.06.008

Fei, L., Gill, J. S., McKenna, W. J., and Camm, A. J. (1993). Effects of propafenone on calcium currents in single ventricular myocytes of guinea-pig. *Br. J. Pharmacol.* 109, 178–182. doi: 10.1111/j.1476-5381.1993.tb13550.x

Franqueza, L., Valenzuela, C., Delpón, E., Longobardo, M., Caballero, R., and Tamargo, J. (1998). Effects of propafenone and 5-hydroxy-propafenone on hKv1.5 channels. *Br. J. Pharmacol.* 125, 969–978. doi: 10.1038/sj.bjp.0702129

Frea, S., Giustetto, C., Capriolo, M., Scrocco, C., Fornengo, C., Benedetto, S., et al. (2015). New echocardiographic insights in short QT syndrome: more than a channelopathy? *Heart Rhythm.* 12, 2096–2105. doi: 10.1016/j.hrthm.2015.05.024

Gaita, F., Giustetto, C., Bianchi, F., Schimpf, R., Haissaguerre, M., Cal,ò, L., et al. (2004). Short QT syndrome: pharmacological treatment. *J. Am. Coll. Cardiol.* 43, 1494–1499. doi: 10.1016/j.jacc.2004.02.034

Giustetto, C. (2006). "Quinidine to treat short QT syndrome: a real alternative to ICD?," in *Cardiac Arrhythmias 2005*, ed. A. R. MD (Milan: Springer), 333–335.

Giustetto, C., Schimpf, R., Mazzanti, A., Scrocco, C., Maury, P., Anttonen, O., et al. (2011). Long-term follow-Up of patients with short QT syndrome. *J. Am. Coll. Cardiol.* 58, 587–595. doi: 10.1016/j.jacc.2011.03.038

Gross, G. J., and Castle, N. A. (1998). Propafenone inhibition of human atrial myocyte repolarizing currents. *J. Mol. Cell. Cardiol.* 30, 783–793. doi: 10.1006/jmcc.1998.0643

Hancox, J. C., and Mitcheson, J. S. (1997). Inhibition of L-type calcium current by propafenone in single myocytes isolated from the rabbit atrioventricular node. *Br. J. Pharmacol.* 121, 7–14. doi: 10.1038/sj.bjp.0701086

Hancox, J. C., Whittaker, D. G., Du, C., Stuart, A. G., and Zhang, H. (2018). Emerging therapeutic targets in the short QT syndrome. *Expert Opin. Ther. Targets* 22:439–51. doi: 10.1080/14728222.2018.1470621

Harmer, A. R., Abi-Gerges, N., Easter, A., Woods, A., Lawrence, C. L., Small, B. G., et al. (2008). Optimisation and validation of a medium-throughput electrophysiology-based hNav1.5 assay using IonWorks^{TM}. *J. Pharmacol. Toxicol. Methods* 57, 30–41. doi: 10.1016/j.vascn.2007.09.002

Hong, K., Bjerregaard, P., Gussak, I., and Brugada, R. (2005). Short QT syndrome and atrial fibrillation caused by mutation in KCNH2. *J. Cardiovasc. Electrophysiol.* 16, 394–396. doi: 10.1046/j.1540-8167.2005.40621.x

Hu, D., Li, Y., Zhang, J., Pfeiffer, R., Gollob, M. H., Healey, J., et al. (2017). The phenotypic spectrum of a mutation hotspot responsible for the short QT syndrome. *JACC. Clin. Electrophysiol.* 3, 727–43. doi: 10.1016/j.jacep.2016.11.013

Katoh, H., Shinozaki, T., Baba, S., Satoh, S., Kagaya, Y., Watanabe, J., et al. (2005). Monophasic action potential duration at the crista terminalis in patients with sinus node disease. *Circ. J.* 69, 1361–1367. doi: 10.1253/circj.69.1361

Kim, B.-S., Kim, Y.-H., Hwang, G.-S., Pak, H.-N., Lee, S. C., Shim, W. J., et al. (2002). Action potential duration restitution kinetics in human atrial fibrillation. *J. Am. Coll. Cardiol.* 39, 1329–1336. doi: 10.1016/S0735-1097(02)01760-6

Koumi, S., Sato, R., Katori, R., Hisatome, I., Nagasawa, K., and Hayakawa, H. (1992). Sodium channel states control binding and unbinding behaviour of antiarrhythmic drugs in cardiac myocytes from the guinea pig. *Cardiovasc. Res.* 26, 1199–1205. doi: 10.1093/cvr/26.12.1199

Krueger, M. W., Schmidt, V., Tobón, C., Weber, F. M., Lorenz, C., Keller, D. U. J., et al. (eds.). (2011). "Modeling atrial fiber orientation in patient-specific geometries: a semi-automatic rule-based approach," in *Functional Imaging and Modeling of the Heart Lecture Notes in Computer Science.* (Springer, Berlin, Heidelberg), 223–232.

Kumagai, K., Ogawa, M., Noguchi, H., Yasuda, T., Nakashima, H., and Saku, K. (2004). Electrophysiologic properties of pulmonary veins assessed using a multielectrode basket catheter. *J. Am. Coll. Cardiol.* 43, 2281–2289. doi: 10.1016/j.jacc.2004.01.051

Lazar, S., Dixit, S., Marchlinski, F. E., Callans, D. J., and Gerstenfeld, E. P. (2004). Presence of left-to-right atrial frequency gradient in paroxysmal but not persistent atrial fibrillation in humans. *Circulation* 110, 3181–3186. doi: 10.1161/01.CIR.0000147279.91094.5E

Lee, G., Sanders, P., and Kalman, J. M. (2012). Catheter ablation of atrial arrhythmias: state of the art. *Lancet* 380, 1509–1519. doi: 10.1016/S0140-6736(12)61463-9

Lemery, R., Birnie, D., Tang, A. S., l., Green, M., Gollob, M., Hendry, M., et al. (2007). Normal atrial activation and voltage during sinus rhythm in the human heart: an endocardial and epicardial mapping study in patients with a history of atrial fibrillation. *J. Cardiovasc. Electrophysiol.* 18, 402–408. doi: 10.1111/j.1540-8167.2007.00762.x

Loewe, A., Lutz, Y., Wilhelms, M., Sinnecker, D., Barthel, P., Scholz, E. P., et al. (2014a). *In-silico* assessment of the dynamic effects of amiodarone and dronedarone on human atrial patho-electrophysiology. *Europace* 16, iv30–iv38. doi: 10.1093/europace/euu230

Loewe, A., Wilhelms, M., Fischer, F., Scholz, E. P., Dössel, O., and Seemann, G. (2014b). Arrhythmic potency of human ether-à-go-go-related gene mutations L532P and N588K in a computational model of human atrial myocytes. *Europace* 16, 435–443. doi: 10.1093/europace/eut375

Mandapati, R., Skanes, A., Chen, J., Berenfeld, O., and Jalife, J. (2000). Stable microreentrant sources as a mechanism of atrial fibrillation in the isolated sheep heart. *Circulation* 101, 194–199. doi: 10.1161/01.CIR.101.2.194

McLeod, A. A., Stiles, G. L., and Shand, D. G. (1984). Demonstration of beta adrenoceptor blockade by propafenone hydrochloride: clinical pharmacologic, radioligand binding and adenylate cyclase activation studies. *J. Pharmacol. Exp. Ther.* 228, 461–466.

McPate, M. J., Duncan, R. S., Hancox, J. C., and Witchel, H. J. (2008). Pharmacology of the short QT syndrome N588K-hERG K+ channel mutation: differential impact on selected class I and class III antiarrhythmic drugs. *Br. J. Pharmacol.* 155, 957–966. doi: 10.1038/bjp.2008.325

McPate, M. J., Duncan, R. S., Milnes, J. T., Witchel, H. J., and Hancox, J. C. (2005). The N588K-HERG K^+ channel mutation in the 'short QT syndrome': mechanism of gain-in-function determined at 37 °C. *Biochem. Biophys. Res. Commun.* 334, 441–449. doi: 10.1016/j.bbrc.2005.06.112

Mizobuchi, M., Enjoji, Y., Yamamoto, R., Ono, T., Funatsu, A., Kambayashi, D., et al. (2008). Nifekalant and disopyramide in a patient with short QT syndrome: evaluation of pharmacological effects and electrophysiological properties. *Pacing Clin. Electrophysiol.* 31, 1229–1232. doi: 10.1111/j.1540-8159.2008.01169.x

Moreno, J. D., Lewis, T. J., and Clancy, C. E. (2016). Parameterization for *in-silico* modeling of ion channel interactions with drugs. *PLoS ONE* 11:e0150761. doi: 10.1371/journal.pone.0150761

Nakajima, T., Kurachi, Y., Ito, H., Takikawa, R., and Sugimoto, T. (1989). Anti-cholinergic effects of quinidine, disopyramide, and procainamide in isolated atrial myocytes: mediation by different molecular mechanisms. *Circ. Res.* 64, 297–303. doi: 10.1161/01.RES.64.2.297

Nenov, N. I., Crumb, W. J., Pigott, J. D., Harrison, L. H., and Clarkson, C. W. (1998). Quinidine interactions with human atrial potassium channels. *Circ. Res.* 83, 1224–1231. doi: 10.1161/01.RES.83.12.1224.

Ni, H., Whittaker, D. G., Wang, W., Giles, W. R., Narayan, S. M., and Zhang, H. (2017). Synergistic anti-arrhythmic effects in human atria with combined use of sodium blockers and acacetin. *Front. Physiol.* 8:946. doi: 10.3389/fphys.2017.00946

Nof, E., Burashnikov, A., and Antzelevitch, C. (2010). Cellular basis for atrial fibrillation in an experimental model of short QT1: Implications for a pharmacological approach to therapy. *Heart Rhythm* 7, 251–257. doi: 10.1016/j.hrthm.2009.10.017

O'Hara, T., Virág, L., Varr,ó, A., and Rudy, Y. (2011). Simulation of the undiseased human cardiac ventricular action potential: model formulation and experimental validation. *PLoS Comput. Biol.* 7:e1002061. doi: 10.1371/journal.pcbi.1002061

Patel, C., and Antzelevitch, C. (2008). Cellular basis for arrhythmogenesis in an experimental model of the SQT1 form of the short QT syndrome. *Heart Rhythm* 5, 585–590. doi: 10.1016/j.hrthm.2008.01.022

Pau, D., Workman, A. J., Kane, K. A., and Rankin, A. C. (2007). Electrophysiological and arrhythmogenic effects of 5-hydroxytryptamine on human atrial cells are reduced in atrial fibrillation. *J. Mol. Cell. Cardiol.* 42, 54–62. doi: 10.1016/j.yjmcc.2006.08.007

Paul, A. A., Witchel, H. J., and Hancox, J. C. (2002). Inhibition of the current of heterologously expressed HERG potassium channels by flecainide and comparison with quinidine, propafenone and lignocaine. *Br. J. Pharmacol.* 136, 717–729. doi: 10.1038/sj.bjp.0704784

Redpath, C. J., Rankin, A. C., Kane, K. A., and Workman, A. J. (2006). Anti-adrenergic effects of endothelin on human atrial action potentials are potentially anti-arrhythmic. *J. Mol. Cell. Cardiol.* 40, 717–724. doi: 10.1016/j.yjmcc.2006.01.012

Roden, D. M. (2014). Pharmacology and toxicology of Nav1.5-class 1 anti-arrhythmic drugs. *Card. Electrophysiol. Clin.* 6, 695–704. doi: 10.1016/j.ccep.2014.07.003

Schimpf, R., Veltmann, C., Giustetto, C., Gaita, F., Borggrefe, M., and Wolpert, C. (2007). *In vivo* effects of mutant HERG K+ channel inhibition by disopyramide in patients with a short QT-1 syndrome: a pilot study. *J. Cardiovasc. Electrophysiol.* 18, 1157–1160. doi: 10.1111/j.1540-8167.2007.00925.x

Schimpf, R., Wolpert, C., Gaita, F., Giustetto, C., and Borggrefe, M. (2005). Short QT syndrome. *Cardiovasc. Res.* 67, 357–366. doi: 10.1016/j.cardiores.2005.03.026

Seemann, G., Höper, C., Sachse, F. B., Dössel, O., Holden, A. V., and Zhang, H. (2006). Heterogeneous three-dimensional anatomical and electrophysiological model of human atria. *Philos. Trans. R. Soc. Lond. Math. Phys. Eng. Sci.* 364, 1465–1481. doi: 10.1098/rsta.2006.1781

Seki, A., Hagiwara, N., and Kasanuki, H. (1999). Effects of propafenone on K currents in human atrial myocytes. *Br. J. Pharmacol.* 126, 1153–1162. doi: 10.1038/sj.bjp.0702428

Slawsky, M. T., and Castle, N. A. (1994). K+ channel blocking actions of flecainide compared with those of propafenone and quinidine in adult rat ventricular myocytes. *J. Pharmacol. Exp. Ther.* 269, 66–74.

Starmer, C. F., Grant, A. O., and Strauss, H. C. (1984). Mechanisms of use-dependent block of sodium channels in excitable membranes by local anesthetics. *Biophys. J.* 46, 15–27. doi: 10.1016/S0006-3495(84)83994-6

Stephenson, R. S., Atkinson, A., Kottas, P., Perde, F., Jafarzadeh, F., Bateman, M., et al. (2017). High resolution 3-Dimensional imaging of the human cardiac conduction system from microanatomy to mathematical modeling. *Sci. Rep.* 7:7188. doi: 10.1038/s41598-017-07694-8

ten Tusscher, K. H., and Panfilov, A. V. (2006). Alternans and spiral breakup in a human ventricular tissue model. *Am. J. Physiol. - Heart Circ. Physiol.* 291, H1088–H1100. doi: 10.1152/ajpheart.00109.2006

Varela, M., Colman, M. A., Hancox, J. C., and Aslanidi, O. V. (2016). Atrial heterogeneity generates re-entrant substrate during atrial fibrillation and anti-arrhythmic drug action: mechanistic insights from canine atrial models. *PLOS. Comput. Biol.* 12:e1005245. doi: 10.1371/journal.pcbi.1005245.

Voigt, N., Trausch, A., Knaut, M., Matschke, K., Varró, A., Wagoner, D. R. V., et al. (2010). Left-to-right atrial inward rectifier potassium current gradients in patients with paroxysmal versus chronic atrial fibrillationclinical perspective. *Circ. Arrhythm. Electrophysiol.* 3, 472–480. doi: 10.1161/CIRCEP.110.954636

Whittaker, D. G., Colman, M. A., Ni, H., Hancox, J. C., and Zhang, H. (2015). *In silico* investigation of short QT syndrome-linked potassium channel mutations on electro-mechanical function of human atrial cells. *Comput. Cardiol. Conference* 2015, 853–856. doi: 10.1109/CIC.2015.7411045.

Whittaker, D. G., Colman, M. A., Ni, H., Hancox, J. C., and Zhang, H. (2018). Human atrial arrhythmogenesis and sinus bradycardia in KCNQ1-linked short QT syndrome: insights from computational modelling. *Front. Physiol.* 9:1402. doi: 10.3389/fphys.2018.01402

Whittaker, D. G., Ni, H., Benson, A. P., Hancox, J. C., and Zhang, H. (2017a). Computational analysis of the mode of action of disopyramide and quinidine on hERG-linked short QT syndrome in human ventricles. *Front. Physiol.* 8:759. doi: 10.3389/fphys.2017.00759

Whittaker, D. G., Ni, H., Harchi, A. E., Hancox, J. C., and Zhang, H. (2017b). Atrial arrhythmogenicity of KCNJ2 mutations in short QT syndrome: insights from virtual human atria. *PLOS. Comput. Biol.* 13:e1005593. doi: 10.1371/journal.pcbi.1005593

Wilhelms, M., Hettmann, H., Maleckar, M. M., Koivumäki, J. T., Dössel, O., and Seemann, G. (2013). Benchmarking electrophysiological models of human atrial myocytes. *Front. Physiol.* 3:487. doi: 10.3389/fphys.2012.00487

Workman, A. J., Smith, G. L., and Rankin, A. C. (2011). Mechanisms of termination and prevention of atrial fibrillation by drug therapy. *Pharmacol. Ther.* 131, 221–241. doi: 10.1016/j.pharmthera.2011.02.002

Yuan, Y., Bai, X., Luo, C., Wang, K., and Zhang, H. (2015). The virtual heart as a platform for screening drug cardiotoxicity. *Br. J. Pharmacol.* 172, 5531–5547. doi: 10.1111/bph.12996

Zhang, H., and Hancox, J. C. (2004). *In silico* study of action potential and QT interval shortening due to loss of inactivation of the cardiac rapid delayed rectifier potassium current. *Biochem. Biophys. Res. Commun.* 322, 693–699. doi: 10.1016/j.bbrc.2004.07.176

Zhou, J., Augelli-Szafran, C. E., Bradley, J. A., Chen, X., Koci, B. J., Volberg, W. A., et al. (2005). Novel potent human ether-à-Go-Go-related gene (hERG) potassium channel enhancers and their *in vitro* antiarrhythmic activity. *Mol. Pharmacol.* 68, 876–884. doi: 10.1124/mol.105.014035

9

Sensitivity of Ablation Targets Prediction to Electrophysiological Parameter Variability in Image-Based Computational Models of Ventricular Tachycardia in Post-Infarction Patients

*Dongdong Deng[1,2], Adityo Prakosa[1], Julie Shade[1], Plamen Nikolov[1] and Natalia A. Trayanova[1]**

[1] Department of Biomedical Engineering, Johns Hopkins University, Baltimore, MD, United States, [2] School of Biomedical Engineering, Dalian University of Technology, Dalian, China

***Correspondence:**
Natalia A. Trayanova
ntrayanova@jhu.edu

Ventricular tachycardia (VT), which could lead to sudden cardiac death, occurs frequently in patients with myocardial infarction. Computational modeling has emerged as a powerful platform for the non-invasive investigation of lethal heart rhythm disorders in post-infarction patients and for guiding patient VT ablation. However, it remains unclear how VT dynamics and predicted ablation targets are influenced by inter-patient variability in action potential duration (APD) and conduction velocity (CV). The goal of this study was to systematically assess the effect of changes in the electrophysiological parameters on the induced VTs and predicted ablation targets in personalized models of post-infarction hearts. Simulations were conducted in 5 patient-specific left ventricular models reconstructed from late gadolinium-enhanced magnetic resonance imaging scans. We comprehensively characterized all possible pre-ablation and post-ablation VTs in simulations conducted with either an "average human VT"-based electrophysiological representation (i.e., EP_{avg}) or with $\pm$10% APD or CV (i.e., EP_{var}); additional simulations were also executed in some models for an extended range of these parameters. The results showed that: (1) a subset of reentries (76.2–100%, depending on EP parameter set) conducted with $\pm$10% APD/CV was observed in approximately the same locations as reentries observed in EP_{avg} cases; (2) emergent VTs could be induced sometimes after ablation in EP_{avg} models, and these emergent VTs often corresponded to the pre-ablation reentries in simulations with EP_{var} parameter sets. These findings demonstrate that the VT ablation target uncertainty in patient-specific ventricular models with an average representation of VT-remodeled electrophysiology is relatively low and the ablation targets stable, as the localization of the induced VTs was primarily driven by the remodeled structural substrate. Thus, personalized ventricular modeling with an average representation of infarct-remodeled electrophysiology may uncover most targets for VT ablation.

Keywords: ventricular tachycardia, patient-specific modeling, ablation, uncertainty, LGE-MRI

INTRODUCTION

Ventricular tachycardia (VT), a life-threatening fast heart rhythm, occurs frequently in patients with myocardial infarction, and leading to sudden cardiac death. Although increased utilization of pre-procedural imaging (Fernandez-Armenta et al., 2013), high-density mapping (Anter et al., 2016), epicardial access (d'Avila et al., 2006), and more extensive ablation strategies (Di Biase et al., 2012; Jais et al., 2012) have all contributed to improved procedure outcome, a high efficacy of treatment for VT in the electrophysiology (EP) laboratory has not yet been achieved. At present, catheter ablation is the most effective method to eliminate VT, however, it only has modest success, 50–88% (Aliot et al., 2009). This is the result of limitations in current techniques for mapping the electrical functioning of the heart and identifying the targets for VT ablation.

Computational modeling has emerged as a powerful platform for the non-invasive investigation of lethal heart rhythm disorders and their treatment (Behradfar et al., 2014; Pathmanathan and Gray, 2014; Grandi and Maleckar, 2016; Loewe et al., 2018; Roney et al., 2018a,b); it has been used for risk stratification in patients with myocardial infarction (MI) (Vadakkumpadan et al., 2014; Arevalo et al., 2016; Deng et al., 2016) and prediction of reentry location (Ashikaga et al., 2013; Deng et al., 2015; Zahid et al., 2016). Computational technology has also been recently developed to guide patient ablation (the Virtual-heart Arrhythmia Ablation Targeting, or VAAT), and even used prospectively, as a prove of feasibility of the approach, in a small number of patients (Prakosa et al., 2018). In these models, the personalized element is limited to information that is extracted from non-invasive late gadolinium-enhanced magnetic resonance imaging (LGE-MRI) scans, which is the patient-specific ventricular geometry, and the spatial distribution of infarcted-remodeled tissue. Cell- and tissue scale EP in these models, while reflecting the fact that the substrate in VT patients involves EP ventricular remodeling (Dangman et al., 1982; Dun et al., 2004; Mendonca Costa et al., 2018), is derived from an average human set of EP parameters (i.e., EP_{avg}) to represent non-infarcted tissue and remodeled gray zone (GZ). Clearly, an ideal option would be to use personalized EP in each model, however acquisition of such information is invasive, in contrast to the VAAT approach, which offers a non-invasive prediction of the ablation targets. Thus, the ablation targets that are predicted to terminate VT in post-MI patients using the VAAT approach might have a level of uncertainty associated with the fact that pre-determined EP is used.

Similar issues had previously arisen in using patient-specific models of persistent atrial fibrillation (AF) in patients with fibrotic remodeling (Trayanova, 2014; Zahid et al., 2016; Deng et al., 2017; Hakim et al., 2018). As the intention is that such models be used in the future to predict the patient-specific targets for AF, in a series of papers we sought to assess the level of uncertainty in such predictions (Deng et al., 2017; Hakim et al., 2018). Research in these studies demonstrated that while not always the same ablation targets are predicted under the examined variable EP conditions (Deng et al., 2017), the majority of the targets that were not predicted under the average EP conditions manifested themselves upon repeating the pacing protocol post-ablation (Hakim et al., 2018).

While persistent AF in the fibrotic substrate and VT post-MI have very different arrhythmia dynamics, they both result from a combination of remodeled structural substrate interacting with a remodeled EP. Thus, in this study, we aimed to systematically assess the effect of changes in the electrophysiological parameter set on the induced VTs and predicted ablation targets in personalized models of post-MI patient hearts.

MATERIALS AND METHODS

Post-infarction Human Heart Models

For this retrospective study, we used data from 5 patients who were referred for catheter ablation of VT; their MRI data are used for model reconstruction. Details regarding patient information and model construction can be found in our previous publication (Prakosa et al., 2018). Briefly, the myocardium boundaries were semi-automatically segmented and regions of gray zone (GZ), core scar, and non-infarcted tissue were segmented from LGE-MRI by means of signal thresholding (Arevalo et al., 2016; Deng et al., 2016). Tetrahedral meshes were constructed directly from the segmented images using a previously described approach (Prassl et al., 2009), which uses the dual mesh of an octree applied directly to the segmented 3D image stacks. Fiber orientations in the mesh were assigned using a previously validated rule-based method (Bayer et al., 2012). In order to be able to conduct this research in a tractable manner, as it involves a very large number of simulations (see below), we conducted simulations in the left ventricle (LV) only in all these 5 models. The rationale for this choice is based on the fact that human infarcts resulting in VT are typically located in the LV (Cano et al., 2017; Martin et al., 2018); the LV was also the location where all the clinical VTs in these patients were sustained.

Modeling Cell- and Tissue-Scale Variability of Ventricle

Electrophysiology properties were assigned in the model as previously described (Prakosa et al., 2018). Briefly, the mathematical description of electrical conduction in cardiac tissue was based on the monodomain representation (Plank et al., 2008). Core scar was modeled as passive tissue. Non-infarcted tissue and GZ were assigned human ventricular myocyte action potential dynamics (ten Tusscher et al., 2004). The values of the non-infarcted tissue conductivities used in this study were 0.255 and 0.0775 S/m in the longitudinal and transverse directions, respectively. Tissue in the GZ region was characterized with a 90% decrease in transverse conductivity to reflect connexin-43 remodeling in the infarct border zone (Yao et al., 2003).

To establish baseline reentry dynamics in the absence of variability in the electrophysiological component of the infarcted substrate, we first conducted simulations under average human VT EP, as in previous studies (Arevalo et al., 2016; Deng et al., 2016). For brevity, these conditions are referred to as EP_{avg}. We then ran simulations in ventricular models with the same geometric structure and infarcted tissue distribution to assess the effects of APD and CV variability. For simulations with APD variability, specific ionic currents were modified to achieve ±10% APD (**Figures 1A,B**), while minimally altering other AP properties, including resting membrane potential [V_m], AP amplitude, and restitution curve slope (**Figure 1C**). To simplify ionic current parameters selection process, I_{Kr} and I_{Ks} were modified simultaneously in 10% increments from −90 to 300%, and the current values that resulted in APD closest to the target APD (i.e., ±10% or ±20% APD) in each case were used in this study (**Table 1**). For simulations with CV variability, the longitudinal and transverse components of the conductivity tensor were modified to achieve ±10% CV. To avoid biasing effects from the complex infarcted structure in ventricular models, CV values were calibrated by simulating wavefront propagation following stimulation of the center point in a slab model (6 cm × 6 cm × 2.7 mm) with uniform fiber orientations, and conductivity tensor values were adjusted until the desired longitudinal and transverse CVs were observed. In both families of cases (i.e., $APD_{\pm 10\%}$ and $CV_{\pm 10\%}$ conditions), parameter changes required to achieve the desired emergent property were different for non-infarcted and GZ tissues. Complete details about these changes and the resulting variability in APD and CV are presented in **Tables 1, 2**, respectively.

As experimental measurements (Britton et al., 2013) have shown that APD and CV could vary in a larger range, we conducted additional simulations in two models only (for computational tractability) with $APD_{\pm 20\%}$ and $CV_{\pm 25\%}$, and in one model, with a combination of $APD_{\pm 20\%}$ and $CV_{\pm 25\%}$. The parameter changes were listed in **Tables 1, 2**. We chose $APD_{\pm 20\%}$ instead of $APD_{\pm 25\%}$ because $APD_{+25\%}$ resulted in longer APD

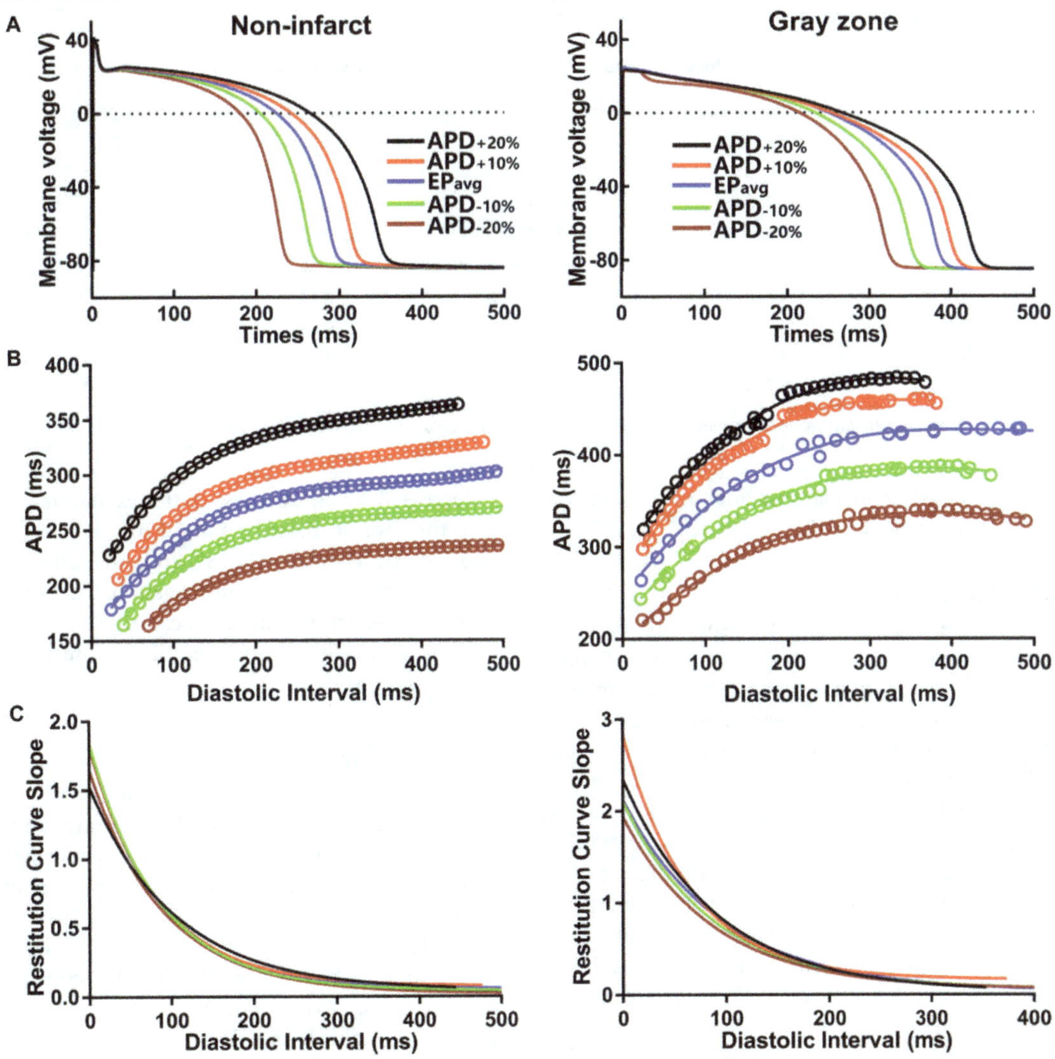

FIGURE 1 | (A) Action potential (AP) traces for simulated normal (non-infarcted) (left) and GZ (right) ventricular myocytes, paced to steady-state (1000 stimuli at basic CL = 600 ms) under average human VT electrophysiology (EP_{avg}) conditions, and with AP duration (APD_{90}) variability (±10% and ±20%). **(B)** APD restitution relationships for the respective cell types shown in A. Fit lines obtained via exponential regression. **(C)** Plots showing APD restitution curve slope values for different diastolic intervals.

TABLE 1 | Cell-scale electrophysiological model parameters modified to achieve ±10% and ±20% action potential duration (APD) in non-infarcted and GZ tissues.

		Parameters changed		APD_{target} (ms)	APD_{actual} (ms)	Percentage of APD changed	APA (mV)	V_{rest} (mV)
Non-infarcted	$APD_{-20\%}$	+80% I_{Kr}	+80% I_{Ks}	230.8	233.28	−20.8%	126.3	−84.8
	$APD_{-10\%}$	+30% I_{Kr}	+30% I_{Ks}	263.8	262.44	−9.5%	126.1	−84.8
	EP_{avg}	...	...	291.6	291.6	...	126.0	−84.7
	$APD_{+10\%}$	−20% I_{Kr}	−20% I_{Ks}	315.9	320.76	8.3%	126.0	−84.7
	$APD_{+20\%}$	−40% I_{Kr}	−40% I_{Ks}	348.5	349.92	19.5%	126.0	−84.6
Gray zone	$APD_{-20\%}$	+80% I_{Kr}	+80% I_{Ks}	309.7	306.24	−19.1%	110.1	−85.3
	$APD_{-10\%}$	+30% I_{Kr}	+30% I_{Ks}	348.1	344.52	−9.1%	109.9	−85.3
	EP_{avg}	...	...	382.8	382.8	...	109.9	−85.2
	$APD_{+10\%}$	−20% I_{Kr}	−20% I_{Ks}	409.4	421.08	7.0%	109.3	−85.2
	$APD_{+20\%}$	−30% I_{Kr}	−30% I_{Ks}	454.2	459.36	18.7%	108.7	−85.1

"..." indicates no change. EP_{avg}, average human VT electrophysiology; APA, action potential amplitude; V_{rest}, resting membrane potential; I_{Ks}, slow delayed rectifier potassium current; I_{Kr}, rapid delayed rectifier potassium current. APD_{90} was used to calculate APD. APD_{target}: The target APD (±10% or ±20% APD). APD_{actual}: It represents the actual value of APD (closest to the target) obtained by altering I_{Kr} and I_{Ks} simultaneously (see section "Materials and Methods).

TABLE 2 | Tissue-scale electrophysiological model parameters modified to achieve ±10% and ±25% longitudinal and transverse conduction velocities (CV_L and CV_T, respectively) in non-fibrotic and fibrotic atrial tissues.

		Parameters changed		CV_L (cm/s)	CV_T (cm/s)	CV_L:CV_T
Non-infarcted	$CV_{-25\%}$	−47.6% σ_{iL}	−47.6% σ_{iT}	41.1	26.2	1.57
	$CV_{-10\%}$	−22.2% σ_{iL}	−22.1% σ_{iT}	49.3	30.7	1.61
	EP_{avg}	...	...	54.8	33.5	1.63
	$CV_{+10\%}$	+28.5% σ_{iL}	+28.1% σ_{iT}	60.3	36.6	1.65
	$CV_{+25\%}$	+86.4% σ_{iL}	+86.5% σ_{iT}	68.5	41.3	1.66
Gray zone	$CV_{-25\%}$	−46.1% σ_{iL}	−46.1% σ_{iT}	32.6	15.3	2.13
	$CV_{-10\%}$	−21.4% σ_{iL}	−21.3% σ_{iT}	39.1	17.5	2.23
	EP_{avg}	...	...	43.4	18.8	2.42
	$CV_{+10\%}$	+25.6% σ_{iL}	+25.5% σ_{iT}	47.7	20.0	2.39
	$CV_{+25\%}$	+81.2% σ_{iL}	+81.4% σ_{iT}	54.6	21.9	2.49

"..." indicates no change. σ_{iL} and σ_{iT}, longitudinal and transverse conductivity tensor values; EP_{avg}, average human VT electrophysiology.

than the upper limit of APD in experimental measurements (364 ms vs. 340 ms) (Britton et al., 2013).

Stimulation Protocol

All simulations were performed using the software package CARP[1] on a parallel computing platform (Vigmond et al., 2003). A programmed electrical stimulation protocol similar to standard clinical stimulation protocols was performed to examine the arrhythmogenic propensity of the post-MI ventricular models (Cheng et al., 2013). All models were paced from 7 locations, optimized for maximum likelihood of VT induction, for 6 beats (S1) at a cycle length (CL) of 600 ms followed by a premature stimulus (S2) initially given at 90% of S1 CL. The timing between S1 and S2 was progressively shortened until reentry was induced. If reentry was not induced, a second premature stimulus (S3) was delivered after S2. If VT was still not induced, a third premature stimulus (S4) was delivered after S3. Three seconds of VT were simulated.

The smallest S1-S2 coupling interval was determined in the fowling way: Six stimulus of S1 (CL = 600 ms) were delivered; then S2 was given at 250 ms. If excitation was elicited, then we decreased S2 to 200 ms. If the excitation could propagate again, then we decreased S2 in 10 ms intervals until excitation could not be elicited. The S2 coupling interval was the last one that elicited excitation propagation. The same protocol was applied to determine the smallest S2-S3 and S3-S4 intervals. If reentry was induced after the S2 stimulus, then no addition stimulus was given.

Ablation Strategy

First, the reentrant circuit was identified in all models with EP_{avg} through analysis of the 3D reentrant wave propagation. *In silico* ablation was performed by rendering the tissue in the narrowest region of the reentrant circuit [typically a channel in the scar as in (Prakosa et al., 2018)] non-excitable. Each virtual ablation lesion was of radius in our simulation was 3.5 mm, which is similar to the clinical catheter size (Narayan et al., 2012). The VT induction protocol was then repeated to establish that VT was no longer inducible in the ablated LV substrate. If a new VT arose in the post-ablation model, then the new VT circuit was analyzed and additional ablation targets were determined and implemented in the model, and the pacing protocol was repeated until VT was no longer inducible.

[1]https://carpentry.medunigraz.at/carputils/

All simulations were then repeated in the family of models with EP_{var} ($APD_{\pm 10\%}$ and $CV_{\pm 10\%}$, 20 additional 3D LV models; 25 3D LV models in total for this study). For VTs induced in each of these models, if the reentry morphology was the same or similar to VT induced in the corresponding EP_{avg} model, the ablation lesion from the EP_{avg} model was applied to the same location in the EP_{var} model. By similar reentry morphology we refer to reentries that have the same wavefront conduction pathway, with the same critical conduction channels (or conduction isthmus), but could have different CL, and even different reentry direction. If VT in the EP_{var} model was terminated, the ablation lesions in EP_{var} and EP_{avg} models were considered "overlapping." If VT persisted in the EP_{var} model despite the ablation, then these two VTs were considered non-overlapping. Then ablation in the EP_{avg} model proceeded as described above. Finally, the number of ablation lesions was compared between EP_{avg} and EP_{var} models.

RESULTS

For simulations conducted under EP_{avg} conditions, rapid pacing induced sustained VTs in all 5 patient-specific ventricular models. **Table 3** summarized the results of simulations conducted in EP_{avg} models. A total of 16 distinct reentries were induced in five models under the EP_{avg} condition, and after ablation, only one new distinct reentry was induced. The average amount of ablated ventricular tissue under EP_{avg} condition was 0.92%. Before ablation, there were 2–4 different sustained VTs (3.2 ± 0.8) induced in each model, and the organizing centers of all 16 VTs perpetuated in distinct locations. Ablation, as described in Section "Materials and Methods," did not always render the remodeled substrate non-inducible for VT; in some cases, new VTs could arise. Specifically, after ablation, 4 patient models did not have emergent VTs, while 1 patient model had one emergent VT at a location different from those before ablation. The volume of the simulated ablation lesions that terminated the VTs, both original and emergent, in each model was $0.92 \pm 0.83\%$ of the total ventricular volume (min: 0.1%, max: 2.1%).

Comprehensive summary data for the VTs induced in simulations conducted in all 5 ventricular models under the 5 different APD/$CV_{\pm 10\%}$ conditions each (EP_{avg}, $APD_{\pm 10\%}$, and $CV_{\pm 10\%}$) are provided in **Table 4** and **Supplementary Tables S1–S4**. Of all 25 3D LV models used in this study, VT could be induced in 24. The only model in which VT could not be induced is that of patient 2 with $CV_{+10\%}$ parameters. In terms of the total number of VTs, 22 unique VTs were induced in the 24 inducible models. Eight of the VTs were induced under all five electrophysiological conditions; these were for patients 1, 3, 4, and 5. The activation maps of these 8 VTs are shown in **Figures 2** and **Supplementary Figures S1–S3**. The VT in model 2 that was induced under 4 of the 5 EP parameter sets (and not under the CV_{+10}) is shown in **Figure 3**. Of the 4 varied parameter sets ($APD_{\pm 10\%}$ and $CV_{\pm 10\%}$), $APD_{\pm 10\%}$, and $CV_{+10\%}$ resulted in less VTs, while $CV_{-10\%}$ resulted in more VTs compared with the EP_{avg} conditions.

There were 10 distinct reentries induced in models with the $APD_{+10\%}$ parameter set before ablation, and all of them corresponded to VTs under EP_{avg} conditions (**Table 4** and **Supplementary Table S1**). There were no emergent reentries after ablation under these electrophysiological conditions. For the $CV_{+10\%}$ parameter set (**Table 4** and **Supplementary Table S3**), there were 9 distinct VTs induced before ablation, and they all also matched the VTs in EP_{avg}. Under the $APD_{-10\%}$ conditions (**Table 4** and **Supplementary Table S2**), there were 11 distinct VTs before ablation, and 9 of them corresponded to those under EP_{avg} conditions. Only for patient 2 there was one emergent VT after ablation, which was different from any VT under EP_{avg} conditions before and after ablation (the blue lesion in Panel B of **Figure 3**). In patient 1, two reentries were new and different from any VT under EP_{avg} conditions before ablation, but one of them was induced under EP_{avg} conditions after ablation (Panel B in **Supplementary Figure S1**). Thus overall, for the $APD_{-10\%}$ parameter set, 10 out of 12 VTs had matching reentries under EP_{avg} conditions, while the remaining 2 VTs were new, and different from the reentries in EP_{avg}.

For the $CV_{-10\%}$ parameter set (**Table 4** and **Supplementary Table S4**), there were 20 distinct VTs induced before ablation, and 14 of them had corresponding reentries under EP_{avg} conditions. After ablation, there was only one emergent VT in patient 2 (Panel B in **Figure 3**), but 2 of the VTs induced before ablation were also induced under EP_{avg} conditions, so 16 out of 21 VTs in the $CV_{-10\%}$ parameter set models had matching VTs under EP_{avg} after ablation.

The results for one example model (patient 5) under all 5 EP parameter sets are shown in **Figure 2**. There were 3 distinct VTs induced under EP_{avg}, one located at the septum (**Figure 2C**, Morphology 1 in EP_{avg}), another one at the LV lateral wall (**Figure 2C**, Morphology 2 in EP_{avg}), and the third one located at the posterior wall (morphology not shown). For the $APD_{\pm 10\%}$ and $CV_{\pm 10\%}$ parameter sets, both resulted in two reentries being induced, which were located at the septum and the LV lateral wall. Under $CV_{-10\%}$ conditions, there were 5 distinct VTs induced, and 3 of them had matching reentries in EP_{avg} models (ablation lesions in Panel B of **Figure 2**).

For the 2 VTs induced under all 5 conditions, the morphology and location were very similar for across all models. For morphology 1 (first row in **Figure 2C**), the reentry was circular, with the only difference being the CL, which varied from 195 ms to 380 ms. After ablating the narrowest channel region in VT morphology 1, the reentry was terminated. After applying the ablation lesions from EP_{avg} to the other 4 conditions (light blue lesions on the left side of **Figure 2B**), and the reentry

TABLE 3 | Summary of results for simulations conducted in EP_{avg} models.

ID	# reentries pre-ablation	# reentries post-ablation	Extent of ablated tissue (%)
P01	4	1	1.3
P02	3	0	0.2
P03	2	0	0.1
P04	4	0	2.1
P05	3	0	0.9

TABLE 4 | Summary of simulation results regarding the number of VTs obtained for the EP_{avg} and EP_{var} ($APD_{\pm10\%}$ and $CV_{\pm10\%}$) models with the 5 patient-specific ventricular geometries.

		Total number of VTs	Number of VTs in EP_{avg} models	Percentage of VTs in EP_{var} models that were also present in EP_{avg} (%) models (%)
# of induced VTs in EP_{avg}	Pre- ablation	16	–	–
	Post-ablation	17	–	–
# of induced VTs in $APD_{+10\%}$	Pre- ablation	10	10	100
	Post-ablation	10	10	100
# of induced VTs in $APD_{-10\%}$	Pre- ablation	11	9	81.8
	Post-ablation	12	10	83.3
# of induced VTs in $CV_{+10\%}$	Pre- ablation	9	9	100
	Post-ablation	9	9	100
# of induced VTs in $CV_{-10\%}$	Pre- ablation	20	14	70
	Post-ablation	21	16	76.2
# of induced VTs in $APD_{+20\%}$*	Pre- ablation	3	3	100
	Post-ablation	3	3	100
# of induced VTs in $APD_{-20\%}$*	Pre- ablation	3	3	100
	Post-ablation	4	3	75
# of induced VTs in $CV_{+25\%}$*	Pre- ablation	3	3	100
	Post-ablation	3	3	100
# of induced VTs in $CV_{-25\%}$*	Pre- ablation	6	5	83.3
	Post-ablation	7	5	71.4
# of induced VTs in $APD_{+20\%}$ & $CV_{+25\%}$**	Pre- ablation	0	0	0
	Post-ablation	0	0	0
# of induced VTs in $APD_{-20\%}$ & $CV_{+25\%}$**	Pre- ablation	0	0	0
	Post-ablation	0	0	0
# of induced VTs in $APD_{+20\%}$ & $CV_{-25\%}$**	Pre- ablation	1	1	100
	Post-ablation	1	1	100
# of induced VTs in $APD_{-20\%}$ & $CV_{-25\%}$**	Pre- ablation	3	3	100
	Post-ablation	4	3	75

*"Number of VTs in EP_{avg} models" represents the number of reentry morphologies induced in each set of modified conditions with similar or same reentry morphologies induced under the EP_{avg} condition. The last column in **Table 4** is calculated as "Number of VTs in EPavg models"/" Total number of VTs", which represents how many reentry morphologies induced under each of the modified condition corresponded to the reentry morphologies induced under EP_{avg}. *, only 2 models were used with this EP parameter set; **, only 1 model was used with this EP parameter set.*

at that region was terminated in all 4 conditions too. For morphology 2, the reentry was circular in all 5 conditions, but the conduction pathway in $CV_{-10\%}$ condition showed differences. Under EP_{avg}, $APD_{\pm10\%}$ and $CV_{+10\%}$ conditions, there was only one conduction pathway, but under the $CV_{-10\%}$ condition, the reentry had two condition pathways, one of which, the one close to posterior wall, was the same under the other 4 conditions. After ablating the narrowest channel region in morphology 2 in EP_{avg}, the reentry was terminated. Then applying the ablation lesion from EP_{avg} to the four other EP versions (light blue lesions on the right side of **Figure 2B**), the reentry under $APD_{\pm10\%}$, and $CV_{+10\%}$ conditions was terminated. But applying the ablation lesions from EP_{avg} didn't terminate the reentry induced in $CV_{-10\%}$. After ablating the narrowest parts of both conducting pathways under $CV_{-10\%}$ conditions, reentry was terminated (the light blue and blue on the right-most side of $CV_{-10\%}$ in **Figure 2B**). The VTs induced at the posterior wall in EP_{avg} could not be induced under $APD_{\pm10\%}$ and $CV_{+10\%}$ conditions; the ablation lesion for that reentry is shown in purple in the first 3 panels of **Figure 2B**. The 3 VTs induced in EP_{avg} were all induced in $CV_{-10\%}$ (light blue lesions in $CV_{-10\%}$ panel of **Figure 2B**), but there were 2 new VTs induced in $CV_{-10\%}$, of which the 2 ablation lesions are shown as blue in the $CV_{-10\%}$ panel in **Figure 2B**.

Figure 3 shows the results for another patient model (patient 2) for the 5 EP parameter sets. There were 3 VTs induced in EP_{avg}, with two of them being on the anterior wall, and the third on septum. For $CV_{+10\%}$, there was no reentry induced, and this is the only model variant of all 25 model variants in 5 the patients in which no reentry could be induced. Before ablation, the models with $APD_{\pm10\%}$ parameters had only one reentry induced, on the anterior middle wall (**Figure 3C**), and this reentry is similar to the one induced in EP_{avg} (first panel in **Figure 3C**). In $CV_{-10\%}$, there were 3 VTs induced, and two of them had matching reentries in EP_{avg}. But the one on the middle anterior wall had minor differences compared to the corresponding one in EP_{avg}: it had 2 conduction pathways ($CV_{-10\%}$ panel in **Figure 3C**), with the pathway on the right matching the one in EP_{avg}, but the left side was a new pathway. Applying the lesions determined from EP_{avg}, the middle anterior wall VT could not be terminated in $CV_{-10\%}$ (light blue lesion in the $CV_{-10\%}$ panel of the first row

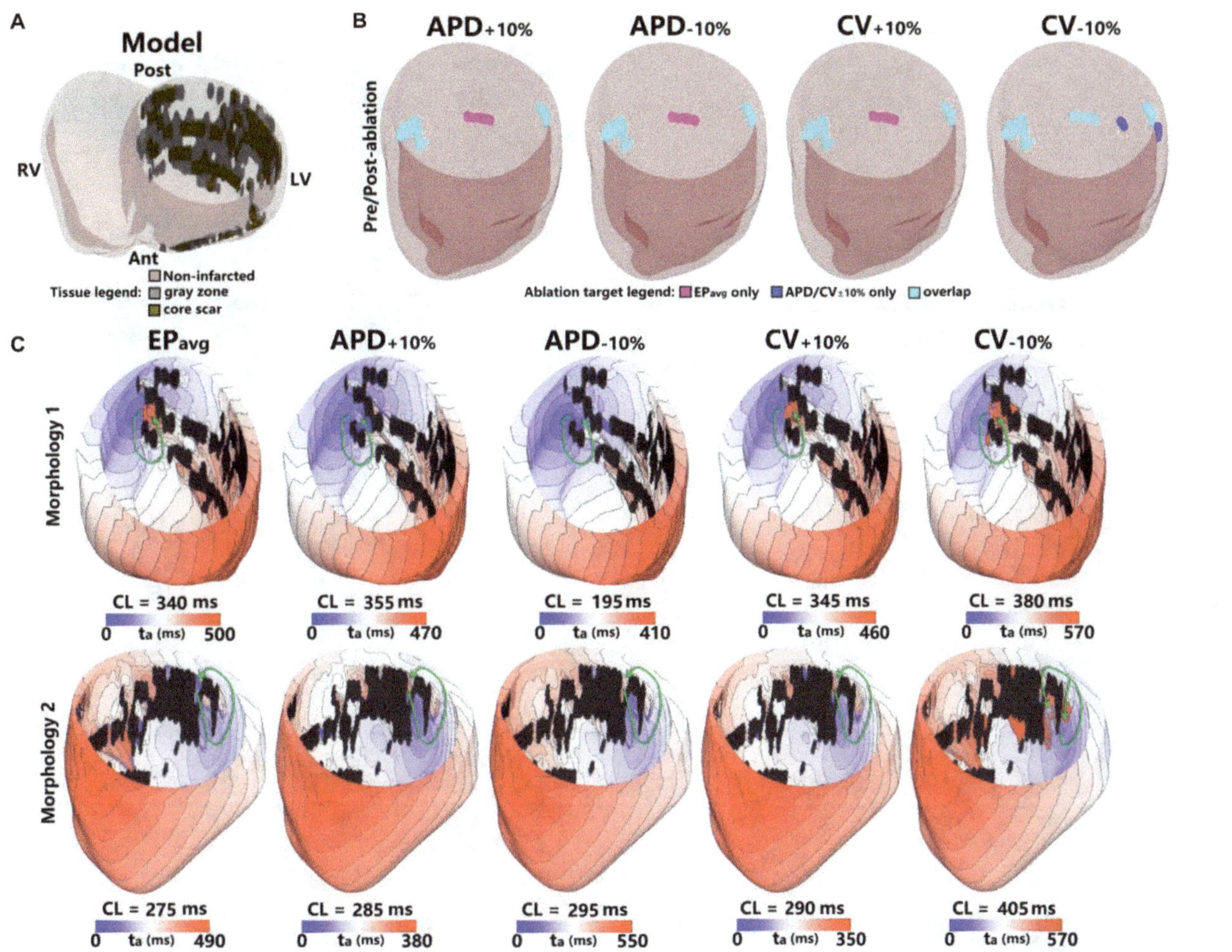

FIGURE 2 | Geometry and simulated activation maps and ablation lesions under average human VT EP_{avg} and variable APD/CV conditions for model 5. **(A)** Geometric model of the infarcted heart of patient model 5. **(B)** Ablation lesions for simulations with the 5 different parameter sets. **(C)** Highlighting two VT morphologies in which the same pacing sequence applied in the same model led to the initiation of VT driven by an RD in the same ventricular region, regardless of the variability in APD/CV. t_a, activation time. The black areas in panel C for all figures are core scar – there is no electrical activation there.

in **Figure 3B**), and an additional lesion had to be applied to narrowest portion of the left condition pathway in $CV_{-10\%}$ to terminate the reentry on the anterior middle wall (blue lesion in the $CV_{-10\%}$ panel of the first row in **Figure 3B**). After ablation, no reentry could be induced in EP_{avg} and $APD_{+10\%}$, but in $APD_{-10\%}$, a new VT emerged at the vicinity of the ablation lesion on the anterior wall; the condition pathway of this RD is very similar to the left side pathway of the VT induced in $CV_{-10\%}$. Applying the EP_{avg} ablation lesions to $CV_{-10\%}$ terminated the VT. In $CV_{-10\%}$ condition, after ablation, there was an emergent VT, which matched the VT on the left side of the anterior wall in EP_{avg}; applying the ablation lesion from EP_{avg} terminated the emergent reentry in $CV_{-10\%}$. Results of the study for the other 3 patients are shown in **Supplementary Figures S1–S3**. Vann diagrams summarizing the results of simulations for all above cases are presented in **Figure 4**.

Next, we present results of simulations with the additional EP parameter sets (from the extended parameter range) in the limited number of models, as described in Section "Materials and Methods." Results from simulations with model 2 are presented in **Figure 3**. Upon change of APD from +10% to +20% and from −10 to −20%, there was no difference in reentry morphology and reentry location. When changing CV from ±10 to ±25%, there was a difference between results for the $CV_{+10\%}$ and $CV_{+25\%}$ cases: no reentry was induced in $CV_{+10\%}$ simulations, and there was one reentry induced in $CV_{+25\%}$. There was no difference between the cases of $CV_{-10\%}$ and $CV_{-25\%}$. Results for model 3 and the same parameter range are presented in **Supplementary Figure S2**. For this model, there was no difference between results for the $APD_{\pm 20\%}$ and $CV_{+25\%}$ conditions, but under the $CV_{-25\%}$ condition, one new reentry emerged (panel D of **Supplementary Figure S2**) that was not present for the other modified APD and CV cases. Thus, based on the simulation results for the 2 patients with $APD_{\pm 20\%}$ and $CV_{\pm 25\%}$, we conclude that APD changes within the range of ±20% had no additional effects on reentry location. Changing CV in the range

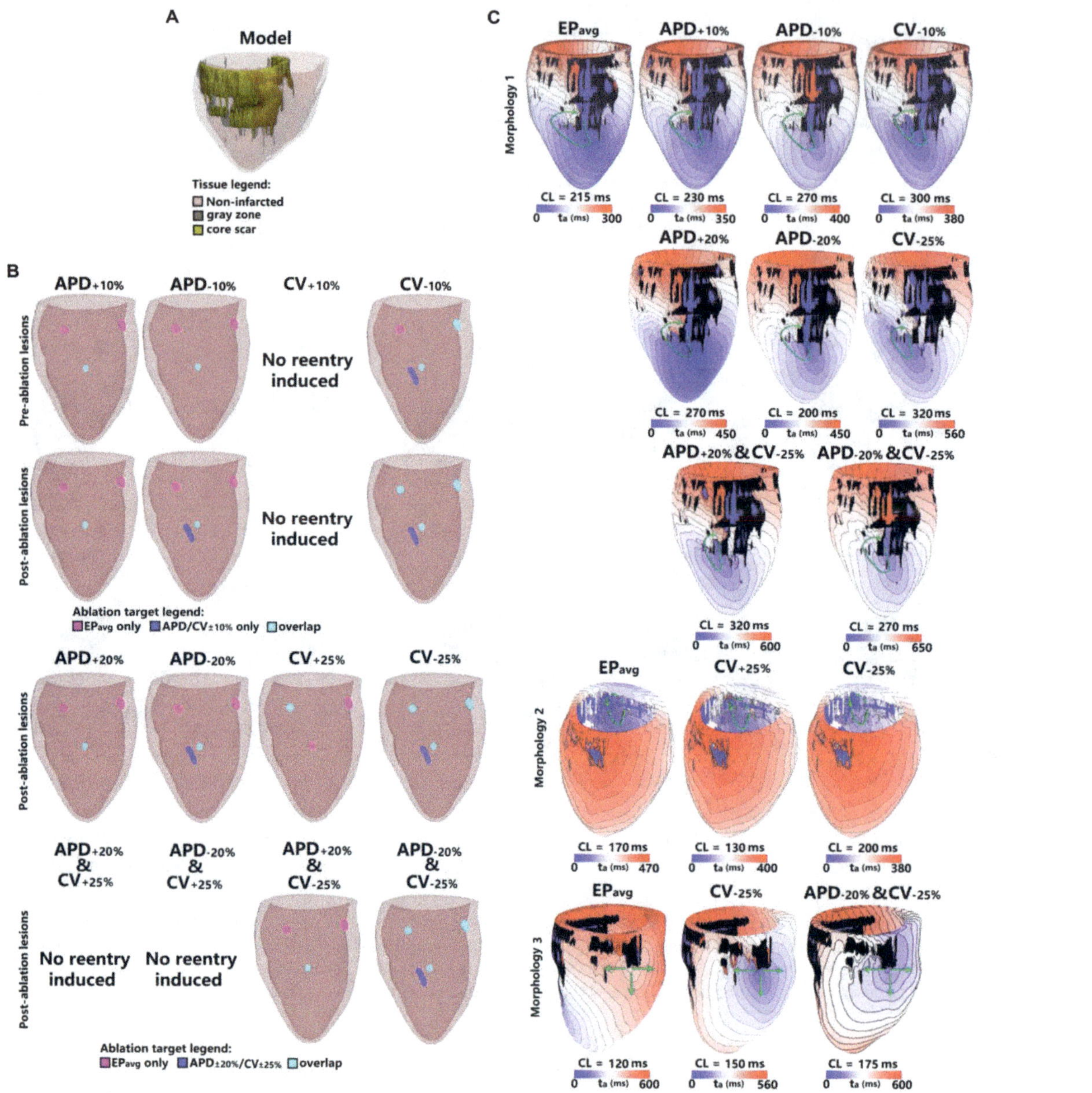

FIGURE 3 | Geometry and simulated activation maps and ablation lesions under average human VT EP_{avg} and variable APD/CV conditions for model 2. **(A)** Geometric model of the infarcted heart of patient model 2. **(B)** Ablation lesions for simulations for the 13 different parameter sets. **(C)** Highlighting one VT morphology in which the same pacing sequence applied in the same model led to the initiation of VT driven by an RD in the same ventricular region, regardless of the variability in APD/CV. t_a, activation time. The black areas in panel C for all figures represent core scar – there is no electrical activation there.

(±25%) resulted in changes in reentry location only when CV was at the boundaries of that range. A Venn diagram of these results is provided in **Figure 4**.

Finally we executed simulations in one model with a combination of parameter changes, as described in Section "Materials and Methods." Conducting simulations with model 2, the combinations of $APD_{+20\%}$ & $CV_{+25\%}$ and $APD_{-20\%}$ & $CV_{+25\%}$ conditions did not result in reentry. There were two reentries induced under the $APD_{+20\%}$ & $CV_{-25\%}$ condition, one of which corresponded to the reentry morphology in EP_{avg} (see **Figure 3**), and the other one was a new VT morphology with respect to the EP_{avg} case. There were four VT morphologies induced in the $APD_{-20\%}$ & $CV_{-25\%}$ condition, 3 of which corresponded to EP_{avg}, and one was new. The combined reduction/increase of CV and APD produced only one different VT morphology as compared to EP_{avg}. This VT morphology was the same as the ones induced for cases where only APD or only CV was changed. Thus we conclude, based on the simulations in model 2, that combined reduction/increase of CV and APD within the range of ±20%

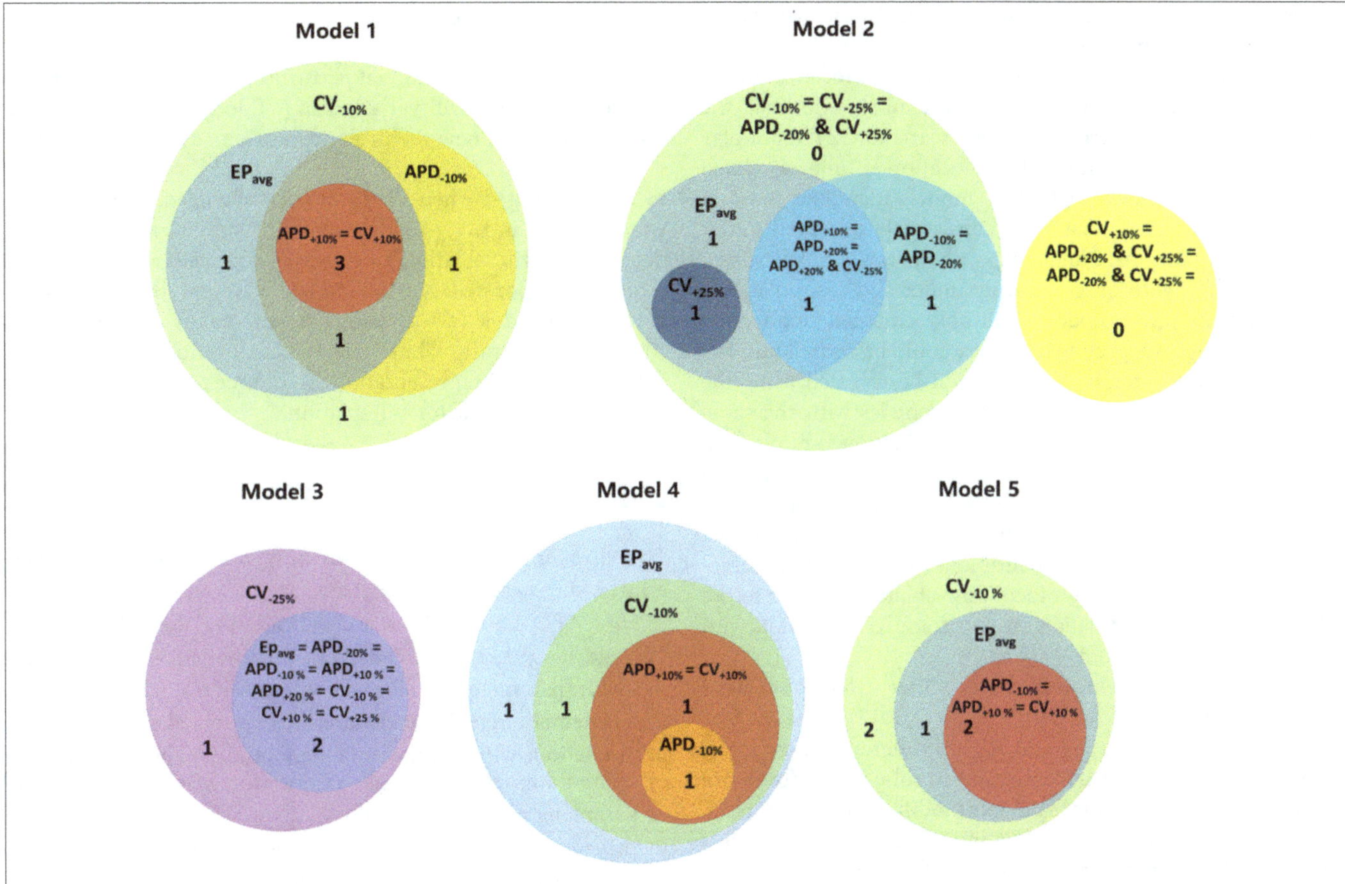

FIGURE 4 | Venn diagrams for each models under average human VT EP_{avg} and variable APD/CV conditions. Numbers represent the number of distinct reentries in each case.

or ±25% had no additional effects on VTs compared with only changing APD or CV.

DISCUSSION

In this study, we used computational models reconstructed from LGE-MRI scans of the infarcted ventricle of individuals with VT to assess the sensitivity of VT localization to variability in cell- and tissue-scale electrophysiological parameters. We showed that: (1) in simulations conducted with ±10% APD/CV, a subset of VTs (76.2–100%, depending on the EP parameter set) were observed in approximately the same locations as those in the EP_{avg} case; (2) EP_{avg} conditions resulted in more VTs (5–8) than in $APD_{\pm 10\%}$ and $CV_{+10\%}$, and in less reentries than in $CV_{-10\%}$; (3) Emergent VTs were induced sometimes post-ablation, and the emergent reentries often matched the pre-ablation VTs in models with other parameter sets. (4) Where the VTs were robust to APD/CV variability, there were differences, as expected, in macroscopic arrhythmia features such as CL and total activation time.

About 53% (9/17) of the reentries that occurred in EP_{avg} were also induced in all other four parameter set models (±10% APD/CV), and the remainder of reentries were induced in at least one of the four parameter set models. Interestingly, all the reentries induced in $APD_{+10\%}$ and $CV_{+10\%}$ models had matching reentries in the EP_{avg} models. The models with EP_{avg} were more inducible than the $APD_{+10\%}$ and $CV_{+10\%}$ models, as the wavelength in the former case was smaller, allowing for more space for the reentry to propagate and be sustained. While there were new VTs induced in models with $APD_{-10\%}$ and $CV_{-10\%}$, more than 76% of the VTs occurred also in models with EP_{avg}. The models with $APD_{-10\%}$ had a smaller number of induced VTs than the corresponding EP_{avg} models. A possible explanation for this finding is that APD in the EP_{avg} parameter set falls in the arrhythmogenesis susceptibility window of APD (Clayton and Holden, 2005), where there is a unidirectional block of electrical conduction through a VT-sustaining channel. Upon further reduction of APD, the VT channel conducts bi-directionally, resulting in a smaller number of included reentries.

In the additional simulations with the extended range of APD and CV and their combination, the results with the combined reduction/increase of CV and APD were very similar, in terms of reentry location, and pathway to those when varying APD or CV independently. Furthermore, $APD_{\pm 20\%}$ and $CV_{\pm 25\%}$ cases had similar outcomes to those with $APD_{\pm 10\%}$ and $CV_{\pm 10\%}$. Thus, simulating only ±10% APD or ±10% CV changes may be sufficient in representing the results from simulations with larger electrophysiological parameters variations.

These findings present evidence that VT localization is fairly robust to electrophysiological variability, and that the distribution of the infarcted tissue (core scar and GZ) might play a dominant role in determining the location of infarct-related VTs. Our results suggest that EP_{avg} models identified most of the VT ablation targets that were consistently observed under different EP conditions. Nonetheless, there was a small subset of reentries that were observed only under EP_{avg} simulations. Furthermore, in some models, VTs only emerged upon APD and/or CV change, suggesting that there could be a small number of potential ablation targets that may not be revealed using the EP_{avg} parameter set. Furthermore, for reentries with the same morphology and location of the critical conduction isthmus (and thus the same ablation target) we observed differences in CL, total activation time and in rare cases, even direction of propagation. Finally, we demonstrated that majority of ablation targets that were not predicted under EP_{avg} conditions manifested themselves upon repeating the pacing protocol post-ablation, similar to the findings in modeling of ablation for persistent AF in patients with fibrotic remodeling (Hakim et al., 2018).

The results shown in this paper differ from our atrial sensitivity analysis study (Deng et al., 2017) because the mechanism of reentry in VT and AF are different. In the atrial models, there is only non-fibrotic and fibrotic tissue (both are excitable tissues, but fibrotic tissue has modified EP). In contrast, in the ventricular models, there is additionally a core scar. Thus reentries in the atrial models had a larger functional component and their morphologies and locations could be affected, by somewhat larger degree, by changes in APD or CV. In infarct-related VT, most of the reentries were anchored to core scar or included conduction through channels, consistent with published data (Martin et al., 2018).

Patient-specific computational modeling of VT has been proposed as a new approach to non-invasively predict personalized VT ablation targets in post-MI patients (Prakosa et al., 2018). The present study demonstrates that simulations conducted under EP_{avg} conditions identified most of VTs that were consistently observed under multiple different EP conditions. The uncertainty in the post-MI VT ablation targets under EP_{avg} is further mitigated by the design of the pipeline for determining the optimal set of targets [as in the VAAT approach (Prakosa et al., 2018)], where the protocol is repeated post-ablation with virtual targets incorporated, until the remodeled substrate is no longer capable of sustaining VT. This allows the protocol to reveal additional VTs under EP_{avg} that are not manifested following the initial pacing protocol prior to virtual ablation, but appear right away in simulations using models with different EP properties.

CONCLUSION

In conclusion, we showed that perturbing APD and CV by $\pm$10% caused relatively small variation in VT localization. In a small number of cases, new reentries at locations distinct from those in EP_{avg} emerged when EP parameters changed. Most of those were revealed in EP_{avg} models when the simulation protocol for determining the ablation targets was repeated with the initial targets incorporated in the models. Overall, the localization of the induced VTs was primarily driven by the remodeled structural substrate. Thus, personalized ventricular modeling with an average representation of infarct-remodeled EP may uncover most targets for VT ablation.

LIMITATIONS

The first limitation is that we only considered a relatively limited subset of the parameter space of four discrete changes ($\pm$10% APD and $\pm$10% CV). Considering the relatively low CV and long APD in GZ used in our model, further changes in these parameters will make these values fall out of the experimental range. Furthermore, we conducted a large number of simulations with 25 different 3D LV models. The sheer amount of computational time makes exploration of additional ranges of parameter values technically difficult. The second limitation in this study is that in order to achieve different APD values, we only changed I_{Kr} and I_{Ks} currents in our single cell models. We did not alter the Ca current as it would not only affect APD restitution, but would also have impact on other single cell properties and thus making the organ scale modeling too complicated to analyze. Furthermore, as the goal of this study was to provide a sensitivity analysis of ablation targeting, we did not explore the mechanisms of all the observed phenomena, including arrhythmogenesis arising from locally reduced APD. Finally, our model did not consider the influence of Purkinje system, the role of the right ventricle, and potential alterations in fiber orientation that cannot be captures by our patient-specific rule-based approach.

AUTHOR CONTRIBUTIONS

DD, AP, and PN performed the LGE-MRI scan segmentation and model creation. DD performed the simulations of VT in all models. DD, AP, and NT analyzed the data. DD, JS, and NT wrote the manuscript. All authors discussed the results and commented on the manuscript.

REFERENCES

Aliot, E. M., Stevenson, W. G., Almendral-Garrote, J. M., Bogun, F., Calkins, C. H., Delacretaz, E., et al. (2009). Registered Branch of the European Society of, C., Heart Rhythm, S., American College of, C., and American Heart, A. EHRA/HRS Expert Consensus on Catheter Ablation of Ventricular Arrhythmias: developed in a partnership with the European Heart Rhythm Association (EHRA), a Registered Branch of the European Society of Cardiology (ESC), and the Heart Rhythm Society (HRS); in collaboration with the American College of Cardiology (ACC) and the American Heart Association (AHA). *Heart Rhythm* 6, 886–933. doi: 10.1016/j.hrthm.2009.04.030

Anter, E., Tschabrunn, C. M., Buxton, A. E., and Josephson, M. E. (2016). High-resolution mapping of postinfarction reentrant ventricular tachycardia: electrophysiological characterization of the circuit. *Circulation* 134, 314–327. doi: 10.1161/CIRCULATIONAHA.116.021955

Arevalo, H. J., Vadakkumpadan, F., Guallar, E., Jebb, A., Malamas, P., Wu, K. C., et al. (2016). Arrhythmia risk stratification of patients after myocardial infarction using personalized heart models. *Nat. Commun.* 7:11437. doi: 10.1038/ncomms11437

Ashikaga, H., Arevalo, H., Vadakkumpadan, F., Blake, R. C., Bayer, J. D., Nazarian, S., et al. (2013). Feasibility of image-based simulation to estimate ablation target in human ventricular arrhythmia. *Heart Rhythm* 10, 1109–1116. doi: 10.1016/j.hrthm.2013.04.015

Bayer, J. D., Blake, R. C., Plank, G., and Trayanova, N. A. (2012). A novel rule-based algorithm for assigning myocardial fiber orientation to computational heart models. *Ann. Biomed. Eng.* 40, 2243–2254. doi: 10.1007/s10439-012-0593-5

Behradfar, E., Nygren, A., and Vigmond, E. J. (2014). The role of Purkinje-myocardial coupling during ventricular arrhythmia: a modeling study. *PLoS One* 9:e88000. doi: 10.1371/journal.pone.0088000

Britton, O. J., Bueno-Orovio, A., Van Ammel, K., Lu, H. R., Towart, R., Gallacher, D. J., et al. (2013). Experimentally calibrated population of models predicts and explains intersubject variability in cardiac cellular electrophysiology. *Proc. Natl. Acad. Sci. U.S.A.* 110, E2098–E2105. doi: 10.1073/pnas.1304382110

Cano, O., Plaza, D., Sauri, A., Osca, J., Alonso, P., Andres, A., et al. (2017). Utility of high density multielectrode mapping during ablation of scar-related ventricular tachycardia. *J. Cardiovasc. Electrophysiol.* 28, 1306–1315. doi: 10.1111/jce.13302

Cheng, A., Dalal, D., Butcher, B., Norgard, S., Zhang, Y. Y., Dickfeld, T., et al. (2013). Prospective observational study of implantable cardioverter-defibrillators in primary prevention of sudden cardiac death: study design and cohort description. *J. Am. Heart Assoc.* 2:e000083. doi: 10.1161/JAHA.112.000083

Clayton, R. H., and Holden, A. V. (2005). Dispersion of cardiac action potential duration and the initiation of re-entry: a computational study. *Biomed. Eng. Online* 4:11.

Dangman, K. H., Danilo, P., Hordof, A. J., Maryrabine, L., Reder, R. F., and Rosen, M. R. (1982). Electrophysiologic characteristics of human ventricular and purkinje-Fibers. *Circulation* 65, 362–368. doi: 10.1161/01.cir.65.2.362

d'Avila, A., Scanavacca, M., and Sosa, E. (2006). Transthoracic epicardial catheter ablation of ventricular tachycardia. *Heart Rhythm* 3, 1110–1111. doi: 10.1016/j.hrthm.2006.03.029

Deng, D., Arevalo, H. J., Prakosa, A., Callans, D. J., and Trayanova, N. A. (2016). A feasibility study of arrhythmia risk prediction in patients with myocardial infarction and preserved ejection fraction. *Europace* 18(Suppl. 4), iv60–iv66. doi: 10.1093/europace/euw351

Deng, D., Murphy, M. J., Hakim, J. B., Franceschi, W. H., Zahid, S., Pashakhanloo, F., et al. (2017). Sensitivity of reentrant driver localization to electrophysiological parameter variability in image-based computational models of persistent atrial fibrillation sustained by a fibrotic substrate. *Chaos* 27:093932. doi: 10.1063/1.5003340

Deng, D. D., Arevalo, H., Pashakhanloo, F., Prakosa, A., Ashikaga, H., McVeigh, E., et al. (2015). Accuracy of prediction of infarct-related arrhythmic circuits from image-based models reconstructed from low and high resolution MRI. *Front. Physiol.* 6:282. doi: 10.3389/fphys.2015.00282

Di Biase, L., Santangeli, P., Burkhardt, D. J., Bai, R., Mohanty, P., Carbucicchio, C., et al. (2012). Endo-epicardial homogenization of the scar versus limited substrate ablation for the treatment of electrical storms in patients with ischemic cardiomyopathy. *J. Am. Coll. Cardiol.* 60, 132–141. doi: 10.1016/j.jacc.2012.03.044

Dun, W., Baba, S. G., Yagi, T., and Boyden, A. (2004). Dynamic remodeling of K+ and Ca2+ currents in cells that survived in the epicardial border zone of canine healed infarcted heart. *Am. J. Physiol. Heart Circ. Physiol.* 287, H1046–H1054.

Fernandez-Armenta, J., Berruezo, A., Andreu, D., Camara, O., Silva, E., Serra, L., et al. (2013). Three-dimensional architecture of scar and conducting channels based on high resolution ce-cmr: insights for ventricular tachycardia ablation. *Circ. Arrhythm. Electrophysiol.* 6, 528–537. doi: 10.1161/CIRCEP.113.000264

Grandi, E., and Maleckar, M. M. (2016). Anti-arrhythmic strategies for atrial fibrillation: the role of computational modeling in discovery, development, and optimization. *Pharmacol. Ther.* 168, 126–142. doi: 10.1016/j.pharmthera.2016.09.012

Hakim, J. B., Murphy, M. J., Trayanova, N. A., and Boyle, M. (2018). Arrhythmia dynamics in computational models of the atria following virtual ablation of re-entrant drivers. *Europace* 20(Suppl. 3), iii45–iii54. doi: 10.1093/europace/euy234

Jais, P., Maury, P., Khairy, P., Sacher, F., Nault, I., Komatsu, Y., et al. (2012). Elimination of local abnormal ventricular activities: a new end point for substrate modification in patients with scar-related ventricular tachycardia. *Circulation* 125, 2184–2196. doi: 10.1161/CIRCULATIONAHA.111.043216

Loewe, A., Poremba, E., Oesterlein, T., Luik, A., Schmitt, C., Seemann, G., et al. (2018). Patient-specific identification of atrial flutter vulnerability-a computational approach to reveal latent reentry pathways. *Front. Physiol.* 9:1910. doi: 10.3389/fphys.2018.01910

Martin, R., Maury, P., Bisceglia, C., Wong, T., Estner, H., Meyer, C., et al. (2018). Characteristics of scar-related ventricular tachycardia circuits using ultra-high-density mapping: a multi-center study. *Circ. Arrhythm. Electrophysiol.* 11:e006569.

Mendonca Costa, C., Plank, G., Rinaldi, C. A., Niederer, S. A., and Bishop, M. J. (2018). Modeling the electrophysiological properties of the infarct border zone. *Front. Physiol.* 9:356. doi: 10.3389/fphys.2018.00356

Narayan, S. M., Krummen, D. E., Shivkumar, K., Clopton, P., Rappel, W. J., and Miller, J. M. (2012). Treatment of atrial fibrillation by the ablation of localized sources confirm (conventional ablation for atrial fibrillation with or without focal impulse and rotor modulation) trial. *JACC* 60, 628–636. doi: 10.1016/j.jacc.2012.05.022

Pathmanathan, P., and Gray, R. A. (2014). Verification of computational models of cardiac electro-physiology. *Int. J. Numer. Method Biomed. Eng.* 30, 525–544. doi: 10.1002/cnm.2615

Plank, G., Zhou, L., Greenstein, J. L., Cortassa, S., Winslow, R. L., O'Rourke, B., et al. (2008). From mitochondrial ion channels to arrhythmias in the heart: computational techniques to bridge the spatio-temporal scales. *Philos. Trans. A Math. Phys. Eng. Sci.* 366, 3381–3409. doi: 10.1098/rsta.2008.0112

Prakosa, A., Arevalo, H. J., Deng, D., Boyle, M., Nikolov, P., Ashikaga, H., et al. (2018). Personalized virtual-heart technology for guiding the ablation of infarct-related ventricular tachycardia. *Nat. Biomed. Eng.* 2, 732–740. doi: 10.1038/s41551-018-0282-2

Prassl, A. J., Kickinger, F., Ahammer, H., Grau, V., Schneider, J. E., Hofer, E., et al. (2009). Automatically generated, anatomically accurate meshes for cardiac electrophysiology problems. *IEEE Trans. Biomed. Eng.* 56, 1318–1330. doi: 10.1109/tbme.2009.2014243

Roney, C. H., Bayer, J. D., Cochet, H., Meo, M., Dubois, R., Jais, P., et al. (2018a). Variability in pulmonary vein electrophysiology and fibrosis determines arrhythmia susceptibility and dynamics. *PLoS Comput. Biol.* 14:e1006166. doi: 10.1371/journal.pcbi.1006166

Roney, C. H., Williams, S. E., Cochet, H., Mukherjee, R. K., O'Neill, L., Sim, I., et al. (2018b). Patient-specific simulations predict efficacy of ablation of interatrial connections for treatment of persistent atrial fibrillation. *Europace* 20(Suppl. 3), iii55–iii68. doi: 10.1093/europace/euy232

ten Tusscher, K. H. W. J., Noble, D., Noble, J., and Panfilov, A. V. (2004). A model for human ventricular tissue. *Am. J. Physiol. Heart Circ. Physiol.* 286, H1573–H1589.

Trayanova, N. A. (2014). Mathematical approaches to understanding and imaging atrial fibrillation significance for mechanisms and management. *Circ. Res.* 114, 1516–1531. doi: 10.1161/CIRCRESAHA.114.302240

Vadakkumpadan, F., Trayanova, N., and Wu, K. C. (2014). Image-based left ventricular shape analysis for sudden cardiac death risk stratification. *Heart Rhythm* 11, 1693–1700. doi: 10.1016/j.hrthm.2014.05.018

Vigmond, E. J., Hughes, M., Plank, G., and Leon, L. J. (2003). Computational tools for modeling electrical activity in cardiac tissue. *J. Electrocardiol.* 36(Suppl.), 69–74. doi: 10.1016/j.jelectrocard.2003.09.017

Yao, J. A., Hussain, W., Patel, P., Peters, N. S., Boyden, A., and Wit, A. L. (2003). Remodeling of gap junctional channel function in epicardial border zone of healing canine infarcts. *Circ. Res.* 92, 437–443. doi: 10.1161/01.res.0000059301.81035.06

Zahid, S., Cochet, H., Boyle, M., Schwarz, E. L., Whyte, K. N., Vigmond, E. J., et al. (2016). Patient-derived models link re-entrant driver localization in atrial fibrillation to fibrosis spatial pattern. *Cardiovasc. Res.* 110, 443–454. doi: 10.1093/cvr/cvw073

10

Investigating the Complex Arrhythmic Phenotype Caused by the Gain-of-Function Mutation KCNQ1-G229D

Xin Zhou[1], Alfonso Bueno-Orovio[1], Richard J. Schilling[2], Claire Kirkby[2], Chris Denning[3], Divya Rajamohan[3], Kevin Burrage[1,4,5], Andrew Tinker[6], Blanca Rodriguez[1] and Stephen C. Harmer[6*†]*

[1] Department of Computer Science, British Heart Foundation Centre of Research Excellence, University of Oxford, Oxford, United Kingdom, [2] St Bartholomew's Hospital, London, United Kingdom, [3] Department of Stem Cell Biology, Centre for Biomolecular Sciences, University of Nottingham, Nottingham, United Kingdom, [4] Australian Research Council Centre of Excellence for Mathematical and Statistical Frontiers, Queensland University of Technology, Brisbane, QLD, Australia, [5] School of Mathematical Sciences, Queensland University of Technology, Brisbane, QLD, Australia, [6] The William Harvey Research Institute, Barts and The London School of Medicine and Dentistry, Queen Mary University of London, London, United Kingdom

***Correspondence:**
Blanca Rodriguez
blanca.rodriguez@cs.ox.ac.uk
Stephen C. Harmer
s.c.harmer@bristol.ac.uk

†Present address:
Stephen C. Harmer,
School of Physiology, Pharmacology and Neuroscience, University of Bristol, Bristol, United Kingdom

The congenital long QT syndrome (LQTS) is a cardiac electrophysiological disorder that can cause sudden cardiac death. LQT1 is a subtype of LQTS caused by mutations in KCNQ1, affecting the slow delayed-rectifier potassium current (I_{Ks}), which is essential for cardiac repolarization. Paradoxically, gain-of-function mutations in KCNQ1 have been reported to cause borderline QT prolongation, atrial fibrillation (AF), sinus bradycardia, and sudden death, however, the mechanisms are not well understood. The goal of the study is to investigate the ionic, cellular and tissue mechanisms underlying the complex phenotype of a gain-of-function mutation in KCNQ1, c.686G > A (p.G229D) using computer modeling and simulations informed by *in vitro* measurements. Previous studies have shown this mutation to cause AF and borderline QT prolongation. We report a clinical description of a family that carry this mutation and that a member of the family died suddenly during sleep at 21 years old. Using patch-clamp experiments, we confirm that KCNQ1-G229D causes a significant gain in channel function. We introduce the effect of the mutation in populations of atrial, ventricular and sinus node (SN) cell models to investigate mechanisms underlying phenotypic variability. In a population of human atrial and ventricular cell models and tissue, the presence of KCNQ1-G229D predominantly shortens atrial action potential duration (APD). However, in a subset of models, KCNQ1-G229D can act to prolong ventricular APD by up to 7% (19 ms) and underlie depolarization abnormalities, which could promote QT prolongation and conduction delays. Interestingly, APD prolongations were predominantly seen at slow pacing cycle lengths (CL > 1,000 ms), which suggests a greater arrhythmic risk during bradycardia, and is consistent with the observed sudden death during sleep. In a population of human SN cell models, the KCNQ1-G229D mutation results in slow/abnormal sinus rhythm, and we identify that a stronger L-type calcium current enables the SN to be more robust to the mutation. In conclusion, our computational modeling experiments provide novel mechanistic explanations for the observed borderline QT prolongation, and predict that KCNQ1-G229D could underlie SN dysfunction and conduction delays. The mechanisms revealed in the study can potentially inform management and treatment of KCNQ1 gain-of-function mutation carriers.

Keywords: KCNQ1, long QT syndrome, gain-of-function, arrhythmia, sinus node, computational biology

INTRODUCTION

Long QT Syndrome (LQTS) is a type of cardiac disorder that is often related to syncope and sudden cardiac death. LQT1, which is the most common form of LQTS, is caused by mutations in the KCNQ1 gene, affecting the slow delayed-rectifier repolarizing current (I_{Ks}) (Barhanin et al., 1996; Sanguinetti et al., 1996). Loss-of-function mutations in KCNQ1 can reduce I_{Ks} and underlie the inherited form of long QT syndrome (LQT1) (Wang et al., 1996), while gain-of-function mutations in KCNQ1 can act to increase channel opening, resulting in enhanced I_{Ks} (Chen et al., 2003; Hong et al., 2005; Lundby et al., 2007; Das et al., 2009; Bartos et al., 2011, 2013; Ki et al., 2014; Moreno et al., 2015).

Gain-of-function mutations in KCNQ1 associate with complex phenotypes. To date, eight gain-of-function mutations in KCNQ1 have been identified that underlie persistent familial atrial fibrillation (AF) (Hancox et al., 2014; Hasegawa et al., 2014), and four have been reported to cause short QT syndrome type 2 (SQT2) (Bellocq et al., 2004; Hong et al., 2005; Moreno et al., 2015; Wu et al., 2015). Some of these gain-of-function mutations are additionally associated with sinus bradycardia [S140G (Chen et al., 2003), V141M (Hong et al., 2005), R231C (Henrion et al., 2012), V241F (Ki et al., 2014), and F279I (Moreno et al., 2015)], and paradoxically, some KCNQ1 gain-of-function mutations have been linked to QT prolongation (borderline LQT) [S140G (Chen et al., 2003), Q147R (Lundby et al., 2007), R231C (Bartos et al., 2011; Henrion et al., 2012) and R231H (Bartos et al., 2013)]. The mechanisms underlying how certain KCNQ1 gain-of-function mutations cause AF and SQT2 have been revealed by *in silico* studies. In general, the gain in I_{Ks} function acts to shorten the refractory period and stabilize re-entrant waves, therefore promoting AF and ventricular arrhythmia (Kharche et al., 2012; Zulfa et al., 2016; Adeniran et al., 2017). In addition, the effects of several gain-of-function KCNQ1 mutations (V141M, R231C, and V241F) on sinus bradycardia have recently been explored using human *in silico* models of the sinus node (SN) (Fabbri et al., 2017; Whittaker et al., 2018). However, the mechanisms that underlie why certain KCNQ1 gain-of-function mutations are associated with borderline LQT and the factors that may explain phenotypic variability remain unclear.

The goal of this study is to investigate the ionic, cellular and tissue mechanisms underlying the complex phenotype of a gain-of-function mutation in KCNQ1, p.G229D (c.686G > A), (KCNQ1-G229D) using human atrial, ventricular and SN models informed by *in vitro* patch-clamp measurements. This mutation was first reported in 2014 in a 16-year-old boy with AF (Hasegawa et al., 2014). Interestingly, after radiofrequency catheter ablation therapy sinus rhythm was maintained, but the boy represented with borderline LQT (Hasegawa et al., 2014). Here, we report the clinical features of members of a British family affected by the same mutation. In addition to AF and borderline LQT, sudden death also happened in this family. By using a population of models approach, we investigate how natural variations in ionic current density could underlie variability in the phenotype of mutation carriers. In particular, we focus on the mechanisms that underlie the associated borderline LQT, which has also been reported for other KCNQ1 gain-of-function mutations but has not been explored. In addition, we investigate potential effects on the SN, based on the SN dysfunction caused by other KCNQ1 gain-of-function mutations.

MATERIALS AND METHODS

Clinical Data and QT Interval Duration Assessment

The clinical characterisation of the family carrying the G229D mutation was carried out in accordance with the recommendations of the National Health Service (NHS) Health Research Authority. The protocol was approved by the National Research Ethics Service (NRES Committee) East Midlands - Nottingham 2 [Research Ethics Committee (REC) reference: 09/H0508/74]. All subjects gave written informed consent in accordance with the Declaration of Helsinki. QT interval duration was measured on resting electrocardiograms (ECGs) using lead V5 or II (**Figure 1**). In patients in sinus rhythm an average of three consecutive beats was calculated. In patients with AF an average of six consecutive beats was calculated. The Bazett formula (Bazett, 1920) was used to correct QT according to heart rate (QTc).

Molecular Biology and Cell Culture

We characterized the effects of the G229D mutation on KCNQ1/KCNE1 (I_{Ks}) channel function by whole-cell patch-clamp in a heterologous expression system [Chinese Hamster Ovary-K1 (CHO-K1) cells]. KCNQ1 (GenBank® accession number AF000571) and KCNE1 are as described in Harmer et al. (2014). pEGFP-N1 was from Clontech. The patient-identified G229D mutation (c.686G > A) was introduced into KCNQ1 using site-directed mutagenesis [Quikchange II XL (Agilent Technologies)].

CHO-K1 cells (Sigma-Aldrich, 85051005) were cultured as described in Harmer et al. (2014). To analyze the effects of G229D, cells were transfected with 250 ng of wild-type (WT) KCNQ1 or LQT1 mutant cDNA and 500 ng of KCNE1 (+50 ng pEGFP-N1) (I_{Ks}-WT or I_{Ks}-G229D, respectively). To mimic the heterozygous patient phenotype (I_{Ks}-HET), cells were transfected with 125 ng of wild-type channel + 125 ng of mutant channel and 500 ng KCNE1 (+50 ng pEGFP-N1). Transfections were performed as described in Harmer et al. (2014). After transfection, cells were split at low density onto 10 mm glass coverslips and transfected cells (identified by fluorescence) were patched 48 h later.

Patch-Clamp Electrophysiological Recording and Analysis

Whole-cell currents were recorded using an Axopatch 200B amplifier (Axon Instruments/Molecular Devices). Data acquisition was performed using pCLAMP10 software through a Digidata 1440A (Axon Instruments/Molecular Devices). Data digitization (sampling) rates were 0.5 kHz and recordings were lowpass Bessel filtered at 1 kHz.

Whole-Cell Patch-Clamp

For the experiments detailed in **Figure 2** whole-cell patch-clamp recording was performed at room temperature (22°C) as described in Thomas et al. (2011). The intracellular (pipette) solution contained: (mmol/L) 150 KCl, 10 HEPES, 5 EGTA, 2 $MgCl_2$, 1 $CaCl_2$ and 5 $(Na)_2ATP$ (pH 7.2 with KOH). The extracellular (bath) solution contained: (mmol/L) 150 NaCl, 5 KCl, 10 HEPES, 2 $MgCl_2$, and 1 $CaCl_2$ (pH 7.4 with NaOH). Pipette resistances were, once filled with intracellular solution, between 2 and 3 mega-ohms (MΩ). Pipette capacitance was reduced by coating the pipette tip with SigmaCote (SL2, Sigma). Once the whole-cell configuration had been achieved cells were dialyzed for 2 min before recording. Series resistance (R_{series}) was compensated by at least 70% using the amplifier circuitry. The liquid junction potential [calculated using the Junction Potential tool in pCLAMP (Axon Instruments/Molecular Devices)] was relatively small (+4.3 mV) and therefore post-recording adjustments of membrane potential were not performed. The voltage protocol used is outlined in **Figure 2** and the cycle length for this protocol was 0.1 Hz.

Patch-Clamp Recording Analysis

Data were analyzed using Clampfit (Molecular Devices) and GraphPad Prism. As previously described in Thomas et al. (2011) current-voltage relationships were generated by normalizing the maximal current densities at the end of each pulse-potential to cell capacitance. Peak-tail current density (PTCD) was analyzed by normalizing the peak tail currents (in response to the prior test potential) to cell capacitance. The voltage-dependence of channel activation (or steady-state of activation) was determined by fitting the normalized peak tail current amplitudes (y/y_{max}) versus a test potential (V_t) with a Boltzmann function [$y/y_{max} = 1/(1 + \exp[(V_{0.5} - V_t)/k])$] ($k$ indicates the slope factor). The $V_{0.5}$ value indicates the potential at which channel activation is half-maximal.

Computational Modeling of the Effects of the G229D Mutation on KCNQ1/KCNE1 Channel Function

The I_{Ks} formulation from the human ventricular O'Hara-Rudy dynamic model (ORd) model (O'Hara et al., 2011) was used to replicate the patch-clamp data (**Supplementary Material**). Least square curve fitting (lsqcurvefit) was combined with the Multi-Start algorithm in Matlab to find the parameters with optimized fitting results for the mutated I_{Ks}. Additional fitting details including model formulation are presented in the **Supplementary Material**. The optimized fitting results for I_{Ks}-HET (KCNQ1 + G229D + KCNE1) and I_{Ks}-G229D (G229D + KCNE1) were inserted into the I_{Ks} current formulation of the ORd model, the human atrial (Grandi et al., 2011) and (Maleckar et al., 2009) and Fabbri human SN models (Fabbri et al., 2017).

To test whether the effects of our I_{Ks}-HET formulation on action potential duration (APD) and SN were stable, we also used the I_{Ks}/I_{Ks}-HET formulations of Hasegawa et al. (2014) to check the robustness of our results. Action Potential (AP) clamp simulations using three AP traces with different plateau levels were used to examine whether the effect of AP plateau on rapid delayed rectifier potassium current (I_{Kr}) was model specific by comparing the ORd, Maleckar, and Grandi models.

In silico Populations of Human Ventricular Cell and One-Dimensional (1D) Tissue Fibers Models

A population of 2326 ORd-derived models calibrated with human *in vivo* data was used to account for the effect of human electrophysiological variability as in Zhou et al. (2016). An initial population of 10,000 models was constructed by varying the main ionic conductances by up to ±100% using Latin Hypercube Sampling, including fast sodium current conductance (G_{Na}), late sodium current conductance (G_{NaL}), transient outward potassium current conductance (G_{to}), L-type calcium current conductance (G_{CaL}), rapid delayed rectifier potassium current conductance (G_{Kr}), slow delayed rectifier potassium current conductance (G_{Ks}), inward rectifier potassium current conductance (G_{K1}), sodium-potassium pump current conductance (G_{NaK}), sodium-calcium exchange current conductance (G_{NaCa}), sarcoplasmic reticulum (SR) calcium release permeability (P_{Jrel}) and SR calcium re-uptake permeability (P_{Jup}). The initial population of 10,000 models was calibrated using the human *in vivo* measurements described in Zhou et al. (2016). The advantage of using a population of models rather than just a standard baseline model is that it provides scenarios of natural variability (Muszkiewicz et al., 2016), in particular for investigations on multiple disease phenotypes and variable penetrance (Passini et al., 2016).

In the ORd model, the level of G_{Ks} is greatest in epicardial cells. Therefore, in order to evaluate the strongest possible effects in ventricles, we simulated the effect of the KCNQ1-G229D mutation in epicardial fibers. A population of monodomain homogeneous epicardial 1D fibers of 2 cm was derived from the

ORd single cell population. Pseudo-ECG signals were computed as the integral of spatial gradient of transmembrane potentials from all the points in the fibers (Gima and Rudy, 2002). The tissue simulations and pseudo-ECG calculations were conducted in the open-source software CHASTE (Pitt-Francis et al., 2009) for 50 beats with a conductivity of 3.92 mS/cm to obtain a conduction velocity of 69 cm/s in the baseline ORd epicardial fiber. Transmural fibers consisting of 80% of endocardial cells and 20% of epicardial cells were also simulated for some representative cases with a conductivity of 1.19 mS/cm to obtain a transmural conduction velocity of 40 cm/s in the baseline ORd model.

Construction and Calibration of Human Atrial Cell Population of Models

Using a similar methodology as in Britton et al. (2013), the nine current conductances of the Grandi atrial cell models (Grandi et al., 2011) were varied by up to ±100% using Latin Hypercube Sampling to generate an initial candidate population of 5,000 models: G_{Na}, G_{NaL}, G_{to}, G_{CaL}, G_{Kr}, G_{Ks}, G_{K1}, ultrarapid delayed rectifier potassium current conductance (G_{Kur}), G_{NaK}, and G_{NaCa}. These currents were chosen based on their direct contributions to the regulation of APDs, and intracellular calcium fluxes were not varied due to their relatively small effects on APD (Muszkiewicz et al., 2018). After pacing each model under CL = 1,000 ms for 500 beats, the experimental biomarker ranges from human atrial cells were used to select the models in range with the experimental data reported in Sanchez et al. (2014). The models accepted under cycle length (CL) = 1,000 ms were then paced under CL = 2,000 ms and CL = 500 ms. The 917 models that did not display delayed afterdepolarizations, early afterdepolarizations or depolarization failure under all three CLs were accepted for further analysis.

Construction and Calibration of Human Sinus Node Cell Population of Models

An initial population of 5,000 models was generated from the baseline Fabbri model (Fabbri et al., 2017) by using Latin hypercube sampling to introduce up to ±100% variations to 12 current conductances and ion flux magnitudes: funny current conductance (G_f), G_{CaL}, T-type calcium current conductance (G_{CaT}), G_{Kr}, G_{Ks}, G_{to}, G_{Na}, G_{NaK}, G_{NaCa}, G_{Kur}, P_{Jrel}, and P_{Jup}. These currents were chosen because both sarcolemmal currents and calcium handling affect spontaneous depolarization. After simulating each model for 1,000 s, 1046 models with a basic cycle length between 600 and 1,000 ms (heart rate between 60 and 100 bpm) and a positive overshoot membrane potential were accepted for further analysis. The effects of I_{Ks}-HET in human SN models were classified into three categories: Robust (heart rate between 60 and 100 bpm and a positive overshoot potential), Bradycardia (a positive overshoot potential and heart rate slower than 60 bpm), and Pacemaking failure (a negative maximum potential or a loss of spontaneous activity).

Statistical Analysis

Patch-clamp experimental data was compared/analyzed using a one-way ANOVA with Bonferroni *post hoc* test for multiple comparisons. Patch-clamp data was considered significantly different if $P < 0.05$. Statistical analysis of *in silico* modeling was conducted with Wilcoxon rank-sum test using Matlab, using a standard $P < 0.05$, and differences in current conductances are reported in the figures and visualized as the differences of the medians of the distributions.

RESULTS

Clinical Description of KCNQ1-G229D Mutation Carriers

Patient A was seen after her daughter (Patient C) died unexpectedly whilst sleeping at 21 years of age (**Figure 1A**). Patient A reported that as a teenager she had occasional periods of fainting but no reported exertional syncope. Her ECG was in sinus rhythm at 68 bpm (**Figures 1B,C**) and her QTc was 465 ms. It was noted following an ectopic beat that her QTc prolonged to 490 ms.

On the basis of the borderline QT prolongation and the death of her daughter she was genetically tested. Genetic testing found a previously reported pathogenic variant in *KCNQ1* c.686G > A (p.G229D) (Hasegawa et al., 2014). Based on this finding, other members of the family were genetically screened. Screening revealed that her mother (Patient B) and granddaughter (Patient D) are carriers of the *KCNQ1* c.686G > A (p.G229D) mutation. Genetic testing for Patient C was not performed during autopsy but her relationship in the family proves that she was an obligate carrier. Clinical details for Patient D are unavailable. Patient B was first diagnosed with AF at 60 years of age and does not have a history of syncope. Her QTc values, measured in the presence of AF, were 440–446 ms (**Figure 1C**). Our clinical data, and that reported by (Hasegawa et al., 2014) and (Moreton et al., 2013), indicate that *KCNQ1* c.686G > A (p.G229D) has high penetrance and that it is associated with AF, borderline LQT and sudden cardiac death.

Effect of the G229D Mutation on I_{Ks} Channel Function *in vitro* and *in silico*

Patch clamp measurements show that G229D co-expression with KCNE1 (I_{Ks}-G229D) produced currents with marked instantaneous activation and tail currents that failed to deactivate (**Figure 2A**). To mimic the patient phenotype KCNQ1 and G229D were co-expressed (with KCNE1) in heterozygous form (I_{Ks}-HET). The currents produced by I_{Ks}-HET possessed both instantaneous and slow activation components reflecting a combined phenotype (**Figure 2A**) and the presence of G229D acted to shift the voltage-dependence of channel activation ($V_{0.5}$) by approximately −35 mV (**Figure 2D**).

Overall, our observed effects of G229D on channel function correlate well with the gain-of-function effect first reported by (Hasegawa et al., 2014). Using the electrophysiological data from the patch-clamp studies, we then modeled *in silico* the effects of the G229D mutation on channel function. The fitting details for I_{Ks}-G229D and I_{Ks}-HET are shown in **Supplementary Figures S1–S3**. The resulting I_{Ks}-G229D and I_{Ks}-HET models

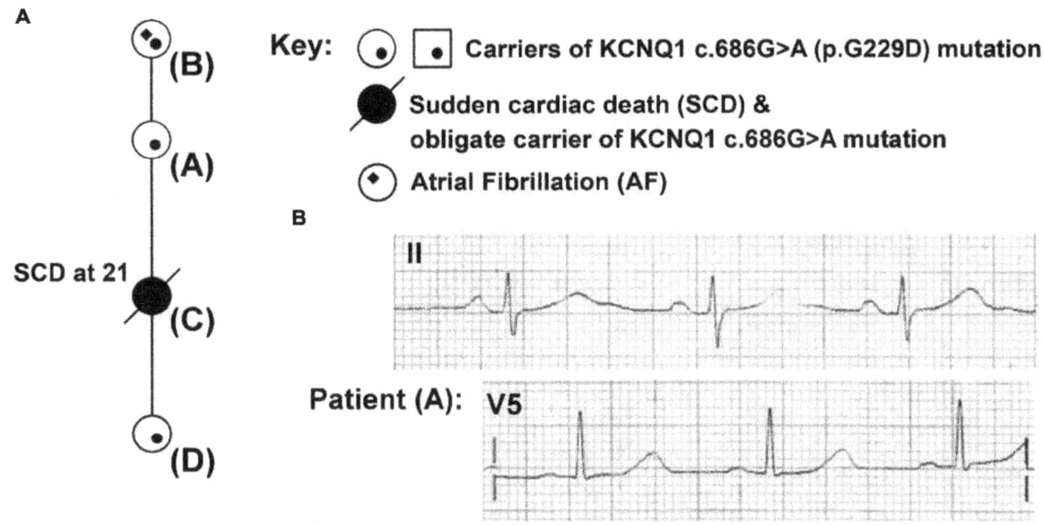

C

Patient	Age at last clinic visit	Mutation carrier	Atrial fibrillation	Sinus node dysfunction	QT interval (ms)	Heart rate (bpm) (resting ECG)
(A)	61	Yes	No	No	QTc 460-465	68
(B)	81	Yes	Yes	NK	QTc 440-446	78
(C)	Sudden death age 21	Yes*	NK	NK	NA	NA
(D)	8	Yes	NK	NK	NA	NA

FIGURE 1 | Partial pedigree and clinical information for members of a family carrying the KCNQ1 mutation G229D (c.686G>A). **(A)** Partial mini pedigree of a British family that present with a complex arrhythmic phenotype that includes sudden cardiac death (SCD), atrial fibrillation (AF), and borderline QT prolongation. Circles indicate female family members. **(B)** Lead II and V5 electrocardiograms (ECGs) from Patient (A) with borderline QT prolongation but not AF. **(C)** Clinical characteristics of carriers of the KCNQ1-G229D mutation. * = Not genetically tested but obligate carrier of the KCNQ1-G229D mutation (c.686G>A) based on position in the family. Please refer to **(A)** for the location of each patient in the pedigree. NK, not known; NA, not available.

were then incorporated into the populations of human atrial, ventricular and sino-atrial cell models to investigate the complex electrophysiological consequences of the mutation.

The Predominant Effect of I_{Ks} Gain-of-Function G229D Mutation Is APD Shortening in Both the Atria and Ventricle

In the baseline human atrial Grandi model, I_{Ks}-HET caused significant reductions in APD (14.22%) and weakened the AP upstroke (**Figure 3A**), in agreement with (Hasegawa et al., 2014). Similarly, in the baseline ventricular ORd model, the presence of I_{Ks}-HET also weakened the AP upstroke and led to AP shortening by 9.83%. Both APD shortenings occurred because I_{Ks}-HET produced a much stronger current during the whole AP, and therefore repolarization proceeded more quickly. The degree of shortening in the Grandi atrial model was greater than in the ventricular model (**Figures 3A,B**), and even greater shortening of APD was seen in the Maleckar human atrial model (33.23% reduction, **Supplementary Figure S4**). Therefore, the more significant APD shortening observed in human atrial models is not model-dependent.

We investigated potential variability in the effect of I_{Ks}-HET formulations when inserted in populations of human ventricular and atrial models with variable ionic profiles. As an accumulation of I_{Ks} during increases in heart rate may be important for repolarization (Viswanathan et al., 1999), we applied both slow and fast pacing CLs (2,000, 1,000, 500, and 333 ms). For both populations of models, the most common effect of the mutation was APD shortening (**Supplementary Figure S5** and **Figures 3C,D**). Under CL = 1,000 ms, the median APD shortening in the human ventricular cell population was 22 ms, while in the human atrial cell population, the median shortening was 29 ms (**Figures 3C,D**). Thus, when considering ionic variability in the population, the G229D mutation induced greater APD shortening in human atria than in the ventricular models. Since the baseline Maleckar atrial model already showed an even greater APD shortening than the Grandi atrial model under the mutation, we did not construct a population of Maleckar atrial models to verify this phenomenon. Further analysis showed that the conductances of I_{Kr}, I_{Ks}, and I_{CaL} were the main determinants for the extent of ventricular APD shortening caused by I_{Ks}-HET (**Figure 3E**). Models with weak G_{CaL} and G_{Kr} and strong G_{Ks} tended to present with more significant APD shortening under I_{Ks}-HET (**Figure 3F**). In the atrial population of models, a greater number of currents played roles in the regulation of APD shortening, and the most important factor was G_{Ks} (**Figure 3E**). Stronger G_{Ks},

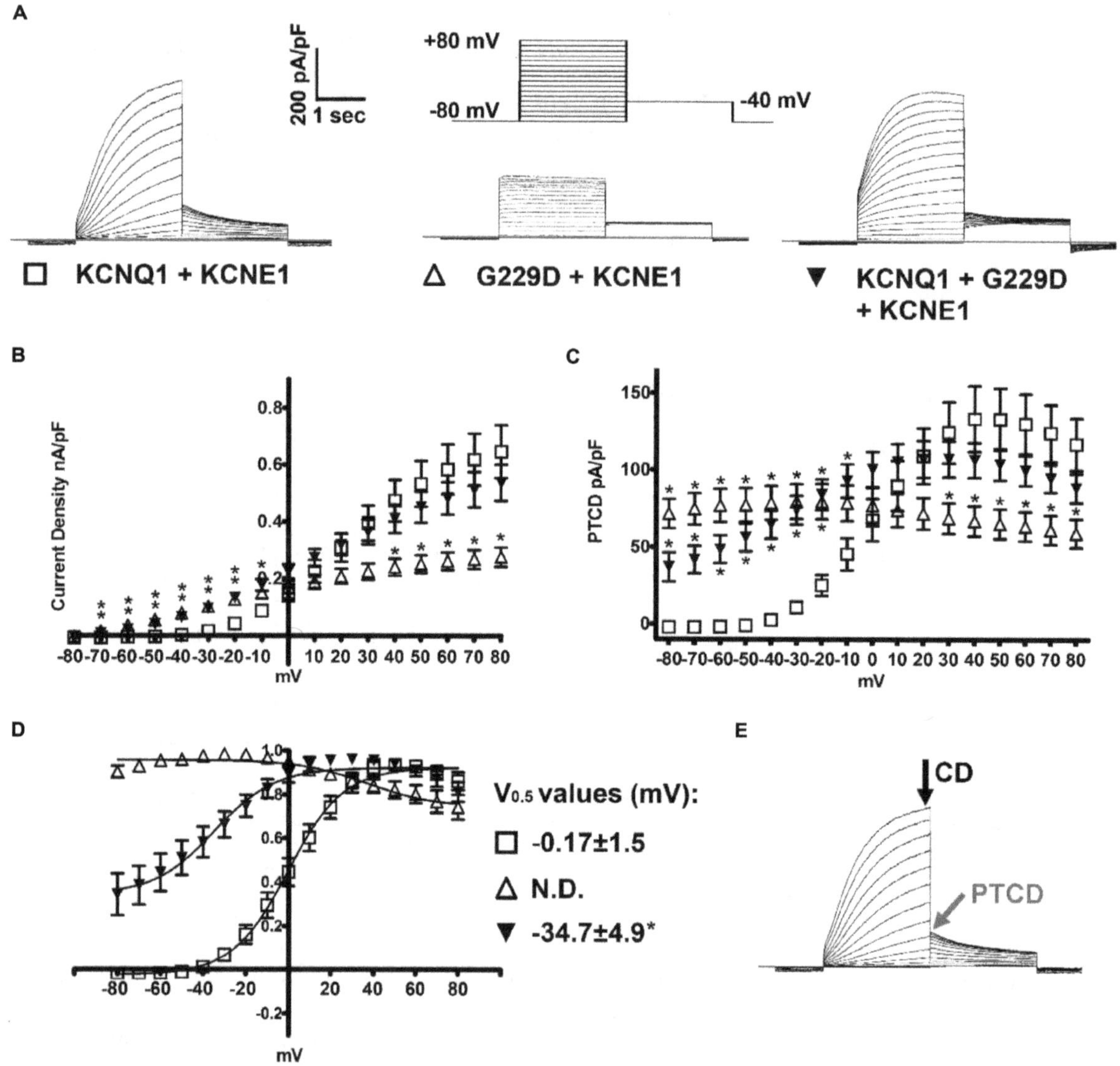

FIGURE 2 | KCNQ1-G229D dramatically alters the biophysical properties of the KCNQ1/KCNE1 (I_{Ks}) channel. **(A)** Representative traces of the currents produced by wild-type (WT) KCNQ1 (KCNQ1 + KCNE1: I_{Ks}-WT) or G229D when expressed homozygously (G229D + KCNE1: I_{Ks}-G229D) or in heterozygous fashion (KCNQ1 + G229D + KCNE1: I_{Ks}-HET). The effect of the G229D mutation on channel function, in CHO-K1 cells, was analyzed by whole-cell patch-clamp. In all cases, to recapitulate the I_{Ks} current, KCNE1 was co-expressed. The zero-current level (0 pA) is indicated by the gray line. The voltage protocol used to elicit these currents is inset in **(A)**. **(B)** Mean current-voltage relationships (current density). **(C)** Peak-tail current density (PTCD). **(D)** Normalized voltage-dependent activation curves ($V_{0.5}$) (in mV). The activation curves are fit with Boltzmann functions (solid lines). **(E)** Black and gray arrows indicate the points where the current density signals [current density (CD)] and PTCD were used to calculate the corresponding biomarkers for analysis and fitting. Data are presented as mean ± SEM. (n = 8–12). N.D., not determined. * indicates significantly different from WT control value (P < 0.05) (One-way ANOVA analysis with Bonferroni *post hoc* test).

G_{NaK}, and G_{CaL}, and weaker G_{K1}, G_{to}, G_{Kur}, and G_{Kr} were associated with more significant APD shortening in the atrial cells (**Figure 3E**).

Borderline APD Prolongation May Occur Due to the Interplay Between I_{Kr} and I_{Ks}-HET

Although APD shortening was consistently observed under four pacing CLs (**Supplementary Figure S5**), some human ventricular models in the population resulted in APD prolongation in the presence of I_{Ks}-HET, especially at slower pacing rates (**Figure 4A**). Furthermore, the number of ventricular cell models that showed obvious APD prolongation (>5 ms) was also increased as pacing rates became slower (no models under CL = 500/333 ms, 5 models under CL = 1,000 ms and 25 models under CL = 2,000 ms). Therefore, in the presence of KCNQ1-G229D, APD prolongation occurred more often at slower pacing rates.

There was no significant difference between the WT APDs between the prolongation models and other models in the population. However, the AP peak membrane voltage was

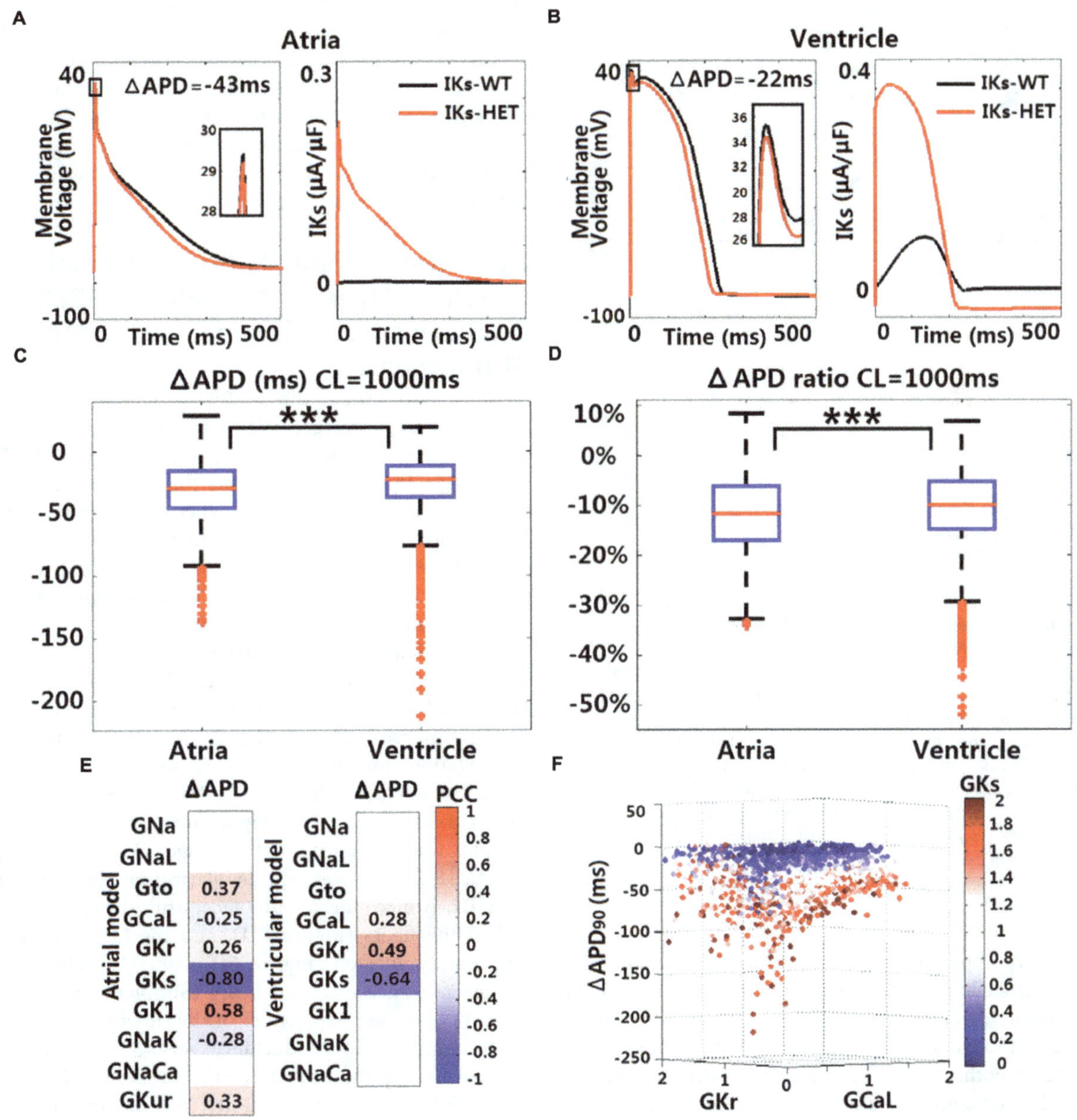

FIGURE 3 | *In silico* simulations of the effects of KCNQ1-G229D on human ventricular and atrial action potentials. The effect of the G229D mutation on membrane voltage (V_m, mV, insets showing peak upstroke) and I_{Ks} (µA/µF) in the Grandi human atrial cell model **(A)** and the ORd human ventricular epicardial cell model **(B)**. Comparison of absolute APD change (ΔAPD = APD-I_{Ks}-HET – APD-I_{Ks}-WT, **C)** and relative APD change (ΔAPD/APD-I_{Ks}-WT, **D)** after introducing I_{Ks}-HET between Grandi atrial population of models and ORd ventricular population of models at CL = 1,000 ms (***$P < 0.001$) (Wilcoxon rank-sum test). **(E)** Partial correlation analysis between ΔAPD at CL = 1,000 ms and current conductances in the population of atrial and ventricular models. The partial correlation coefficients (PCC) are indicated by the color scale, where red implies a strong positive correlation and blue implies a strong negative correlation. **(F)** Relationship between the conductances of I_{Kr}, I_{Ks}, and I_{CaL} and the ΔAPD in the ORd population. 0–2 represent the scaling factors for the baseline conductances in the ±100% range.

significantly reduced (**Figure 4B**) due to smaller baseline depolarization current conductances (G_{Na} and G_{CaL}) in the models displaying APD prolongation (**Figure 4C**). In addition, stronger baseline G_{Kr} was found in the models displaying APD prolongation at CL = 1,000 or 2,000 ms (**Figure 4C**). In the subgroup of models producing APD prolongation at CL = 1,000 ms, replacing our I_{Ks}/I_{Ks}-HET formulations with the I_{Ks}/I_{Ks}-HET formulations of Hasegawa et al. (2014) also generated consistent APD prolongation, supporting the robustness of these phenomena (**Supplementary Figure S6**).

To understand the ionic mechanisms underlying APD prolongation/shortening, we analyzed the change of individual currents induced by the presence of the G229D mutation. The biggest differences in ionic currents for both prolongation and shortening were the increase of I_{Ks} (**Figures 5A,B**, middle panels) and the secondary decrease of I_{Kr} (**Figures 5A,B**, right panels).

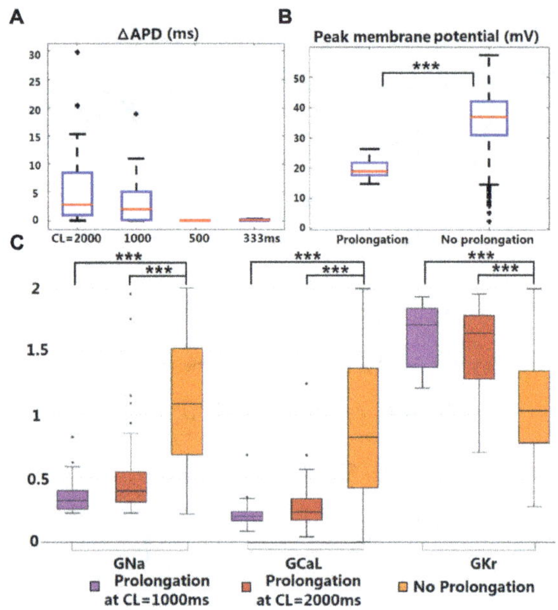

FIGURE 4 | KCNQ1-G229D can lead to ventricular APD prolongation at slow pacing rates. **(A)** APD prolongations under four pacing rates (ΔAPD = APD-I_{Ks}-HET – APD-I_{Ks}-WT). **(B)** Comparison of the WT peak membrane voltage between the models that showed or did not show APD prolongation under I_{Ks}-HET at CL = 1,000 ms. **(C)** Parameter comparison between models that showed APD prolongation at CL = 1,000 or 2,000 ms and those that did not show APD prolongation under I_{Ks}-HET. The *y*-axis represents the scaling factors in the ±100% range (0–2) to the original baseline ORd model current conductances (***P < 0.001) (Wilcoxon rank-sum test). Black points indicate extreme values that lie more than 1.5 times the interquartile range away from the top (the 75th percentile) or bottom (the 25th percentile) of the box.

We selected two representative ventricular cell models with similar AP upstroke but one displaying shortening and the other prolongation with I_{Ks}-HET. The presence of I_{Ks}-HET affected the AP upstroke and led to a smaller peak membrane voltage and a lower plateau in both models. The reduction in I_{Kr} magnitude after G229D introduction was likely due to the reduced phase 2 AP plateau (**Figures 5A,B**, left panels).

To verify whether this was model-specific, we conducted AP clamp simulations using different human I_{Kr} models. The I_{Kr} magnitude was consistently weaker under a smaller phase 2 AP plateau in all models tested (**Supplementary Figure S7**). For the human ventricular model displaying APD prolongation with I_{Ks}-HET, the decrease of I_{Kr} amplitude was slightly bigger than the increase of I_{Ks} amplitude under the I_{Ks}-HET condition (**Figure 5A**, middle and right panels). In contrast, in the human ventricular model displaying APD shortening, the augmentation of I_{Ks} was more significant than the inhibition of I_{Kr} (**Figure 5B**, middle and right panels).

Therefore, our explanation was that if the inhibition of I_{Kr} can overcome the augmentation of I_{Ks}, the presence of the G229D mutation could lead to an overall weaker repolarization, and therefore a prolonged APD. Importantly, the prolongation models tended to have stronger I_{Kr} (**Figure 4C**), which was crucial for I_{Kr} reduction to be dominant under I_{Ks}-HET. We also noticed that under slow pacing, the magnitude of I_{Ks} decreased, whereas I_{Kr} increased (**Supplementary Figure S8**), which explained the increased number of models with APD prolongation at slow pacing. Overall, these findings further highlight that in the presence of the G229D mutation, ventricular APD prolongation is more likely to occur during bradycardia, particularly for strong I_{Kr} models.

By Counteracting Action Potential Upstroke Dynamics KCNQ1-G229D Could Promote Tissue Conduction Abnormalities

As illustrated earlier, the G229D mutation can reduce peak AP membrane voltage. We hypothesized that I_{Ks}-HET by counteracting AP upstroke dynamics (**Figures 3A,B, 5A,B**) could have important effects on the safety of conduction. In addition, we need to confirm whether the ionic mechanisms underlying APD prolongation in single cells hold true at the tissue level. Therefore, we investigated conduction and repolarization patterns in the presence of I_{Ks}-HET on the population of human ventricular one-dimensional (1D) fibers.

The original ventricular 1D fiber showed a shorter QT interval with the G229D mutation (**Figure 6A**). In the population of 1D fibers, both significant QT prolongation and QT shortening can be observed (**Figure 6B**). 36 I_{Ks}-HET fibers showed QT prolongation compared to the corresponding I_{Ks}-WT fibers. In the QT prolongation fibers, the AP upstroke was delayed at the end of the I_{Ks}-HET fiber (**Figure 6C**). In these cases, the QRS complex was wider, leading to a longer QT interval (**Figure 6C**, insert). 18 fibers developed depolarization abnormalities under I_{Ks}-HET, which meant no successful depolarization at the end of the fibers (**Figure 6D**), and the QT interval was also significantly affected (**Figure 6D**, insert). Similar results were obtained using transmural fibers (**Supplementary Figure S9**). By comparing the parameters of the different groups of fibers, we found that the conductances of I_{Na}, I_{CaL}, I_{Kr}, I_{Ks}, I_{K1}, I_{NaCa} were significantly different. In both QT prolongation and depolarization abnormalities, the baseline I_{Na} was weak (**Figure 6E**). Models exhibiting depolarization abnormalities also tended to have weak baseline I_{CaL}, I_{K1}, I_{NaCa} and relatively strong I_{Ks}, which explained the danger of G229D mutation presence in their conduction (**Figure 6E**). The fibers showing QT prolongation had the strongest baseline I_{Kr}, which was consistent with the results from the cellular simulations.

In silico Simulations Predict That KCNQ1-G229D Is Capable of Promoting SN Dysfunction by Perturbing Diastolic Depolarization

Sinus node dysfunction and bradycardia has been reported for carriers of different KCNQ1 gain-of-function mutations [S140G (Chen et al., 2003), V141M (Hong et al., 2005), R231C (Henrion et al., 2012), V241F (Ki et al., 2014), and F279I (Moreno et al., 2015)]. Even though SN dysfunction has not been associated

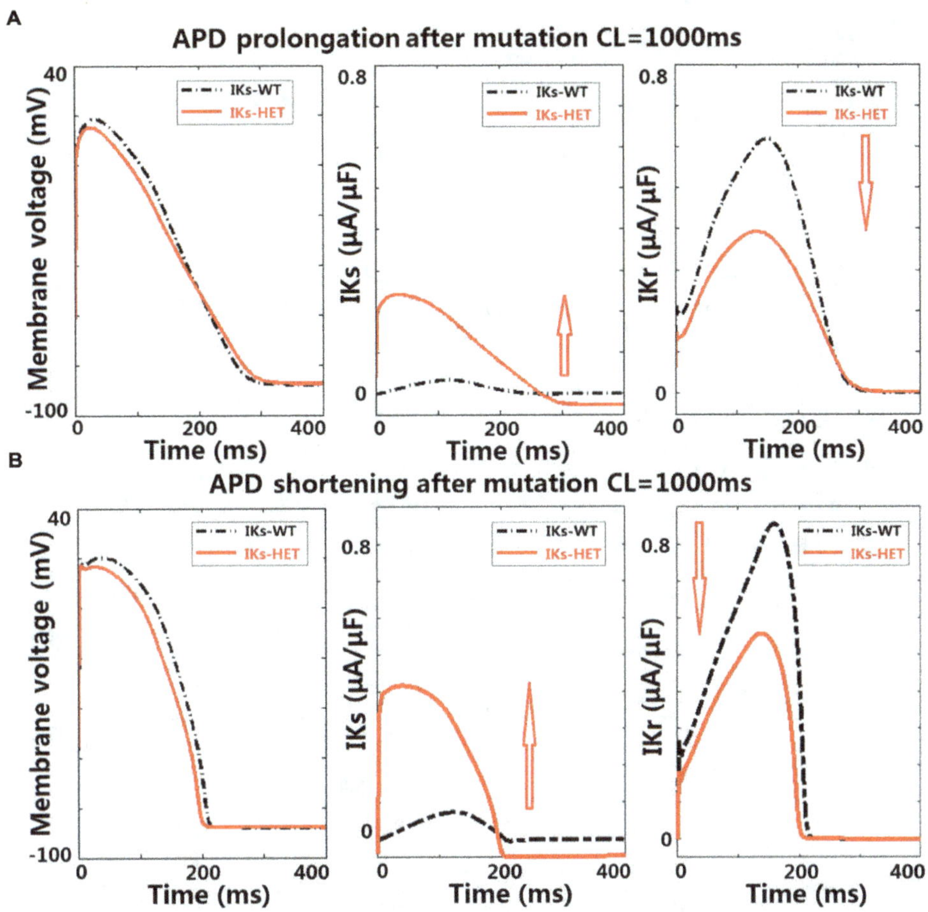

FIGURE 5 | KCNQ1-G229D can lead to ventricular APD prolongation by altering the interplay between I_{Kr} and I_{Ks}. Effects of KCNQ1-G229D mutation (I_{Ks}-HET) on I_{Kr} and I_{Ks} in representative models displaying **(A)** APD prolongation and **(B)** APD shortening, at CL = 1,000 ms. The arrows indicate the change of current magnitude after introducing G229D. In **(A)**, the decrease of I_{Kr} is more significant than the increase of I_{Ks}, while in **(B)** the opposite occurs.

with KCNQ1-G229D (Hasegawa et al., 2014) or in the mutation carriers reported here, the effects of V141M on channel gating (Hong et al., 2005) are similar to those induced by the G229D mutation [this study and (Hasegawa et al., 2014)]. Therefore, we investigated whether the G229D mutation can cause SN dysfunction in populations of sino-atrial node cells. In a recently published human SN model (Fabbri et al., 2017), the normal SN model had a stable heart rate (HR) around 73.7 beats per minute (bpm) (**Figure 7A**). Starting from the same initial condition, when introduced I_{Ks}-HET produced an increasingly stronger I_{Ks} and slower HR, and the sinus rhythm was terminated after 625 s (**Figure 7A**). Plugging the I_{Ks}-HET model developed by (Hasegawa et al., 2014) into the simulation was confirmatory, as this model also led to sinus rhythm termination after 135 s (**Supplementary Figure S10**).

Sinus node activity was related to the interplay between the calcium subsystem and membrane potential in agreement with (Lakatta et al., 2010). For successful spontaneous SN activation, a positive feedback loop between subsarcolemmal calcium (Ca_{sub}) and V_m was needed for the diastolic depolarization. I_{CaL} and I_{NaCa} provided the biggest depolarization current during the upstroke phase, and the net current excluding I_{CaL} and I_{NaCa} was always positive (**Supplementary Figures S11, S12**). The activation of I_{NaCa} was regulated by Ca_{sub}, and during diastolic depolarization, I_{CaL} provided the biggest contribution for the initial accumulation of Ca_{sub} (**Supplementary Figure S13**). During normal diastolic depolarization, the total net current was inward, leading to very slow/limited activation of I_{CaL}, accumulation of Ca_{sub} and enhancement of I_{NaCa} (**Figure 7B**, left columns). At the end of diastolic depolarization, the augmentation of I_{NaCa} was strong enough to result in a significant increase in V_m that further activated I_{CaL}, promoting faster depolarization in a positive feedback manner to initiate the upstroke phase (**Figure 7B**, left columns).

In the SN cell model I_{Ks}-HET produced a much stronger repolarization current to counteract the diastolic depolarization process. At the time of diastolic depolarization interruption (time = 628.5 s), I_{Ks} became so strong that the overall total current became outward. The membrane potential then started to decrease, along with the slow decay of I_{CaL}, Ca_{sub}, and I_{NaCa} activity (**Figure 7B**, right columns). Consequently, positive feedback during the depolarization phase was interrupted.

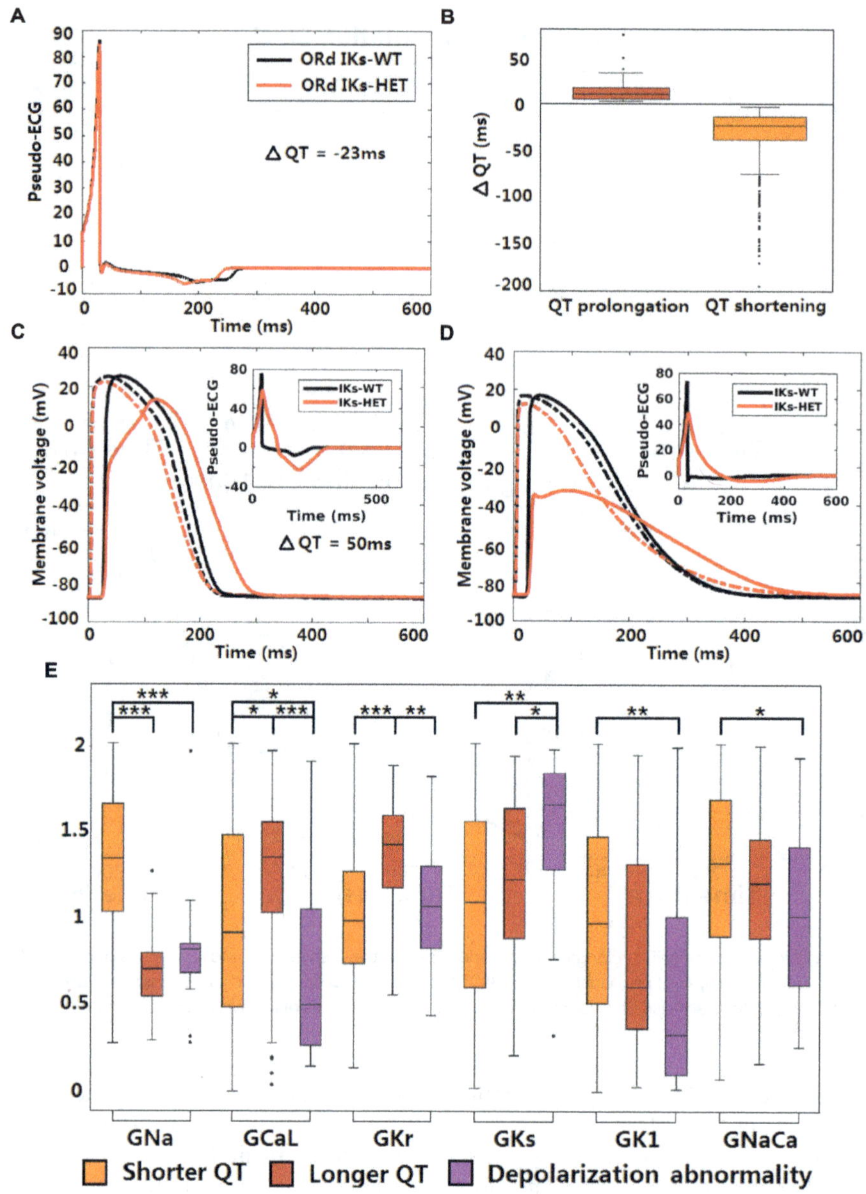

FIGURE 6 | KCNQ1-G229D can impair conduction safety by counteracting action potential upstroke. **(A)** Pseudo-ECG of the original ORd human homogeneous epicardial 1D fiber. **(B)** Longer and shorter QT intervals are possible in the presence of the G229D mutation (I_{Ks}-HET) in Pseudo-ECGs of the population of human epicardial 1D fiber. **(C)** APs of a fiber that showed slower conduction in the presence of the G229D mutation, with the corresponding pseudo-ECG as an insert. **(D)** APs of a fiber that showed a depolarization abnormality in the presence of the G229D mutation, with the corresponding pseudo-ECG as an insert. **(C,D)** There are 100 nodes in the whole fiber, and Node 20 (dashed lines) and Node 80 (solid lines) are at sites near the beginning and the end of the fiber. **(E)** Comparisons of ionic current conductances between the fibers that showed shorter QT, longer QT and depolarization abnormalities in the presence of G229D (***$P < 0.001$, **$P < 0.01$, *$P < 0.05$) (Wilcoxon rank-sum test). Black points indicate extreme values that lie more than 1.5 times the interquartile range away from the top (the 75th percentile) or bottom (the 25th percentile) of the box.

To understand why the carriers of KCNQ1-G229D described in our study and those reported by (Hasegawa et al., 2014) do not present with bradycardia, we used a population of human SN models to explore the effects of heterogeneity in ion channel expression. In the 1,046 human SN cell models, 168 models are robust to I_{Ks}-HET, 153 models became bradycardic, and the rest (725 models) displayed pacemaking failure. By comparing the parameters, we identified differences in I_{Ks}, I_{CaL}, I_{NaCa}, I_{NaK}, and I_{Kr} conductances between models displaying different phenotypes (**Figure 7C**). As expected, the Pacemaking failure group had the highest level of I_{Ks}-HET. A stronger I_{CaL} in the Robust and Bradycardia groups can counteract the changes caused by I_{Ks}-HET and enable safer spontaneous activation. In the Robust group, a stronger inward I_{NaCa} and a weaker outward I_{NaK} contributed to maintaining negative total current during diastolic depolarization. In addition, a stronger I_{Kr} in Robust and

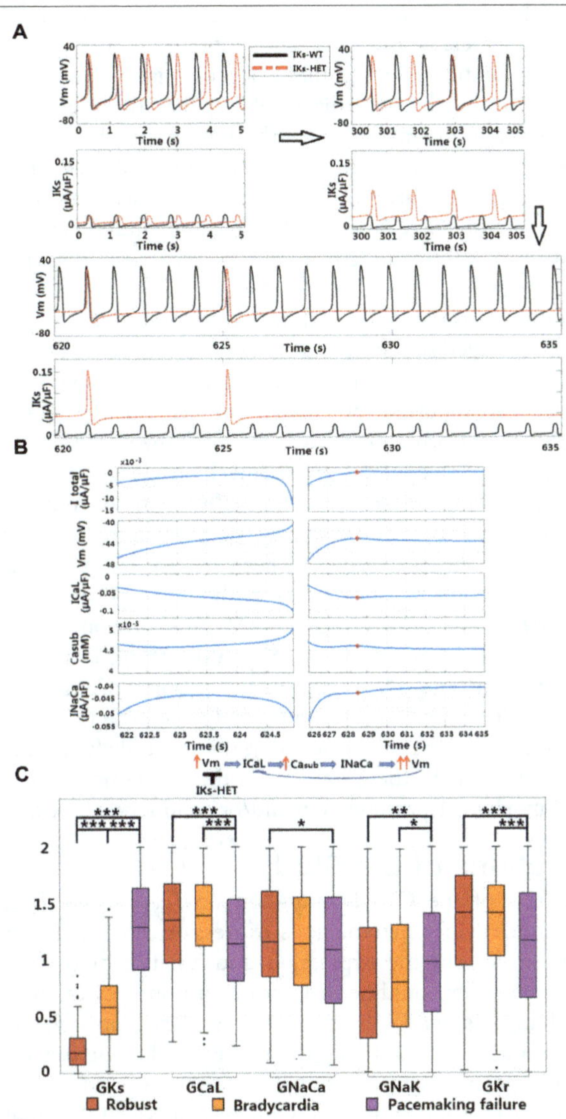

FIGURE 7 | KCNQ1-G229D can cause sinus node dysfunction. **(A)** I_{Ks}-HET presence results in a loss of sinus rhythm. **(B)** Comparison between the last spontaneous activated beat and the failing process under I_{Ks}-HET. The red circles in the right columns indicate the time = 628.5 s when diastolic depolarization was interrupted, and membrane potential started to decrease. **(C)** Parameter comparison between Robust, Bradycardia, and Pacemaking failure groups under I_{Ks}-HET (***$P < 0.001$, **$P < 0.01$, *$P < 0.05$) (Wilcoxon rank-sum test). Black points indicate extreme values that lie more than 1.5 times the interquartile range away from the top (the 75th percentile) or bottom (the 25th percentile) of the box.

Bradycardia groups can counteract the effect of high level I_{CaL}, preventing excessive APD prolongation (**Figure 7C**).

DISCUSSION

In this present study, we investigate the complex phenotypic implications of a gain-of-function mutation in I_{Ks} (KCNQ1-G229D) through a combination of computational modeling and simulation and patch clamp experimental characterization, as well as clinical presentation. We describe members of a family that carry KCNQ1-G229D and report that this mutation underlies a complex phenotype characterized by AF, borderline LQT and sudden death. Our clinical findings correlate well with those reported by Moreton et al. (2013) and Hasegawa et al. (2014). We explored the pathogenic role of this mutation using a combination of *in vitro* experiments and *in silico* simulations in human SN, atrial and ventricular models. In addition to providing further evidence supporting the role of G229D in promoting AF as shown in previous studies, we expand our knowledge of G229D and other gain-of-function KCNQ1 mutations in additional ways. Firstly, we present the first mechanistic investigation into why the G229D mutation (and perhaps other KCNQ1 gain-of function mutations) could be associated with a borderline LQT phenotype. Secondly, we demonstrate that the gain-of-function mutation could promote pro-arrhythmic conduction abnormalities by counteracting the AP depolarization phase and reducing conduction safety. This could be a critical mechanism of sudden cardiac death. Thirdly, we utilize populations of human SN models to provide detailed mechanistic predictions which highlight that KCNQ1-G229D could underlie SN dysfunction. Finally, our findings provide plausible reasons for observed phenotypic variability and insights for the clinical management of these patients.

A Potential Explanation for G229D Associated QT Prolongation

The mechanisms underlying the presence of borderline LQT in G229D carriers [(Moreton et al., 2013; Hasegawa et al., 2014) and this study] and other KCNQ1 gain-of-function mutations (particularly S140G) (Chen et al., 2003; Lundby et al., 2007; Bartos et al., 2011, 2013) are unclear. We used a population of human ventricular cell models to investigate the complex interactions between different currents in the presence of G229D. In addition to APD shortening produced by the standard ventricular model, a subset of the models in the population exhibited APD prolongation. We found that APD prolongation was caused by an interplay between a decrease in I_{Kr} activity and increase in I_{Ks} activity at slow pacing. Based on our simulations, the instantaneous current component produced by KCNQ1-G229D reduces the magnitude of the AP upstroke which leads to a smaller peak membrane voltage and a lower plateau. Consequently, the presence of a lower plateau acts to decrease the activity of I_{Kr} which, in turn, acts to prolong APD. In our fibers showing QT prolongation at the tissue level, I_{Kr} tended to be stronger, suggesting that the I_{Kr}/I_{Ks} interplay mechanism, originally identified in single cells, also holds true at the tissue level.

KCNQ1-G229D May Induce Defects in Conduction

The 1D fiber results also indicate that the presence of KCNQ1-G229D could impair myocardial conduction. Although QRS widening in fibers was not observed clinically in mutation carriers, whole ventricle simulations have shown that QRS width is more sensitive to the activation pattern in the conduction system rather than myocardial propagation (Cardone-Noott et al., 2016). Therefore, local conduction abnormalities in the myocardium may still be present even with normal QRS width. Local or regional conduction abnormalities may also occur due to heterogeneous expression of KCNQ1/G229D throughout the ventricles (Liu and Antzelevitch, 1995; Viswanathan et al., 1999). Although the fiber simulations we used do not account for the full heterogeneity known to span the human ventricles, they do provide a rough approximation of tissue behavior. Despite these potential limitations, our findings emphasize that G229D could enhance regional differences in conduction and this could contribute to the substrate required for the formation of a lethal arrhythmia.

In silico Modeling Using Human Models Provides Explanations for SN and Atrial Dysfunction

Our human SN model simulations predict that the G229D mutation is likely to underlie SN dysfunction and that this could increase the risk of sinus arrest. By examining variations in ionic current density, our population of SN models may also provide plausible explanations as to why a dysfunctional SN phenotype was not seen by Hasegawa et al. (2014) or in the mutation carriers we report. Based on the mechanisms revealed in this study and those of Fabbri et al. (2017) and Whittaker et al. (2018), disturbed SN activity could be a general action of KCNQ1 gain-of-function mutations that alter channel gating in a similar fashion.

Mechanistically, the G229D mutation has been postulated to cause AF by promoting atrial APD shortening (Hasegawa et al., 2014) and two and three-dimensional tissue models have described that this mutation promotes the sustainment of re-entrant waves thereby increasing susceptibility to atrial arrhythmia (Zulfa et al., 2016). In our baseline and population of models, the G229D mutation results in atrial and ventricular AP shortening, but the average degree of shortening is less for ventricular than atrial APs, which agrees with the findings of Hasegawa et al. (2014) and implies a more prominent effect of the mutation on the human atria.

Clinical Implications for KCNQ1-G229D Carriers

KCNQ1-G229D presents in adults largely as AF, and Class I drugs such as flecainide and quinidine may be prescribed. Based on our simulation results, KCNQ1-G229D could impair conduction by counteracting AP upstroke, and class I sodium channel blockers could exacerbate this. Furthermore, our simulations predict that this mutation could underlie SN dysfunction which has been postulated to act as a substrate for the development of AF (Duhme et al., 2013). Indeed, a trend in disease progression from bradycardia in to persistent AF has been reported for patients that carry the KCNQ1 gain-of-function mutation V241F (Ki et al., 2014). As revealed by our SN simulations, I_{CaL} played a crucial role in the maintenance of normal sinus rhythm in the presence of the G229D mutation. Therefore, drugs with class IV calcium channel blocking actions could unravel bradycardia in G229D mutation carriers with normal sinus rhythm.

Our simulations showed that QT prolongation was primarily observed during bradycardia implying that the prevention of bradycardia to maintain sinus rhythm should be considered in the management of mutation carriers. The use of drugs with a negative chronotropic effect, such as beta-blockers, should therefore be reviewed and device implantation considered for KCNQ1 gain-of-function mutation carriers that present with bradycardia.

Another intriguing observation is that some G229D mutation carriers have died suddenly whilst sleeping [reported in this study and (Moreton et al., 2013)]. Sudden cardiac arrest during sleep has also been reported for a carrier of KCNQ1-R231H (Bartos et al., 2013). Unfortunately, we do not have the necessary clinical information to establish the precise mechanisms underlying these deaths. In LQT1, cardiac arrest normally occurs during exercise and sudden cardiac death during sleep is more a feature of LQT3 (Schwartz et al., 2001). Therefore, we can propose two possible mechanisms: sinus arrest without escape rhythms or a lethal arrhythmia caused by severe QT prolongation. It is worth noting that sinus arrest, due to SN dysfunction, is an unusual cause of death and SN disease in the absence of symptoms is not generally considered prognostically important. In view of these considerations we suspect that the most likely mechanism of sudden death in these patients is the promotion of a lethal arrhythmia by QT prolongation and/or conduction block.

Limitations of the Study

The effects of the G229D mutation on I_{Ks} channel function were modeled in a heterologous expression system. Therefore, it is possible that the expression and kinetics of the mutant channel complex could be distinct in cardiomyocytes. We were limited to this model because: (1) it is not possible to use mice or rats as a model as these species do not use I_{Ks} for cardiac repolarization in adult life (Nerbonne, 2014). (2) The generation of transgenic rabbit models of KCNQ1 mutations (Brunner et al., 2008), would be prohibitively expensive and the higher heart rate of this species would likely confound modeling the effects of the mutation on the SN. (3) The current utility of human induced pluripotent stem derived cardiomyocytes (hiPSC-CMs) for examining I_{Ks} function has been questioned and this may relate to their relative immaturity (Christ et al., 2015). We would also like to highlight that although we propose an explanation for the borderline LQT seen in carriers of the G229D mutation the observed APD prolongations in the population of models subset were relatively mild. This could relate to the potential differences between the function of the mutant channel complex in the heterologous expression system versus in cardiomyocytes or alternatively it could imply that other mechanisms contributing to QT prolongation exist. In the future, the validation of our *in silico* predictions in a physiological system is warranted. hiPSC-CM technology is rapidly advancing, and we hope that in time we will be able to use this model to study the effects of the G229D mutation in human cardiomyocytes that possess adult-like and chamber/region specific electrophysiological properties.

CONCLUSION

By using a combined *in vitro* and *in silico* approach we have explored how the KCNQ1 mutation G229D can underlie the reported phenotype of AF and borderline QT prolongation. In addition, our modeling results suggest that the G229D mutation can cause conduction abnormalities, and can underlie SN dysfunction. Importantly, our results suggest that for G229D mutation carriers (and perhaps for other KCNQ1 gain-of-function mutation carriers), the prescription of beta-blockers, class I sodium channel blockers and compounds with class IV calcium channel blocking properties should be used with caution.

AUTHOR CONTRIBUTIONS

XZ conducted the *in silico* simulations, took part in the design, analysis and interpretation of the modeling results. AB-O contributed to the design, interpretation, and discussion of the *in silico* results. RS, CK, CD, and DR were involved in collation of patient data and clinical interpretation. KB contributed to the design of the model fitting process. BR took part in the design, interpretation, discussion, and provided the funding for the modeling work. AT and SH conducted the *in vitro* experimentation, overviewed the project design, interpretation and discussion, and provided funding for the *in vitro* experiments. All authors contributed to writing the manuscript.

ACKNOWLEDGMENTS

The authors would like to acknowledge the helpful discussions with Dr. Alan Fabbri. This work used the ARCHER UK National Supercomputing Service (http://www.archer.ac.uk).

REFERENCES

Adeniran, I., Whittaker, D. G., El Harchi, A., Hancox, J. C., and Zhang, H. (2017). 'In silico investigation of a KCNQ1 mutation associated with short QT syndrome'. *Sci. Rep.* 7:8469. doi: 10.1038/s41598-017-08367-2

Barhanin, J., Lesage, F., Guillemare, E., Fink, M., Lazdunski, M., and Romey, G. (1996). 'K(V)LQT1 and lsK (minK) proteins associate to form the I(Ks) cardiac potassium current'. *Nature* 384, 78–80. doi: 10.1038/384078a0

Bartos, D. C., Anderson, J. B., Bastiaenen, R., Johnson, J. N., Gollob, M. H., Tester, D. J., et al. (2013). 'A KCNQ1 mutation causes a high penetrance for familial atrial fibrillation'. *J. Cardiovasc. Electrophysiol.* 24, 562–569. doi: 10.1111/jce.12068

Bartos, D. C., Duchatelet, S., Burgess, D. E., Klug, D., Denjoy, I., Peat, R., et al. (2011). 'R231C mutation in KCNQ1 causes long QT syndrome type 1 and familial atrial fibrillation'. *Heart Rhythm* 8, 48–55. doi: 10.1016/j.hrthm.2010.09.010

Bazett, H. C. (1920). 'An analysis of the time-relations of electrocardiograms.'. *Heart J. Study Circ.* 7, 353–370.

Bellocq, C., van Ginneken, A. C., Bezzina, C. R., Alders, M., Escande, D., Mannens, M. M., et al. (2004). 'Mutation in the KCNQ1 gene leading to the short QT-interval syndrome'. *Circulation* 109, 2394–2397. doi: 10.1161/01.CIR.0000130409.72142.FE

Britton, O. J., Bueno-Orovio, A., Van Ammel, K., Lu, H. R., Towart, R., Gallacher, D. J., et al. (2013). 'Experimentally calibrated population of models predicts and explains intersubject variability in cardiac cellular electrophysiology'. *Proc. Natl. Acad. Sci. U.S.A.* 110, E2098–E2105. doi: 10.1073/pnas.1304382110

Brunner, M., Peng, X., Liu, G. X., Ren, X. Q., Ziv, O., Choi, B. R., et al. (2008). 'Mechanisms of cardiac arrhythmias and sudden death in transgenic rabbits with long QT syndrome'. *J. Clin. Invest.* 118, 2246–2259. doi: 10.1172/JCI33578

Cardone-Noott, L., Bueno-Orovio, A., Minchole, A., Zemzemi, N., and Rodriguez, B. (2016). 'Human ventricular activation sequence and the simulation of the electrocardiographic QRS complex and its variability in healthy and intraventricular block conditions'. *Europace* 18, iv4–iv15. doi: 10.1093/europace/euw346

Chen, Y. H., Xu, S. J., Bendahhou, S., Wang, X. L., Wang, Y., Xu, W. Y., et al. (2003). 'KCNQ1 gain-of-function mutation in familial atrial fibrillation'. *Science* 299, 251–254. doi: 10.1126/science.1077771

Christ, T., Horvath, A., and Eschenhagen, T. (2015). 'LQT1-phenotypes in hiPSC: are we measuring the right thing?'. *Proc. Natl. Acad. Sci. U.S.A.* 112:E1968. doi: 10.1073/pnas.1503347112

Das, S., Makino, S., Melman, Y. F., Shea, M. A., Goyal, S. B., Rosenzweig, A., et al. (2009). 'Mutation in the S3 segment of KCNQ1 results in familial lone atrial fibrillation'. *Heart Rhythm* 6, 1146–1153. doi: 10.1016/j.hrthm.2009.04.015

Duhme, N., Schweizer, P. A., Thomas, D., Becker, R., Schroter, J., Barends, T. R., et al. (2013). 'Altered HCN4 channel C-linker interaction is associated with familial tachycardia-bradycardia syndrome and atrial fibrillation'. *Eur. Heart J.* 34, 2768–2775. doi: 10.1093/eurheartj/ehs391

Fabbri, A., Fantini, M., Wilders, R., and Severi, S. (2017). 'Computational analysis of the human sinus node action potential: model development and effects of mutations'. *J. Physiol.* 595, 2365–2396. doi: 10.1113/JP273259

Gima, K., and Rudy, Y. (2002). 'Ionic current basis of electrocardiographic waveforms: a model study'. *Circ. Res.* 90, 889–896. doi: 10.1161/01.RES.0000016960.61087.86

Grandi, E., Pandit, S. V., Voigt, N., Workman, A. J., Dobrev, D., Jalife, J., et al. (2011). 'Human atrial action potential and Ca2+ model: sinus rhythm and chronic atrial fibrillation'. *Circ. Res.* 109, 1055–1066. doi: 10.1161/CIRCRESAHA.111.253955

Hancox, J. C., Kharche, S., El Harchi, A., Stott, J., Law, P., and Zhang, H. (2014). 'In silico investigation of a KCNQ1 mutation associated with familial atrial fibrillation'. *J. Electrocardiol.* 47, 158–165. doi: 10.1016/j.jelectrocard.2013.12.004

Harmer, S. C., Mohal, J. S., Royal, A. A., McKenna, W. J., Lambiase, P. D., and Tinker, A. (2014). 'Cellular mechanisms underlying the increased disease severity seen for patients with long QT syndrome caused by compound mutations in KCNQ1'. *Biochem. J.* 462, 133–142. doi: 10.1042/BJ20140425

Hasegawa, K., Ohno, S., Ashihara, T., Itoh, H., Ding, W. G., Toyoda, F., et al. (2014). 'A novel KCNQ1 missense mutation identified in a patient with juvenile-onset atrial fibrillation causes constitutively open IKs channels'. *Heart Rhythm* 11, 67–75. doi: 10.1016/j.hrthm.2013.09.073

Henrion, U., Zumhagen, S., Steinke, K., Strutz-Seebohm, N., Stallmeyer, B., Lang, F., et al. (2012). 'Overlapping cardiac phenotype associated with a familial mutation in the voltage sensor of the KCNQ1 channel'. *Cell Physiol. Biochem.* 29, 809–818. doi: 10.1159/000178470

Hong, K., Piper, D. R., Diaz-Valdecantos, A., Brugada, J., Oliva, A., Burashnikov, E., et al. (2005). 'De novo KCNQ1 mutation responsible for atrial fibrillation and short QT syndrome in utero'. *Cardiovasc. Res.* 68, 433–440. doi: 10.1016/j.cardiores.2005.06.023

Kharche, S., Adeniran, I., Stott, J., Law, P., Boyett, M. R., Hancox, J. C., et al. (2012). 'Pro-arrhythmogenic effects of the S140G KCNQ1 mutation in human atrial fibrillation - insights from modelling'. *J. Physiol.* 590, 4501–4514. doi: 10.1113/jphysiol.2012.229146

Ki, C. S., Jung, C. L., Kim, H. J., Baek, K. H., Park, S. J., On, Y. K., et al. (2014). 'A KCNQ1 mutation causes age-dependant bradycardia and persistent atrial fibrillation'. *Pflug. Arch.* 466, 529–540. doi: 10.1007/s00424-013-1337-6

Lakatta, E. G., Maltsev, V. A., and Vinogradova, T. M. (2010). 'A coupled SYSTEM of intracellular Ca2+ clocks and surface membrane voltage clocks controls the timekeeping mechanism of the heart's pacemaker'. *Circ. Res.* 106, 659–673. doi: 10.1161/CIRCRESAHA.109.206078

Liu, D. W., and Antzelevitch, C. (1995). 'Characteristics of the delayed rectifier current (IKr and IKs) in canine ventricular epicardial, midmyocardial, and endocardial myocytes. a weaker IKs contributes to the longer action potential of the M cell. *Circ. Res.* 76, 351–365. doi: 10.1161/01.RES.76.3.351

Lundby, A., Ravn, L. S., Svendsen, J. H., Olesen, S. P., and Schmitt, N. (2007). 'KCNQ1 mutation Q147R is associated with atrial fibrillation and prolonged QT interval'. *Heart Rhythm* 4, 1532–1541. doi: 10.1016/j.hrthm.2007.07.022

Maleckar, M. M., Greenstein, J. L., Giles, W. R., and Trayanova, N. A. (2009). 'K+ current changes account for the rate dependence of the action potential in the human atrial myocyte'. *Am. J. Physiol. Heart Circ. Physiol.* 297, H1398–H1410. doi: 10.1152/ajpheart.00411.2009

Moreno, C., Oliveras, A., de la Cruz, A., Bartolucci, C., Munoz, C., Salar, E., et al. (2015). 'A new KCNQ1 mutation at the S5 segment that impairs its association with KCNE1 is responsible for short QT syndrome'. *Cardiovasc. Res.* 107, 613–623. doi: 10.1093/cvr/cvv196

Moreton, N., Venetucci, L., Garratt, C. J., Newman, W., and Metcalfe, K. (2013). *'Atrial Fibrillation, Long QT Syndrome and Sudden Cardiac Death Found in an Extended Family With KCNQ1 C.686G > A (P.G229D).* Available at: http://www.genomicmedicine.org/wp-content/uploads/2014/01/Cardiovascular-Genetics-Symposium-Abstracts.pdf

Muszkiewicz, A., Britton, O. J., Gemmell, P., Passini, E., Sanchez, C., Zhou, X., et al. (2016). 'Variability in cardiac electrophysiology: using experimentally-calibrated populations of models to move beyond the single virtual physiological human paradigm'. *Prog. Biophys. Mol. Biol.* 120, 115–127. doi: 10.1016/j.pbiomolbio.2015.12.002

Muszkiewicz, A., Liu, X., Bueno-Orovio, A., Lawson, B. A. J., Burrage, K., Casadei, B., et al. (2018). 'From ionic to cellular variability in human atrial myocytes: an integrative computational and experimental study. *Am. J. Physiol. Heart Circ. Physiol.* 314, H895–H916. doi: 10.1152/ajpheart.00477.2017

Nerbonne, J. M. (2014). 'Mouse models of arrhythmogenic cardiovascular disease: challenges and opportunities'. *Curr. Opin. Pharmacol.* 15, 107–114. doi: 10.1016/j.coph.2014.02.003

O'Hara, T., Virag, L., Varro, A., and Rudy, Y. (2011). 'Simulation of the undiseased human cardiac ventricular action potential: model formulation and experimental validation'. *PLoS Comput. Biol.* 7:e1002061. doi: 10.1371/journal.pcbi.1002061

Passini, E., Minchole, A., Coppini, R., Cerbai, E., Rodriguez, B., Severi, S., et al. (2016). 'Mechanisms of pro-arrhythmic abnormalities in ventricular repolarisation and anti-arrhythmic therapies in human hypertrophic cardiomyopathy'. *J. Mol. Cell Cardiol.* 96, 72–81. doi: 10.1016/j.yjmcc.2015.09.003

Pitt-Francis, J., Pathmanathan, P., Bernabeu, M. O., Bordas, R., Cooper, J., Fletcher, A. G., et al. (2009). 'Chaste: a test-driven approach to software development for biological modelling'. *Comp. Phys. Commun.* 180, 2452–2471. doi: 10.1016/j.cpc.2009.07.019

Sanchez, C., Bueno-Orovio, A., Wettwer, E., Loose, S., Simon, J., Ravens, U., et al. (2014). 'Inter-subject variability in human atrial action potential in sinus rhythm versus chronic atrial fibrillation. *PLoS One* 9:e105897. doi: 10.1371/journal.pone.0105897

Sanguinetti, M. C., Curran, M. E., Zou, A., Shen, J., Spector, P. S., Atkinson, D. L., et al. (1996). 'Coassembly of K(V)LQT1 and minK (IsK) proteins to form cardiac I(Ks) potassium channel'. *Nature* 384, 80–83. doi: 10.1038/384080a0

Schwartz, P. J., Priori, S. G., Spazzolini, C., Moss, A. J., Vincent, G. M., Napolitano, C., et al. (2001). 'Genotype-phenotype correlation in the long-QT syndrome: gene-specific triggers for life-threatening arrhythmias'. *Circulation* 103, 89–95. doi: 10.1161/01.CIR.103.1.89

Thomas, A. M., Harmer, S. C., Khambra, T., and Tinker, A. (2011). 'Characterization of a binding site for anionic phospholipids on KCNQ1'. *J. Biol. Chem.* 286, 2088–2100. doi: 10.1074/jbc.M110.153551

Viswanathan, P. C., Shaw, R. M., and Rudy, Y. (1999). 'Effects of IKr and IKs heterogeneity on action potential duration and its rate dependence: a simulation study'. *Circulation* 99, 2466–2474. doi: 10.1161/01.CIR.99.18.2466

Wang, Q., Curran, M. E., Splawski, I., Burn, T. C., Millholland, J. M., VanRaay, T. J., et al. (1996). 'Positional cloning of a novel potassium channel gene: KVLQT1 mutations cause cardiac arrhythmias'. *Nat. Genet.* 12, 17–23. doi: 10.1038/ng0196-17

Whittaker, D. G., Colman, M. A., Ni, H., Hancox, J. C., and Zhang, H. (2018). 'Human atrial arrhythmogenesis and sinus bradycardia in KCNQ1-linked short QT syndrome: insights from computational modelling'. *Front. Physiol.* 9:1402. doi: 10.3389/fphys.2018.01402

Wu, Z. J., Huang, Y., Fu, Y. C., Zhao, X. J., Zhu, C., Zhang, Y., et al. (2015). 'Characterization of a chinese KCNQ1 mutation (R259H) that shortens repolarization and causes short QT syndrome 2'. *J. Geriatr. Cardiol.* 12, 394–401. doi: 10.11909/j.issn.1671-5411.2015.04.002

Zhou, X., Bueno-Orovio, A., Orini, M., Hanson, B., Hayward, M., Taggart, P., et al. (2016). 'In vivo and in silico investigation into mechanisms of frequency dependence of repolarization alternans in human ventricular cardiomyocytes'. *Circ. Res.* 118, 266–278. doi: 10.1161/CIRCRESAHA.115.307836

Zulfa, I., Shim, E. B., Song, K. S., and Lim, K. M. (2016). 'Computational simulations of the effects of the G229D KCNQ1 mutation on human atrial fibrillation'. *J. Physiol. Sci.* 66, 407–415. doi: 10.1007/s12576-016-0438-3

11

A Heart for Diversity: Simulating Variability in Cardiac Arrhythmia Research

*Haibo Ni, Stefano Morotti and Eleonora Grandi**

Department of Pharmacology, University of California, Davis, Davis, CA, United States

***Correspondence:**
Eleonora Grandi
ele.grandi@gmail.com

In cardiac electrophysiology, there exist many sources of inter- and intra-personal variability. These include variability in conditions and environment, and genotypic and molecular diversity, including differences in expression and behavior of ion channels and transporters, which lead to phenotypic diversity (e.g., variable integrated responses at the cell, tissue, and organ levels). These variabilities play an important role in progression of heart disease and arrhythmia syndromes and outcomes of therapeutic interventions. Yet, the traditional *in silico* framework for investigating cardiac arrhythmias is built upon a parameter/property-averaging approach that typically overlooks the physiological diversity. Inspired by work done in genetics and neuroscience, new modeling frameworks of cardiac electrophysiology have been recently developed that take advantage of modern computational capabilities and approaches, and account for the variance in the biological data they are intended to illuminate. In this review, we outline the recent advances in statistical and computational techniques that take into account physiological variability, and move beyond the traditional cardiac model-building scheme that involves averaging over samples from many individuals in the construction of a highly tuned composite model. We discuss how these advanced methods have harnessed the power of big (simulated) data to study the mechanisms of cardiac arrhythmias, with a special emphasis on atrial fibrillation, and improve the assessment of proarrhythmic risk and drug response. The challenges of using *in silico* approaches with variability are also addressed and future directions are proposed.

Keywords: cardiac electrophysiology, physiological variability, computational modeling, arrhythmia mechanisms, big data

INTRODUCTION

Beginning with the seminal paper by Hodgkin and Huxley, 1952, mathematical models of electrophysiology have proven to be valuable tools for better understanding many physiological processes, especially in cardiac arrhythmia research (Noble et al., 2012; Dibb et al., 2015). Fifty-six years after publication of the first cardiac model (Noble, 1962), there is currently a computational model for almost every cell type of the heart, including nodal, atrial, ventricular, and Purkinje cells (Beeler and Reuter, 1977; Difrancesco and Noble, 1985; Luo and Rudy, 1991; Inada et al., 2009; Maltsev and Lakatta, 2009; Sampson et al., 2010; Grandi et al., 2011; O'Hara et al., 2011), for numerous species, and for various levels of complexity across multiple spatial scales (e.g., inclusion of disease-associated remodeling, drug action, contractile, energetics, and signaling modules) (Fink et al., 2011). Most of these models use average data from voltage-clamp experiments of individual ionic membrane currents, and while they have led to many important advances in studies of cardiac electrophysiology and pathology, especially cardiac arrhythmias (Sepulveda et al., 1989; Courtemanche and Winfree, 1991; Panfilov and Holden, 1991; Gray et al., 1995; Krogh-Madsen and Christini, 2012; Roberts et al., 2012; Bueno-Orovio et al., 2014), they typically represent the average behavior of a particular cell type. Because these models ignore evident inter- and intra-personal variability, they can fail to capture the properties of any given individual cell or cells in a given patient (Golowasch et al., 2002; Dokos and Lovell, 2004; Sarkar and Sobie, 2010; Marder, 2011; Zaniboni, 2011; Groenendaal et al., 2015; Pathmanathan et al., 2015). This is in part because incorporating variance that reflects biological data into cardiac models requires significant computational capacity, particularly as compared to what was available when mathematical modeling of electrophysiology first emerged. Given ever-increasing computational capabilities, new modeling approaches have been developed to reproduce and analyze the immense physiological diversity observed in electrophysiology.

In this review, we discuss the importance of accounting for variability when building models of cardiac electrophysiology in both physiological and diseased conditions, and describe new tools being developed to address the limitations of traditional modeling approaches. In particular, we focus on two computational approaches that have emerged as leading methodologies for studying variability in cardiac electrophysiology, which we will refer to as (1) population-based modeling and (2) sample-specific modeling. Both methodologies have provided valuable insights in the fields of neuroscience, cardiology, and pharmacology. Here we review how they have advanced our understanding of the basic mechanisms of cardiac arrhythmias, and particularly atrial fibrillation (AF). As these *in silico* approaches have led to important insights into arrhythmia risks, mechanisms of arrhythmogenesis, and variable response to drugs, they should be considered when determining the regulatory requirements for the proarrhythmia assessment and drug efficacy and safety evaluation of candidate compounds.

Abbreviations: AF, atrial fibrillation; AP, action potential; APD, AP duration; cAF, chronic AF; CaT, Ca^{2+} transient; CiPA, Comprehensive *in vitro* Proarrhythmia Assay; DAD, delayed afterdepolarization; diLQTS, drug-induced long QT syndrome; EAD, early afterdepolarization; ECG, electrocardiogram; FRD, forward rate dependence; GA, genetic algorithm; hERG, human *ether-à-go-go*-related gene; hMSCs, human mesenchymal stem cells; I_{CaL}, L-type Ca^{2+} current; I_{to}, transient outward K^+ current; I_{Kur}, ultra-rapid delayed-rectifier K^+ current; I_{Kr}, rapid delayed-rectifier K^+ current; I_{Ks}, slow delayed-rectifier K^+ current; I_{K1}, inward rectifier K^+ current; I_{Na}, fast Na^+ current; I_{NaL}, late Na^+ current; iPSC-CM, induced pluripotent stem-cell-derived cardiomyocyte; LHS, latin hypercube sampling; LQT3, long QT syndrome type 3; NCX, Na^+/Ca^{2+} exchanger; nSR, normal sinus rhythm; SERCA, sarco/endoplasmic reticulum Ca^{2+}-ATPase; TdP, torsades de pointes.

IMPORTANCE OF TAKING INTO ACCOUNT VARIABILITY IN CARDIAC ELECTROPHYSIOLOGY

Sources of variability in cardiac electrophysiology encompass multiple spatial and temporal scales, and include inter-species (Sham et al., 1995; Su et al., 2003), inter-ethnic (Lau et al., 2012; Fender et al., 2014), inter-subject (Taneja et al., 2001; Batchvarov et al., 2002), regional (Feng et al., 1998; Yan et al., 1998), and temporal (Jeyaraj et al., 2012) differences. Variability in experimental electrophysiological data does not only represent natural physiological diversity, but also reflects, in part, differences in the experimental conditions in which electrophysiological measurements are performed (Groenendaal et al., 2015). These conditions can vary from laboratory to laboratory (Niederer et al., 2009; Fink et al., 2011), experiment to experiment, or during the same experiment, e.g., due to deterioration of the experimental preparations over time (Fink et al., 2011). There is also instrument noise (Mirams et al., 2016), artifacts, and use of non-physiological temperatures and solutions (Groenendaal et al., 2015), all of which impact the structure and function of the cellular or tissue components being studied. These sources of variation are difficult to control even for experienced electrophysiologists and are equally as challenging to account for by modelers.

Mathematical cardiomyocyte models have remained useful tools for unraveling physiological and pathophysiological mechanisms, including mechanisms of arrhythmia, and identifying antiarrhythmic strategies without accounting for variability (Sepulveda et al., 1989; Courtemanche and Winfree, 1991; Clancy and Rudy, 1999, 2002; Clancy et al., 2002; Rivolta et al., 2002; Gong et al., 2007; Noble et al., 2007; Tsujimae et al., 2007; Zhang et al., 2007; Zhu and Clancy, 2007; Campbell et al., 2008; Comtois et al., 2008; Kharche et al., 2008; Sale et al., 2008; Ahrens-Nicklas et al., 2009; Butters et al., 2010; Adeniran et al., 2012; Edwards et al., 2014; Grandi and Maleckar, 2016; Morotti et al., 2016; Ni et al., 2017). Although average models have also been successfully applied to the study of sources of variability, such as sexual and hormonal factors (Yang et al., 2010, 2017; Yang and Clancy, 2012), age (Behar and Yaniv, 2017), and circadian regulation (Fotiadis and Forger, 2013), the rationale for developing novel computational approaches that specifically account for electrophysiological variability can be summarized by two main reasons.

Average Data May Not Accurately Represent Any Specific Individual or Behavior Well

The traditional cardiac model-building scheme involves averaging over samples from multiple experiments from many individuals, both to parameterize the model and validate it, which may not represent any specific measured physiological behavior very well. This "failure of averaging" has been demonstrated in many fields, most recently in neuroscience (Golowasch et al., 2002; Marder, 2011), and was particularly well-documented in 1952, the same year that the seminal Hodgkin and Huxley paper was published, when Lt. Gilbert S. Daniels of the U.S. Air Force published a Technical Note that highlighted the fundamental problem with fitting data to the mean (Daniels, 1952; Rose, 2017). Using data from 4,063 pilots, Lt. Daniels calculated the average of 10 physical dimensions believed to be most relevant for design of the cockpit on a plane, including a pilot's height, chest circumference, and sleeve length. Surprisingly, he found that a total of zero individuals fit within the middle 30% of the range of values for each dimension, and less than 3.5% of pilots would be average sized on any three dimensions. After this finding, the U.S. Air Force completely moved from standardizing all dimensions to an "average pilot," to making all the dimensions adjustable to each individual pilot, which immediately and drastically improved performance and was soon adopted by all branches of the American military. Modeling of electrophysiology is undergoing a similar evolution, which will likely improve the translational significance of the models.

Variability Has Implications on Genesis and Treatment of Arrhythmia

Variability plays an important role in arrhythmia generation and treatment, as exemplified by AF. The atria are characterized by a high degree of phenotypic variability in physiological properties, with broad and diverging distributions of biomarkers in patients in normal sinus rhythm (nSR) or chronic AF (cAF, **Figure 1A**) (Ravens et al., 2015), likely due to innate variability of the ionic currents (perhaps due to stochastic gating) that can affect whole cell and/or tissue proarrhythmic behavior (Pueyo et al., 2011; Heijman et al., 2013). This phenotypic variability can be captured by adding variability in the conductance parameters of a mathematical model of the action potential (AP, **Figures 1B,C**). In some circumstances, physiological variability itself can be the substrate for arrhythmia. For example, increased heterogeneity of refractoriness is important for the maintenance of AF (Moe et al., 1964; Boutjdir et al., 1986; Misier et al., 1992; Sato et al., 1992; Wang et al., 1995, 1996; Gaspo et al., 1997; Liu and Nattel, 1997; Ramirez et al., 2000), and regional differences in atrial ionic currents play a significant role in atrial arrhythmia initiation (Feng et al., 1998; Gaborit et al., 2007; Colman et al., 2013). Consequently, pharmacotherapy that increases dispersion of refractoriness is an adverse side effect of drugs for the treatment of AF (Ramanna et al., 2001; Soylu et al., 2003).

It is well-known that individuals may present largely different responses to same pharmacological interventions. As an example, it has been shown that drugs that block the hERG (human *ether-à-go-go*-related gene) channel are generally responsible for drug-induced long QT syndrome (diLQTS), but in a population this adverse response is highly variable, from minimum changes in the electrocardiogram (ECG) to induction of lethal ventricular arrhythmias (Singh et al., 2000; Kannankeril et al., 2011). Accounting for physiological variability may help better understand why some individuals display adverse side effects, while others do not. Given the different etiologies of many cardiac arrhythmias, such as AF, computational approaches that take into account variability may help us identify subpopulations in which a particular antiarrhythmic therapy will be effective and safe, or toxic. Furthermore, when assessing the efficacy and safety of a drug administration for heart conditions, it is important to take into account physiological and pathological variabilities to make sure that results are quantified and valid at the population level. Such approaches will potentially be more clinically useful in simulating the effects of drugs and aiding the design of safer and more effective therapies (Britton et al., 2013, 2017a; Passini et al., 2016; Yang et al., 2016).

APPROACHES AND INSIGHT ON THE IMPACT OF VARIABILITY ON CARDIAC ELECTROPHYSIOLOGY

Although many methods have been developed, two families of approaches have emerged as leading methodologies to account for variability in cardiac electrophysiology: (1) population-based and (2) sample-specific modeling (**Figure 2**). Both methods generally start with the building or use of a baseline cardiac cell model, which has been parameterized and validated to average data. Population-based approaches generate model variants of the baseline model that fit given experimental distributions of electrophysiological outcomes or biomarkers, while sample-specific modeling approaches re-parameterize the baseline model based on cell- or patient-specific datasets (**Figure 2**). Because their implementation requires computational power, the advancements in computing capabilities and techniques (Pitt-Francis et al., 2006; Abramson et al., 2010), especially in parallel computing (Wang et al., 2011), have helped these methods gain traction in the last decade.

Population-Based Modeling

Population-based modeling approaches have been developed and employed to obtain results at the population level, which led to many novel insights into physiological and pathophysiological variabilities, and variable responses to drug administration. We refer the readers to a recent review from the Rodriguez group (Muszkiewicz et al., 2016), where this methodology is described in detail. Here, we briefly describe the general approach of population-based modeling, and summarize how it has contributed to advancing the field as exemplified by some important studies.

Creating Populations of AP Models

Populations of models are generally created by modifying sets of parameters in a baseline model (**Figure 2**). This process involves determination of the parameters to be varied, over what range, and a sampling method to select the parameter values. Frequently, maximal conductances or maximum transport rates of ion channels, pumps and transporters in AP models are selected to vary. The parameter space over which these model parameters vary can be chosen either to reflect the experimental range, when available, or theoretical upper and lower bounds. Then, populations of parameter sets are created by sampling the parameters within the predefined parameter spaces. Typically, four types of sampling methods have been applied to obtain the populations of parameter sets: uniform-interval sampling

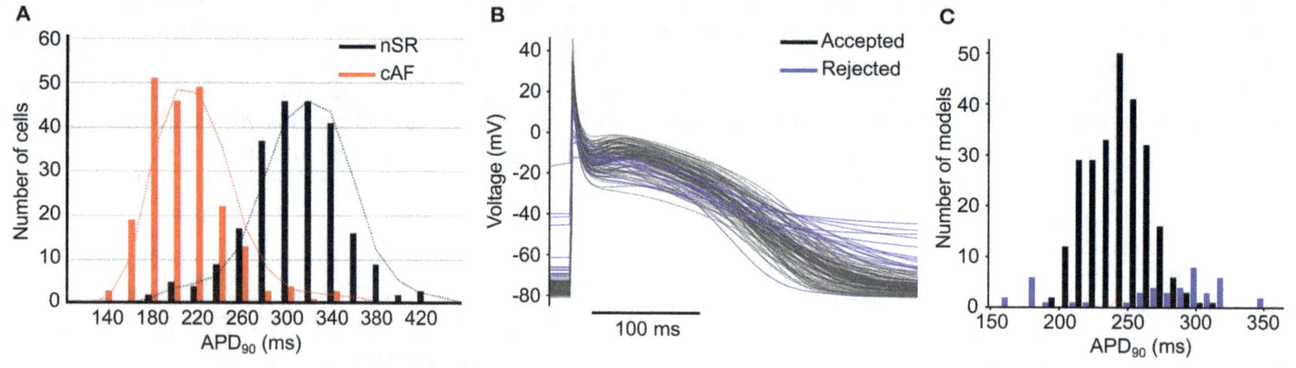

FIGURE 1 | Variability in cardiac electrophysiology. **(A)** Histograms of AP duration at 90% repolarization (APD_{90}) for patients in nSR (*black*) and cAF (*red*) show substantial variability. Reproduced from Ravens et al. (2015) with permission. **(B)** Example of APs and **(C)** histogram of APD_{90} produced using models incorporating variability in conductances of ionic currents; some models (*in blue*) are rejected due to non-physiological behaviors.

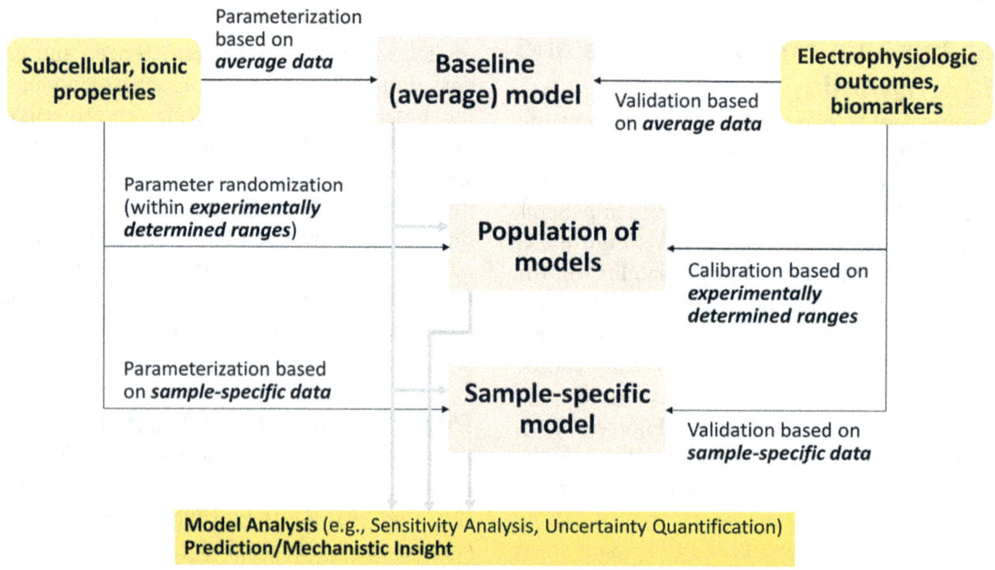

FIGURE 2 | Flowchart connecting traditional cardiac modeling approach to the new methodologies that account for variability.

(Romero et al., 2009, 2011; Corrias et al., 2011), log-normal sampling (Sobie, 2009; Sadrieh et al., 2013; Ellinwood et al., 2017a; Morotti and Grandi, 2017), Latin hypercube sampling (LHS) (Britton et al., 2013) and its variants such as orthogonal sampling (Burrage et al., 2015; Donovan et al., 2018), and sequential Monte Carlo sampling (Muszkiewicz et al., 2017).

After generating hundreds or thousands of model variants, calibration can be performed to exclude models that display non-physiological behaviors (**Figure 2**). This can be done, for example, by removing models showing repolarization failure (Sobie, 2009), or exhibiting AP duration (APD) more than three standard deviations from the population mean (Devenyi and Sobie, 2016). Population of models are also calibrated to measured data from patient samples, whereby model variants are selected based on simulated electrophysiological properties, such as APD, upstroke velocity, resting membrane potential and/or Ca^{2+} transient (CaT) (Britton et al., 2013, 2017a; Sanchez et al., 2014; Passini et al., 2016; Rees et al., 2018). Other studies use additional information such as ionic current data (Muszkiewicz et al., 2017), or ECG data (Mann et al., 2016). This calibration step is meant to ensure that (1) variants displaying non-physiological properties are discarded before analysis, and (2) the simulated electrophysiological properties of models in a given population are in the same range as experimental data, or, more recently, correspond to the same distribution of observed experimental biomarkers (Lawson et al., 2018), thus possibly making inferences from *in silico* experiments more physiologically relevant.

Analyzing Populations of AP Models

Once a population of cardiac AP models is generated, and electrophysiological simulations have been performed corresponding to the scientific question at hand, mechanistic insights can be obtained using various analysis techniques. These analyses have contributed to our understanding of the relative role of the underlying parameters in modulating the physiological properties of interest (i.e., sensitivity analysis), or revealing association of certain parameter ranges or properties with specific physiological behaviors (e.g., repolarization abnormalities, ectopic activity, drug response). Many relevant examples have recently been reviewed (Muszkiewicz et al., 2016). Here we highlight new recent developments and discuss details of parameter sensitivity analysis.

Performing parameter sensitivity analysis

A common systematic analysis of populations of models is sensitivity analysis. It assesses how model outputs, which typically represent whole cell behavior (e.g., APD), are sensitive to changes in model parameters, (e.g., conductances and maximum transport rates). Because many parameters are often varied to generate the populations of models, multivariable linear regression (Hair et al., 2010; Draper and Smith, 2014) has emerged as a frequently utilized tool to perform sensitivity analysis in cardiac electrophysiology. Moreover, as the number of independent parameters varied is used to predict a smaller set of dependent variables, sensitivity analysis is typically performed using partial least squares regression (Geladi and Kowalski, 1986; Sobie, 2009), as compared to standard multivariable regression. The result of linear regression is a set of coefficients (forming a "regression model") describing how perturbing a particular parameter influences an output of interest. This method has been successfully utilized in other fields such as molecular biology (Janes et al., 2005) and neuroscience (Weaver and Wearne, 2008), and was first used in cardiac electrophysiology by Sobie (2009), who applied it to study sensitivities of properties such as APD and pacing rate threshold for inducing AP alternans. Since the regression model represents a linear approximation of a highly non-linear system, it is important to always check the goodness of fit. Several papers by the Sobie's group have indeed shown that the linear approximation actually provides a very good fit of the AP biomarkers, which was not trivially predictable (Sarkar et al., 2012).

The approach of varying multiple ionic conductances at once in a systematic fashion (as opposed to one at a time) and employing sensitivity analysis using multivariable regression has led to many important insights in cardiac electrophysiology (Sarkar and Sobie, 2011; Mann et al., 2012; Heijman et al., 2013; Walmsley et al., 2013), some of which have been confirmed experimentally (Lee et al., 2013; Devenyi and Sobie, 2016; Devenyi et al., 2017). For example, it has been used to study how different diseased conditions affect the sensitivities of given electrophysiological properties (Sadrieh et al., 2013; Ellinwood et al., 2017a; Vagos et al., 2017; Koivumaki et al., 2018), mechanisms of physiological phenomena (Lee et al., 2013), and for constraining free parameters (Sarkar and Sobie, 2010). Through sensitivity analysis, Cummins et al. identified multiple potential ionic targets mediating forward rate dependence (FRD) of AP, and demonstrated that modulation of the inward rectifier K^+ current (I_{K1}) or the Na^+/K^+ pump current was more likely to produce FRD (Cummins et al., 2014). Devenyi and Sobie performed sensitivity analysis of rat ventricular myocyte models, and quantitatively compared the modulatory role of transient outward K^+ current (I_{to}) and sarco/endoplasmic reticulum Ca^{2+}-ATPase (SERCA) in CaT amplitude. They found that in rat epicardial cells I_{to} plays a more important role than SERCA in regulating CaT amplitude, and this was analogous to human atrial cells, where both I_{to} and ultra-rapid delayed-rectifier K^+ current (I_{Kur}) had greater impacts on CaT amplitude than did SERCA (Devenyi and Sobie, 2016). These studies highlight how sensitivity analysis can be applied to compare and contrast roles of different ionic processes and Ca^{2+} handling in regulating physiological properties and behaviors between cell types and species. Sensitivity analysis has also been used to compare the dependence of AP biomarkers on ionic processes in healthy and diseased conditions. For example, Lee et al. compared the impact of ionic processes on APD in control and AF-remodeled cells and found that the Na^+/Ca^{2+} exchanger (NCX) current has little influence on APD in control cells but more markedly impacts AF cells; the analysis also revealed that I_{K1} upregulation plays a dominant role in APD shortening in AF, and that the L-type Ca^{2+} current (I_{CaL}) significantly contributes to rate-dependent APD changes in both control and AF myocytes (Lee Y. S. et al., 2016). Most recently, Gong and Sobie described a novel use of regression models, cross-cell regression, to predict adult myocyte drug responses from induced pluripotent stem-cell-derived cardiomyocytes (iPSC-CMs) behaviors (Gong and Sobie, 2018).

Multivariable linear regression is used if the physiological output of interest is continuous, but, for the study of arrhythmia mechanisms, another particularly useful and efficient regression technique is logistic regression, which is used when the outcome of interest is Boolean (i.e., yes/no, true/false). Applying logistic regression in studies of physiology is well-described by Lee et al. who examined Ca^{2+} spark triggering (an all-or-none event), and demonstrated the accuracy of logistic regression using receiver operator characteristic curves (Lee et al., 2013). This method has since been used to study the probability that a certain arrhythmic event such as early afterdepolarizations (EADs) will occur and suggest underlying factors (Morotti and Grandi, 2017).

The main limitation of regression (both linear and logistic) analysis is that it only highlights how inputs are correlated to outputs, so the conclusions drawn from the analysis can be misleading if only a few outputs are considered. For example, it has been shown that completely different parameter combinations could produce essentially identical AP shapes but substantially different CaT amplitudes (**Figure 3**) (Sarkar and Sobie, 2010). However, sensitivity analysis can still help determine whether the relationships between inputs and outputs in computational models match experimental findings and assumptions, and whether there are particularly influential parameters that can be exploited therapeutically or targeted to better understand a given physiological phenomena (e.g., arrhythmia mechanism).

Comparing subpopulations of models

Comparing subgroups in a population of models (often using statistical difference tests of parameters of interest) can help identify underlying determinants of different phenotypes, behaviors, and pathological conditions (Sanchez et al., 2014;

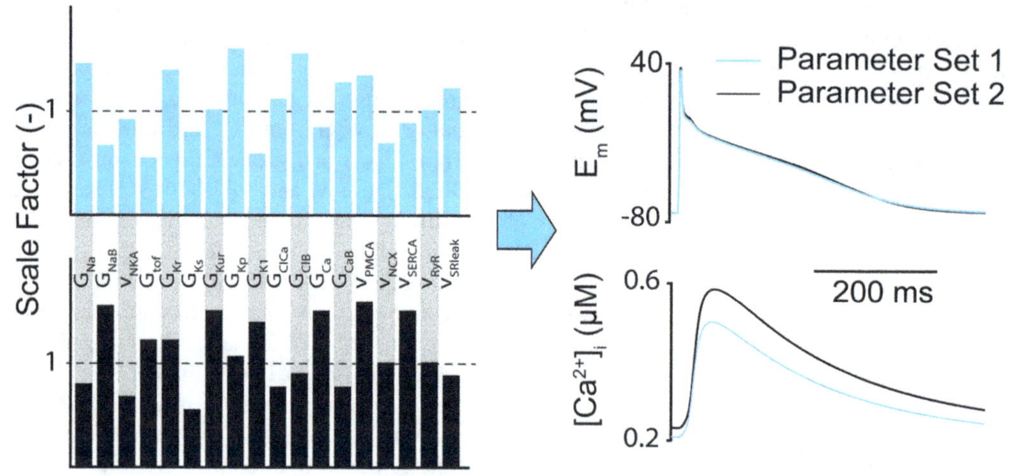

FIGURE 3 | Different subcellular parameter combinations can lead to same AP shape. Example of how different model parameter combinations (e.g., ion channel conductances and maximum transport rates) can produce nearly identical atrial AP morphologies, but notably different CaTs.

Zhou et al., 2016; Britton et al., 2017b; Muszkiewicz et al., 2017; Vagos et al., 2017; Lawson et al., 2018). For example, through characterizing ionic parameters of models that are prone to repolarization abnormalities, Britton et al. found that the electrogenic Na^+/K^+ pump is a key determinant of susceptibility to repolarization abnormalities in human ventricular cardiomyocytes by applying arrhythmia-provoking conditions to a population of experimentally-calibrated cardiac cells (Britton et al., 2017b). A population-based approach has also been used to tease out the ionic mechanisms underlying variability in iPSC-CMs (Paci et al., 2017). By calibrating generated subpopulations of human atrial myocyte models to ranges of experimental data from a large number of patients with nSR or cAF, Sanchez et al. characterized potential ionic determinants of inter-subject variability in AP biomarkers, and identified similar changes in I_{K1}, I_{Kur}, and I_{to} in cAF vs. nSR subpopulations that were consistent with experimentally reported AF-induced remodeling effects (Sanchez et al., 2014). In a more recent study, instead of calibrating population of models to the range of experimental dataset, Lawson et al. proposed a novel method to calibrate these models to the distributions of multiple experimentally measured biomarkers (Lawson et al., 2018), which led to an improved characterization of ionic differences between nSR and cAF. These studies focused on AP biomarkers at a fixed pacing rate. In a different study, Vagos et al. expanded the use of population of models to compare the steady state and dynamic restitution behaviors of AP in nSR and cAF populations (Vagos et al., 2017). By combining population-based modeling and experiments, Muszkiewicz et al. characterized variability in AP and ionic densities and their impact on CaT in atrial cells from right atrial appendage of patients exhibiting nSR (Muszkiewicz et al., 2017). In addition to calibrating model outputs to measured AP biomarkers, they also extended the experimental calibration of population of human atrial models to model parameter (inputs) by using experimental data of major ionic currents.

Quantifying drug modulatory effects, understanding variability in drug response, and identifying phenotype-specific therapy

By using a population of models that incorporate variabilities, drug modulatory effects on electrophysiological properties can be interpreted at a whole population level, which also contributes to limiting potential model-dependent results. For example, Yang et al. used a population-based approach to simulate effects of late Na^+ current (I_{NaL}) and hERG block and found that the selective I_{NaL} blocker GS-458967 could suppress proarrhythmic markers after hERG block in ventricular myocytes (Yang et al., 2016). Population-based modeling has also allowed for more rigorous quantitative comparison of modulatory effects between multiple drugs. A recent study by Britton et al. calibrated populations of ventricular models to specific individuals using data from human trabeculae (Britton et al., 2017a). They then assessed the effects of four different (selective and non-selective) blockers of the rapid delayed-rectifier K^+ current (I_{Kr}), dofetilide, sotalol, quinidine, and verapamil, to quantitatively compare changes in AP biomarkers, and demonstrated good agreement with experiments for the selective I_{Kr} blockers (dofetilide and sotalol) but not for the non-selective I_{Kr} inhibitors (quinidine and verapamil). Paci et al. utilized populations of *in silico* iPSC-CMs to evaluate antiarrhythmic effects of mexiletine and ranolazine to treat iPSC-CM long QT syndrome type 3 (LQT3) mutants and demonstrated that mexilitine stops spontaneous APs in more LQT3 models than ranolazine due to its stronger effects on the fast Na^+ current (I_{Na}) (Paci et al., 2017). In contrast to the traditional modeling approach using a single model, the population-based modeling can gain insights into the physiologically relevant variability of predictions made *in silico*, as demonstrated in these studies.

By taking a step further, simulations using populations of models incorporating variabilities can also help recognize the contributing factors underlying the variability observed in response to drugs. One relevant example is the variable outcomes of hERG inhibition, which is frequently linked with diLQTS. Population-based modeling has offered insights into the mechanisms underlying the fact that individuals will not exhibit the same degree of QT interval prolongation after hERG block (Singh et al., 2000; Kannankeril et al., 2011; Weeke et al., 2014). Employing a population of models of ventricular myocytes, Sobie and Sarkar attributed the variable outcomes to the different ionic properties of the cells (Sarkar and Sobie, 2011). In another interesting application, Passini et al. implemented an *in silico* drug trial using experimentally-calibrated populations of AP models to investigate the risk of drug-induced arrhythmias, and to identify specific subpopulations at higher risk for proarrhythmic cardiotoxicity (Passini et al., 2017). Their methodology not only demonstrated higher accuracy than animal models in predicting arrhythmia risk, but also provided mechanistic insight into the underlying ionic contributors to repolarization/depolarization abnormalities.

Understanding the bases of variability in electrophysiological behavior and arrhythmia proclivity may also allow developing specific antiarrhythmic therapies for different disease phenotypes. For example, Liberos et al. compared AF models that had self-sustained vs. self-terminating reentries (Liberos et al., 2016). They found that AF maintenance was correlated with high I_{CaL} and I_{Na}, and that I_{CaL} block could be an effective treatment depending on the basal availability of Na^+ and Ca^{2+} ion channel conductivities (I_{Na} depression increased efficacy). Mayourian et al. employed a comprehensive integrated approach to study the mechanisms of cardiac contractility and arrhythmogenicity using experimentally-calibrated human mesenchymal stem cells (hMSCs) (Mayourian et al., 2017). In simulations testing proarrhythmic effects, they found that hMSCs paracrine signaling protected such adverse effects of heterocellular coupling at various levels of engraftment. This work highlights that antiarrhythmic strategies can move beyond simply considering repolarization abnormalities.

Sample-Specific Modeling

Instead of taking a baseline cardiac model and introducing variability by randomly varying the ionic conductances, optimization and statistical techniques can also be used to tailor the baseline model to describe a specific experimental sample. Depending on the characteristics of the dataset at hand, sample-specific models can be representative of either individual myocytes or a particular group of cells. The former approach, cell-specific modeling, can be helpful when integrating mathematical modeling into an experimental setup. For example, Ravagli et al. characterized the role of the "funny" current I_f in sinoatrial myocytes using the dynamic clamp technique by adapting the extent of injected I_f in a cell-specific fashion, i.e., based on the basal firing rate measured in each individual cell (Ravagli et al., 2016). Despite the use of average data, sample-specific models built from a group of cells (e.g., a cell line developed in a certain laboratory, myocytes isolated from disease models, iPSC-CMs derived from a single patient) can allow for specific characterization of conditions that are far from the average, or even of personalized physiology (Barichello et al., 2018). For example, monophasic AP data recorded in AF patients undergoing ablation procedures have been used to construct atrial cell models that capture patient-specific electrophysiological properties (Lombardo et al., 2016). This approach has the promise of making patient-specific predictions given interventions such as arrhythmia-provoking protocols or drug application. Here we summarize methodologies for building and improving sample-specific cell models. For more detail, we refer the readers to a previous review on the topic (Krogh-Madsen et al., 2016).

Fitting Sample-Specific Models

Sample-specific models can be constructed by fitting the parameters of a baseline model so that the model outputs match the corresponding physiological behaviors seen in a single patient or myocyte (**Figure 2**). Cardiac electrophysiology models can be optimized using many different fitness functions (Druckmann et al., 2007; Tomaiuolo et al., 2012), such as global search heuristics (Vanier and Bower, 1999; Dokos and Lovell, 2004; Bueno-Orovio et al., 2008; Guo et al., 2010). Recently, many sample-specific models are generated using the genetic algorithm (GA), which traces its beginnings to evolutionary biology (Fraser and Burnell, 1970; Crosby, 1982), but is still being applied in new ways today (Chen and Guan, 2004; Hussein and El-Ghazaly, 2004; Leung et al., 2004; Vieira et al., 2004). Its use for optimization of ionic models is relatively new in both neuroscience (Achard and De Schutter, 2006; Gurkiewicz and Korngreen, 2007; Hobbs and Hooper, 2008; Ben-Shalom et al., 2012) and cardiac electrophysiology (Syed et al., 2005; Bot et al., 2012; Kaur et al., 2014; Groenendaal et al., 2015). Syed et al. demonstrated its feasibility for atrial cell models when they proved they could fit two different cell models (Courtemanche et al., 1998; Nygren et al., 1998) to any given atrial AP (Syed et al., 2005). Essentially, the GA optimization procedure is initialized in the same way as for the population-based approach (varying maximal conductance and/or transport rates), and then it iteratively evolves toward better solutions in generations, while the underlying parameters can be varied, swapped, or discarded. Sensitivity analysis can be used in conjunction with generating sample-specific models as it can inform the design of the error function (i.e., weights) by revealing the conductances that more significantly impact the electrophysiological outputs used for fitting. For example, Krogh-Madsen et al. recently combined sensitivity analysis and global optimization (using a GA) of a ventricular myocyte model to clinical long QT data and intracellular Ca^{2+} and Na^+ concentrations, to better constrain the model parameters (Krogh-Madsen et al., 2017). They found that this improved prediction of drug-induced *torsades de pointes* (TdP), especially in eliminating false-positive outcomes generated by the baseline model parameters.

Improving Fidelity of Sample-Specific Models

The final solution of an optimization procedure using some fitness function may not match experimental data well if only fitting to a single electrophysiological output such as a single AP, because multiple parameter combinations can potentially produce the same AP (**Figure 3**) (Syed et al., 2005; Druckmann et al., 2007; Sarkar and Sobie, 2010; Guo et al., 2013; Kaur et al., 2014; Groenendaal et al., 2015). In this case, although fitness function itself can be improved, for example, by increasing the population size or diversity for GAs can improve the fit of a sample-specific model, it may not necessarily guarantee that the final solution relates to the global minimum. To address this issue, many methods have been developed using (1) additional electrophysiological properties for fitting and/or (2) more complex electrophysiological protocols to improve model fidelity. It has been shown that model faithfulness can be improved by adding membrane resistance as an objective (Kaur et al., 2014), by optimizing to Ca^{2+} handling (Dokos and Lovell, 2004; Sarkar and Sobie, 2010; Rees et al., 2018), or by accounting for experimental data generated from multiple pacing frequencies (Syed et al., 2005; Lombardo et al., 2016) or irregular pacing protocols (Guo et al., 2013; Groenendaal et al., 2015).

In addition to using multiple electrophysiological properties to improve the fit of sample-specific models, more intricate voltage-clamp protocols that capture complex and rich electrophysiological dynamics have been employed, as first demonstrated to improve the fit of Markov models of ionic currents with many parameters (Dokos and Lovell, 2004; Zhou et al., 2009; Beattie et al., 2018). These can be implemented over a short time frame and may be used to emphasize certain currents over others. In the absence of pharmacological isolation, Groenendaal et al. used only a 6-s protocol that effectively isolated I_{K1}, I_{CaL}, and slow delayed-rectifier K^+ current (I_{Ks}) given their disproportionately large contribution at voltage steps of −120, +20, +40, and −30 mV, respectively (Groenendaal et al., 2015). They found that using this protocol alone cannot isolate all ionic currents, and when used in combination with a stochastic pacing protocol there was a considerable improvement in parameter estimation. Developing short but information-rich protocols is useful especially when trying to improve the results of an optimization procedure for cell-specific modeling, because longer protocols take longer to implement experimentally and thus are difficult to perform in a single cell. In a recent study, Beattie et al. proposed an innovative experimental and mathematical modeling method that allows to concisely measure the dominant processes involved in hERG channel gating by applying a short (8-s long) "sum of sinusoids" voltage-clamp protocol (Beattie et al., 2018). The sinusoidal waves were able to provoke a wider range of non-equilibrium behavior than traditional square voltage steps, thus allowing rich and complete characterization of hERG channel kinetics in the same cell and efficient model fitting (**Figure 4A**).

The final step in improving fidelity of sample-specific models is to directly experimentally test the predictions of the model given new protocols (Groenendaal et al., 2015; Devenyi et al., 2017; Beattie et al., 2018). **Figure 4B** reports an example of such validation experiments, where predictions obtained with cell-specific I_{Kr} models (identified applying the sinusoidal protocol in **Figure 4A** in 9 cells) are compared to the I_{Kr}-voltage relationships experimentally determined in each cell (Beattie et al., 2018). The order of the panels in **Figure 4B** is based on an index of recording stability (lowest to highest difference in leak resistance between the vehicle and dofetilide recordings) that is associated to "data quality". Cell-specific predictions are excellent for cells 1–5 (higher data quality), but less accurate for cells 6–9 (lower data quality). The analysis also shows that cell-specific models provide better predictions than the average model for the cells with the highest data quality (cells 1–5). Experimental validation is an important last step in improving cell-specific models, as generating cell-specific models is potentially more susceptible to observational error. Devenyi et al. used a GA to re-parameterize the Livshitz-Rudy model of the guinea pig ventricular cardiomyocyte (Livshitz and Rudy, 2009), and predicted an increase in I_{Kr} and a drastic decrease in I_{Ks} given a dynamic clamp protocol as compared to the original model, and this was validated experimentally (Devenyi et al., 2017). Their adjusted model predicted that I_{Ks} can stabilize the AP and EADs better as compared to I_{Kr}—which improved the ability to assess arrhythmia risk, given the baseline model did not produce physiological behaviors that were quantitatively similar to their experiments.

Models of Patient-Specific Anatomy

While a detailed discussion of patient-specific anatomical models is beyond the scope of our review, recent studies have begun investigating how inter-patient differences in myocardial structure affects atrial arrhythmia, as reviewed by Barichello et al. (2018). For example, Zhao et al. developed a 3D human heart-specific atrial computer model integrating 3D high resolution structural and functional mapping data to test the impact of wall thickness, fibrosis, and myofiber orientation on AF induction, maintenance, and ablation strategies (Zhao et al., 2017). Deng et al. demonstrated that reentrant driver localization dynamics are influenced by inter-patient variability in the spatial distribution of atrial fibrosis, APD, and conduction velocity (Deng et al., 2017). This suggests that incorporating patient-specific electrophysiological models in patient-specific geometries might enhance their predictive value. We discuss the computational challenges associated to this task in the section entitled "Arrhythmia Research Requires Understanding Variability at Larger Spatial Scales". Furthermore, obtaining patient-specific electrophysiological data might constitute another logistical roadblock.

Overall, methods that incorporate variability are particularly useful for (1) analyzing variability in cardiac electrophysiology, (2) assessing proarrhythmic risk, (3) determining the underlying factors contributing to variable drug response, and (4) identifying phenotype-specific (and in the future patient-specific) antiarrhythmic targets. **Table 1** summarizes applications of these approaches and new insights provided by the studies (shaded areas indicate atrial studies).

CHALLENGES AND FUTURE DIRECTIONS

We reviewed the most common methods used to account for variability in cardiac electrophysiology, which largely fall into the two categories of (1) population-based modeling and (2) sample-specific modeling. These methods complement each other well, as population-based methods can help characterize behavior in a particular patient group (healthy, diseased, stressed, etc.), and sample-specific modeling shows significant promise to

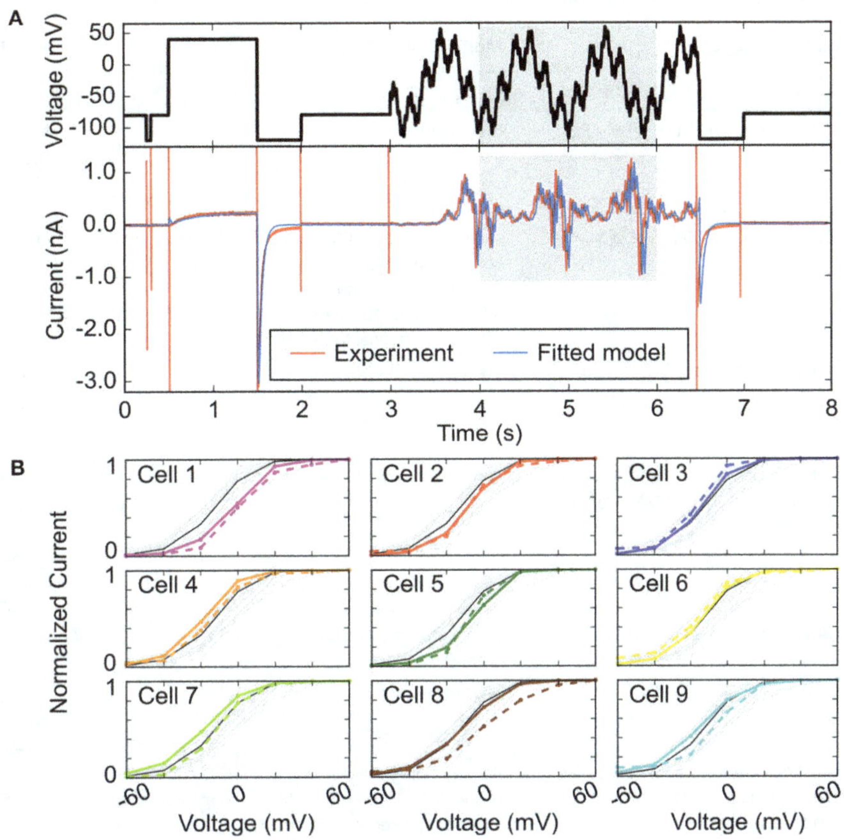

FIGURE 4 | Improving fit of sample-specific models. **(A)** Experimental and simulated I_{Kr} time courses (bottom) evoked in response to an efficient, information-rich sum-of-sinusoid voltage protocol (top) that allows rapid characterization of I_{Kr} behavior. **(B)** Steady-state peak I_{Kr}-voltage curves comparing cell-specific model predictions (bold, colored) to cell-specific experimental recordings (dashed, colored). The black lines in each plot are from the model calibrated to averaged sinusoidal data from all the cells (light gray). Reproduced from Beattie et al. (2018) with permission.

develop personalized medical approaches for individual patients. Both methods have led to many important insights into the mechanisms of arrhythmogenesis and antiarrhythmic strategies. However, there are several important limitations to consider, which suggest potential future developments in modeling of cardiac electrophysiology.

Analysis of Electrophysiology From Populations of Models May Require Different Statistical Methods

As opposed to the traditional approach of producing a single value from a single baseline model, models that incorporate variability have allowed statistical methods to be applied that can either ask new scientific questions or quantify the impact of variability on electrophysiological outputs, as performed in experimental studies. While the statistical analysis methods used in experimental studies can be directly applied in the *in silico* population-based studies, differences in the nature of experimental and simulation studies may need to be considered. For example, some population-based techniques generate model population sizes (often sample sizes in the 1000s) that are much greater than could be achieved by experiments (often sample sizes of 3–12) or the traditional cardiac modeling approach alone. Therefore, given similar effects, results produced in the population-based simulations have greater statistical power to detect differences. Furthermore, because even very small effects can reach statistical significance with large samples, physiological significance should be assessed (White et al., 2014). Additionally, when evaluating drug effects on electrophysiology, in simulations of the same virtual cell (a single model out of the population-models) can be used to perform both control and with-drug studies, allowing for paired comparisons, which is often not practical in experimental studies. The methodologies for analyzing and interpreting the "big data" produced by the population of models should be carefully considered and standards should be established going forward.

Variability Does Not Fully Account for Uncertainty

Physiologic variability should be thought of in the context of the broader umbrella of uncertainty, which is the confidence (or precision) with which a quantity, such as an electrophysiological output, can be given a value (Mirams et al., 2016). While here we reviewed how cardiac electrophysiology models have

TABLE 1 | Applications and main findings of computational methods incorporating cardiac electrophysiological variability (**shaded areas indicate atrial studies).

Author, Year	Baseline Model	Model Generation	Approach	Insight
ANALYZING VARIABILITY				
Sobie, 2009	MVMMs: Luo and Rudy, 1991; Fox et al., 2002; Kurata et al., 2005	Sampled from LND	MLR	New method to rapidly identify ionic mechanisms shaping AP properties, CaT, and alternans
Sanchez et al., 2014	HAMMs: Courtemanche et al., 1998; Maleckar et al., 2009; Grandi et al., 2011	Sampled over a ±100% variation range around their baseline values as described by Marino et al. (2008); calibrated to AP recordings in atrial trabecula	Statistical difference tests	Ionic determinants of variability in human AP in nSR vs. cAF
Lee Y. S. et al., 2016	HAMM: Courtemanche et al., 1998	Sampled from LND	MLR	Comparison of parameter sensitivity between nSR and AF condition. Ionic contributions to rate-dependence and spiral wave dynamics in AF
Devenyi and Sobie, 2016	HAMM: Grandi et al., 2011; HVMM: Grandi et al., 2010; RVMM: Pandit et al., 2001	Sampled from LND	MLR	In human atrial myocytes, both I_{to} and I_{Kur} had greater impacts on CaT amplitude than did SERCA. This was similar in rat left ventricular epicardial cells, where I_{to} played a more important role than SERCA
Vagos et al., 2017	HAMM: Skibsbye et al., 2016	Sampled from Gaussian distribution	MLR	Ionic determinants of unstable behaviors in nSR vs. cAF
Ellinwood et al., 2017b	HAMM: Grandi et al., 2011	Sampled from LND	MLR	I_{Kur} impacts APD and effective refractory period more in cAF (even though it is downregulated) vs. nSR
Muszkiewicz et al., 2017	HAMMs: Courtemanche et al., 1998; Maleckar et al., 2009; Grandi et al., 2011	Sampled using LHS and sequential MC; calibrated to experimental recordings	PCCs, statistical difference tests	Ionic determinants of electrophysiological and CaT properties
Lawson et al., 2018	HAMM: Courtemanche et al., 1998	Sampled over a ±100% variation range around their baseline values; sequential MC; model calibrated based on distributions of biomarkers estimated from multivariate kernel density estimation	Statistical difference tests	Accurate identification of inherent variability within the experimental population and improved characterization of ionic differences between nSR and cAF
ASSESSING ARRHYTHMIA RISK				
Walmsley et al., 2013	HVMM: O'Hara et al., 2011	MC sampling from a uniform distribution (±30%); calibrated to mRNA expression data in failing and non-failing hearts	MLR	Combination of low SERCA activity and high I_{CaL} conductance impacted the formation of alternans the most in the non-failing heart population, but low hERG conductance was the main contributor to alternans in the failing heart population
Zhou et al., 2016	HVMM: O'Hara et al., 2011	Sampled using LHS; calibrated to *in vivo* recordings	PCCs, statistical difference tests	I_{CaL} and NCX current determine the cell-to-cell differences in repolarization alternans through intracellular and sarcoplasmic Ca^{2+} regulation
Britton et al., 2017b	HVMM: O'Hara et al., 2011	Sampled using LHS; calibrated to data in human ventricular trabeculae	Logistic regression, PCCs, statistical difference tests	Na^+/K^+ pump is a key determinant of repolarization abnormality susceptibility
Morotti and Grandi, 2017	HAMM: Grandi et al., 2011	Sampled from LND	Logistic regression	EADs are particularly sensitive to conductances of I_{Na}, acetylcholine-sensitive and ultra-rapid K^+ channels, and NCX transport rate
Devenyi et al., 2017	Guinea pig left ventricular myocyte model Livshitz and Rudy, 2009	Fit using GA; sampled from LND	Dynamic clamp data for fitting, MLR	I_{Ks} is more capable to stabilize AP and EADs as compared to I_{Kr}

(Continued)

TABLE 1 | Continued

Author, Year	Baseline Model	Model Generation	Approach	Insight
IDENTIFYING ANTIARRHYTHMIC TARGETS				
Cummins et al., 2014	MVMMs: Luo and Rudy, 1991; Fox et al., 2002; Hund and Rudy, 2004; Ten Tusscher et al., 2004; Ten Tusscher and Panfilov, 2006; Livshitz and Rudy, 2009; O'Hara et al., 2011	Sampled from LND	MLR	I_{K1} and Na^+/K^+ pump currents favor forward rate dependence
Liberos et al., 2016	HAMM: Skibsbye et al., 2016	Sampled using LHS; calibrated to AP recordings in atrial trabeculae in patients with AF	PCCs, statistical difference tests	AF maintenance was correlated to high I_{CaL} and I_{Na}, and I_{CaL} block could be an effective treatment depending on the basal availability of Na^+ and Ca^{2+} channel conductivities
Passini et al., 2016	HVMM: O'Hara et al., 2011	Sampled using LHS; calibrated to non-diseased and HCM myocytes AP recordings	Analysis of repolarization properties	I_{CaL} re-activation is the key mechanism for repolarization abnormalities in HCM myocytes, and combined NCX, I_{NaL} and I_{CaL} block is effective to partially reverse the HCM phenotype
Yang et al., 2016	Rabbit ventricular myocyte model Soltis and Saucerman, 2010	Randomly selected within ±10% of nominal value (uniform distribution)	Analysis of TRIaD pro-arrhythmic markers	GS-458967 suppressed proarrhythmic markers following hERG block
ASSESSING THE VARIABLE RESPONSE TO DRUGS				
Sarkar and Sobie, 2011	MVMMs: Fox et al., 2002; Hund and Rudy, 2004; Ten Tusscher et al., 2004; Kurata et al., 2005; Grandi et al., 2010	Sampled from LND	MLR	Individuals do not exhibit the same degree of QT interval prolongation due to different ionic ensembles
Britton et al., 2013	Adapted rabbit Purkinje cell model Corrias et al., 2011	Sampled using LHS; calibrated to experimental data	PCCs	Quantitatively predicted the arrhythmia risk of four concentrations of the K^+ channel blocker dofetilide; baseline I_{Kr} conductance is the primary determinant of APD prolongation caused by dofetilide
Lancaster and Sobie, 2016	HVMMs: Ten Tusscher et al., 2004; Grandi et al., 2010; O'Hara et al., 2011	Sampled from LND; calibrated to experimental data	PCA, ROC curves, TdP risk scores	TdP risk assessment could be improved by quantifying the impact of multiple cardiac ion channels (even those not typically considered to affect risk)
Britton et al., 2017a	HVMM: Adapted O'Hara et al., 2011	Sampled using LHS, calibrated to heart-specific *ex vivo* measurements	Coefficients of variation	Good agreement with experiments for selective I_{Kr} blockers, but notable differences for the non-selective I_{Kr} inhibitors
Passini et al., 2017	HVMM: O'Hara et al., 2011	Sampled using LHS; calibrated to experimental data	TdP scoring system	*In silico* drug trial demonstrated higher accuracy than animal models in predicting arrhythmia risk (89%); underlying ionic contributions to repolarization/depolarization abnormalities
Krogh-Madsen et al., 2017	HVMM: O'Hara et al., 2011	Fit using GA; optimized to clinical data	TdP risk prediction	TdP risk assessment could be improved by using global optimization methods and multi-variable objectives
Gong and Sobie, 2018	HVMM O'Hara et al., 2011 and human iPSC-CM models Paci et al., 2017	Sampled from LND	Cross-cell MLR	Cross-cell regression predicted adult ventricular myocyte drug responses from the behaviors of an iPSC-CM *in silico* population

HAMM, human atrial myocyte model; HCM, hypertrophic cardiomyopathy; HVMM, human ventricular myocyte model; LHS, Latin hypercube sampling; LND, log-normal distribution; MLR, multivariable linear regression; MVMM, mammalian ventricular myocyte model; RVMM, rat ventricular myocyte model; PCA, principal component analysis; PCC, partial correlation coefficient; ROC, receiver operator characteristic; MC, Monte Carlo; TRIaD, Triangulation, Reverse use dependence, beat-to-beat Instability of action potential duration, and temporal and spatial action potential duration Dispersion.

begun to account for physiological and experimental variability, uncertainty analysis should determine whether the baseline model itself is a valid representation of its physical system. The extent and rigor of validation during model development affects uncertainty, whereby the broader the set of constraints, e.g., the model recapitulates both voltage and Ca^{2+} responses, their pacing rate-dependence, short- and long-term behavior, the lesser the uncertainty in the obtained parameters. Uncertainty analysis should also verify that the experiments used to construct the model are appropriate. For example, in experiments, voltage-clamp protocols used to characterize ionic currents are often done using non-selective pharmacological block which may have unidentified effects, over a range narrower than the entire physiological range, or on larger cells that are easier to patch-clamp with intrinsically greater than normal maximal conductances (Courtemanche et al., 1998). All of these would lead to uncertainties in the initial parameters and conditions due to experimental error and lack of knowledge. Likewise, the choice of the computational methods or resources used to perform the model parameterization and simulations can produce uncertainty in model results. This is because cardiac models may use different mathematical equations to describe the same physiological process, perhaps based on different analyses or assumptions on the physical-world process. Using more than one (e.g., cell) model to confirm predictions or validate the mechanistic understanding of a process is therefore a useful strategy (see for example Sarkar and Sobie, 2011; Sanchez et al., 2014; Lancaster and Sobie, 2016; Muszkiewicz et al., 2017). Additionally, even the choice of the numerical solver used by the software can lead to variability in model outputs, i.e., simulator uncertainty (Pathmanathan et al., 2012). Moreover, uncertainty in model outputs may arise if the code has not been verified to truly represent the mathematical equations in the computational model (Niederer et al., 2011a). Finally, optimization procedures can also introduce uncertainty, whereby the choice of whether to optimize simplified models with few parameters (Bueno-Orovio et al., 2008; Al Abed et al., 2013; Guo et al., 2013) or detailed models but only a few properties (e.g., focusing on specific currents) (Zhou et al., 2009; Fink et al., 2011) can lead to multiple distinct models given the same experimental data.

Used in conjunction with the approaches discussed in this review that take into account electrophysiological variability, new methods have been developed that try to quantify uncertainty more generally (Marino et al., 2008). Uncertainty quantification methods aim to quantify uncertainties in model inputs and propagation through the model to see how they affect model predictions (Pathmanathan et al., 2015; Mirams et al., 2016). This is typically done by assigning probability distribution functions, rather than fixed values to model parameters, as done for example by Pathmanathan et al. and applied to the study of I_{Na} steady-state inactivation (Pathmanathan et al., 2015). However, this process can be slow and tedious (requiring lots of simulations), especially if using a Monte Carlo sampling method that chooses input values from a statistical distribution. Also, in some cases, this statistical distribution of input parameters can be difficult to obtain or justify experimentally. To solve this issue, uncertainty quantification analysis has developed surrogate models or emulators (e.g., polynomial chaos expansions, and Gaussian process emulators; Chang et al., 2015), which are fast-running statistical approximations of the computational models and are quite powerful when fit to carefully constructed training data. Formal studies using uncertainty quantification in cardiac models are still limited, given the huge number of parameters in cardiac models, and may require the development of new methods or computational techniques (Johnstone et al., 2016).

Potential Covariance in Ionic Conductances Challenges the Current Method of Incorporating Variability

Currently, populations of cardiac models and sample-specific models typically calibrate or fit to maximal conductance values or transport rates of channels or receptors, based on the observation that changes in expression levels of ion channels and transport proteins are the primary contributors to (inter-species) variability (Rosati et al., 2008). However, this approach does not take into account that the expression of ion channels will vary over relatively short time scales given changes in transcription, translation, degradation, or even circadian rhythm. Moreover, with a few exceptions (Sarkar and Sobie, 2011; Cummins et al., 2014) these methods do not typically account for variability in ion channel kinetics, which is known to change especially in response to drugs (Clancy et al., 2007). The methods discussed in this review can attempt to account for these properties using additional parameters.

Although the correlation between parameters (i.e., maximal conductances) is assessed sometimes (Britton et al., 2013), neither population-based nor the sample-specific approaches account for possible covariance in ion channel conductances, despite the fact it has been observed in neurons (Schulz et al., 2006, 2007; Tobin et al., 2009) and cardiac tissue (Schram et al., 2002; Rosati and Mckinnon, 2004; Deschenes et al., 2008; Xiao et al., 2008; Banyasz et al., 2011; Milstein et al., 2012). The exact mechanisms responsible for these covariances are still being explored. Xiao et al. found that sustained reductions in I_{Kr} may lead to compensatory upregulation of I_{Ks} through post-transcriptional upregulation of underlying subunits (Xiao et al., 2008), which potentially underlie the observed phenomenon of repolarization reserve (Roden, 2008). Macromolecular complexes or post-transcriptional modifications could also facilitate coregulation of ionic conductances, as demonstrated by the observed structural or functional complex between I_{to} and I_{Na} (Deschenes et al., 2008). Rees et al. recently argued that sensing of aggregate CaT may be sufficient in itself to regulate ionic conductances (of K^+ and inward Ca^{2+}) to maintain normal Ca^{2+} handling (Rees et al., 2018). Moreover, knockout and knockdown studies are consistent with the idea that cardiac cells have compensatory mechanisms to maintain AP or CaTs (perhaps to prevent arrhythmias) (Guo et al., 1999; Zhou et al., 2003). The covariance of ionic conductance can have significant implications for both calibrating populations of models or fitting sample-specific models, because it could propose additional constraints for how the underlying parameters of the computational model can be varied. Thus, new methods have begun to be developed that measure all ionic conductances at once, and can not only tease out how ionic conductances are correlated, but the extent to which they vary between cells (Banyasz et al., 2011; Groenendaal et al., 2015).

Arrhythmia Research Requires Understanding Variability at Larger Spatial Scales

Accounting for variability at tissue and organ-level scales is a logical, but not trivial (Elshrif and Cherry, 2014), next step. A thorough investigation of variability would first require including differences among the cells in the same tissue, and evaluating the impact of diverse geometrical distributions. One should also account for patient-specific structural differences, based on measures of tissue conductivity and anatomic properties, including heterogeneity in signaling due to non-uniform innervation. This last step can be particularly problematic when investigating diseased conditions affected by pronounced structural remodeling, such as fibrosis, organ dilation, and alterations in gap junction coupling. Where there has been meaningful progress in accounting for variability is in developing personalized atrial model structures based on medical images (Dossel et al., 2012; Trayanova, 2014). These methods have shown some promise in developing personalized ablation strategies (Mcdowell et al., 2015). For example, recently, Soor et al. implemented a modeling approach to optimize ablation times based on patient-specific atrial geometries to create lesions for a given atrial wall thickness (Soor et al., 2016). Combining these methods that utilize medical images with the methods described here, could significantly improve the clinical value of both methods alone (Hansen et al., 2017; Zhao et al., 2017). For example, Arevalo et al. developed personalized heart models based on cardiac imaging and published patch-clamp data to better predict arrhythmic events and possibly avoid unnecessary implantable cardioverter defibrillators (Arevalo et al., 2016). Developing multi-scale frameworks that account for variability is the next frontier in cardiac modeling that will greatly benefit from further advancements in computing capabilities. Beyond the availability of large experimental and clinical datasets, the development of novel techniques to speed model derivations and to integrate automation will be crucial to capture variability for different cell types and conditions at various scales.

Safety Pharmacology Requires Complementary Electrophysiological Experimental Methods

The *in silico* approaches described here are being combined with other state-of-the-art tools to improve the evaluation of drug safety. Of significance, these approaches can help further the mission of the CiPA (Comprehensive *in vitro* Proarrhythmia Assay) initiative, which aspires to develop better methods to predict TdP. Beyond exclusively using steady-state hERG block as the main predictor of arrhythmia and not at all using QT interval prolongation, the CiPA initiative attempts to gain a more comprehensive understanding of proarrhythmic risk by combining (1) mechanistically-based *in vitro* assays, (2) *in silico* reconstructions of cardiac electrophysiology, and (3) confirmation using human iPSC-CMs (Colatsky et al., 2016). The methods described in this review are being utilized to help meet the mission of the CiPA initiative (Cummins et al., 2014; Lancaster and Sobie, 2016; Britton et al., 2017a; Passini et al., 2017). Most of the methods described here that assess the effects of drugs on populations of cardiac myocytes use simple pore block schemes. However, it is also clear that the sole use of steady-state hERG block assays is insufficient to predict arrhythmia risk, and thus studies are beginning to simulate the effects drug-binding kinetics and state-specific binding, which have been shown to affect electrophysiological outcomes (Lee W. et al., 2016; Dutta et al., 2017; Ellinwood et al., 2017b; Li et al., 2017). Incorporating more detailed drug-binding effects may allow studying the effects of populations of drugs characteristics (e.g., state-dependent block and kinetics) on populations of cardiomyocytes.

CONCLUSION

Computational approaches that have been developed over the past decade to account for variability in cardiac electrophysiology have led to important insights into mechanisms of arrhythmogenesis, etiology of disease, and variable response to drugs. The approaches outlined in this review are used in basic research studies, i.e., quite separately from actual clinical workflows, where decisions are made sometimes for a particular patient within minutes. Advanced computing facilities now allow near real-time simulations of anatomically realistic, biophysically detailed models of human cardiac electrophysiology (Niederer et al., 2011b; Okada et al., 2015, 2017). Such massively parallel processes could be optimized to run personalized cardiac simulations pre-determined to have clinical value. However, implementing these approaches more comprehensively into clinical workflows still presents challenges and simulation of variability may not find immediate application.

AUTHOR CONTRIBUTIONS

HN, SM, and EG reviewed the literature and wrote the manuscript.

ACKNOWLEDGMENTS

This work was supported by the American Heart Association grant 15SDG24910015 (EG); the National Institutes of Health (NIH) Stimulating Peripheral Activity to Relieve Conditions grant 1OT2OD023848-01 (EG), the National Heart, Lung, and Blood Institute R01HL131517 and R01HL141214 grants (EG) and K99HL138160 award (SM); and the Heart Rhythm Society post-doctoral fellowship 16OA9HRS (SM). An early version of this article was drafted by Dr. Nicholas Ellinwood.

REFERENCES

Abramson, D., Bernabeu, M. O., Bethwaite, B., Burrage, K., Corrias, A., Enticott, C., et al. (2010). High-throughput cardiac science on the Grid. *Philos. Trans. A Math. Phys. Eng. Sci.* 368, 3907–3923. doi: 10.1098/rsta.2010.0170

Achard, P., and De Schutter, E. (2006). Complex parameter landscape for a complex neuron model. *PLoS. Comput. Biol.* 2:e94. doi: 10.1371/journal.pcbi.0020094

Adeniran, I., El Harchi, A., Hancox, J. C., and Zhang, H. (2012). Proarrhythmia in KCNJ2-linked short QT syndrome: insights from modelling. *Cardiovasc. Res.* 94, 66–76. doi: 10.1093/cvr/cvs082

Ahrens-Nicklas, R. C., Clancy, C. E., and Christini, D. J. (2009). Re-evaluating the efficacy of beta-adrenergic agonists and antagonists in long QT-3 syndrome through computational modelling. *Cardiovasc. Res.* 82, 439–447. doi: 10.1093/cvr/cvp083

Al Abed, A., Guo, T., Lovell, N. H., and Dokos, S. (2013). Optimisation of ionic models to fit tissue action potentials: application to 3D atrial modelling. *Comput. Math. Methods Med.* 2013:951234. doi: 10.1155/2013/951234

Arevalo, H. J., Vadakkumpadan, F., Guallar, E., Jebb, A., Malamas, P., Wu, K. C., et al. (2016). Arrhythmia risk stratification of patients after myocardial infarction using personalized heart models. *Nat. Commun.* 7:11437. doi: 10.1038/ncomms11437

Banyasz, T., Horvath, B., Jian, Z., Izu, L. T., and Chen-Izu, Y. (2011). Sequential dissection of multiple ionic currents in single cardiac myocytes under action potential-clamp. *J. Mol. Cell. Cardiol.* 50, 578–581. doi: 10.1016/j.yjmcc.2010.12.020

Barichello, S., Roberts, J. D., Backx, P., Boyle, P. M., and Laksman, Z. (2018). Personalizing therapy for atrial fibrillation: the role of stem cell and *in silico* disease models. *Cardiovasc. Res.* 114, 931–943. doi: 10.1093/cvr/cvy090

Batchvarov, V. N., Ghuran, A., Smetana, P., Hnatkova, K., Harries, M., Dilaveris, P., et al. (2002). QT-RR relationship in healthy subjects exhibits substantial intersubject variability and high intrasubject stability. *Am. J. Physiol. Heart Circ. Physiol.* 282, H2356–H2363. doi: 10.1152/ajpheart.00860.2001

Beattie, K. A., Hill, A. P., Bardenet, R., Cui, Y., Vandenberg, J. I., Gavaghan, D. J., et al. (2018). Sinusoidal voltage protocols for rapid characterisation of ion channel kinetics. *J. Physiol.* 596, 1813–1828. doi: 10.1113/JP275733

Beeler, G. W., and Reuter, H. (1977). Reconstruction of the action potential of ventricular myocardial fibres. *J. Physiol.* 268, 177–210. doi: 10.1113/jphysiol.1977.sp011853

Behar, J., and Yaniv, Y. (2017). Age-related pacemaker deterioration is due to impaired intracellular and membrane mechanisms: insights from numerical modeling. *J. Gen. Physiol.* 149, 935–949. doi: 10.1085/jgp.2017 11792

Ben-Shalom, R., Aviv, A., Razon, B., and Korngreen, A. (2012). Optimizing ion channel models using a parallel genetic algorithm on graphical processors. *J. Neurosci. Methods* 206, 183–194. doi: 10.1016/j.jneumeth.2012.02.024

Bot, C. T., Kherlopian, A. R., Ortega, F. A., Christini, D. J., and Krogh-Madsen, T. (2012). Rapid genetic algorithm optimization of a mouse computational model: benefits for anthropomorphization of neonatal mouse cardiomyocytes. *Front. Physiol.* 3:421. doi: 10.3389/fphys.2012.00421

Boutjdir, M., Le Heuzey, J. Y., Lavergne, T., Chauvaud, S., Guize, L., Carpentier, A., et al. (1986). Inhomogeneity of cellular refractoriness in human atrium: factor of arrhythmia? *Pacing Clin. Electrophysiol.* 9, 1095–1100. doi: 10.1111/j.1540-8159.1986.tb06676.x

Britton, O. J., Abi-Gerges, N., Page, G., Ghetti, A., Miller, P. E., and Rodriguez, B. (2017a). Quantitative comparison of effects of dofetilide, sotalol, quinidine, and verapamil between human *ex vivo* trabeculae and *in silico* ventricular models incorporating inter-individual action potential variability. *Front. Physiol.* 8:597. doi: 10.3389/fphys.2017.00597

Britton, O. J., Bueno-Orovio, A., Van Ammel, K., Lu, H. R., Towart, R., Gallacher, D. J., et al. (2013). Experimentally calibrated population of models predicts and explains intersubject variability in cardiac cellular electrophysiology. *Proc. Natl. Acad. Sci. U.S.A.* 110, E2098–E2105. doi: 10.1073/pnas.13043 82110

Britton, O. J., Bueno-Orovio, A., Virag, L., Varro, A., and Rodriguez, B. (2017b). The Electrogenic Na(+)/K(+) Pump is a key determinant of repolarization abnormality susceptibility in human ventricular cardiomyocytes: a population-based simulation study. *Front. Physiol.* 8:278. doi: 10.3389/fphys.2017.00278

Bueno-Orovio, A., Cherry, E. M., and Fenton, F. H. (2008). Minimal model for human ventricular action potentials in tissue. *J. Theor. Biol.* 253, 544–560. doi: 10.1016/j.jtbi.2008.03.029

Bueno-Orovio, A., Sánchez, C., Pueyo, E., and Rodriguez, B. (2014). Na/K pump regulation of cardiac repolarization: insights from a systems biology approach. *Pflugers Arch.* 466, 183–193. doi: 10.1007/s00424-013-1293-1

Burrage, K., Burrage, P., Donovan, D., and Thompson, B. (2015). Populations of models, experimental designs and coverage of parameter space by latin hypercube and orthogonal sampling. *Procedia Comp. Sci.* 51, 1762–1771. doi: 10.1016/j.procs.2015.05.383

Butters, T. D., Aslanidi, O. V., Inada, S., Boyett, M. R., Hancox, J. C., Lei, M., et al. (2010). Mechanistic links between Na+ channel (SCN5A) mutations and impaired cardiac pacemaking in sick sinus syndrome. *Circ. Res.* 107, 126–137. doi: 10.1161/CIRCRESAHA.110.219949

Campbell, S. G., Flaim, S. N., Leem, C. H., and Mcculloch, A. D. (2008). Mechanisms of transmurally varying myocyte electromechanics in an integrated computational model. *Philos. Trans. A Math. Phys. Eng. Sci.* 366, 3361–3380. doi: 10.1098/rsta.2008.0088

Chang, E. T., Strong, M., and Clayton, R. H. (2015). Bayesian sensitivity analysis of a cardiac cell model using a gaussian process emulator. *PLoS ONE* 10: e0130252. doi: 10.1371/journal.pone.0130252

Chen, Q., and Guan, S. U. (2004). Incremental multiple objective genetic algorithms. *IEEE. Trans. Syst. Man. Cybern. B Cybern.* 34, 1325–1334. doi: 10.1109/TSMCB.2003.822958

Clancy, C. E., and Rudy, Y. (1999). Linking a genetic defect to its cellular phenotype in a cardiac arrhythmia. *Nature* 400, 566–569. doi: 10.1038/23034

Clancy, C. E., and Rudy, Y. (2002). Na(+) channel mutation that causes both Brugada and long-QT syndrome phenotypes: a simulation study of mechanism. *Circulation* 105, 1208–1213. doi: 10.1161/hc1002.105183

Clancy, C. E., Tateyama, M., and Kass, R. S. (2002). Insights into the molecular mechanisms of bradycardia-triggered arrhythmias in long QT-3 syndrome. *J. Clin. Invest.* 110, 1251–1262. doi: 10.1172/JCI0215928

Clancy, C. E., Zhu, Z. I., and Rudy, Y. (2007). Pharmacogenetics and anti-arrhythmic drug therapy: a theoretical investigation. *Am. J. Physiol. Heart Circ. Physiol.* 292, H66–H75. doi: 10.1152/ajpheart.00312.2006

Colatsky, T., Fermini, B., Gintant, G., Pierson, J. B., Sager, P., Sekino, Y., et al. (2016). The Comprehensive *in Vitro* Proarrhythmia Assay (CiPA) initiative - Update on progress. *J. Pharmacol. Toxicol. Methods* 81, 15–20. doi: 10.1016/j.vascn.2016.06.002

Colman, M. A., Aslanidi, O. V., Kharche, S., Boyett, M. R., Garratt, C., Hancox, J. C., et al. (2013). Pro-arrhythmogenic effects of atrial fibrillation-induced electrical remodelling: insights from the three-dimensional virtual human atria. *J. Physiol.* 591, 4249–4272. doi: 10.1113/jphysiol.2013. 254987

Comtois, P., Sakabe, M., Vigmond, E. J., Munoz, M., Texier, A., Shiroshita-Takeshita, A., et al. (2008). Mechanisms of atrial fibrillation termination by rapidly unbinding Na+ channel blockers: insights from mathematical models and experimental correlates. *Am. J. Physiol. Heart. Circ. Physiol.* 295, H1489–H1504. doi: 10.1152/ajpheart.01054.2007

Corrias, A., Giles, W., and Rodriguez, B. (2011). Ionic mechanisms of electrophysiological properties and repolarization abnormalities in rabbit Purkinje fibers. *Am. J. Physiol. Heart Circ. Physiol.* 300, H1806–H1813. doi: 10.1152/ajpheart.01170.2010

Courtemanche, M., Ramirez, R. J., and Nattel, S. (1998). Ionic mechanisms underlying human atrial action potential properties: insights from a mathematical model. *Am. J. Physiol.* 275, H301–H321. doi: 10.1152/ajpheart.1998.275.1.H301

Courtemanche, M., and Winfree, A. T. (1991). Re-entrant rotating waves in a beeler-reuter based model of two-dimensional cardiac electrical activity. *Int. J. Bifurcation Chaos* 1, 431–444. doi: 10.1142/S0218127491000336

Crosby, J. L. (1982). *Computer Simulation in Genetics*. London, New York, NY: John Wiley.

Cummins, M. A., Dalal, P. J., Bugana, M., Severi, S., and Sobie, E. A. (2014). Comprehensive analyses of ventricular myocyte models identify targets exhibiting favorable rate dependence. *PLoS. Comput. Biol.* 10:e1003543. doi: 10.1371/journal.pcbi.1003543

Daniels, G. S. (1952). *The Average Man?* Technical Note WCRD53-7, Wright Air Development Center, Ohio AD-10203.

Deng, D., Murphy, M. J., Hakim, J. B., Franceschi, W. H., Zahid, S., Pashakhanloo, F., et al. (2017). Sensitivity of reentrant driver localization to electrophysiological parameter variability in image-based computational models of persistent atrial fibrillation sustained by a fibrotic substrate. *Chaos* 27, 093932. doi: 10.1063/1.5003340

Deschênes, I., Armoundas, A. A., Jones, S. P., and Tomaselli, G. F. (2008). Post-transcriptional gene silencing of KChIP2 and Navbeta1 in neonatal rat cardiac myocytes reveals a functional association between Na and Ito currents. *J. Mol. Cell. Cardiol.* 45, 336–346. doi: 10.1016/j.yjmcc.2008.05.001

Devenyi, R. A., Ortega, F. A., Groenendaal, W., Krogh-Madsen, T., Christini, D. J., and Sobie, E. A. (2017). Differential roles of two delayed rectifier potassium currents in regulation of ventricular action potential duration and arrhythmia susceptibility. *J. Physiol.* 595, 2301–2317. doi: 10.1113/JP273191

Devenyi, R. A., and Sobie, E. A. (2016). There and back again: iterating between population-based modeling and experiments reveals surprising regulation of calcium transients in rat cardiac myocytes. *J. Mol. Cell. Cardiol.* 96, 38–48. doi: 10.1016/j.yjmcc.2015.07.016

Dibb, K., Trafford, A., Zhang, H., and Eisner, D. (2015). A model model: a commentary on DiFrancesco and Noble (1985) 'A model of cardiac electrical activity incorporating ionic pumps and concentration changes'. *Philos. Trans. R Soc. Lond. B Biol. Sci.* 370:20140316. doi: 10.1098/rstb.2014.0316

Difrancesco, D., and Noble, D. (1985). A model of cardiac electrical activity incorporating ionic pumps and concentration changes. *Philos. Trans. R Soc. Lond. B Biol. Sci.* 307, 353–398. doi: 10.1098/rstb.1985.0001

Dokos, S., and Lovell, N. H. (2004). Parameter estimation in cardiac ionic models. *Prog. Biophys. Mol. Biol.* 85, 407–431. doi: 10.1016/j.pbiomolbio.2004.02.002

Donovan, D., Burrage, K., Burrage, P., Mccourt, T. A., Thompson, B., and Yazici, E. S. (2018). Estimates of the coverage of parameter space by latin hypercube and orthogonal array-based sampling. *Appl. Math. Model.* 57, 553–564. doi: 10.1016/j.apm.2017.11.036

Dössel, O., Krueger, M. W., Weber, F. M., Wilhelms, M., and Seemann, G. (2012). Computational modeling of the human atrial anatomy and electrophysiology. *Med. Biol. Eng. Comput.* 50, 773–799. doi: 10.1007/s11517-012-0924-6

Draper, N. R., and Smith, H. (2014). *Applied Regression Analysis.* Hoboken; Somerset, NJ: John Wiley and Sons.

Druckmann, S., Banitt, Y., Gidon, A., Schürmann, F., Markram, H., and Segev, I. (2007). A novel multiple objective optimization framework for constraining conductance-based neuron models by experimental data. *Front. Neurosci.* 1, 7–18. doi: 10.3389/neuro.01.1.1.001.2007

Dutta, S., Chang, K. C., Beattie, K. A., Sheng, J., Tran, P. N., Wu, W. W., et al. (2017). Optimization of an *in silico* cardiac cell model for proarrhythmia risk assessment. *Front. Physiol.* 8:616. doi: 10.3389/fphys.2017.00616

Edwards, A. G., Grandi, E., Hake, J. E., Patel, S., Li, P., Miyamoto, S., et al. (2014). Nonequilibrium reactivation of Na+ current drives early afterdepolarizations in mouse ventricle. *Circ. Arrhythm Electrophysiol.* 7, 1205–1213. doi: 10.1161/CIRCEP.113.001666

Ellinwood, N., Dobrev, D., Morotti, S., and Grandi, E. (2017a). *In silico* assessment of efficacy and safety of IKur inhibitors in chronic atrial fibrillation: role of kinetics and state-dependence of drug binding. *Front. Pharmacol.* 8, 799. doi: 10.3389/fphar.2017.00799

Ellinwood, N., Dobrev, D., Morotti, S., and Grandi, E. (2017b). Revealing kinetics and state-dependent binding properties of IKur-targeting drugs that maximize atrial fibrillation selectivity. *Chaos* 27, 093918. doi: 10.1063/1.5000226

Elshrif, M. M., and Cherry, E. M. (2014). A quantitative comparison of the behavior of human ventricular cardiac electrophysiology models in tissue. *PLoS ONE* 9:e84401. doi: 10.1371/journal.pone.0084401

Fender, E. A., Henrikson, C. A., and Tereshchenko, L. (2014). Racial differences in sudden cardiac death. *J. Electrocardiol.* 47, 815–818. doi: 10.1016/j.jelectrocard.2014.07.023

Feng, J., Yue, L., Wang, Z., and Nattel, S. (1998). Ionic mechanisms of regional action potential heterogeneity in the canine right atrium. *Circ. Res.* 83, 541–551. doi: 10.1161/01.RES.83.5.541

Fink, M., Niederer, S. A., Cherry, E. M., Fenton, F. H., Koivumäki, J. T., Seemann, G., et al. (2011). Cardiac cell modelling: observations from the heart of the cardiac physiome project. *Prog. Biophys. Mol. Biol.* 104, 2–21. doi: 10.1016/j.pbiomolbio.2010.03.002

Fotiadis, P., and Forger, D. B. (2013). Modeling the effects of the circadian clock on cardiac electrophysiology. *J. Biol. Rhythms* 28, 69–78. doi: 10.1177/0748730412469499

Fox, J. J., Mcharg, J. L., and Gilmour, R. F. (2002). Ionic mechanism of electrical alternans. *Am. J. Physiol. Heart Circ. Physiol.* 282, H516–H530. doi: 10.1152/ajpheart.00612.2001

Fraser, A., and Burnell, D. (1970). *Computer Models in Genetics.* New York, NY: McGraw-Hill.

Gaborit, N., Le Bouter, S., Szuts, V., Varro, A., Escande, D., Nattel, S., et al. (2007). Regional and tissue specific transcript signatures of ion channel genes in the non-diseased human heart. *J. Physiol.* 582, 675–693. doi: 10.1113/jphysiol.2006.126714

Gaspo, R., Bosch, R. F., Talajic, M., and Nattel, S. (1997). Functional mechanisms underlying tachycardia-induced sustained atrial fibrillation in a chronic dog model. *Circulation* 96, 4027–4035. doi: 10.1161/01.CIR.96.11.4027

Geladi, P., and Kowalski, B. R. (1986). Partial least-squares regression - a tutorial. *Anal. Chim. Acta* 185, 1–17. doi: 10.1016/0003-2670(86)80028-9

Golowasch, J., Goldman, M. S., Abbott, L. F., and Marder, E. (2002). Failure of averaging in the construction of a conductance-based neuron model. *J. Neurophys.* 87, 1129–1131. doi: 10.1152/jn.00412.2001

Gong, J. Q. X., and Sobie, E. A. (2018). Population-based mechanistic modeling allows for quantitative predictions of drug responses across cell types. *NPJ. Syst. Biol. Appl.* 4, 11. doi: 10.1038/s41540-018-0047-2

Gong, Y., Xie, F., Stein, K. M., Garfinkel, A., Culianu, C. A., Lerman, B. B., et al. (2007). Mechanism underlying initiation of paroxysmal atrial flutter/atrial fibrillation by ectopic foci: a simulation study. *Circulation* 115, 2094–2102. doi: 10.1161/CIRCULATIONAHA.106.656504

Grandi, E., and Maleckar, M. M. (2016). Anti-arrhythmic strategies for atrial fibrillation: the role of computational modeling in discovery, development, and optimization. *Pharmacol. Ther.* 168, 126–142. doi: 10.1016/j.pharmthera.2016.09.012

Grandi, E., Pandit, S. V., Voigt, N., Workman, A. J., Dobrev, D., Jalife, J., et al. (2011). Human atrial action potential and Ca^{2+} model: sinus rhythm and chronic atrial fibrillation. *Circ. Res.* 109, 1055–1066. doi: 10.1161/CIRCRESAHA.111.253955

Grandi, E., Pasqualini, F. S., and Bers, D. M. (2010). A novel computational model of the human ventricular action potential and Ca transient. *J. Mol. Cell. Cardiol.* 48, 112–121. doi: 10.1016/j.yjmcc.2009.09.019

Gray, R. A., Jalife, J., Panfilov, A., Baxter, W. T., Cabo, C., Davidenko, J. M., et al. (1995). Nonstationary vortexlike reentrant activity as a mechanism of polymorphic ventricular tachycardia in the isolated rabbit heart. *Circulation* 91, 2454–2469. doi: 10.1161/01.CIR.91.9.2454

Groenendaal, W., Ortega, F. A., Kherlopian, A. R., Zygmunt, A. C., Krogh-Madsen, T., and Christini, D. J. (2015). Cell-specific cardiac electrophysiology models. *PLoS Comput. Biol.* 11:e1004242. doi: 10.1371/journal.pcbi.1004242

Guo, T., Abed, A. A., Lovell, N. H., and Dokos, S. (2010). A generic ionic model of cardiac action potentials. *Conf. Proc. IEEE. Eng. Med. Biol. Soc.* 2010, 1465–1468. doi: 10.1109/IEMBS.2010.5626853

Guo, T., Al Abed, A., Lovell, N. H., and Dokos, S. (2013). Optimisation of a generic ionic model of cardiac myocyte electrical activity. *Comput. Math. Methods Med.* 2013:706195. doi: 10.1155/2013/706195

Guo, W., Xu, H., London, B., and Nerbonne, J. M. (1999). Molecular basis of transient outward K+ current diversity in mouse ventricular myocytes. *J. Physiol.* 521(Pt 3), 587–599. doi: 10.1111/j.1469-7793.1999.00587.x

Gurkiewicz, M., and Korngreen, A. (2007). A numerical approach to ion channel modelling using whole-cell voltage-clamp recordings and a genetic algorithm. *PLoS Comput. Biol.* 3:e169. doi: 10.1371/journal.pcbi.0030169

Hair, J. F., Black, W. C., Babin, B. J., and Anderson, R. E. (2010). *Multivariate Data Analysis.* Upper Saddle River, NJ: Pearson Prentice Hall.

Hansen, B. J., Zhao, J., and Fedorov, V. V. (2017). Fibrosis and atrial fibrillation: computerized and optical mapping; a view into the human atria at submillimeter resolution. *JACC Clin. Electrophysiol.* 3, 531–546. doi: 10.1016/j.jacep.2017.05.002

Heijman, J., Zaza, A., Johnson, D. M., Rudy, Y., Peeters, R. L., Volders, P. G., et al. (2013). Determinants of beat-to-beat variability of repolarization duration in the canine ventricular myocyte: a computational analysis. *PLoS Comput. Biol.* 9:e1003202. doi: 10.1371/journal.pcbi.1003202

Hobbs, K. H., and Hooper, S. L. (2008). Using complicated, wide dynamic range driving to develop models of single neurons in single recording sessions. *J. Neurophysiol.* 99, 1871–1883. doi: 10.1152/jn.00032.2008

Hodgkin, A. L., and Huxley, A. F. (1952). A quantitative description of membrane current and its application to conduction and excitation in nerve. *J. Physiol.* 117, 500–544. doi: 10.1113/jphysiol.1952.sp004764

Hund, T. J., and Rudy, Y. (2004). Rate dependence and regulation of action potential and calcium transient in a canine cardiac ventricular cell model. *Circulation* 110, 3168–3174. doi: 10.1161/01.CIR.0000147231.69595.D3

Hussein, Y. A., and El-Ghazaly, S. M. (2004). Modeling and optimization of microwave devices and circuits using genetic algorithms. *IEEE Trans. Microwave Theory Tech.* 52, 329–336. doi: 10.1109/TMTT.2003.820899

Inada, S., Hancox, J. C., Zhang, H., and Boyett, M. R. (2009). One-dimensional mathematical model of the atrioventricular node including atrio-nodal, nodal, and nodal-his cells. *Biophys. J.* 97, 2117–2127. doi: 10.1016/j.bpj.2009.06.056

Janes, K. A., Albeck, J. G., Gaudet, S., Sorger, P. K., Lauffenburger, D. A., and Yaffe, M. B. (2005). A systems model of signaling identifies a molecular basis set for cytokine-induced apoptosis. *Science* 310, 1646–1653. doi: 10.1126/science.1116598

Jeyaraj, D., Haldar, S. M., Wan, X., Mccauley, M. D., Ripperger, J. A., Hu, K., et al. (2012). Circadian rhythms govern cardiac repolarization and arrhythmogenesis. *Nature* 483, 96–99. doi: 10.1038/nature10852

Johnstone, R. H., Chang, E. T. Y., Bardenet, R., de Boer, T. P., Gavaghan, D. J., Pathmanathan, P., et al. (2016). Uncertainty and variability in models of the cardiac action potential: can we build trustworthy models? *J. Mol. Cell. Cardiol.* 96, 49–62. doi: 10.1016/j.yjmcc.2015.11.018

Kannankeril, P. J., Norris, K. J., Carter, S., and Roden, D. M. (2011). Factors affecting the degree of QT prolongation with drug challenge in a large cohort of normal volunteers. *Heart Rhythm* 8, 1530–1534. doi: 10.1016/j.hrthm.2011.03.042

Kaur, J., Nygren, A., and Vigmond, E. J. (2014). Fitting membrane resistance along with action potential shape in cardiac myocytes improves convergence: application of a multi-objective parallel genetic algorithm. *PLoS ONE* 9:e107984. doi: 10.1371/journal.pone.0107984

Kharche, S., Garratt, C. J., Boyett, M. R., Inada, S., Holden, A. V., Hancox, J. C., et al. (2008). Atrial proarrhythmia due to increased inward rectifier current (I(K1)) arising from KCNJ2 mutation–a simulation study. *Prog. Biophys. Mol. Biol.* 98, 186–197. doi: 10.1016/j.pbiomolbio.2008.10.010

Koivumäki, J. T., Naumenko, N., Tuomainen, T., Takalo, J., Oksanen, M., Puttonen, K. A., et al. (2018). Structural immaturity of human iPSC-Derived cardiomyocytes: *in silico* investigation of effects on function and disease modeling. *Front. Physiol.* 9:80. doi: 10.3389/fphys.2018.00080

Krogh-Madsen, T., and Christini, D. J. (2012). Nonlinear dynamics in cardiology. *Annu. Rev. Biomed. Eng.* 14, 179–203. doi: 10.1146/annurev-bioeng-071811-150106

Krogh-Madsen, T., Jacobson, A. F., Ortega, F. A., and Christini, D. J. (2017). Global optimization of ventricular myocyte model to multi-variable objective improves predictions of drug-induced torsades de pointes. *Front. Physiol.* 8:1059. doi: 10.3389/fphys.2017.01059

Krogh-Madsen, T., Sobie, E. A., and Christini, D. J. (2016). Improving cardiomyocyte model fidelity and utility via dynamic electrophysiology protocols and optimization algorithms. *J. Physiol.* 594, 2525–2536. doi: 10.1113/JP270618

Kurata, Y., Hisatome, I., Matsuda, H., and Shibamoto, T. (2005). Dynamical mechanisms of pacemaker generation in IK1-downregulated human ventricular myocytes: insights from bifurcation analyses of a mathematical model. *Biophys. J.* 89, 2865–2887. doi: 10.1529/biophysj.105.060830

Lancaster, M. C., and Sobie, E. A. (2016). Improved prediction of drug-induced torsades de pointes through simulations of dynamics and machine learning algorithms. *Clin. Pharmacol. Ther.* 100, 371–379. doi: 10.1002/cpt.367

Lau, C. P., Tse, H. F., Siu, C. W., and Gbadebo, D. (2012). Atrial electrical and structural remodeling: implications for racial differences in atrial fibrillation. *J. Cardiovasc. Electrophysiol.* 23(Suppl. 1), S36–S40. doi: 10.1111/jce.12022

Lawson, B. A. J., Drovandi, C. C., Cusimano, N., Burrage, P., Rodriguez, B., and Burrage, K. (2018). Unlocking data sets by calibrating populations of models to data density: a study in atrial electrophysiology. *Sci. Adv.* 4:e1701676. doi: 10.1126/sciadv.1701676

Lee, W., Mann, S. A., Windley, M. J., Imtiaz, M. S., Vandenberg, J. I., and Hill, A. P. (2016). *In silico* assessment of kinetics and state dependent binding properties of drugs causing acquired LQTS. *Prog. Biophys. Mol. Biol.* 120, 89–99. doi: 10.1016/j.pbiomolbio.2015.12.005

Lee, Y. S., Hwang, M., Song, J. S., Li, C., Joung, B., Sobie, E. A., et al. (2016). The contribution of ionic currents to rate-dependent action potential duration and pattern of reentry in a mathematical model of human atrial fibrillation. *PLoS ONE* 11:e0150779. doi: 10.1371/journal.pone.0150779

Lee, Y. S., Liu, O. Z., Hwang, H. S., Knollmann, B. C., and Sobie, E. A. (2013). Parameter sensitivity analysis of stochastic models provides insights into cardiac calcium sparks. *Biophys. J.* 104, 1142–1150. doi: 10.1016/j.bpj.2012.12.055

Leung, F. H. F., Lam, H. K., Ling, S. H., and Tam, P. K. S. (2004). Optimal and stable fuzzy controllers for nonlinear systems based on an improved genetic algorithm. *IEEE Trans. Indus. Electron.* 51, 172–182. doi: 10.1109/TIE.2003.821898

Li, Z., Dutta, S., Sheng, J., Tran, P. N., Wu, W., Chang, K., et al. (2017). Improving the *in silico* assessment of proarrhythmia risk by combining herg (human ether-a-go-go-related gene) channel-drug binding kinetics and multichannel pharmacology. *Circ. Arrhythm. Electrophysiol.* 10:e004628. doi: 10.1161/CIRCEP.116.004628

Liberos, A., Bueno-Orovio, A., Rodrigo, M., Ravens, U., Hernandez-Romero, I., Fernandez-Aviles, F., et al. (2016). Balance between sodium and calcium currents underlying chronic atrial fibrillation termination: an *in silico* intersubject variability study. *Heart Rhythm* 13, 2358–2365. doi: 10.1016/j.hrthm.2016.08.028

Liu, L., and Nattel, S. (1997). Differing sympathetic and vagal effects on atrial fibrillation in dogs: role of refractoriness heterogeneity. *Am. J. Physiol.* 273, H805–H816. doi: 10.1152/ajpheart.1997.273.2.H805

Livshitz, L., and Rudy, Y. (2009). Uniqueness and stability of action potential models during rest, pacing, and conduction using problem-solving environment. *Biophys. J.* 97, 1265–1276. doi: 10.1016/j.bpj.2009.05.062

Lombardo, D. M., Fenton, F. H., Narayan, S. M., and Rappel, W. J. (2016). Comparison of detailed and simplified models of human atrial myocytes to recapitulate patient specific properties. *PLoS Comput. Biol.* 12:e1005060. doi: 10.1371/journal.pcbi.1005060

Luo, C. H., and Rudy, Y. (1991). A model of the ventricular cardiac action potential. Depolarization, repolarization, and their interaction. *Circ. Res.* 68, 1501–1526. doi: 10.1161/01.RES.68.6.1501

Maleckar, M. M., Greenstein, J. L., Giles, W. R., and Trayanova, N. A. (2009). K+ current changes account for the rate dependence of the action potential in the human atrial myocyte. *Am. J. Physiol. Heart Circ. Physiol.* 297, H1398–H1410. doi: 10.1152/ajpheart.00411.2009

Maltsev, V. A., and Lakatta, E. G. (2009). Synergism of coupled subsarcolemmal Ca2+ clocks and sarcolemmal voltage clocks confers robust and flexible pacemaker function in a novel pacemaker cell model. *Am. J. Physiol. Heart Circ. Physiol.* 296, H594–H615. doi: 10.1152/ajpheart.01118.2008

Mann, S. A., Imtiaz, M., Winbo, A., Rydberg, A., Perry, M. D., Couderc, J. P., et al. (2016). Convergence of models of human ventricular myocyte electrophysiology after global optimization to recapitulate clinical long QT phenotypes. *J. Mol. Cell. Cardiol.* 100, 25–34. doi: 10.1016/j.yjmcc.2016.09.011

Mann, S. A., Otway, R., Guo, G., Soka, M., Karlsdotter, L., Trivedi, G., et al. (2012). Epistatic effects of potassium channel variation on cardiac repolarization and atrial fibrillation risk. *J. Am. Coll. Cardiol.* 59, 1017–1025. doi: 10.1016/j.jacc.2011.11.039

Marder, E. (2011). Variability, compensation, and modulation in neurons and circuits. *Proc. Natl. Acad. Sci. U.S.A.* 108(Suppl. 3), 15542–15548. doi: 10.1073/pnas.1010674108

Marino, S., Hogue, I. B., Ray, C. J., and Kirschner, D. E. (2008). A methodology for performing global uncertainty and sensitivity analysis in systems biology. *J. Theor. Biol.* 254, 178–196. doi: 10.1016/j.jtbi.2008.04.011

Mayourian, J., Cashman, T. J., Ceholski, D. K., Johnson, B. V., Sachs, D., Kaji, D. A., et al. (2017). Experimental and computational insight into human mesenchymal stem cell paracrine signaling and heterocellular coupling effects on cardiac contractility and arrhythmogenicity. *Circ. Res.* 121, 411–423. doi: 10.1161/CIRCRESAHA.117.310796

McDowell, K. S., Zahid, S., Vadakkumpadan, F., Blauer, J., Macleod, R. S., and Trayanova, N. A. (2015). Virtual electrophysiological study of atrial fibrillation in fibrotic remodeling. *PLoS ONE* 10:e0117110. doi: 10.1371/journal.pone.0117110

Milstein, M. L., Musa, H., Balbuena, D. P., Anumonwo, J. M., Auerbach, D. S., Furspan, P. B., et al. (2012). Dynamic reciprocity of sodium and potassium channel expression in a macromolecular complex controls cardiac excitability and arrhythmia. *Proc. Natl. Acad. Sci. U.S.A.* 109, E2134–E2143. doi: 10.1073/pnas.1109370109

Mirams, G. R., Pathmanathan, P., Gray, R. A., Challenor, P., and Clayton, R. H. (2016). Uncertainty and variability in computational and mathematical models of cardiac physiology. *J. Physiol.* 594, 6833–6847. doi: 10.1113/JP271671

Misier, A. R., Opthof, T., Van Hemel, N. M., Defauw, J. J., de Bakker, J. M., Janse, M. J., et al. (1992). Increased dispersion of "refractoriness" in patients with idiopathic paroxysmal atrial fibrillation. *J. Am. Coll. Cardiol.* 19, 1531–1535. doi: 10.1016/0735-1097(92)90614-S

Moe, G. K., Rheinboldt, W. C., And Abildskov, J. A. (1964). A computer model of atrial fibrillation. *Am. Heart J.* 67, 200–220. doi: 10.1016/0002-8703(64)90371-0

Morotti, S., and Grandi, E. (2017). Logistic regression analysis of populations of electrophysiological models to assess proarrythmic risk. *MethodsX* 4, 25–34. doi: 10.1016/j.mex.2016.12.002

Morotti, S., Mcculloch, A. D., Bers, D. M., Edwards, A. G., and Grandi, E. (2016). Atrial-selective targeting of arrhythmogenic phase-3 early afterdepolarizations in human myocytes. *J. Mol. Cell. Cardiol.* 96, 63–71. doi: 10.1016/j.yjmcc.2015.07.030

Muszkiewicz, A., Britton, O. J., Gemmell, P., Passini, E., Sánchez, C., Zhou, X., et al. (2016). Variability in cardiac electrophysiology: using experimentally-calibrated populations of models to move beyond the single virtual physiological human paradigm. *Prog. Biophys. Mol. Biol.* 120, 115–127. doi: 10.1016/j.pbiomolbio.2015.12.002

Muszkiewicz, A., Liu, X., Bueno-Orovio, A., Lawson, B. A. J., Burrage, K., Casadei, B., et al. (2017). From ionic to cellular variability in human atrial myocytes: an integrative computational and experimental study. *Am. J. Physiol. Heart Circ. Physiol.* 314, H895–H916. doi: 10.1152/ajpheart.00477.2017

Ni, H., Whittaker, D. G., Wang, W., Giles, W. R., Narayan, S. M., and Zhang, H. (2017). Synergistic anti-arrhythmic effects in human atria with combined use of sodium blockers and acacetin. *Front. Physiol.* 8:946. doi: 10.3389/fphys.2017.00946

Niederer, S. A., Fink, M., Noble, D., and Smith, N. P. (2009). A meta-analysis of cardiac electrophysiology computational models. *Exp. Physiol.* 94, 486–495. doi: 10.1113/expphysiol.2008.044610

Niederer, S. A., Kerfoot, E., Benson, A. P., Bernabeu, M. O., Bernus, O., Bradley, C., et al. (2011a). Verification of cardiac tissue electrophysiology simulators using an N-version benchmark. *Philos. Trans. R. Soc. Math. Phys. Eng. Sci.* 369, 4331–4351. doi: 10.1098/rsta.2011.0139

Niederer, S., Mitchell, L., Smith, N., and Plank, G. (2011b). Simulating human cardiac electrophysiology on clinical time-scales. *Front. Physiol.* 2:14. doi: 10.3389/fphys.2011.00014

Noble, D. (1962). A modification of the Hodgkin–Huxley equations applicable to Purkinje fibre action and pace-maker potentials. *J. Physiol.* 160, 317–352. doi: 10.1113/jphysiol.1962.sp006849

Noble, D., Garny, A., and Noble, P. J. (2012). How the Hodgkin-Huxley equations inspired the Cardiac Physiome Project. *J. Physiol. Lond.* 590, 2613–2628. doi: 10.1113/jphysiol.2011.224238

Noble, D., Sarai, N., Noble, P. J., Kobayashi, T., Matsuoka, S., and Noma, A. (2007). Resistance of cardiac cells to NCX knockout: a model study. *Ann. N. Y. Acad. Sci.* 1099, 306–309. doi: 10.1196/annals.1387.018

Nygren, A., Fiset, C., Firek, L., Clark, J. W., Lindblad, D. S., Clark, R. B., et al. (1998). Mathematical model of an adult human atrial cell: the role of K+ currents in repolarization. *Circ. Res.* 82, 63–81. doi: 10.1161/01.RES.82.1.63

O'Hara, T., Virág, L., Varró, A., and Rudy, Y. (2011). Simulation of the undiseased human cardiac ventricular action potential: model formulation and experimental validation. *PLoS Comput. Biol.* 7:e1002061. doi: 10.1371/journal.pcbi.1002061

Okada, J. I., Washio, T., Nakagawa, M., Watanabe, M., Kadooka, Y., Kariya, T., et al. (2017). Multi-scale, tailor-made heart simulation can predict the effect of cardiac resynchronization therapy. *J. Mol. Cell. Cardiol.* 108, 17–23. doi: 10.1016/j.yjmcc.2017.05.006

Okada, J., Yoshinaga, T., Kurokawa, J., Washio, T., Furukawa, T., Sawada, K., et al. (2015). Screening system for drug-induced arrhythmogenic risk combining a patch clamp and heart simulator. *Sci. Adv.* 1:e1400142. doi: 10.1126/sciadv.1400142

Paci, M., Passini, E., Severi, S., Hyttinen, J., and Rodriguez, B. (2017). Phenotypic variability in LQT3 human induced pluripotent stem cell-derived cardiomyocytes and their response to antiarrhythmic pharmacologic therapy: an *in silico* approach. *Heart Rhythm* 14, 1704–1712. doi: 10.1016/j.hrthm.2017.07.026

Pandit, S. V., Clark, R. B., Giles, W. R., and Demir, S. S. (2001). A mathematical model of action potential heterogeneity in adult rat left ventricular myocytes. *Biophys. J.* 81, 3029–3051. doi: 10.1016/S0006-3495(01)75943-7

Panfilov, A. V., and Holden, A. V. (1991). Spatiotemporal irregularity in a two-dimensional model of cardiac tissue. *Int. J. Bifurcation Chaos* 1, 219–225. doi: 10.1142/S0218127491000142

Passini, E., Britton, O. J., Lu, H. R., Rohrbacher, J., Hermans, A. N., Gallacher, D. J., et al. (2017). Human *in silico* drug trials demonstrate higher accuracy than animal models in predicting clinical pro-arrhythmic cardiotoxicity. *Front. Physiol.* 8:668. doi: 10.3389/fphys.2017.00668

Passini, E., Mincholé, A., Coppini, R., Cerbai, E., Rodriguez, B., Severi, S., et al. (2016). Mechanisms of pro-arrhythmic abnormalities in ventricular repolarisation and anti-arrhythmic therapies in human hypertrophic cardiomyopathy. *J. Mol. Cell. Cardiol.* 96, 72–81. doi: 10.1016/j.yjmcc.2015.09.003

Pathmanathan, P., Bernabeu, M. O., Niederer, S. A., Gavaghan, D. J., and Kay, D. (2012). Computational modelling of cardiac electrophysiology: explanation of the variability of results from different numerical solvers. *Int. J. Numer. Methods Biomed. Eng.* 28, 890–903. doi: 10.1002/cnm.2467

Pathmanathan, P., Shotwell, M. S., Gavaghan, D. J., Cordeiro, J. M., and Gray, R. A. (2015). Uncertainty quantification of fast sodium current steady-state inactivation for multi-scale models of cardiac electrophysiology. *Prog. Biophys. Mol. Biol.* 117, 4–18. doi: 10.1016/j.pbiomolbio.2015.01.008

Pitt-Francis, J., Garny, A., and Gavaghan, D. (2006). Enabling computer models of the heart for high-performance computers and the grid. *Philos. Trans. A Math. Phys. Eng. Sci.* 364, 1501–1516. doi: 10.1098/rsta.2006.1783

Pueyo, E., Corrias, A., Virág, L., Jost, N., Szél, T., Varró, A., et al. (2011). A multiscale investigation of repolarization variability and its role in cardiac arrhythmogenesis. *Biophys. J.* 101, 2892–2902. doi: 10.1016/j.bpj.2011.09.060

Ramanna, H., Elvan, A., Wittkampf, F. H., de Bakker, J. M., Hauer, R. N., and Robles de Medina, E. O. (2001). Increased dispersion and shortened refractoriness caused by verapamil in chronic atrial fibrillation. *J. Am. Coll. Cardiol.* 37, 1403–1407. doi: 10.1016/S0735-1097(01)01132-9

Ramirez, R. J., Nattel, S., and Courtemanche, M. (2000). Mathematical analysis of canine atrial action potentials: rate, regional factors, and electrical remodeling. *Am. J. Physiol. Heart Circ. Physiol.* 279, H1767–H1785. doi: 10.1152/ajpheart.2000.279.4.H1767

Ravagli, E., Bucchi, A., Bartolucci, C., Paina, M., Baruscotti, M., DiFrancesco, D., et al. (2016). Cell-specific Dynamic Clamp analysis of the role of funny If current in cardiac pacemaking. *Prog. Biophys. Mol. Biol.* 120, 50–66. doi: 10.1016/j.pbiomolbio.2015.12.004

Ravens, U., Katircioglu-Öztürk, D., Wettwer, E., Christ, T., Dobrev, D., Voigt, N., et al. (2015). Application of the RIMARC algorithm to a large data set of action potentials and clinical parameters for risk prediction of atrial fibrillation. *Med. Biol. Eng. Comput.* 53, 263–273. doi: 10.1007/s11517-014-1232-0

Rees, C., Yang, J.-H., Santolini, M., Lusis, A. J., Weiss, J. N., and Karma, A. (2018). Variability and compensation of cardiomycoyte ionic conductances at the population level. *bioRxiv* [Preprint]. doi: 10.1101/283275

Rivolta, I., Clancy, C. E., Tateyama, M., Liu, H., Priori, S. G., and Kass, R. S. (2002). A novel SCN5A mutation associated with long QT-3: altered inactivation kinetics and channel dysfunction. *Physiol. Genomics* 10, 191–197. doi: 10.1152/physiolgenomics.00039.2002

Roberts, B. N., Yang, P. C., Behrens, S. B., Moreno, J. D., and Clancy, C. E. (2012). Computational approaches to understand cardiac electrophysiology and arrhythmias. *Am. J. Physiol. Heart Circ. Physiol.* 303, H766–H783. doi: 10.1152/ajpheart.01081.2011

Roden, D. M. (2008). Repolarization reserve: a moving target. *Circulation* 118, 981–982. doi: 10.1161/CIRCULATIONAHA.108.798918

Romero, L., Carbonell, B., Trenor, B., Rodríguez, B., Saiz, J., and Ferrero, J. M. (2011). Systematic characterization of the ionic basis of rabbit cellular electrophysiology using two ventricular models. *Prog. Biophys. Mol. Biol.* 107, 60–73. doi: 10.1016/j.pbiomolbio.2011.06.012

Romero, L., Pueyo, E., Fink, M., and Rodríguez, B. (2009). Impact of ionic current variability on human ventricular cellular electrophysiology. *Am. J. Physiol. Heart Circ. Physiol.* 297, H1436–H1445. doi: 10.1152/ajpheart.00263.2009

Rosati, B., Dong, M., Cheng, L., Liou, S. R., Yan, Q., Park, J. Y., et al. (2008). Evolution of ventricular myocyte electrophysiology. *Physiol. Genomics* 35, 262–272. doi: 10.1152/physiolgenomics.00159.2007

Rosati, B., and Mckinnon, D. (2004). Regulation of ion channel expression. *Circ. Res.* 94, 874–883. doi: 10.1161/01.RES.0000124921.81025.1F

Rose, T. (2017). *End of Average.* London: Penguin Books.

Sadrieh, A., Mann, S. A., Subbiah, R. N., Domanski, L., Taylor, J. A., Vandenberg, J. I., et al. (2013). Quantifying the origins of population variability in cardiac electrical activity through sensitivity analysis of the electrocardiogram. *J. Physiol.* 591, 4207–4222. doi: 10.1113/jphysiol.2013.251710

Sale, H., Wang, J., O'Hara, T. J., Tester, D. J., Phartiyal, P., He, J. Q., et al. (2008). Physiological properties of hERG 1a/1b heteromeric currents and a hERG 1b-specific mutation associated with Long-QT syndrome. *Circ. Res.* 103, e81–95. doi: 10.1161/CIRCRESAHA.108.185249

Sampson, K. J., Iyer, V., Marks, A. R., and Kass, R. S. (2010). A computational model of Purkinje fibre single cell electrophysiology: implications for the long QT syndrome. *J. Physiol.* 588, 2643–2655. doi: 10.1113/jphysiol.2010.187328

Sánchez, C., Bueno-Orovio, A., Wettwer, E., Loose, S., Simon, J., Ravens, U., et al. (2014). Inter-subject variability in human atrial action potential in sinus rhythm versus chronic atrial fibrillation. *PLoS ONE* 9:e105897. doi: 10.1371/journal.pone.0105897

Sarkar, A. X., Christini, D. J., and Sobie, E. A. (2012). Exploiting mathematical models to illuminate electrophysiological variability between individuals. *J. Physiol.* 590, 2555–2567. doi: 10.1113/jphysiol.2011.223313

Sarkar, A. X., and Sobie, E. A. (2010). Regression analysis for constraining free parameters in electrophysiological models of cardiac cells. *PLoS Comput. Biol.* 6:e1000914. doi: 10.1371/journal.pcbi.1000914

Sarkar, A. X., and Sobie, E. A. (2011). Quantification of repolarization reserve to understand interpatient variability in the response to proarrhythmic drugs: a computational analysis. *Heart Rhythm* 8, 1749–1755. doi: 10.1016/j.hrthm.2011.05.023

Sato, S., Yamauchi, S., Schuessler, R. B., Boineau, J. P., Matsunaga, Y., and Cox, J. L. (1992). The effect of augmented atrial hypothermia on atrial refractory period, conduction, and atrial flutter/fibrillation in the canine heart. *J. Thorac. Cardiovasc. Surg.* 104, 297–306.

Schram, G., Pourrier, M., Melnyk, P., and Nattel, S. (2002). Differential distribution of cardiac ion channel expression as a basis for regional specialization in electrical function. *Circ. Res.* 90, 939–950. doi: 10.1161/01.RES.0000018627.89528.6F

Schulz, D. J., Goaillard, J. M., and Marder, E. (2006). Variable channel expression in identified single and electrically coupled neurons in different animals. *Nat. Neurosci.* 9, 356–362. doi: 10.1038/nn1639

Schulz, D. J., Goaillard, J. M., and Marder, E. E. (2007). Quantitative expression profiling of identified neurons reveals cell-specific constraints on highly variable levels of gene expression. *Proc. Natl. Acad. Sci. U.S.A.* 104, 13187–13191. doi: 10.1073/pnas.0705827104

Sepulveda, N. G., Roth, B. J., and Wikswo, J. P. (1989). Current injection into a two-dimensional anisotropic bidomain. *Biophys. J.* 55, 987–999. doi: 10.1016/S0006-3495(89)82897-8

Sham, J. S., Hatem, S. N., and Morad, M. (1995). Species differences in the activity of the Na(+)-Ca2+ exchanger in mammalian cardiac myocytes. *J. Physiol.* 488 (Pt 3), 623–631. doi: 10.1113/jphysiol.1995.sp020995

Singh, S., Zoble, R. G., Yellen, L., Brodsky, M. A., Feld, G. K., Berk, M., et al. (2000). Efficacy and safety of oral dofetilide in converting to and maintaining sinus rhythm in patients with chronic atrial fibrillation or atrial flutter: the symptomatic atrial fibrillation investigative research on dofetilide (SAFIRE-D) study. *Circulation* 102, 2385–2390. doi: 10.1161/01.CIR.102.19.2385

Skibsbye, L., Jespersen, T., Christ, T., Maleckar, M. M., Van den Brink, J., Tavi, P., et al. (2016). Refractoriness in human atria: time and voltage dependence of sodium channel availability. *J. Mol. Cell. Cardiol.* 101, 26–34. doi: 10.1016/j.yjmcc.2016.10.009

Sobie, E. A. (2009). Parameter sensitivity analysis in electrophysiological models using multivariable regression. *Biophys. J.* 96, 1264–1274. doi: 10.1016/j.bpj.2008.10.056

Soltis, A. R., and Saucerman, J. J. (2010). Synergy between CaMKII Substrates and beta-Adrenergic Signaling in Regulation of Cardiac Myocyte Ca^{2+} Handling. *Biophys. J.* 99, 2038–2047. doi: 10.1016/j.bpj.2010.08.016

Soor, N., Morgan, R., Varela, M., and Aslanidi, O. V. (2016). Towards patient-specific modelling of lesion formation during radiofrequency catheter ablation for atrial fibrillation. *Conf. Proc. IEEE Eng. Med. Biol. Soc.* 2016, 489–492. doi: 10.1109/EMBC.2016.7590746

Soylu, M., Demir, A. D., Ozdemir, O., Soylu, O., Topaloglu, S., Kunt, A., et al. (2003). Increased dispersion of refractoriness in patients with atrial fibrillation in the early postoperative period after coronary artery bypass grafting. *J. Cardiovasc. Electrophysiol.* 14, 28–31. doi: 10.1046/j.1540-8167.2003.02218.x

Su, Z., Li, F., Spitzer, K. W., Yao, A., Ritter, M., and Barry, W. H. (2003). Comparison of sarcoplasmic reticulum Ca^{2+}-ATPase function in human, dog, rabbit, and mouse ventricular myocytes. *J. Mol. Cell. Cardiol.* 35, 761–767. doi: 10.1016/S0022-2828(03)00119-6

Syed, Z., Vigmond, E., Nattel, S., and Leon, L. J. (2005). Atrial cell action potential parameter fitting using genetic algorithms. *Med. Biol. Eng. Comput.* 43, 561–571. doi: 10.1007/BF02351029

Taneja, T., Mahnert, B. W., Passman, R., Goldberger, J., and Kadish, A. (2001). Effects of sex and age on electrocardiographic and cardiac electrophysiological properties in adults. *Pacing Clin. Electrophysiol.* 24, 16–21. doi: 10.1046/j.1460-9592.2001.00016.x

ten Tusscher, K. H., Noble, D., Noble, P. J., and Panfilov, A. V. (2004). A model for human ventricular tissue. *Am. J. Physiol. Heart Circ. Physiol.* 286, H1573–H1589. doi: 10.1152/ajpheart.00794.2003

ten Tusscher, K. H., and Panfilov, A. V. (2006). Alternans and spiral breakup in a human ventricular tissue model. *Am. J. Physiol. Heart Circ. Physiol.* 291, H1088–H1100. doi: 10.1152/ajpheart.00109.2006

Tobin, A. E., Cruz-Bermúdez, N. D., Marder, E., and Schulz, D. J. (2009). Correlations in ion channel mRNA in rhythmically active neurons. *PLoS ONE* 4:e6742. doi: 10.1371/journal.pone.0006742

Tomaiuolo, M., Bertram, R., Leng, G., and Tabak, J. (2012). Models of electrical activity: calibration and prediction testing on the same cell. *Biophys. J.* 103, 2021–2032. doi: 10.1016/j.bpj.2012.09.034

Trayanova, N. A. (2014). Mathematical approaches to understanding and imaging atrial fibrillation significance for mechanisms and management. *Circ. Res.* 114, 1516–1531. doi: 10.1161/CIRCRESAHA.114.302240

Tsujimae, K., Suzuki, S., Murakami, S., and Kurachi, Y. (2007). Frequency-dependent effects of various IKr blockers on cardiac action potential duration in a human atrial model. *Am. J. Physiol. Heart Circ. Physiol.* 293, H660–H669. doi: 10.1152/ajpheart.01083.2006

Vagos, M. R., Arevalo, H., de Oliveira, B. L., Sundnes, J., and Maleckar, M. M. (2017). A computational framework for testing arrhythmia marker sensitivities to model parameters in functionally calibrated populations of atrial cells. *Chaos* 27, 093941. doi: 10.1063/1.4999476

Vanier, M. C., and Bower, J. M. (1999). A comparative survey of automated parameter-search methods for compartmental neural models. *J. Comput. Neurosci.* 7, 149–171. doi: 10.1023/A:1008972005316

Vieira, D.,a,.G., Adriano, R. L. S., Vasconcelos, J. A., and Krahenbuhl, L. (2004). Treating constraints as objectives in multiobjective optimization problems using niched pareto genetic algorithm. *IEEE Trans. Magn.* 40, 1188–1191. doi: 10.1109/TMAG.2004.825006

Walmsley, J., Rodriguez, J. F., Mirams, G. R., Burrage, K., Efimov, I. R., and Rodriguez, B. (2013). mRNA expression levels in failing human hearts predict cellular electrophysiological remodeling: a population-based simulation study. *PLoS ONE* 8:e56359. doi: 10.1371/journal.pone.0056359

Wang, J., Liu, L., Feng, J., and Nattel, S. (1996). Regional and functional factors determining induction and maintenance of atrial fibrillation in dogs. *Am. J. Physiol.* 271, H148–H158. doi: 10.1152/ajpheart.1996.271.1.H148

Wang, W., Huang, H. H., Kay, M., and Cavazos, J. (2011). GPGPU accelerated cardiac arrhythmia simulations. *Conf. Proc. IEEE Eng. Med. Biol. Soc.* 2011, 724–727. doi: 10.1109/IEMBS.2011.6090164

Wang, Z., Feng, J., and Nattel, S. (1995). Idiopathic atrial fibrillation in dogs: electrophysiologic determinants and mechanisms of antiarrhythmic action of flecainide. *J. Am. Coll. Cardiol.* 26, 277–286. doi: 10.1016/0735-1097(95)90845-F

Weaver, C. M., and Wearne, S. L. (2008). Neuronal firing sensitivity to morphologic and active membrane parameters. *PLoS Comput. Biol.* 4:e11. doi: 10.1371/journal.pcbi.0040011

Weeke, P., Mosley, J. D., Hanna, D., Delaney, J. T., Shaffer, C., Wells, Q. S., et al. (2014). Exome sequencing implicates an increased burden of rare potassium channel variants in the risk of drug-induced long QT interval syndrome. *J. Am. Coll. Cardiol.* 63, 1430–1437. doi: 10.1016/j.jacc.2014.01.031

White, J. W., Rassweiler, A., Samhouri, J. F., Stier, A. C., and White, C. (2014). Ecologists should not use statistical significance tests to interpret simulation model results. *Oikos* 123, 385–388. doi: 10.1111/j.1600-0706.2013.01073.x

Xiao, L., Xiao, J., Luo, X., Lin, H., Wang, Z., and Nattel, S. (2008). Feedback remodeling of cardiac potassium current expression: a novel potential mechanism for control of repolarization reserve. *Circulation* 118, 983–992. doi: 10.1161/CIRCULATIONAHA.107.758672

Yan, G. X., Shimizu, W., and Antzelevitch, C. (1998). Characteristics and distribution of M cells in arterially perfused canine left ventricular wedge preparations. *Circulation* 98, 1921–1927. doi: 10.1161/01.CIR.98.18.1921

Yang, P. C., and Clancy, C. E. (2012). *In silico* prediction of sex-based differences in human susceptibility to cardiac ventricular tachyarrhythmias. *Front. Physiol.* 3:360. doi: 10.3389/fphys.2012.00360

Yang, P. C., El-Bizri, N., Romero, L., Giles, W. R., Rajamani, S., Belardinelli, L., et al. (2016). A computational model predicts adjunctive pharmacotherapy for cardiac safety via selective inhibition of the late cardiac Na current. *J. Mol. Cell. Cardiol.* 99, 151–161. doi: 10.1016/j.yjmcc.2016.08.011

Yang, P. C., Kurokawa, J., Furukawa, T., and Clancy, C. E. (2010). Acute effects of sex steroid hormones on susceptibility to cardiac arrhythmias: a simulation study. *PLoS Comput. Biol.* 6:e1000658. doi: 10.1371/journal.pcbi.1000658

Yang, P. C., Perissinotti, L. L., López-Redondo, F., Wang, Y., Demarco, K. R., Jeng, M. T., et al. (2017). A multiscale computational modelling approach predicts mechanisms of female sex risk in the setting of arousal-induced arrhythmias. *J. Physiol.* 595, 4695–4723. doi: 10.1113/JP273142

Zaniboni, M. (2011). 3D current-voltage-time surfaces unveil critical repolarization differences underlying similar cardiac action potentials: a model study. *Math. Biosci.* 233, 98–110. doi: 10.1016/j.mbs.2011.06.008

Zhang, Z. S., Tranquillo, J., Neplioueva, V., Bursac, N., and Grant, A. O. (2007). Sodium channel kinetic changes that produce Brugada syndrome or progressive cardiac conduction system disease. *Am. J. Physiol. Heart Circ. Physiol.* 292, H399–H407. doi: 10.1152/ajpheart.01025.2005

Zhao, J., Hansen, B. J., Wang, Y., Csepe, T. A., Sul, L. V., Tang, A., et al. (2017). Three-dimensional integrated functional, structural, and computational mapping to define the structural "fingerprints" of heart-specific atrial fibrillation drivers in human heart *ex vivo*. *J. Am. Heart. Assoc.* 6:e005922. doi: 10.1161/JAHA.117.005922

Zhou, J., Kodirov, S., Murata, M., Buckett, P. D., Nerbonne, J. M., and Koren, G. (2003). Regional upregulation of Kv2.1-encoded current, IK,slow2, in Kv1DN mice is abolished by crossbreeding with Kv2DN mice. *Am. J. Physiol. Heart Circ. Physiol.* 284, H491–H500. doi: 10.1152/ajpheart.00576.2002

Zhou, Q., Zygmunt, A. C., Cordeiro, J. M., Siso-Nadal, F., Miller, R. E., Buzzard, G. T., et al. (2009). Identification of Ikr kinetics and drug binding in native myocytes. *Ann. Biomed. Eng.* 37, 1294–1309. doi: 10.1007/s10439-009-9690-5

Zhou, X., Bueno-Orovio, A., Orini, M., Hanson, B., Hayward, M., Taggart, P., et al. (2016). *In vivo* and *in silico* investigation into mechanisms of frequency dependence of repolarization alternans in human ventricular cardiomyocytes. *Circ. Res.* 118, 266–278. doi: 10.1161/CIRCRESAHA.115.307836

Zhu, Z. I., and Clancy, C. E. (2007). Genetic mutations and arrhythmia: simulation from DNA to electrocardiogram. *J. Electrocardiol.* 40, S47–50. doi: 10.1016/j.jelectrocard.2007.05.033

12

Sudden Cardiac Death in Dialysis: Arrhythmic Mechanisms and the Value of Non-Invasive Electrophysiology

Dimitrios Poulikakos[1,2], Katerina Hnatkova[3], Sofia Skampardoni[1,2], Darren Green[1,2], Philip Kalra[1,2] and Marek Malik[3]*

[1] Renal Department, Salford Royal NHS Foundation Trust, Salford, United Kingdom, [2] Centre for Cardiac Research, Institute of Cardiovascular Sciences, The University of Manchester, Manchester, United Kingdom, [3] National Heart and Lung Institute, Imperial College London, London, United Kingdom

***Correspondence:**
Dimitrios Poulikakos
dimitrios.poulikakos@srft.nhs.uk;
dempoulikakos@hotmail.com

Sudden Cardiac Death (SCD) is the leading cause of cardiovascular death in dialysis patients. This review discusses potential underlying arrhythmic mechanisms of SCD in the dialysis population. It examines recent evidence from studies using implantable loop recorders and from electrophysiological studies in experimental animal models of chronic kidney disease. The review summarizes advances in the field of non-invasive electrophysiology for risk prediction in dialysis patients focusing on the predictive value of the QRS-T angle and of the assessments of autonomic imbalance by means of heart rate variability analysis. Future research directions in non-invasive electrophysiology are identified to advance the understanding of the arrhythmic mechanisms. A suggestion is made of incorporation of non-invasive electrophysiology procedures into clinical practice.

Key Concepts:

- Large prospective studies in dialysis patients with continuous ECG monitoring are required to clarify the underlying arrhythmic mechanisms of SCD in dialysis patients.
- Obstructive sleep apnoea may be associated with brady-arrhythmias in dialysis patients. Studies are needed to elucidate the burden and impact of sleeping disorders on arrhythmic complications in dialysis patients.
- The QRS-T angle has the potential to be used as a descriptor of uremic cardiomyopathy.
- The QRS-T angle can be calculated from routine collected surface ECGs. Multicenter collaboration is required to establish best methodological approach and normal values.
- Heart Rate Variability provides indirect assessment of cardiac modulation that may be relevant for cardiac risk prediction in dialysis patients. Short-term recordings with autonomic provocations are likely to overcome the limitations of out of hospital 24-h recordings and should be prospectively assessed.

Keywords: sudden cardiac death, arrhythmias, dialysis, QRS-T angle, TCRT, heart rate variability, implantable loop recorders

INTRODUCTION

Chronic kidney disease affects 5–7% of the global population and is associated with a 10-fold increase in cardiovascular mortality. Over 2 million people worldwide are on renal replacement therapy (Couser et al., 2011). Despite technological advances in the field of renal replacement therapy, the long-term survival of patients receiving chronic dialysis remains poor, comparable with survival in some forms of cancer (United States Renal Data System, 2012). Cardiovascular disease and infections account for most of these deaths. SCD accounts for a large proportion of cardiovascular deaths and almost one fourth of the overall mortality in these patients as evidenced from registry data (United States Renal Data System, 2012) and from prospective trials with death adjudication (Cheung et al., 2004; Wanner et al., 2005). High risk of SCD is present even at early stages of CKD but it increases substantially when patients are on HD. This high risk is aggravated by the fluctuations in volume and electrolyte status induced by the intermittent pattern of the treatment (Poulikakos et al., 2014a).

It has been shown that renal dysfunction increases the risk of ventricular arrhythmias in patients with underlying ischaemic heart disease. After a first myocardial infarction, the presence of CKD stage 3 was found to be associated with a sixfold increase in odds of developing VF independently of traditional cardiovascular risk factors (Dalal et al., 2012). Advanced CKD has been shown to be a strong predictor of appropriate delivery of shock therapies for ventricular arrhythmias in implantable cardioverter defibrillator recipients (Robin et al., 2006; Cuculich et al., 2007). In these patients, advanced CKD has also been associated with decreased time to the first appropriate shock (Hreybe et al., 2006). However, the implantation of cardioverter defibrillators based on existing guidance has not been associated with survival benefit in retrospective studies in this high-risk population (Charytan et al., 2011; Pun et al., 2015).

Although CKD often coexists with coronary artery disease (Herzog et al., 2011), SCD is also highly prevalent in dialysis patients without a history of coronary artery disease or impaired left ventricular ejection fraction (Baigent et al., 2011). Possible mechanisms that increase cardiovascular risk related to advanced CKD include the ensuing bone mineral abnormalities and vascular calcification (London et al., 2003), endothelial dysfunction (Poulikakos et al., 2014d), electrolyte fluxes (Wang et al., 2018), chronic inflammation (Nowak and Chonchol, 2018), insulin resistance (Semple et al., 2011), increased levels of FGF 23 (Gutiérrez et al., 2009; Isakova et al., 2011) and autonomic imbalance (Converse et al., 1992b). Based on epidemiological data, it has also been postulated that heritable factors contribute to the risk of cardiac arrest in patients receiving dialysis (Chan et al., 2015). However, the exact pathogenic mechanisms that interlink these factors and lead to the high risk cardiovascular phenotype in CKD remain elusive.

Furthermore, whereas the increased risk of ventricular arrhythmias due to advanced CKD in the context of severe ischaemic cardiomyopathy has been confirmed (Robin et al., 2006; Cuculich et al., 2007; Dalal et al., 2012; Wan et al., 2014), the underlying arrhythmic mechanisms leading to SCD in dialysis patients with preserved left ventricular function are not well understood. Recent studies that used ILR in small cohorts of asymptomatic HD patients have shown increased rates of bradyarrhythmic events and deaths (Kalra et al., 2018).

Risk stratification strategies to identify dialysis individuals who are at high risk of SCD are lacking. This is despite them attending hospital or satellite facilities for their dialysis treatment three times weekly and having clinical observations and blood tests more often than any other out-patient group. Because of this, it is recognized that non-invasive electrophysiology could serve the unmet clinical need for risk prediction in this population (Skampardoni et al., 2018b). Descriptors of repolarization aberration and autonomic dysregulation can be assessed by applying advanced computerized analysis of snapshot and/or continuous ECGs and can be used for this purpose. There is accumulating evidence that increased QRS-T angle is a good descriptor of the arrhythmogenic myocardial substrate and predicts cardiovascular risk in this population (Skampardoni et al., 2018b). Furthermore, measurements of cardiac autonomic regulation by HRV have also shown promising results in cardiac risk assessment in dialysis patients.

This review summarizes the recent evidence from the use of ILRs in HD patients and electrophysiological studies in animal models of CKD, exploring the potential underlying arrhythmic mechanisms. It also presents the evidence from the use of non-invasive electrocardiography in dialysis patients focusing on QRS-T angle and HRV and concludes with suggestions for future directions of research.

Arrhythmic Patterns in Dialysis Patients. Insight From Studies Involving Continuous ECG Monitoring From Implantable Loop Recorders

Since 2015, five studies using ILR in asymptomatic HD patients have been published (Silva et al., 2015; Wong M.C. et al., 2015; Roberts et al., 2017; Roy-Chaudhury et al., 2018; Sacher et al., 2018) (**Table 1**). Collectively, they included 317 prevalent HD patients with largely preserved left ventricular ejection fraction. The age ranged from 56 $\pm$ 12 (Roy-Chaudhury et al., 2018) to 68 $\pm$ 12 (Roberts et al., 2017) years and follow up time ranged from 6 (Roy-Chaudhury et al., 2018) to 21 $\pm$ 7 (Sacher et al., 2018) months. In total, there were 52 deaths (15%) of which 21 (6.6% of patients, 40% of deaths) were classified as SCD. ILRs revealed bradyarrhythmia or asystole as the terminal rhythm in the majority (13) of SCD deaths. SCD cases in the 5 studies ranged from 83% (Wong M.C.G. et al., 2015) to 25% (Roberts et al., 2017) of all deaths and bradycardia as the terminal SCD rhythm was reported in 42% (Silva et al., 2015) to 100% (Sacher et al., 2018) of SCD cases. On the contrary, there were only 4 cases of sustained VT or VF across the 5 studies. In total 9 patients required pacemaker implantation for bradyarrhythmia

---

Abbreviations: AF, atrial fibrillation; CKD, chronic kidney disease; ECG, electrocardiogram; HD, hemodialysis; HRV, heart rate variability; IHD, ischemic heart disease; ILR, implantable loop recorder; SCD, sudden cardiac death; TCRT, total Cosine R To T; VF, ventricular fibrillation; VT, ventricular tachycardia.

TABLE 1 | Studies using implantable loop recorders in HD patients.

Study	Number	Age (years)	IHD	Follow up (months)	SCD/Total mortality (%)	Brady-arrhythmic SCD	VT-VF	Significant arrhythmic events	Comments
Wong M.C.G. et al., 2015	50	67 ± 11	48%	18 ± 4	8/10 (80%)	6	2	**Pacemaker in 1 patient** Bradycardia 30% Sinus arrest 28% 2nd degree atrioventricular block 4% Non-sustained VT 20% AF 28%	All SCDs and increased rates of arrhythmias during long interdialytic interval.
Silva et al., 2015	100	59 ± 8.8	34%	14 ± 4	7/18 (39%)	3	1	Bradycardia 25% Asystole 4% Non-sustained VT 56% AF 13%	Left Ventricular dilatation associated with higher occurrence of non-sustained VT.
Sacher et al., 2018	71	65 ± 9	NR	21 ± 7	4/16 (25%)	4	–	Conduction Abnormalities 14% (patient years) Non-sustained VT 9% (patient years) AF 37% (20% *de novo*)	
Roberts et al., 2017	30	68 ± 12	22%	18 ± 12	2/8 (25%)	0	1	**Pacemakers in 3 patients** (2 dual chamber pacemakers and 1 biventricular pacemaker)	Increased nocturnal bradycardias.
Roy-Chaudhury et al., 2018	66	56 ± 12	48.5%	6	0	–	–	**Pacemakers in 5 patients** Bradycardia 25.8% Asystolic events* 10.6% Non-sustained Ventricular arrhythmias * 77.3% AF* 40.9% (device detected)	Increased rates of bradyarrhythmic events at the end of long interdialytic interval.

AF, atrial fibrillation; IHD, ischemic heart disease; NR, not reported; SCD, sudden cardiac death; VT, ventricular tachycardia; VF, ventricular fibrillation. Table was modified with permission by Kalra et al. (2018).

across the 5 studies [3/30 patients in the study by Roberts et al. (2017), 5/66 in the study by Roy-Chaudhury et al. (2018), and 1/50 in the study by Wong M.C. et al. (2015)]. The temporal pattern of arrhythmias in the detailed study by Roy-Chaudhury et al. (2018) showed an increased rate of clinically significant bradycardias, defined as rate <40 bpm for ≥6 s, toward the latter stages of the long interdialytic interval. One of the studies (Roberts et al., 2017) reported on the circadian pattern of the bradycardic episodes noting an increased rates during night-time. The proportion of patients with at least one episode of severe bradycardia ranged from 20% (Roy-Chaudhury et al., 2018) to 25% (Silva et al., 2015) and asystolic events ranged from 4% (Silva et al., 2015) to 20% (Wong M.C.G. et al., 2015). The studies reported high rates of AF ranging from 13% (Silva et al., 2015) to 40.9% (Roy-Chaudhury et al., 2018).

Although these studies provide novel information, this should be interpreted with caution. The scarcity of available information about the prevalence of bradyarrhythmias from long-term monitoring in asymptomatic patients need to be taken into consideration.

Previous studies using 24-h recordings in healthy individuals have shown a high prevalence of bradycardias (heart rate 40 beats/min or less) during sleep at 24% in males aged 22–27 years (Brodsky et al., 1977). With advancing age, this decreased to 3% in subjects aged 40–79 years (Bjerregaard, 1983) and 2% in the group aged 60–85 years (Fleg and Kennedy, 1982). ILRs are likely to detect more bradycardic events than 24 h Holter monitors (Simantirakis et al., 2004) but have not been used to study healthy populations.

The participants in the HD ILR studies were not young and, despite the lack of knowledge regarding the normal incidence of bradycardias in HD patients and notwithstanding the small number of relatively low cardiovascular risk participants and the heterogeneity amongst the studies, these investigations show a high burden of bradyarrhythmias in HD patients with preserved ejection fraction. This potentially contributes substantially to the overall burden of SCD. Consistent with the HD ILR studies, a recent epidemiological study that investigated registry data of 28,471 dialysis patients (Wang et al., 2016) showed that HD patients had an almost sixfold increased incidence of requiring pacemaker insertion compared to matched patients with normal renal function.

Pathogenesis of Bradycardia

Elucidating the underlying mechanisms of bradycardias and their relationship to SCD has important clinical implications relating to the required routine screening, to the decisions of potential use of beta blockers, and/or to considerations of potential interventions such as pacemaker insertion.

Electrolyte shifts, especially pre-dialysis hyperkalaemia, have been implicated as potential triggers of bradyarrhythmias particularly at the end of the long interdialytic interval in a typical 3 dialysis session week. The electrophysiological role of hyperkalaemia in triggering bradyarrhythmias is likely potentiated by the presence of underlying structural abnormalities in the conduction system and/or abnormal cardiac autonomic regulation of the pacemaker activity that prevent adequate heart rate reactions in response to physiological stress. Cardiac valve calcification may affect the cardiac conduction system and has also been implicated in bradyarrhythmias (Mainigi et al., 2012). It is highly prevalent in HD (Matsuo et al., 2018) and peritoneal dialysis (PD) patients (Wang et al., 2003) and has been associated with increased cardiovascular mortality (Wang et al., 2018). In addition, evidence of impaired cardiac autonomic modulation in dialysis patients has been demonstrated in several HRV studies (Poulikakos et al., 2014a).

The potential contribution of obstructive sleep apnoea to bradyarrhythmias in dialysis patients merits attention. Sleep apnoea is typically characterized by episodes of bradycardia (Zwillich et al., 1982) as shown with long term recordings with ILR in this population (Simantirakis et al., 2004). Sleep apnoea is highly prevalent in HD patients occurring in 34.5% (Tada et al., 2007) to 65% (Sakaguchi et al., 2011) of cases. It is commonly underdiagnosed and its severity has been associated with the magnitude of fluid overload (Ogna et al., 2015). Interestingly, bradyarrhythmias due to sleep apnoea do not seem to be potentiated by the administration of beta blockers (Wolf et al., 2016) and can be successfully treated with continuous positive airway pressure treatment (Simantirakis et al., 2004). No information regarding the presence of sleep apnoea was provided in the publications of the HD ILR studies. However, it can be speculated that it was present in a fair proportion of the participants and that sleep apnoea related bradyarrhythmias would tend to increase during periods of increased fluid retention, i.e., at the end of the long interdialytic interval.

Atrial Fibrillation and Sudden Cardiac Death

The high rate of AF in the HD population is another important finding and may be linked to increased risk of SCD. Evidence suggests that AF may be associated with SCD in cardiac patients (Gronefeld et al., 2000; Berton et al., 2009; Pedersen et al., 2006) and in the general population (Chen et al., 2013). Several mechanisms have been suggested linking AF with SCD (Chen et al., 2014). It has been speculated that fast ventricular rate in the context of atrial tachyarrhythmia can reduce ventricular refractoriness (Denes et al., 1974) thus increasing the vulnerability to ventricular arrhythmias. In addition, AF can lead to short-long-short sequences in the ventricular cycle length that in turn predispose to some types of ventricular arrhythmias (Gronefeld et al., 2000).

ARRHYTHMIC MECHANISMS IN ANIMAL MODELS OF CKD

Animal models have been used to investigate the pre-arrhythmic substrate and the mechanisms of arrhythmias in CKD (**Table 2**).

Hsueh et al. (2014) used a rat cystic kidney disease model (Cy/+ rats) characterized by progressive CKD that reaches terminal uraemia in about 40 weeks. They investigated 12 CKD and 9 normal rats at week 35 with detailed electrophysiological studies including optical mapping and a pacing protocol for VF induction. CKD rats showed increased action potential duration and longer cycle length thresholds to induce action potential duration alterans compared to normal rats, indicating increased vulnerability to ventricular arrhythmias. VF was induced in 9/12 (75%) CKD rats compared to 2/9 (22%) normal rats. Examination of the heart tissue following euthanasia revealed upregulation of pro-fibrotic pathways in CKD animals but did not show significant difference in cardiac fibrosis between the two groups.

Lee et al. (2017) used a rat model of mild CKD (unilateral nephrectomy at 8 weeks) and performed electrophysiological studies 8 weeks after the operation, including surface ECG. After euthanasia, cardiomyocytes were isolated for further electrophysiological recordings of ionic currents and membrane potential. CKD rats exhibited prolonged QTc compared to normal rats. Longer action potential duration at 50 and 90% repolarization of paced cardiomyocytes was observed in epicardiac cardiomyocytes in CKD rats compared to normal rats but there was no difference in endocardial cardiomyocytes. The transient outward potassium current I_{to} was reduced in epicardial cardiomyocytes in CKD rats compared to controls, and associated with decreased transmural gradient of I_{to}. Similar to the previous study, increased heterogeneity of repolarization occurred independently of the cardiac fibrosis that was observed at similar levels in CKD and normal rats (Chang et al., 2015).

(Zhao et al. (2016) used the same CKD model as presented by Hsueh et al. (2014) (Cy/+ rats). The animals were implanted with ECG and subcutaneous nerve activity electrode recorders at 35 weeks. Subcutaneous nerve activity has been shown to correlate with the stellate ganglion nerve activity and was thus used to estimate the sympathetic tone (Robinson et al., 2015). All 6 CKD rats died suddenly 23 ± 14 days after the implantation. All SCDs occurred after the development of atrioventricular block. Terminal rhythms were progressive bradycardia and asystole in 3 rats, VF in 2 rats and VT converted to bradycardia in one rat. In contrast to the previous studies, histology showed fibrosis in all CKD rats, especially surrounding the AV node and in the sub-endocardium, and calcification affecting the conduction system. These findings were not present in normal rats. The magnitude of the increase in heart rate corresponding to increase in subcutaneous nerve activity was smaller in CKD rats 5 days prior to death.

Fontes et al. (2015) used two different mouse models of renal impairment. First model included aged mice that received deoxycorticosterone acetate for 8 weeks and a high-salt diet that continued for 35 weeks. Second model dealt with adult mice that underwent 5/6-subtotal nephrectomy and were treated for 11 weeks with a high-salt diet. *Ex vivo* epicardial mapping was used to assess vulnerability to arrhythmias and hearts were assessed for fibrosis and characterized for connexin 43 (Cx43). Both models demonstrated a high incidence of arrhythmias accompanied by increased interstitial fibrosis and decreased Cx43 expression in the heart.

The first two animal investigations (Hsueh et al., 2014; Lee et al., 2017) suggest that electrophysiological aberrations leading to increased repolarization heterogeneity and vulnerability to

TABLE 2 | Electrophysiological studies in animal models of CKD.

Study	Animal model	Electrophysiological study	Time	Fibrosis assessment	Time	Main findings
Hsueh et al., 2014	Cy/+ rats (12) compared to normal rats (9)	Optical mapping Induced VF via pacing	35 weeks	Picrosirius red staining	35 weeks	Longer action potential duration at 80% repolarization and cycle length thresholds to induce alterans in CKD rats. VF induced in 9/12 CKD rats vs. 2/9 normal rats. Electrical remodeling favoring initiation and maintenance of VTs in CKD rats. No difference in cardiac fibrosis.
Lee et al., 2017	Unilateral nephrectomy at 8 weeks rats (6) compared to sham operated rats (6)	Surface ECG Patch-clamp studies	8 weeks after nephrectomy	Trichrome staining and picrosirius red staining* Cellular hypertrophy based on cellular capacitance in ventricular cardiomyocytes	8 weeks post nephrectomy	Prolonged QTc in CKD rats. Epicardial prolongation of action potential duration in CKD rats and decreased transmural gradient in CKD rats compared to controls. Electronegative LDL may underlie downregulation of KChIP2 protein expression. No difference in fibrosis.
Zhao et al., 2016	Cy/+ rats (6) Compared to normal rats (8)	Continuous ECG Subcutaneous nerve activity recordings	Started at 35 weeks and continued for 23 ± 14 days	Trichrome staining H&E staining	40 weeks for normal rats After sudden death at CKD rats (35 weeks+ 23 ± 14 days)	6 deaths due to bradycardia or atrioventricular block. 3 deaths due to VT/VF. Myocardial calcification involving the conduction system. Blunted response of heart rate to subcutaneous nerve activity increase in CKD rats. Sudden death preceded by reduction in subcutaneous nerve activity.
Fontes et al., 2015	Aged mice deoxycorticosterone acetate and high salt diet ($n = 7$) & 5/6 -subtotal nephrectomy and high salt diet (5) Controls (4)	Programmed electrical stimulation of arrhythmias Conduction velocity from electrocardiograms	68 weeks 11 weeks	Picrosirius red staining	68 weeks 11 weeks	Arrhythmias induced in 86 and 75% in hearts from aged mice and partially nephrectomised mice on high salt diet compared to 0% in control hearts. Cx43 expression was reduced and interstitial fibrosis was increased in both groups with renal dysfunction.

*CKD, chronic kidney disease; Cx43, connexin 43, gap junction protein expressed in the heart; ECG, electrocardiogram; VT, ventricular tachycardia; VF, ventricular fibrillation. *Experiments on cardiac fibrosis were performed in previous study of the same group using the same CKD rat model.*

ventricular arrhythmias occur before the development of overt cardiac fibrosis and calcification which is in turn associated with conduction system disorders and bradyarrhythmias in advanced CKD in rodents. Considering the two studies (Hsueh et al., 2014; Zhao et al., 2016) that used the same Cy/+ CKD models, Hsueh et al. (2014) did not find fibrosis in heart tissue retrieved following euthanasia at 35 weeks whereas Zhao et al. (2016) detected fibrosis and calcification in heart tissue retrieved 3 weeks later (after death), i.e., in animals exposed to CKD for longer.

The observation that the relationship between subcutaneous nerve activity, a surrogate of sympathetic tone, and heart rate was different in CKD rats compared to normal rats is in keeping with human studies describing abnormal autonomic cardiac modulation in CKD.

However, fundamental electrophysiological differences exist between rodents and large mammals (Sallam et al., 2015), making rodents a poor model of human electrophysiology. Furthermore, these animal models did not study the dynamic interactions of the fluctuations in fluid and electrolyte changes. Therefore their contribution in understanding the mechanisms of SCD in dialysis patients is limited. Thus, interpretation and extrapolations from these animal experiments need to be made with caution.

NON-INVASIVE ELECTROPHYSIOLOGY IN DIALYSIS PATIENTS

The standard 12 lead ECG is an essential clinical tool in CKD and dialysis patients (Skampardoni et al., 2018b). It is commonly used for the assessment of the acutely unwell patient. It can also be used as routine investigation for the detection of conduction abnormalities that require clinical intervention such as with medication or dialysis prescription review, further studies and referral for pacemaker implantation. However, the fluctuant fluid and electrolyte status of HD patients may affect the ECG waveform that in turn can influence the automated ECG interpretations including interval calculations (Poulikakos and Malik, 2016). This influence poses challenges in using automated ECG measurements in risk stratification studies. Furthermore, important repolarization abnormalities usually referred to as "non-specific T wave changes" are only subjectively defined and cannot be studied in a quantifiable manner. Advanced computerized analysis of the ECG has the potential to overcome these limitations.

Repolarization Heterogeneity and the Case for QRS-T Angle Assessment in CKD

The QRS-T angle is an established marker of global repolarization heterogeneity (Waks et al., 2016; Hnatkova et al., 2017) that can be measured from a standard 12 lead ECG (**Figure 1**). It is based on three-dimensional vectorial representation of the electrical activity of the heart, that is not affected by impedance changes due to fluid shifts (Vitolo et al., 1987). The QRS-T angle is calculated numerically, is reproducible (Poulikakos et al., 2013; Hnatkova et al., 2017) and thus suitable for risk stratification purposes. A larger QRS-T angle has been shown to predict SCD (de Bie et al., 2013b; Tereshchenko et al., 2016), cardiovascular mortality (Skampardoni et al., 2018a) and all cause mortality (Tereshchenko et al., 2016; de Bie et al., 2013b; Poulikakos et al., 2018) in different cohorts of predominantly African (Tereshchenko et al., 2016) and Caucasian (Sallam et al., 2015; Poulikakos et al., 2018; Skampardoni et al., 2018a) dialysis patients. However, one study in 325 Taiwanese HD patients (Lin et al., 2007) did not find a significant association between magnitude of QRS-T angle and outcomes. Instead, this study reported that T wave residuum, a descriptor of regional repolarization heterogeneity (Zabel and Malik, 2002), was an independent predictor of cardiovascular mortality and SCD. Studies that have investigated the prognostic value of the QRS-T angle in dialysis patients are summarized in **Table 3**.

An increased QRS-T angle has been associated with echocardiographic left ventricular hypertrophy (Tereshchenko et al., 2016), decreased global longitudinal strain (Skampardoni et al., 2018a), lower left ventricular ejection fraction, and with left ventricular systolic dyssynchrony (de Bie et al., 2013a) in different cohorts of HD patients. It has also been associated with increased coronary artery calcium burden, and elevated Troponin T levels in patients receiving peritoneal dialysis (Jaroszynski et al., 2009). The impact of HD treatment on the QRS-T angle has been variable (Jaroszynski et al., 2010; Poulikakos et al., 2013). The intra-subject stability of the QRS-T angle at the start and the end of dialysis has been demonstrated in a cohort of 72 HD patients who underwent five intra-dialytic Holter ECGs at 2-week intervals (Poulikakos et al., 2013). Studies reporting on associations of the QRS-T angle with echocardiographic characteristics and intradialytic changes are presented in **Table 4**. **Figure 2** shows an example of Kaplan–Meier event probability curves of major cardiac events and overall mortality in 72 HD patients (Poulikakos et al., 2018) stratified by QRS-T angle above and below median value.

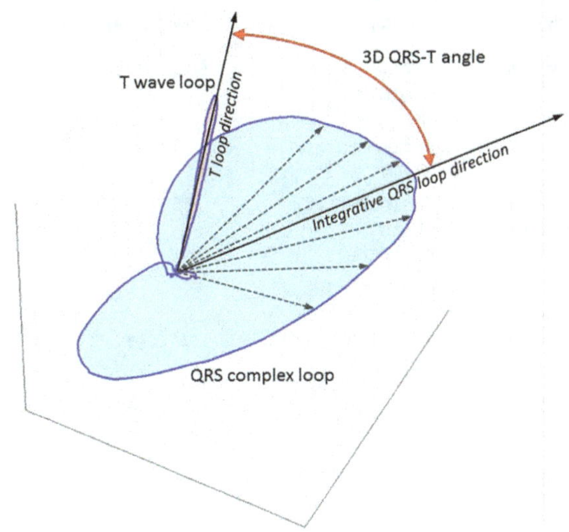

FIGURE 1 | Three-dimensional representation of QRS and T vector loops following computerized analysis of standard 12 lead ECG using singular value decomposition to yield an orthogonal lead system (TCRT method). The little white circle in the middle depicts the loop of the p wave. The curved red line with arrow at both ends depicts the spatial QRS-T angle. The maximal T wave vector magnitude is used for the calculations with this method. TCRT is the averaged cosine of the angles between the T wave vector and all vectors within the QRS complex exceeding a pre-defined level. A different method of QRS-T angle measurement from standard 12 lead digital snapshot ECG uses inverse Dower matrix for vectrographic transformation and calculates the angle between the mean vectors of the QRS and T wave. QRS-T angle has also been calculated from continuous signal averaged ECGs as the angle between the peak QRS vector and the peak T vector.

Methodological Considerations

Different groups have used different methods for the calculation of the QRS-T angle that are summarized in **Table 3**. The methodological differences stem from different approaches in characterizing the spatial deviation between the vectorial loops of depolarization (QRS) and repolarization (T wave). These differences may partially explain the different numerical cut-off values (Hnatkova et al., 2017) used in predicting outcomes in dialysis populations. The challenge lies mainly in the fact that the loops can be irregular and curved in space. It has recently been demonstrated in cardiac patients that the discrepancies between the various methods increase as the angle becomes more abnormal and the distortion of the vectors increases (Hnatkova et al., 2017). In a recent comparative study in cardiac patients, the calculation of the QRS-T angle by the so-called TCRT method was more reliable for cardiac risk prediction. It is thought that the calculation of the sum of the cosines between QRS and T wave vectors increases the ability of depicting the shape and orientation irregularities that accompany increased repolarization heterogeneity.

Racial, and previously described sex differences (Smetana et al., 2002) should also be taken into consideration in studies measuring the QRS-T angle. For example, in the Taiwanese

TABLE 3 | Studies of QRS-T angle for risk prediction in dialysis patients.

Study	Participants	Age (years)	IHD	Calculation	Follow up	Outcome
de Bie et al., 2013b	277 (prevalent) Male 62.1% HD 62.8% Peritoneal dialysis 37.2%	56.3 ± 17.0	24.5%	Inverse Dower matrix from standard 12 lead snapshot ECG. **Measured as angle between mean QRS and T vectors.**	60 months	QRS-T angle independent predictor of all-cause mortality (*N* = 91) and SCD (*N* = 18).
Tereshchenko et al., 2016	358 (incident HD) Male 59% Black 73%	55 ± 13	37%	Calculated from continuous unfiltered averaged *xyz* ECG signal. **Measured as angle between spatial mean QRS vector and spatial peak T vector.**	864.6 person-years of follow-up	QRS-T angle associated with all-cause mortality (*N* = 77) cardiovascular mortality (*N* = 35) and SCD (*N* = 15).
Skampardoni et al., 2018a	178 (prevalent HD) Male 72% Caucasian 80% South Asian 17% Black 3%	67 ± 14	23.5%	Singular value decomposition to standard snapshot 12 lead ECG. **Measured as total cosine R to T.**	36 ± 19 months	TCRT independent predictor of cardiac deaths (*N* = 17) and major cardiac events (*N* = 54).
Poulikakos et al., 2018	72 (prevalent HD) Males 58% Caucasian 44% Black 31% South Asians 25%	61 ± 15	21%	Singular value decomposition to overlapping 10 s segment 12 lead ECGs during continuous monitoring repeated 5 times every 2 weeks. **Measured as total cosine R to T.**	54.8 months	TRCT independent predictor of all-cause mortality (*N* = 16) and major cardiac events (*N* = 9).
Lin et al., 2007	325 (incident) HD Male 44% Taiwanese population	64 ± 13	19%	Singular value decomposition to standard snapshot 12 lead ECG. **Measured as total cosine R to T**	25 ± 22 months	TRCT not associated with all-cause mortality (*N* = 154) cardiovascular mortality (*N* = 79) or arrhythmia related deaths (*N* = 59). T wave residuum independent predictor for all outcomes.

ECG, electrocardiogram; F/up, follow up; HD, hemodialysis; IHD, Ischemic heart disease; SCD, sudden cardiac death; TCRT, Total Cosine R to T.

HD cohort there was no association between QRS-T angle and cardiac outcomes whereas there was with T wave residuum; this may reflect racial differences in repolarization heterogeneity patterns and QRS-T angle. In a previous population study in healthy subjects, the QRS-T angle in Taiwanese individuals was significantly different compared to African, Caucasian and Indian healthy subjects (Elaine and Macfarlane, 2016).

The mechanisms linking abnormal repolarization heterogeneity with clinical outcomes and cardiac structure and function abnormalities remain unclear and will need to be assessed in prospective studies.

Autonomic Dysfunction and Heart Rate Variability in CKD

Sympathetic overactivation has short and long-term proarrhythmogenic effects and may play a role in the pathogenesis of arrhythmic deaths in CKD patients. Sympathetic activation impacts on cellular channel activity increasing repolarization heterogeneity (Vaseghi et al., 2012) and plays a role in the pathogenesis of cardiac fibrosis via α-adrenergic receptor stimulation and via triggering inflammatory responses (Levick et al., 2010). Autonomic imbalance decreases myocardial ability to suppress disorganized electrical activation and may compromise the heart pacemaker response to challenges.

Sympathetic nerve activity, assessed by microneurography of the peroneal nerve, increases with declining renal function (Grassi et al., 2011) and is elevated in patients with end-stage renal disease (Converse et al., 1992b). Potential contributing underlying mechanisms of sympathetic overactivation in CKD (Kaur et al., 2017) include elevated angiotensin 2 levels (Siddiqi et al., 2009) that potentiate norepinephrine release from sympathetic nerve terminals, stimulation of afferent renal nerves and chemoreceptors by adenosine release due to renal ischaemia (Biaggioni et al., 1991; Vallon et al., 2006), and reduced nitric oxide (NO) availability (Jourde-Chiche et al., 2011) potentiated by upregulation of MicroRNA-92a in dialysis patients (Young et al., 2009; Shang et al., 2017).

The baroreflex regulation has also been shown to be impaired in CKD. In dialysis patients, impaired baroreflex sensitivity was shown to be associated with vascular calcification and arterial stiffness (Chesterton et al., 2005) indicating a potential anatomical link between vascular changes and the function of baroreceptors.

Direct measurement of the autonomic system with microneurography poses practical challenges and is not suitable for clinical practice. Nevertheless, indirect measurements are possible by assessing HRV (Task Force of the European Society of Cardiology and North American Society of Pacing and Electrophysiology, 1996). HRV is a non-invasive method based on analysis of tachograms of continuous ECGs. It assesses the cardiac autonomic regulation based on the differences in cardiac pacemaker responses to autonomic activations. HRV can provide an approximation of the cardiac autonomic regulation that integrates multiple feedback systems. In addition to traditional time and frequency domain measurement several different

TABLE 4 | Studies of QRS-T angle reporting on associations with cardiovascular parameters and dialysis procedure.

Study	Participants	Age (years)	IHD	Calculation of QRS-T angle	Findings
de Bie et al., 2013a	101 prevalent Male 76% 66% HD, 44% Peritoneal Dialysis	56.3 ± 17	30%	Inverse Dower matrix from standard 12 lead snapshot ECG. **Measured as angle between mean QRS and T vectors.**	QRS-T angle associated with left ventricular ejection fraction, QRS duration and left ventricular systolic dyssynchrony.
Tereshchenko et al., 2016	358 incident HD Male 59% Black 73%	55 ± 13	37%	Calculated from continuous unfiltered averaged *xyz* ECG signal. **Measured as angle between spatial mean QRS vector and spatial peak T vector.**	QRS-T angle >75° associated with wider QRS and echocardiographic left ventricular hypertrophy defined as left ventricular mass index >51 g/m$^{2.7}$ in men and >47 g/m$^{2.7}$ in women.
Skampardoni et al., 2018a	178 prevalent HD Male 72% Caucasian 80% South Asian 17% Black 3%	67 ± 14	23.5%	Singular value decomposition to standard snapshot 12 lead ECG. **Measured as total cosine R to T.**	QRS-T angle by TCRT correlated with left ventricular mass indexed for height in univariate and Global Longitudinal Strain in multivariate analysis.
Jaroszynski et al., 2009	57 prevalent Peritoneal Dialysis patients 49% male Caucasians	47.7 ± 7.1	Excluded	Inverse Dower matrix from standard 12 lead snapshot ECG. **Measured as angular difference between maximum spatial QRS and T vectors.**	QRS-T angle associated with increased coronary artery calcium burden, atherosclerosis and troponin T elevation.
Jaroszynski et al., 2010	73 prevalent HD 52% male Caucasians	51.5 ± 4.5	Not reported	Inverse Dower matrix from standard 12 lead snapshot ECG. **Measured as angular difference between maximum spatial QRS and T vectors.**	QRS-T angle associated with Troponin T. HD session resulted in increased QRS-T in 59 patients, decreased in 12 patients, and unchanged in 2 patients.
Poulikakos et al., 2013	72 (prevalent HD) Males 70%	61 ± 15	21%	Singular value decomposition to overlapping 10 s segment 12 lead ECGs during continuous monitoring repeated 5 times every 2 weeks. **Measured as total cosine R to T.**	Intra-subject reproducibility confirmed using analysis of variance. Variable effect of HD to TCRT Intradialytic QRS-T change correlated with PTH levels.

ECG, electrocardiogram; HD, hemodialysis; IHD, Ischemic heart disease; TCRT, total Cosine R to T.

methodologies have been developed (Task Force of the European Society of Cardiology and North American Society of Pacing and Electrophysiology, 1996; Sassi et al., 2015).

Many groups have used HRV methodology in dialysis patients. A pubmed search using the terms HRV and dialysis returns 122 studies with the first one published already in 1986 (Forsstrom et al., 1986). Abnormal HRV indices have been associated with all cause (Hayano et al., 1999; Oikawa et al., 2009; Suzuki et al., 2012; Chen et al., 2016; Ng et al., 2017; Poulikakos et al., 2018) and cardiovascular mortality (Hayano et al., 1999; Fukuta et al., 2003; Oikawa et al., 2009; Chen et al., 2016) in east Asian HD patients and in one small study including predominantly Caucasian HD patients (Skampardoni et al., 2018a). Depressed HRV has also been associated with all cause (Pei et al., 2015; Chiang et al., 2016) and cardiovascular (Hayano et al., 1999) mortality in east Asian patients receiving peritoneal dialysis.

Frequent daily HD has been shown to improve components of HRV (Chan et al., 2014). Preserved residual urine output has also been associated with different HRV profiles in peritoneal dialysis patients (Tang et al., 2012) and depressed HRV has been associated with increased PTH (Zhang et al., 2013, 2015; Poulikakos et al., 2014b; Jiang et al., 2016) and FGF 23 levels (Zhang et al., 2015). Depressed HRV has also been associated with increased pulse pressure (Poulikakos et al., 2014c) in patients with end stage renal disease and with increased pulse wave velocity in patients with CKD stages 3–5 (Chandra et al., 2014).

Despite the consistent results confirming the value of HRV in CKD patients, major challenges exist in extrapolating associations from these studies and incorporating HRV measurements into clinical practice. The main challenge is related to the sensitivity of HRV to environmental influences and the need for strict standardization, particularly for 24-h ECG recordings, which is practically impossible when the recording is performed in the outpatient setting.

Short Term HRV Measurements During Autonomic Provocations in HD Patients

For the purposes of standardized assessment, several studies used short term recordings around or during the dialysis procedure, i.e., a period with relatively standardized environment characterized by volume and electrolyte shifts that provoke the autonomic system in a predictable manner. It is known that patients who exhibit excessive intradialytic decline in systolic blood pressure have higher risk of cardiovascular and overall mortality (Chou et al., 2018; Reeves and Mc Causland, 2018). The pathogenesis of intradialytic hypotension is multifactorial (Reeves and Mc Causland, 2018) but it has been postulated that abnormal activation of the sympathetic system plays a central role (Converse et al., 1992a). Some studies have shown that spectral HRV assessment during intradialytic recordings can differentiate patients who are prone to intradialytic hypotension

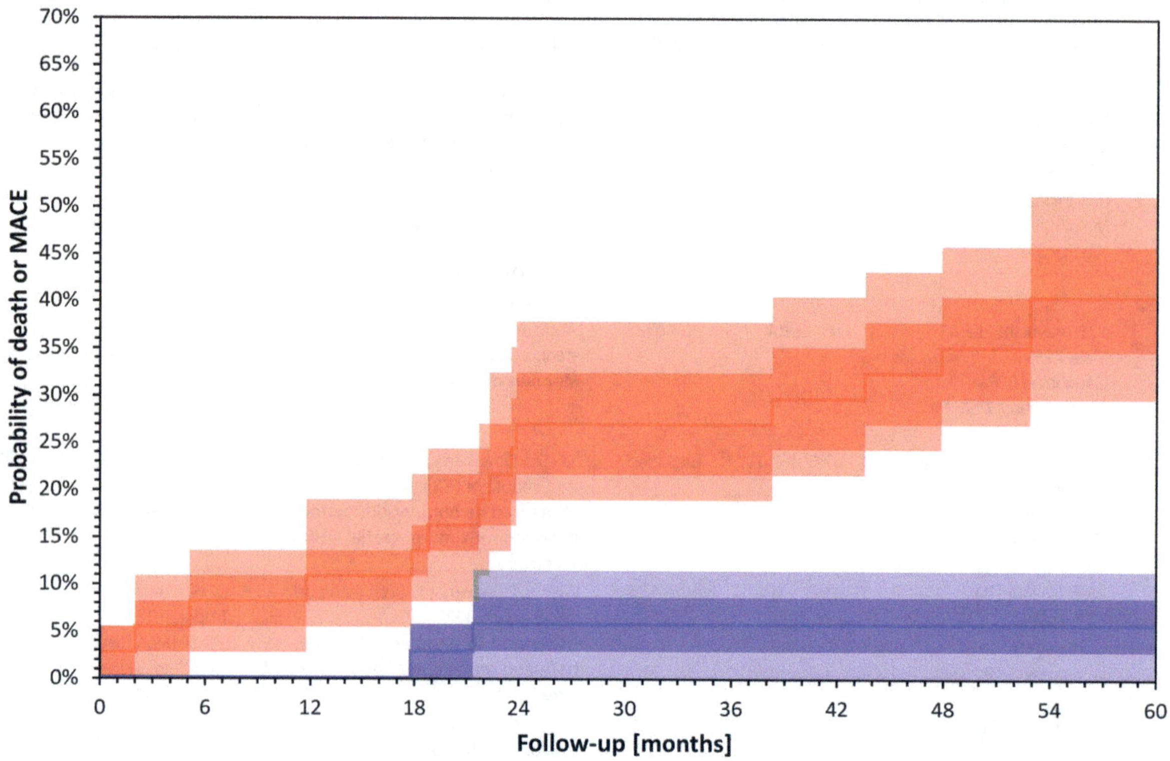

FIGURE 2 | Kaplan–Meier survival curves of total mortality and major cardiac events 72 HD patients included in a recently published study (Poulikakos et al., 2018) stratified by QRS-T angle calculated by TCRT above (red) and below (blue) median value (p = 0.000 Log Rank test). Darker bands depict interquartile ranges and the lighter bands ranges between 10th and 90th percentiles. The calculation of confidence intervals was performed using bootstrap 10,000 repetitions. Major cardiac events were defined as sudden cardiac death, acute coronary syndrome, coronary revascularization or admission due to heart failure or arrhythmia.

(Severi et al., 1997; Hernando et al., 2015). However, Barnas et al. (1999) reported similar intradialytic HRV profiles between hypotension prone and stable patients up to the moment of the hypotensive episode where they observed bradycardia and decline in LF power.

Studies using short term intradialytic ECG monitoring have shown that HRV parameters are influenced by the rate of volume removal during dialysis (Tsuji et al., 2017) and by the dialysis modality between HD and hemofiltration (Genovesi et al., 2007). Two studies also reported associations between short term HRV measurement during dialysis and mortality (Chen et al., 2016; Poulikakos et al., 2018). In a recent study using intradialytic HRV assessment depressed LF/HF over the first hour of treatment predicted overall mortality (Poulikakos et al., 2018). Chen et al. (2016) used spectral HRV assessment before and after HD and showed that decreased difference in LF was associated with increased risk of overall and cardiovascular mortality. **Figure 3** shows an example of Kaplan–Meier event probability curves for major cardiac events and overall mortality in a cohort of 72 HD patients (Poulikakos et al., 2018) stratified by LF/HF ratio above and below median value.

Few studies have used short term HRV assessment during autonomic postural, provocations in HD patients. In the study by Genovesi et al. (2007) postural provocation including 10 min standing before dialysis was performed. Interestingly, whilst active standing was associated with increase in normalized LF and decrease in normalized HF during HD treatment, this was not the case when treatment with hemofiltration was used. Echeverria et al. (2017) showed an increase in LF/HF in response to postural provocations before and after HD treatment.

Genetic differences might contribute to the differences in reported HRV response to autonomic provocations. A recent study in 114 HD patients (Ribas Ribeiro et al., 2018) suggested that genetic polymorphism in the angiotensin converting enzyme, an enzyme that modulates the autonomic system, determines the autonomic response during HD. In this study, an increase in LF and LF/HF through dialysis was observed only in patients with II angiotensin converting enzyme genotype and not in patients with DD genotype. Studies using short term HRV assessment with autonomic provocations are presented in **Table 5**.

Two small studies have reported reasonable reproducibility of HRV measurements from intradialytic recordings (Poulikakos et al., 2014c; da Silva et al., 2016).

CONCLUSION-FUTURE DIRECTIONS

Bradyarrhythmic and Tachyarrhythmic Risk

Recent ILR studies have shown an important relative contribution of bradyarrhythmias to sudden death in

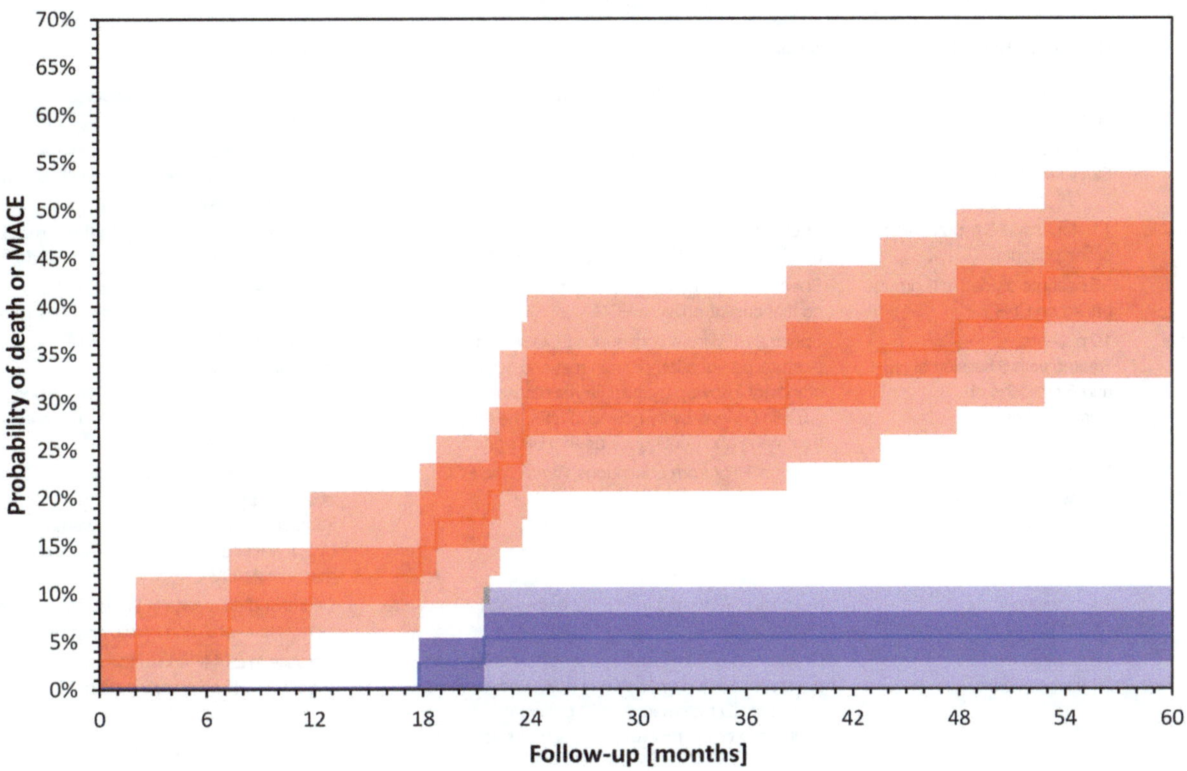

FIGURE 3 | Kaplan–Meier survival curves of total mortality and major cardiac events in 72 HD patients included in a recently published study (Poulikakos et al., 2018) stratified by LF/HF above (blue) and below (red) median value (p = 0.001 Log Rank test). Darker bands depict interquartile ranges and the lighter bands ranges between 10th and 90th percentiles. The calculation of confidence intervals was performed using bootstrap 10,000 repetitions. Major cardiac events were defined as sudden cardiac death, acute coronary syndrome, coronary revascularization or admission due to heart failure or arrhythmia.

dialysis patients. However, these studies did not include incident dialysis patients with high cardiovascular risk that may be more vulnerable to ventricular tachyarrhythmias. Future large studies with long term ECG monitoring in incident dialysis patients are needed to elucidate the precise incidence and underlying arrhythmic mechanisms of SCD. These studies should aim at developing risk stratification strategies for both tachyarrhythmic and bradyarrhythmic risks. Tachyarrhythmic risk is mainly related to static and dynamic ventricular repolarization abnormalities and it is possible that repolarization patterns and changes related dialysis induced fluid and electrolyte shifts prior to the fatal arrhythmias may be important for its prediction. On the contrary, bradyarrhythmic risk is mainly related to cardiac periodicity and is likely to be influenced by autonomic system abnormalities including sleep apnoea.

The ECG signals should be regularly interrogated during the course of such studies and treatment for significant bradyarrhythmias should be offered. Non-invasive surface long term ECG technology with sufficient memory that can record continuous high quality ECG signal could serve the dual purpose of potentially fatal or final rhythm detection and data acquisition for risk profiling for both tachyarrhythmias and bradyarrhythmias. In addition, non-invasive continuous long term ECG monitoring devices that can be attached and exchanged during a dialysis visit may facilitate the recruitment of high risk incident patients who may not wish to attend additional hospital visits or undergo invasive procedures.

Research protocols should include detailed cardiovascular, genetic and sleep disorder phenotyping.

These studies, in addition to clarifying the prevalence of bradyarrhythmias and ventricular arrhythmias, will provide important information about the burden of AF and its potential association with SCD. An association between AF and increased risk of SCD has been shown in cardiac patients (Chen et al., 2014) and may be relevant in the dialysis population given the extremely high burden of AF.

QRS-T Angle-Need for Standardization and Integration Into Clinical Practice

The QRS-T angle assessment has substantial potential to be used as a descriptor of uremic cardiomyopathy. It can also be easily incorporated into clinical practice. In the first instance, the different methodological approaches need to be rigorously tested and compared in existing large ECG databases of CKD and dialysis patients to determine the best methodological approach to the angle expression. This should be based on a multicenter collaboration between clinical

TABLE 5 | Studies using short term Heart Rate Variability assessment with autonomic provocations.

Study	Number of HD patients	Setting	Outcome
Severi et al., 1997	14 stable and 14 hypotension-prone	Spectral HRV from continuous intradialytic ECG.	Spectral HRV different in hypotension prone vs. stable patients.
Hernando et al., 2015	24 patients 52 HD treatment sessions	Spectral HRV from continuous intradialytic ECG and continuous intradialytic arterial BP signal.	Spectral HRV parameters during the first 30 min of the treatment session different in hypotension prone vs. stable patients.
Barnas et al., 1999	11 stable and 9 hypotension prone patients	Spectral HRV from continuous intradialytic ECG and continuous intradialytic arterial BP signal.	No difference in groups up to the point of hypotensive episodes when LF HRV declined
Tsuji et al., 2017	35 patients divided in 3 groups based on UFR	Spectral HRV and approximate entropy from continuous intradialytic ECG.	LF/HF values and approximate entropy increased at the end of HD in patients with UFR >15 ml/h/kg.
Genovesi et al., 2007	10 patients Treated with 6 session of HD and 6 sessions of Hemofiltration	Spectral HRV from continuous ECG during pre-HD postural provocation (10 min rest and 10 min active standing) followed by intradialytic measurements (10 min periods every hour and after the end of treatment) and continuous arterial BP signal.	Normalized LF was higher and HF lower in HF compared to HD. Active standing was associated with increase in normalized LF and decrease in normalized HF in HD but not in Hemofiltration.
Chen et al., 2016	72 patients 5 sessions every 2 weeks	Spectral HRV from continuous intradialytic ECG.	Low LF/HF during the first hour associated with overall mortality. Intrasubject stability of HRV parameters averaged over the first and last hour confirmed by repeated measure ANOVA.
Chen et al., 2016	182 patients	Spectral HRV from 5?min ECG before and 30 min after HD.	Decreased difference in LF associated with increased overall and cardiovascular mortality.
Echeverria et al., 2017	19 stable patients 20 healthy controls	Continuous ECG recording during 16 min in supine position, and during 16 min of active orthostatism pre and post HD treatment for HD patients. Last 5 min of the recording at each position were used for HRV.	Increase in LF/HF and in the short-term scaling exponent (a1) on standing before and after HD.
Ribas Ribeiro et al., 2018	114	HRV from continuous ECG measured for 20 min before, in the second hour and immediately after HD. Assessment of ACE genotypes.	Homozygosity for the II allele of the ACE gene associated with greater increase in LF and LF/HF during HD compared to DD genotype.

ACE, angiotensin converting enzyme; BP, blood pressure; D, deletion; ECG, electrocardiogram; HD, hemodialysis; HF, high frequency; LF, low frequency power; HRV, heart rate variability; I, insertion; UFR, ultrafiltration rate.

research teams and bioengineers. Such collaborative effort can help determine normal reference values and increase our understanding of racial and gender differences in the CKD and dialysis populations.

Furthermore, it is important for the clinical and research community and industry partners in ECG manufacturing to understand the importance of collecting high quality ECGs and storing them in easily accessible formats (Malik et al., 2018) in order to create and maintain open access ECG databases. Such databases would facilitate meaningful research that in turn can inform clinical practice about the possibilities of reducing cardiovascular mortality. The possibility and practical requirements of complementing the existing national and/or international (Goodkin et al., 2001; Perl et al., 2014) renal databases with repositories of routinely collected digital ECG should be explored.

HRV-Methodological Challenges and Clinical Practicality

In the field of HRV and assessment of cardiac autonomic modulation, further research is required to standardize the measurements in dialysis patients. Short-duration tests with autonomic provocations could overcome methodological shortcomings of 24-h outpatient ambulatory ECG recordings. These assessments can be organized around the dialysis treatment in order to minimize a patient's inconvenience and be suitable to be incorporated into regular clinical practice in the future. HRV measurements may be useful for both bradyarrhythmic and tachyarrhythmic risk stratification. The value of cardiac autonomic modulation assessment during standardized autonomic provocations for prediction of significant bradyarrhythmias should be prospectively investigated.

On the other hand, ECG acquisition during autonomic provocations has the potential to yield important prognostic information for tachyarrhythmias, while at the same time characterizing cardiac autonomic regulation measured by HRV and by dynamic repolarization profiles. Short duration continuous ECG measurements with standardized controlled provocations can be used to assess dynamic changes of the QRS-T angle during different stages of cardiac autonomic status; this has been shown to strengthen risk prediction in cardiac patients (Kentta et al., 2012). This type of measurement has the potential to shed more light on the links between autonomic status and cardiac electrical activity and explore the value of combined electrophysiological assessment in this group of patients.

Non-invasive electrophysiology has an important role in CKD patients. Close collaboration across the disciplines of biomedical engineering, clinical cardiology and nephrology is required to bridge the gaps between available technological tools, research efforts and clinical translation in arrhythmic complications of CKD.

AUTHOR CONTRIBUTIONS

DP: concept, design, drafting article, and critical revision of article. KH and SS: critical revision of article. DG and PK: concept and critical revision of article. MM: concept, design, and critical revision of article.

REFERENCES

Baigent, C., Landray, M. J., Reith, C., Emberson, J., Wheeler, D. C., Tomson, C., et al. (2011). The effects of lowering LDL cholesterol with simvastatin plus ezetimibe in patients with chronic kidney disease (Study of Heart and Renal Protection): a randomised placebo-controlled trial. *Lancet* 377, 2181–2192. doi: 10.1016/S0140-6736(11)60739-3

Barnas, M. G., Boer, W. H., and Koomans, H. A. (1999). Hemodynamic patterns and spectral analysis of heart rate variability during dialysis hypotension. *J. Am. Soc. Nephrol.* 10, 2577–2584.

Berton, G., Cordiano, R., Cucchini, F., Cavuto, F., Pellegrinet, M., and Palatini, P. (2009). Atrial fibrillation during acute myocardial infarction: association with all-cause mortality and sudden death after 7-year of follow-up. *Int. J. Clin. Pract.* 63, 712–721. doi: 10.1111/j.1742-1241.2009.02023.x

Biaggioni, I., Killian, T. J., Mosqueda-Garcia, R., Robertson, R. M., and Robertson, D. (1991). Adenosine increases sympathetic nerve traffic in humans. *Circulation* 83, 1668–1675. doi: 10.1161/01.CIR.83.5.1668

Bjerregaard, P. (1983). Mean 24 hour heart rate, minimal heart rate and pauses in healthy subjects 40-79 years of age. *Eur. Heart J.* 4, 44–51. doi: 10.1093/oxfordjournals.eurheartj.a061370

Brodsky, M., Wu, D., Denes, P., Kanakis, C., and Rosen, K. M. (1977). Arrhythmias documented by 24 hour continuous electrocardiographic monitoring in 50 male medical students without apparent heart disease. *Am. J. Cardiol.* 39, 390–395. doi: 10.1016/S0002-9149(77)80094-5

Chan, C. T., Chertow, G. M., Daugirdas, J. T., Greene, T. H., Kotanko, P., Larive, B., et al. (2014). Effects of daily hemodialysis on heart rate variability: results from the Frequent Hemodialysis Network (FHN) Daily Trial. *Nephrol. Dial. Transplant.* 29, 168–178. doi: 10.1093/ndt/gft212

Chan, K. E., Newton-Cheh, C., Gusella, J. F., and Maddux, F. W. (2015). Heritability of risk for sudden cardiac arrest in ESRD. *J. Am. Soc. Nephrol.* 26, 2815–2820. doi: 10.1681/ASN.2014090881

Chandra, P., Sands, R. L., Gillespie, B. W., Levin, N. W., Kotanko, P., Kiser, M., et al. (2014). Relationship between heart rate variability and pulse wave velocity and their association with patient outcomes in chronic kidney disease. *Clin. Nephrol.* 81, 9–19. doi: 10.5414/CN108020

Chang, K. C., Lee, A. S., Chen, W. Y., Lin, Y. N., Hsu, J. F., Chan, H. C., et al. (2015). Increased LDL electronegativity in chronic kidney disease disrupts calcium homeostasis resulting in cardiac dysfunction. *J. Mol. Cell. Cardiol.* 84, 36–44. doi: 10.1016/j.yjmcc.2015.03.016

Charytan, D. M., Patrick, A. R., Liu, J., Setoguchi, S., Herzog, C. A., Brookhart, M. A., et al. (2011). Trends in the use and outcomes of implantable cardioverter-defibrillators in patients undergoing dialysis in the United States. *Am. J. Kidney Dis.* 58, 409–417. doi: 10.1053/j.ajkd.2011.03.026

Chen, L. Y., Benditt, D. G., and Alonso, A. (2014). Atrial fibrillation and its association with sudden cardiac death. *Circ. J.* 78, 2588–2593. doi: 10.1253/circj.CJ-14-0814

Chen, L. Y., Sotoodehnia, N., Buzkova, P., Lopez, F. L., Yee, L. M., Heckbert, S. R., et al. (2013). Atrial fibrillation and the risk of sudden cardiac death: the atherosclerosis risk in communities study and cardiovascular health study. *JAMA Intern. Med.* 173, 29–35. doi: 10.1001/2013.jamainternmed.744

Chen, S. C., Huang, J. C., Tsai, Y. C., Hsiu-Chin Mai, R. N., Jui-Hsin Chen, R. N., Kuo, P. L., et al. (2016). Heart rate variability change before and after hemodialysis is associated with overall and cardiovascular mortality in hemodialysis. *Sci. Rep.* 6:20597. doi: 10.1038/srep20597

Chesterton, L. J., Sigrist, M. K., Bennett, T., Taal, M. W., and McIntyre, C. W. (2005). Reduced baroreflex sensitivity is associated with increased vascular calcification and arterial stiffness. *Nephrol. Dial. Transplant.* 20, 1140–1147. doi: 10.1093/ndt/gfh808

Cheung, A. K., Sarnak, M. J., Yan, G., Berkoben, M., Heyka, R., Kaufman, A., et al. (2004). Cardiac diseases in maintenance hemodialysis patients: results of the HEMO Study. *Kidney Int.* 65, 2380–2389. doi: 10.1111/j.1523-1755.2004.00657.x

Chiang, J. Y., Huang, J. W., Lin, L. Y., Chang, C. H., Chu, F. Y., Lin, Y. H., et al. (2016). Detrended fluctuation analysis of heart rate dynamics is an important prognostic factor in patients with end-stage renal disease receiving peritoneal dialysis. *PLoS One* 11:e0147282. doi: 10.1371/journal.pone.0147282

Chou, J. A., Streja, E., Nguyen, D. V., Rhee, C. M., Obi, Y., Inrig, J. K., et al. (2018). Intradialytic hypotension, blood pressure changes and mortality risk in incident hemodialysis patients. *Nephrol. Dial. Transplant.* 33, 149–159. doi: 10.1093/ndt/gfx037

Converse, R. L. Jr., Jacobsen, T. N., Jost, C. M., Toto, R. D., Grayburn, P. A., Obregon, T. M., et al. (1992a). Paradoxical withdrawal of reflex vasoconstriction as a cause of hemodialysis-induced hypotension. *J. Clin. Invest.* 90, 1657–1665.

Converse, R. L. Jr., Jacobsen, T. N., Toto, R. D., Jost, C. M., Cosentino, F., Fouad-Tarazi, F., et al. (1992b). Sympathetic overactivity in patients with chronic renal failure. *N. Engl. J. Med.* 327, 1912–1918.

Couser, W. G., Remuzzi, G., Mendis, S., and Tonelli, M. (2011). The contribution of chronic kidney disease to the global burden of major noncommunicable diseases. *Kidney Int.* 80, 1258–1270. doi: 10.1038/ki.2011.368

Cuculich, P. S., Sánchez, J. M., Kerzner, R., Greenberg, S. L., Sengupta, J., Chen, J., et al. (2007). Poor prognosis for patients with chronic kidney disease despite ICD therapy for the primary prevention of sudden death. *Pacing Clin. Electrophysiol.* 30, 207–213. doi: 10.1111/j.1540-8159.2007.00651.x

da Silva, D. M., Macedo, M. C., Lemos, L. B., Vieira, F. C., Pirôpo, U. S., Andrade, H. B., et al. (2016). Reliability analysis of the heart autonomic control parameters during hemodialysis sessions. *Biomed. Tech.* 61, 623–630. doi: 10.1515/bmt-2015-0239

Dalal, D., de Jong, J. S., Tjong, F. V., Wang, Y., Bruinsma, N., Dekker, L. R. C., et al. (2012). Mild-to-moderate kidney dysfunction and the risk of sudden cardiac death in the setting of acute myocardial infarction. *Heart Rhythm* 9, 540–545. doi: 10.1016/j.hrthm.2011.11.014

de Bie, M. K., Ajmone Marsan, N., Gaasbeek, A., Bax, J. J., Delgado, V., Rabelink, T. J., et al. (2013a). Echocardiographical determinants of an abnormal spatial QRS-T angle in chronic dialysis patients. *Nephrol. Dial. Transplant.* 28, 3045–3052. doi: 10.1093/ndt/gft347

de Bie, M. K., Koopman, M. G., Gaasbeek, A., Dekker, F. W., Maan, A. C., Swenne, C. A., et al. (2013b). Incremental prognostic value of an abnormal baseline spatial QRS-T angle in chronic dialysis patients. *Europace* 15, 290–296. doi: 10.1093/europace/eus306

Denes, P., Wu, D., Dhingra, R., Pietras, R. J., and Rosen, K. M. (1974). The effects of cycle length on cardiac refractory periods in man. *Circulation* 49, 32–41. doi: 10.1161/01.CIR.49.1.32

Echeverria, J. C., Infante, O., Perez-Grovas, H., Gonzalez, H., Jose, M. V., and Lerma, C. (2017). Effects of orthostatism and hemodialysis on mean heart period and fractal heart rate properties of chronic renal failure patients. *Artif. Organs* 41, 1026–1034. doi: 10.1111/aor.12887

Elaine, C., and Macfarlane, P. W. (2016). "Comparison of spatial QRS-T angle in different healthy racial groups," in *Paper Presented at the 2016 Computing in Cardiology Conference*, Vancouver.

Fleg, J. L., and Kennedy, H. L. (1982). Cardiac arrhythmias in a healthy elderly population: detection by 24-hour ambulatory electrocardiography. *Chest* 81, 302–307. doi: 10.1378/chest.81.3.302

Fontes, M. S., Papazova, D. A., van Koppen, A., de Jong, S., Korte, S. M., Bongartz, L. G., et al. (2015). Arrhythmogenic remodeling in murine models of deoxycorticosterone acetate-salt-induced and 5/6-subtotal nephrectomy-salt-induced cardiorenal disease. *Cardiorenal Med.* 5, 208–218. doi: 10.1159/000430475

Forsstrom, J., Heinonen, E., Valimaki, I., and Antila, K. (1986). Effects of haemodialysis on heart rate variability in chronic renal failure. *Scand. J. Clin. Lab. Invest.* 46, 665–670. doi: 10.3109/00365518609083729

Fukuta, H., Hayano, J., Ishihara, S., Sakata, S., Mukai, S., Ohte, N., et al. (2003). Prognostic value of heart rate variability in patients with end-stage renal disease on chronic haemodialysis. *Nephrol. Dial. Transplant.* 18, 318–325. doi: 10.1093/ndt/18.2.318

Genovesi, S., Bracchi, O., Fabbrini, P., Luisetto, E., Viganò, M. R., Lucini, D., et al. (2007). Differences in heart rate variability during haemodialysis and haemofiltration. *Nephrol. Dial. Transplant.* 22, 2256–2262. doi: 10.1093/ndt/gfm125

Goodkin, D. A., Mapes, D. L., and Held, P. J. (2001). The dialysis outcomes and practice patterns study (DOPPS): how can we improve the care of hemodialysis patients? *Semin. Dial.* 14, 157–159. doi: 10.1046/j.1525-139X.2001.00043.x

Grassi, G., Quarti-Trevano, F., Seravalle, G., Arenare, F., Volpe, M., Furiani, S., et al. (2011). Early sympathetic activation in the initial clinical stages of chronic renal failure. *Hypertension* 57, 846–851. doi: 10.1161/HYPERTENSIONAHA.110.164780

Gronefeld, G. C., Mauss, O., Li, Y. G., Klingenheben, T., and Hohnloser, S. H. (2000). Association between atrial fibrillation and appropriate implantable cardioverter defibrillator therapy: results from a prospective study. *J. Cardiovasc. Electrophysiol.* 11, 1208–1214. doi: 10.1046/j.1540-8167.2000.01208.x

Gutiérrez, O. M., Januzzi, J. L., Isakova, T., Laliberte, K., Smith, K., Collerone, G., et al. (2009). Fibroblast growth factor 23 and left ventricular hypertrophy in chronic kidney disease. *Circulation* 119, 2545–2552. doi: 10.1161/CIRCULATIONAHA.108.844506

Hayano, J., Takahashi, H., Toriyama, T., Mukai, S., Okada, A., Sakata, S., et al. (1999). Prognostic value of heart rate variability during long-term follow-up in chronic haemodialysis patients with end-stage renal disease. *Nephrol. Dial. Transplant.* 14, 1480–1488. doi: 10.1093/ndt/14.6.1480

Hernando, D., Sornmo, L., Sandberg, F., Laguna, P., Llamedo, M., and Bailon, R. (2015). Identification of patients prone to hypotension during hemodialysis based on the analysis of cardiovascular signals. *Med. Eng. Phys.* 37, 1156–1161. doi: 10.1016/j.medengphy.2015.10.003

Herzog, C. A., Asinger, R. W., Berger, A. K., David, M. C., Javier, D., Robert, G. H., et al. (2011). Cardiovascular disease in chronic kidney disease. A clinical update from Kidney Disease: improving Global Outcomes (KDIGO). *Kidney Int.* 80, 572–586. doi: 10.1038/ki.2011.223

Hnatkova, K., Seegers, J., Barthel, P., Novotny, T., Smetana, P., Zabel, M., et al. (2017). Clinical value of different QRS-T angle expressions. *Europace* 20, 1352–1361. doi: 10.1093/europace/eux246

Hreybe, H., Ezzeddine, R., Bedi, M., Barrington, W., Bazaz, R., Ganz, L. I., et al. (2006). Renal insufficiency predicts the time to first appropriate defibrillator shock. *Am. Heart J.* 151, 852–856. doi: 10.1016/j.ahj.2005.06.042

Hsueh, C. H., Chen, N. X., Lin, S. F., Chen, P. S., Gattone, V. H., Allen, M. R., et al. (2014). Pathogenesis of arrhythmias in a model of CKD. *J. Am. Soc. Nephrol.* 25, 2812–2821. doi: 10.1681/ASN.2013121343

Isakova, T., Xie, H., Yang, W., Xie, D., Anderson, A. H., Scialla, J., et al. (2011). Fibroblast growth factor 23 and risks of mortality and end-stage renal disease in patients with chronic kidney disease. *JAMA* 305, 2432–2439. doi: 10.1001/jama.2011.826

Jaroszynski, A., Czekajska-Chechab, E., Drelich-Zbroja, A., Zapolski, T., and Ksiazek, A. (2009). Spatial QRS-T angle in peritoneal dialysis patients: association with carotid artery atherosclerosis, coronary artery calcification and troponin T. *Nephrol. Dial. Transplant.* 24, 1003–1008. doi: 10.1093/ndt/gfn581

Jaroszynski, A., Wysokiński, A., Bednarek-Skublewska, A., Głowniak, A., Książek, P., Sodolski, T., et al. (2010). The effect of a single dialysis session on spatial QRS-T angle in haemodialysis patients. *Nephrol. Dial. Transplant.* 25, 3723–3729. doi: 10.1093/ndt/gfq247

Jiang, Y., Shen, Z., Zhang, J., Xing, C., Zha, X., Shen, C., et al. (2016). Parathyroidectomy increases heart rate variability and leptin levels in patients with stage 5 chronic kidney disease. *Am. J. Nephrol.* 44, 245–254. doi: 10.1159/000449018

Jourde-Chiche, N., Dou, L., Cerini, C., Dignat-George, F., and Brunet, P. (2011). Vascular incompetence in dialysis patients–protein-bound uremic toxins and endothelial dysfunction. *Semin. Dial.* 24, 327–337. doi: 10.1111/j.1525-139X.2011.00925.x

Kalra, P. A., Green, D., and Poulikakos, D. (2018). Arrhythmia in hemodialysis patients and its relation to sudden death. *Kidney Int.* 93, 781–783. doi: 10.1016/j.kint.2017.12.005

Kaur, J., Young, B. E., and Fadel, P. J. (2017). Sympathetic overactivity in chronic kidney disease: consequences and mechanisms. *Int. J. Mol. Sci.* 18:1682. doi: 10.3390/ijms18081682

Kentta, T., Viik, J., Karsikas, M., Seppänen, T., Nieminen, T., Lehtimäki, T., et al. (2012). Postexercise recovery of the spatial QRS/T angle as a predictor of sudden cardiac death. *Heart Rhythm* 9, 1083–1089. doi: 10.1016/j.hrthm.2012.02.030

Lee, A. S., Chen, W. Y., Chan, H. C., Chung, C. H., Peng, H. Y., Chang, C. M., et al. (2017). Electronegative LDL-mediated cardiac electrical remodeling in a rat model of chronic kidney disease. *Sci. Rep.* 7:40676. doi: 10.1038/srep40676

Levick, S. P., Murray, D. B., Janicki, J. S., and Brower, G. L. (2010). Sympathetic nervous system modulation of inflammation and remodeling in the hypertensive heart. *Hypertension* 55, 270–276. doi: 10.1161/HYPERTENSIONAHA.109.142042

Lin, C. Y., Lin, L. Y., and Chen, P. C. (2007). Analysis of T-wave morphology from the 12-lead electrocardiogram for prediction of long-term prognosis in patients initiating haemodialysis. *Nephrol. Dial. Transplant.* 22, 2645–2652. doi: 10.1093/ndt/gfm238

London, G. M., Guérin, A. P., Marchais, S. J., Métivier, F., Pannier, B., and Adda, H. (2003). Arterial media calcification in end-stage renal disease: impact on all-cause and cardiovascular mortality. *Nephrol. Dial. Transplant.* 18, 1731–1740. doi: 10.1093/ndt/gfg414

Mainigi, S. K., Chebrolu, L. H., Romero-Corral, A., Mehta, V., Machado, R. R., Konecny, T., et al. (2012). Prediction of significant conduction disease through noninvasive assessment of cardiac calcification. *Echocardiography* 29, 1017–1021. doi: 10.1111/j.1540-8175.2012.01752.x

Malik, M., Buxton, A. E., Huikuri, H., Lombardi, F., Schmidt, G., and Zabel, M. (2018). Noninvasive electrophysiology in risk assessment and screening. *Heart Rhythm* 15, 803–804. doi: 10.1016/j.hrthm.2018.03.014

Matsuo, H., Dohi, K., Machida, H., Takeuchi, H., Aoki, T., Nishimura, H., et al. (2018). Echocardiographic assessment of cardiac structural and functional abnormalities in patients with end-stage renal disease receiving chronic hemodialysis. *Circ. J.* 82, 586–595. doi: 10.1253/circj.CJ-17-0393

Ng, H. Y., Hsueh, S. K., Lee, Y. T., Chiou, T. T., Huang, P. C., and Lee, C. T. (2017). Synergic impact of vascular calcification and low autonomic tone in mortality of hemodialysis patients. *Nephron* 137, 91–98. doi: 10.1159/000477827

Nowak, K. L., and Chonchol, M. (2018). Does inflammation affect outcomes in dialysis patients? *Semin. Dial.* 31, 388–397. doi: 10.1111/sdi.12686

Ogna, A., Forni Ogna, V., Mihalache, A., Pruijm, M., Halabi, G., Phan, O., et al. (2015). Obstructive sleep apnea severity and overnight body fluid shift before and after hemodialysis. *Clin. J. Am. Soc. Nephrol.* 10, 1002–1010. doi: 10.2215/CJN.08760914

Oikawa, K., Ishihara, R., Maeda, T., Yamaguchi, K., Koike, A., Kawaguchi, H., et al. (2009). Prognostic value of heart rate variability in patients with renal failure on hemodialysis. *Int. J. Cardiol.* 131, 370–377. doi: 10.1016/j.ijcard.2007.10.033

Pedersen, O. D., Abildstrom, S. Z., Ottesen, M. M., Rask-Madsen, C., Bagger, H., Køber, L., et al. (2006). Increased risk of sudden and non-sudden cardiovascular death in patients with atrial fibrillation/flutter following acute myocardial infarction. *Eur. Heart J.* 27, 290–295. doi: 10.1093/eurheartj/ehi629

Pei, J., Tang, W., Li, L. X., Su, C. Y., and Wang, T. (2015). Heart rate variability predicts mortality in peritoneal dialysis patients. *Ren. Fail.* 37, 1132–1137. doi: 10.3109/0886022X.2015.1061729

Perl, J., Robinson, B., and Davies, S. On behalf of the International Society for Peritoneal Dialysis, Arbor Research Collaborative, and the PDOPPS investigators (2014). Update on the peritoneal dialysis outcomes and practice patterns study (PDOPPS). *Perit. Dial. Int.* 34:332. doi: 10.3747/pdi.2014.00162

Poulikakos, D., Banerjee, D., and Malik, M. (2014a). Risk of sudden cardiac death in chronic kidney disease. *J. Cardiovasc. Electrophysiol.* 25, 222–231. doi: 10.1111/jce.12328

Poulikakos, D., Malik, M., and Banerjee, D. (2014b). Parathyroid hormone and heart rate variability in haemodialysis patients. *Nephron Clin. Pract.* 126, 110–115. doi: 10.1159/000360542

Poulikakos, D., Malik, M., and Banerjee, D. (2014c). Sex-dependent association between heart rate variability and pulse pressure in haemodialysis patients. *Nephron Clin. Pract.* 128, 361–366. doi: 10.1159/000368436

Poulikakos, D., Ross, L., Recio-Mayoral, A., Cole, D., Andoh, J., Chitalia, N., et al. (2014d). Left ventricular hypertrophy and endothelial dysfunction in chronic kidney disease. *Eur. Heart J. Cardiovasc. Imaging* 15, 56–61. doi: 10.1093/ehjci/jet120

Poulikakos, D., Banerjee, D., and Malik, M. T. (2013). wave morphology changes during hemodialysis. *J. Electrocardiol.* 46, 492–496. doi: 10.1016/j.jelectrocard.2013.07.006

Poulikakos, D., Hnatkova, K., Banerjee, D., and Malik, M. (2018). Association of QRS-T angle and heart rate variability with major cardiac events and mortality in hemodialysis patients. *Ann. Noninvasive Electrocardiol.* 23:e12570. doi: 10.1111/anec.12570

Poulikakos, D., and Malik, M. (2016). Challenges of ECG monitoring and ECG interpretation in dialysis units. *J. Electrocardiol.* 49, 855–859. doi: 10.1016/j.jelectrocard.2016.07.019

Pun, P. H., Hellkamp, A. S., Sanders, G. D., Middleton, J. P., Hammill, S. C., Al-Khalidi, H. R., et al. (2015). Primary prevention implantable cardioverter defibrillators in end-stage kidney disease patients on dialysis: a matched cohort study. *Nephrol. Dial. Transplant.* 30, 829–835. doi: 10.1093/ndt/gfu274

Reeves, P. B., and Mc Causland, F. R. (2018). Mechanisms, clinical implications, and treatment of intradialytic hypotension. *Clin. J. Am. Soc. Nephrol.* 13, 1297–1303. doi: 10.2215/CJN.12141017

Ribas Ribeiro, L., Flores de Oliveira, J., Bueno Orcy, R., Castilho Barros, C., Damé Hense, J., Santos, F., et al. (2018). Exploring the complexity: the interplay between the angiotensin-converting enzyme insertion/deletion polymorphism and the sympathetic response to hemodialysis. *Am. J. Physiol. Heart Circ. Physiol.* 315, H1002–H1011. doi: 10.1152/ajpheart.00162.2018

Roberts, P. R., Zachariah, D., Morgan, J. M., Yue, A. M., Greenwood, E. F., Phillips, P. C., et al. (2017). Monitoring of arrhythmia and sudden death in a hemodialysis population: the CRASH-ILR study. *PLoS One* 12:e0188713. doi: 10.1371/journal.pone.0188713

Robin, J., Weinberg, K., Tiongson, J., Carnethon, M., Reddy, M., Ciaccio, C., et al. (2006). Renal dialysis as a risk factor for appropriate therapies and mortality in implantable cardioverter-defibrillator recipients. *Heart Rhythm* 3, 1196–1201. doi: 10.1016/j.hrthm.2006.06.013

Robinson, E. A., Rhee, K. S., Doytchinova, A., Kumar, M., Shelton, R., Jiang, Z., et al. (2015). Estimating sympathetic tone by recording subcutaneous nerve activity in ambulatory dogs. *J. Cardiovasc. Electrophysiol.* 26, 70–78. doi: 10.1111/jce.12508

Roy-Chaudhury, P., Tumlin, J. A., Koplan, B. A., Costea, A. I., Kher, V., Williamson, D., et al. (2018). Primary outcomes of the monitoring in dialysis study indicate that clinically significant arrhythmias are common in hemodialysis patients and related to dialytic cycle. *Kidney Int.* 93, 941–951. doi: 10.1016/j.kint.2017.11.019

Sacher, F., Jesel, L., Borni-Duval, C., De Precigout, V., Lavainne, F., Bourdenx, J.-P., et al. (2018). Cardiac rhythm disturbances in hemodialysis patients: early detection using an implantable loop recorder and correlation with biological and dialysis parameters. *JACC Clin. Electrophysiol.* 4, 397–408. doi: 10.1016/j.jacep.2017.08.002

Sakaguchi, Y., Shoji, T., Kawabata, H., Niihata, K., Suzuki, A., Kaneko, T., et al. (2011). High prevalence of obstructive sleep apnea and its association with renal function among nondialysis chronic kidney disease patients in Japan: a cross-sectional study. *Clin. J. Am. Soc. Nephrol.* 6, 995–1000. doi: 10.2215/CJN.08670910

Sallam, K., Li, Y., Sager, P. T., Houser, S. R., and Wu, J. C. (2015). Finding the rhythm of sudden cardiac death: new opportunities using induced pluripotent stem cell-derived cardiomyocytes. *Circ. Res.* 116, 1989–2004. doi: 10.1161/CIRCRESAHA.116.304494

Sassi, R., Cerutti, S., Lombardi, F., Huikuri, H. V., Peng, C. K., Schmidt, G., et al. (2015). Advances in heart rate variability signal analysis: joint position statement by the e-Cardiology ESC Working Group and the European Heart Rhythm Association co-endorsed by the Asia Pacific Heart Rhythm Society. *Europace* 17, 1341–1353. doi: 10.1093/europace/euv015

Semple, D., Smith, K., Bhandari, S., and Seymour, A. M. (2011). Uremic cardiomyopathy and insulin resistance: a critical role for akt? *J. Am. Soc. Nephrol.* 22, 207–215. doi: 10.1681/ASN.2009090900

Severi, S., Cavalcanti, S., and Avanzolini, G. (1997). Heart rate variability spectral indices for haemodynamic classification of haemodialysis patients. *Physiol. Meas.* 18, 339–353. doi: 10.1088/0967-3334/18/4/007

Shang, F., Wang, S. C., Hsu, C. Y., Miao, Y., Martin, M., Yin, Y., et al. (2017). MicroRNA-92a mediates endothelial dysfunction in CKD. *J. Am. Soc. Nephrol.* 28, 3251–3261. doi: 10.1681/ASN.2016111215

Siddiqi, L., Joles, J. A., Grassi, G., and Blankestijn, P. J. (2009). Is kidney ischemia the central mechanism in parallel activation of the renin and sympathetic system? *J. Hypertens.* 27, 1341–1349. doi: 10.1097/HJH.0b013e32832b521b

Silva, R. T., Martinelli Filho, M., Peixoto Gde, L., Lima, J. J., Siqueira, S. F., Costa, R., et al. (2015). Predictors of arrhythmic events detected by implantable loop recorders in renal transplant candidates. *Arq. Bras. Cardiol.* 105, 493–502. doi: 10.5935/abc.20150106

Simantirakis, E. N., Schiza, S. I., Marketou, M. E., Chrysostomakis, S. I., Chlouverakis, G. I., Klapsinos, N. C., et al. (2004). Severe bradyarrhythmias in patients with sleep apnoea: the effect of continuous positive airway pressure treatment: a long-term evaluation using an insertable loop recorder. *Eur. Heart J.* 25, 1070–1076. doi: 10.1016/j.ehj.2004.04.017

Skampardoni, S., Green, D., Hnatkova, K., Malik, M., Kalra, P. A., and Poulikakos, A. D. (2018a). QRS-T angle predicts Cardiac Risk and correlates with Global Longitudinal Strain in Prevalent Hemodialysis Patients. *Front. Physiol.* 10:145. doi: 10.3389/fphys.2019.00145

Skampardoni, S., Poulikakos, D., Malik, M., Green, D., and Kalra, P. A. (2018b). The potential of electrocardiography for cardiac risk prediction in chronic and end-stage kidney disease. *Nephrol. Dial. Transplant.* doi: 10.1093/ndt/gfy255 [Epub ahead of print].

Smetana, P., Batchvarov, V. N., Hnatkova, K., Camm, A. J., and Malik, M. (2002). Sex differences in repolarization homogeneity and its circadian pattern. *Am. J. Physiol. Heart Circ. Physiol.* 282, H1889–H1897. doi: 10.1152/ajpheart.00962.2001

Suzuki, M., Hiroshi, T., Aoyama, T., Tanaka, M., Ishii, H., Kisohara, M., et al. (2012). Nonlinear measures of heart rate variability and mortality risk in hemodialysis patients. *Clin. J. Am. Soc. Nephrol.* 7, 1454–1460. doi: 10.2215/CJN.09430911

Tada, T., Kusano, K. F., Ogawa, A., Iwasaki, J., Sakuragi, S., Kusano, I., et al. (2007). The predictors of central and obstructive sleep apnoea in haemodialysis patients. *Nephrol. Dial. Transplant.* 22, 1190–1197. doi: 10.1093/ndt/gfl748

Tang, W., Li, L. X., Pei, J., and Wang, T. (2012). Heart rate variability in peritoneal dialysis patients: what is the role of residual renal function? *Blood Purif.* 34, 58–66. doi: 10.1159/000338184

Task Force of the European Society of Cardiology and North American Society of Pacing and Electrophysiology (1996). Heart rate variability: standards of measurement, physiological interpretation and clinical use. *Circulation* 93, 1043–1065.

Tereshchenko, L. G., Kim, E. D., Oehler, A., Meoni, L. A., Ghafoori, E., and Rami, T. (2016). Electrophysiologic substrate and risk of mortality in incident hemodialysis. *J. Am. Soc. Nephrol.* 27, 3413–3420. doi: 10.1681/ASN.2015080916

Tsuji, Y., Suzuki, N., Hitomi, Y., Yoshida, T., and Mizuno-Matsumoto, Y. (2017). Quantification of autonomic nervous activity by heart rate variability and approximate entropy in high ultrafiltration rate during hemodialysis. *Clin. Exp. Nephrol.* 21, 524–530. doi: 10.1007/s10157-016-1305-5

United States Renal Data System (2012). *USRDS Annual Data Report: Epidemiology of Kidney Disease in the United States.* Bethesda, MD: National Institutes of Health.

Vallon, V., Muhlbauer, B., and Osswald, H. (2006). Adenosine and kidney function. *Physiol. Rev.* 86, 901–940. doi: 10.1152/physrev.00031.2005

Vaseghi, M., Lux, R. L., Mahajan, A., and Shivkumar, K. (2012). Sympathetic stimulation increases dispersion of repolarization in humans with myocardial infarction. *Am. J. Physiol. Heart Circ. Physiol.* 302, H1838–H1846. doi: 10.1152/ajpheart.01106.2011

Vitolo, E., Madoi, S., Palvarini, M., De Maria, R., Ciró, E., Colombo, A. E., et al. (1987). Relationship between changes in R wave voltage and cardiac volumes. A vectorcardiographic study during hemodialysis. *J. Electrocardiol.* 20, 138–146. doi: 10.1016/S0022-0736(87)80103-6

Waks, J. W., Sitlani, C. M., Soliman, E. Z., Kabir, M., Ghafoori, E., Biggs, M. L., et al. (2016). Global electric heterogeneity risk score for prediction of sudden cardiac death in the general population: the atherosclerosis risk in communities (ARIC) and cardiovascular health (CHS) studies. *Circulation* 133, 2222–2234. doi: 10.1161/CIRCULATIONAHA.116.021306

Wan, C., Herzog, C. A., Zareba, W., and Szymkiewicz, S. J. (2014). Sudden cardiac arrest in hemodialysis patients with wearable cardioverter defibrillator. *Ann. Noninvasive Electrocardiol.* 19, 247–257. doi: 10.1111/anec.12119

Wang, A. Y., Wang, M., Woo, J., Lam, C. W., Li, P. K., Lui, S. F., et al. (2003). Cardiac valve calcification as an important predictor for all-cause mortality and cardiovascular mortality in long-term peritoneal dialysis patients: a prospective study. *J. Am. Soc. Nephrol.* 14, 159–168. doi: 10.1097/01.ASN.0000038685.95946.83

Wang, I. K., Lin, K. H., Lin, S. Y., Lin, C. L., Chang, C. T., Yen, T. H., et al. (2016). Permanent cardiac pacing in patients with end-stage renal disease undergoing dialysis. *Nephrol. Dial. Transplant.* 31, 2115–2122. doi: 10.1093/ndt/gfw302

Wang, Z., Jiang, A., Wei, F., and Chen, H. (2018). Cardiac valve calcification and risk of cardiovascular or all-cause mortality in dialysis patients: a meta-analysis. *BMC Cardiovasc. Disord.* 18:12. doi: 10.1186/s12872-018-0747-y

Wanner, C., Krane, V., März, W., Olschewski, M., Mann, J. F., Ruf, G., et al. (2005). Atorvastatin in patients with type 2 diabetes mellitus undergoing hemodialysis. *N. Engl. J. Med.* 353, 238–248. doi: 10.1056/NEJMoa043545

Wolf, J., Drozdowski, J., Czechowicz, K., Winklewski, P. J., Jassem, E., Kara, T., et al. (2016). Effect of beta-blocker therapy on heart rate response in patients with hypertension and newly diagnosed untreated obstructive sleep apnea syndrome. *Int. J. Cardiol.* 202, 67–72. doi: 10.1016/j.ijcard.2015.08.139

Wong, M. C., Kalman, J. M., Pedagogos, E., Toussaint, N., Vohra, J. K., Sparks, P. B., et al. (2015). Temporal distribution of arrhythmic events in chronic kidney disease: highest incidence in the long interdialytic period. *Heart Rhythm* 12, 2047–2055. doi: 10.1016/j.hrthm.2015.06.033

Wong, M. C. G., Kalman, J. M., Pedagogos, E., Toussaint, N., Vohra, J. K., Sparks, P. B., et al. (2015). Bradycardia and asystole is the predominant mechanism of sudden cardiac death in patients with chronic kidney disease. *J. Am. Coll. Cardiol.* 65, 1263–1265. doi: 10.1016/j.jacc.2014.12.049

Young, C. N., Fisher, J. P., Gallagher, K. M., Whaley-Connell, A., Chaudhary, K., Victor, R. G., et al. (2009). Inhibition of nitric oxide synthase evokes central sympatho-excitation in healthy humans. *J. Physiol.* 587(Pt 20), 4977–4986. doi: 10.1113/jphysiol.2009.177204

Zabel, M., and Malik, M. (2002). Practical use of T wave morphology assessment. *Card. Electrophysiol. Rev.* 6, 316–322. doi: 10.1023/A:1016353714372

Zhang, J., Yu, X., Sun, B., Bai, J., Wei, Y., Zha, X., et al. (2013). Parathyroidectomy and heart rate variability in patients with stage 5 CKD. *Clin. J. Am. Soc. Nephrol.* 8, 1378–1387. doi: 10.2215/CJN.10381012

Zhang, L. N., Yang, G., Cheng, C., Shen, C., Cui, Y. Y., Zhang, J., et al. (2015). Plasma FGF23 levels and heart rate variability in patients with stage 5 CKD. *Osteoporos. Int.* 26, 395–405. doi: 10.1007/s00198-014-2862-7

Zhao, Y., Chen, N. X., Shirazi, J. T., Shen, C., Lin, S. F., Fishbein, M. C., et al. (2016). Subcutaneous nerve activity and mechanisms of sudden death in a rat model of chronic kidney disease. *Heart Rhythm* 13, 1105–1112. doi: 10.1016/j.hrthm.2015.12.040

Zwillich, C., Devlin, T., White, D., Douglas, N., Weil, J., and Martin, R. (1982). Bradycardia during sleep apnea. Characteristics and mechanism. *J. Clin. Invest.* 69, 1286–1292. doi: 10.1172/JCI110568

13

From Genome-Wide Association Studies to Cardiac Electrophysiology: Through the Maze of Biological Complexity

*Koen T. Scholman[1], Veronique M. F. Meijborg[2,3], Carolina Gálvez-Montón[4,5], Elisabeth M. Lodder[2] and Bastiaan J. Boukens[1,2]**

[1] Department of Medical Biology, Amsterdam University Medical Centers, University of Amsterdam, Amsterdam, Netherlands, [2] Department of Experimental Cardiology, Amsterdam University Medical Centers, University of Amsterdam, Amsterdam, Netherlands, [3] Netherlands Heart Institute, Utrecht, Netherlands, [4] ICREC Research Program, Germans Trias i Pujol Health Science Research Institute, Badalona, Spain, [5] CIBERCV, Instituto de Salud Carlos III, Madrid, Spain

***Correspondence:**
Bastiaan J. Boukens
b.j.boukens@amsterdamumc.nl

Genome Wide Association Studies (GWAS) have provided an enormous amount of data on genomic loci associated with cardiac electrophysiology and arrhythmias. Clinical relevance, however, remains unclear since GWAS do not provide a mechanistic explanation for this association. Determining the electrophysiological relevance of variants for arrhythmias would aid development of risk stratification models for patients with arrhythmias. In this review, we give an overview of genetic variants related to ECG intervals and arrhythmogenic pathologies and discuss how these variants may influence cardiac electrophysiology and the occurrence of arrhythmias.

Keywords: GWAS, cardiac electrophysiology, arrhythmias, gene expression, genetics

INTRODUCTION

Genome Wide Association Studies (GWAS) can identify genetic variants associated with phenotypic traits, such as electrocardiographic (ECG) intervals (**Table 1**). Interpretation of GWAS data relies on identification of the target gene affected by the novel discovered variant. Variants can be present in coding DNA, causing amino acid changes affecting protein function – or in non-coding DNA, altering the behavior of regulatory elements, thereby changing expression levels of its target gene(s) (**Figure 1A**). For many highly significant GWAS loci the gene causing the association with ECG intervals has not been identified yet. This is mostly because genes in or near these loci do not have a proven association with the phenotype. Overlaying such loci with publicly available genome wide data sets of gene expression (GTEx Consortium, 2013; Heinig, 2018), cardiac transcriptional elements (van Duijvenboden et al., 2016), genomic conformation Hi-C data sets (Montefiori et al., 2018), and other GWAS results will likely provide more insight into potential novel candidate genes regulating cardiac electrophysiology (van Ouwerkerk et al., 2019).

Upon discovery, the expression of the target gene is often modified in isolated cardiomyocytes (from an animal model or human induced pluripotent stem cells). These cellular models can be used to assess any electrophysiological phenotypes associated with the potential GWAS candidate. However, ECG intervals reflect the complex electrophysiological interaction of the cardiac cells and tissue structures, complicating extrapolation of single cell measurements to ECG intervals (Opthof et al., 1987). Additionally, discovered variants may affect expression of genes in non-cardiomyocytes, further complicating the interpretation of such experiments in isolated cardiomyocytes (Stroud et al., 2016; Veerman et al., 2016).

To overcome these limitations, *in vivo* models such as transgenic mice are most commonly used to investigate the relation between GWAS variants and electrophysiological phenotypes. However, large electrophysiological differences exist between mice and larger mammals such as human (Boukens et al., 2014), which need to be taken into account when interpreting the resulting data.

In this review, we give an overview of genomic loci related to abnormal cardiac electrophysiology and discuss how these variants may directly or indirectly influence ECG intervals and the occurrence of arrhythmias through their expression pattern and regulation within the heart.

GWAS LOCI RELATED TO HEART RATE

The sinus node is located at the border between intercaval area and the right atrium. Action potentials of sinus node cardiomyocytes have low upstroke velocities and occur spontaneously (West, 1955). The mechanism underlying these spontaneous depolarizations is based on the funny current, mediated by the Hyperpolarization-Activated Cyclic Nucleotide-gated channel 4 (*HCN4*), and the calcium clock mediated by e.g., Ryanodine Receptor 2 (*RYR2*) and Phospholamban (*PLN*) (Lakatta and DiFrancesco, 2009). Accordingly, associations between the genetic loci of *HCN4* and *PLN* and heart rate found by GWAS is most likely mediated through variants impacting on the expression and or function of these genes (Eijgelsheim et al., 2010; den Hoed et al., 2013; Nolte et al., 2017). Unfortunately, for the other GWAS loci, the association is not as straightforward. In the proximity of these loci, no genes with a known function in the SAN have been identified. These loci therefore potentially affect SAN function by impacting on other parameters, e.g., electrical coupling with the rest of the atrium and levels of fibrosis (Glukhov et al., 2013).

In smaller mammals – e.g., mice and rabbits – the sinus node is transmural (Bleeker et al., 1980; van Eif et al., 2019), whereas in large mammals – e.g., humans and dogs – it is not (Fedorov et al., 2009, 2010). The geometry of the sinus node affects coupling with atrial myocardium, which influences its electrophysiological behavior (Kirchhof et al., 1987). The delicate interaction between the sinus node and the surrounding atrial myocardium is established by fibrous tissue providing up to five exit pathways in large mammals (**Figure 1B**; Unudurthi et al., 2014; Csepe et al., 2015; Li et al., 2017). A transitional layer of cells within the exit pathways (**Figure 1B**) allows for spontaneous depolarization within the sinus node (Joyner and van Capelle, 1986; Kléber and Rudy, 2004). The identity of the transitional cells may depend on the expression of transcription factor Nkx2-5 and GWAS has found variants near NKX2-5 associating with heart rate (Mommersteeg et al., 2007b; den Hoed et al., 2013; Li et al., 2019). Within the exit pathways, high conductance connexins CX43 and CX40 (*GJA1* and *GJA5*) are lower expressed toward the sinus node, whereas the low conductance CX45 is expressed higher toward the sinus node (Chandler et al., 2009, 2011; Allah et al., 2011). This gradual increase of conductance

TABLE 1 | Level of functional studies for GWAS loci associated with ECG intervals.

Associated gene	G	C	T
AF			
AGBL4	1		
AKAP6	1		
ARHGAP10	1		
ARHGAP26/NR3C1	1		
ASAH1	1		
ATXN1	1	6	
BEST3	1		
ClOorfll	1		
C10orf76	1		
C20orfl66	1		
C6orfl/NUDT3	1		
C9orf3	1		
CAND2	1		13
CASC20/BMP2	1		14
CASZ1	1		
CDK6	1		
CEP68	1		
CGA/ZNF292	1		
COG5	1		
CREB5	1		
CUL4A	1		
CYTH1	1		
DGKB	1		
DNAH10	1		
DPF3	1		
EPHA3	1		
ERBB4	1	25	26
FBN2/SLC27A6	1		
FBRSL1	1		
FBX032	1		
GCOM1	1		
GJA5	1	32	32
GOPC	1		
GORAB/PRRX1	1	35	
GTF2I	1		
GYPC	1		
HAND2	1		
HIP1R	1		
HSPG2/CELA3B	1		
IGF1R	1	38	39
KCND3	1	40	
KCNJ5	1	45	46
KCNN2	1	47	48
KCNN3/PMVK	1	50	51
KDM1B	1		
KIF3C	1		
KRR1/PHLDA1	1		
LHX3	1		
LINC00208/GATA4	1		
LINC00326/EYA4	1		
LINC00540/BASP1P1	1		
LINC00927/ARNT2	1		

(Continued)

TABLE 1 | Continued

Associated gene	G	C	T
LOC100506385	1		
LOC102467213/EFNA5	1		
LRRC74/IRF2BPL	1		
MAPT	1	61	
MBD5	1		
METTL11B/LINC01142	1		
MEX3C	1		
MIR30B	1		
MTSS1/LINC00964	1		
MY018B	1		
NACA	1		
NEURL	1	13	
NUCKS1	1		
OPN1SW	1		
PAK2	1		
PITX2/C4orf32	1	69	69
PKP2	1	70	
POLR2A/TNFSF12	1		
PPFIA4	1		
PPP2R3A	1		
PRDM8/FGF5	1		
PSMB7	1		
PTK2	1		
RBM20	1	81	
REEP1/KDM3A	1		
REEP3	1		
RPS2	1		
SCMH1	1		
SIRT1	1	2	3
SLC24A2/MLLT3	1		
SLC9B1	1		
SLIT3	1		
SMAD7	1		
SNRNP27	1		
SNX6/CFL2	1		
SORL1/MIR100HG	1		
SSPN	1		
SUN1	1		
SYNE2	1		
SYNP02L	1		
TEX41	1		
THRB	1		
TUBA8	1		
UBE4B	1		
USP3	1		
UST	1		
WDR1	1		15
WIPF1/CHRNA1	1		
WNT8A/NME5	1		
XPOI	1		
XP07	1		
XXYLT1	1		
YWHAE/CRK	1		

(Continued)

TABLE 1 | Continued

Associated gene	G	C	T
ZFHX3	1	20	21
ZNF462	1		
ZPBP2	1		
PR			
ALDH18A1/SORBS1	29		
ARHGAP24	29–31		
CCNL1	29		
EFHA1	29		
EOMES	29	34	
EPS15	29		
FAT1	29		
FERMT2	29		
FGFR1	29		
FIGN	29		
ID2	29		37
KRTCAP2	29		
LRCH1	29		
MED13L	29		
MEIS1	29		
MKLN1	29		
MYBPHL	29		52
OBSCN	29		
PAM	29		
PDZRN3	29		
SENP2	29	57	
SH3PXD2A/OBFC1	29		
SKI	29		
SOX5	29	59	60
TMEM182	29		
WNT11	29,31		
XP04	29		
ZFPM2	29		
HR			
ACHE	41	63	64
B3GNT7	41		
CD34	41		
CD46	41		
CHRM2	41		
CPNE8	41		
FADS1	41,42		
FLRT2	41		
FNDC3B	41		
RFX4	41		
SLC12A9	41		
TFPI	41		71
UfSpl	41		
HRV			
NDUFA11	65		
NEOI	65		
PPIL1	65		
RGS6	65	77	78
QRS			
CRIMI	7		

(Continued)

TABLE 1 | Continued

Associated gene	G	C	T
DKK1	7	83	
HAND1/SAP30L	7		
HEATR5B/STRN	7		
IGFBP3	4		
NFIA	4		
SETBP1	4		
TKT/PRKCD/CACNA1D	4	5	5
VTI1A	4		
QT			
ANKRD9	7		
ATP1B1	7	8	
ATP2A2	7	9	10
AZIN1	7		
C30RF75	7		
c6orf204	7		
CNOT1	7,11		12
CREBBP	7		
FEN1/FADS2	7		
GBF1	7		
GFRA3	7		
GMPR	7		
KCNE1	7,11	16	17
KCNQ1	7,11	18	19
LAPTM4B	7		
LIG3	7,11		
LITAF	7,11		
MKL2	7		
NCOA2	7		
NOS1AP	7,11	22	23
RNF207	7,11	24	24
SLC4A4	7	27	
SLC8A1	7	28	28
SMARCAD1	7		
SP3	7		
TCEA3	7		
USP50/TRPM7	7	33	
AF+PR			
CAMK2D	1,29	36	36
FRMD4B	1,29		
MYOCD	1,29		
NAV2	1,29		
PHLDB2	1,29		
TLE3/UACA	1,29		
AF+HR			
GJAI	1,41,42	43	44
GNB4	1,41		
MYH7	1,42	49	
AF+QT			
KCNH2	1,7,11	53	54
KCNJ2/CASC17	1,7	55	56
SPATS2L	1,7		
AF+QRS			
C1orfl85/RNF11/DKN2C/FAF1	1,4		

(Continued)

TABLE 1 | Continued

Associated gene	G	C	T
CASQ2	1,4	58	58
CDKN1A	1,4,30		
GOSR2	1,4		
LRIG1/SLC25A26	1,4		
PR+QRS			
SNORD56B/SIPA1L1	4,29		
TBX20/HERPUD2	4,29	62	
HR+HRV			
GNG11	41,65		
KIAA1755	41,65		
SYT10	41,65		
QRS+QT			
KLF12	4,7		
PRKCA	4,7		
HR+HRV+AF			
HCN4	1,41,65	66	66
HR+SSS+AF			
MYH6	29,30,41,42,67	68	
HR+AF+PR			
NKX2-5/BNIP1	1,29,31,41	72	72
AF+PR+OT			
CAV1/CAV2	1,7,29,31	73	74
AF+PR+QRS			
TBX5/TBX3	1,4,29,30,75	76	76
PR+QRS+QT+AF			
SCN5A/SCN10A/EXOG	1,4,7,11,29,30,75	79	80
HR+AF+PR+QT			
TTN/CCDC141	1,7,29,41		82
HR+HRV+AF+PR			
LINC00477/SOX5/BCAT1	1,29,41,42,65	59	60
HR+AF+QRS+QT			
C6orf204/SLC35F1/PLN/BRD7P3	1,4,7,41,42	84	84

Column G: GWAS reference. Column C: reference with electrophysiological experiments in cells. Column T reference with electrophysiological experiments in tissue. AF, atrial fibrillation; PR, PR interval; HR, heart rate; HRV, heart rate variability; QRS, QRS duration; QT, QT interval; SSS, sick sinus syndrome. [1]Roselli et al., 2018; [2]Vikram et al., 2017; [3]Liu et al., 2016; [4]Sotoodehnia et al., 2010; [5]Zhang et al., 2005; [6]Inoue et al., 2001; [7]Arking et al., 2014; [8]Barwe et al., 2009; [9]Suarez et al., 2004; [10]Shin et al., 2011; [11]Newton-Cheh et al., 2009; [12]Yamaguchi et al., 2018; [13]Sinner et al., 2014; [14]Howden et al., 2013; [15]Huang et al., 2019; [16]Mazhari et al., 2002; [17]Drici et al., 1998; [18]Moreno et al., 2015; [19]Knollmann et al., 2004; [20]Kao et al., 2016; [21]Cheng et al., 2019; [22]Kapoor et al., 2014; [23]Sugiyama et al., 2016; [24]Roder et al., 2014; [25]Yang et al., 2019; [26]Zhou et al., 2018; [27]Myers et al., 2016; [28]Pott et al., 2007; [29]van Setten et al., 2018; [30]Holm et al., 2010; [31]Pfeufer et al., 2010; [32]Noureldin et al., 2018; [33]Sah et al., 2013; [34]Pfeiffer et al., 2018; [35]Tucker et al., 2017; [36]Purohit et al., 2013; [37]Moskowitz et al., 2007; [38]Wang et al., 2014; [39]Sapra et al., 2014; [40]Lugenbiel et al., 2018; [41]den Hoed et al., 2013; [42]Eijgelsheim et al., 2010; [43]Lübkemeier et al., 2013; [44]Tuomi et al., 2011; [45]Bender et al., 2001; [46]Kelly et al., 2014; [47]Li et al., 2009; [48]Yi et al., 2015; [49]Yang et al., 2018; [50]Zhang et al., 2014; [51]Mahida et al., 2014; [52]Barefield et al., 2017; [53]Orvos et al., 2019; [54]Liu et al., 2017; [55]Hattori et al., 2012; [56]Zaritsky et al., 2001; [57]Dustrude et al., 2013; [58]Song et al., 2007; [59]Zheng et al., 2002; [60]Li et al., 2013; [61]Rocher et al., 2010; [62]Caballero et al., 2017; [63]Amend et al., 2019; [64]Masuda and Kawamura, 2003; [65]Nolte et al., 2017; [66]DiFrancesco and Borer, 2007; [67]Holm et al., 2011; [68]Herron et al., 2010; [69]Syeda et al., 2016; [70]Sato et al., 2009; [71]Goldfarb et al., 1998; [72]Li et al., 2019; [73]Barbuti et al., 2012; [74]Park et al., 2002; [75]Smith et al., 2011; [76]Dai et al., 2019; [77]Posokhova et al., 2010; [78]Posokhova et al., 2013; [79]Berecki et al., 2010; [80]Zhang et al., 2007; [81]van den Hoogenhof et al., 2018; [82]Ahlberg et al., 2018; [83]Eldabah et al., 2018; [84]Bai et al., 2013.

from sinus node toward atrial myocardium enables a proper current-to-load match. Therefore, genes involved in sinus node insulation and exit pathway formation are candidates for being associated with sinus node function (or heart rate) in GWAS. Accordingly, a locus near *GJA1* is associated with heart rate in GWAS (den Hoed et al., 2013).

The electrotonic influence of atrial myocardium on sinus node function is important to consider when investigating the relevance of genes provided by GWAS. For instance, common and rare variants in *MYH6* – a component of the sarcomere – are associated with heart rate and sick sinus syndrome (Holm et al., 2010, 2011). However, *MYH6* is more abundantly expressed in the atrial myocardium than in the sinus node (van Eif et al., 2019). *In vitro* experiments in atrial-like cells indicate that mutations in *MYH6* affect conduction velocity (Ishikawa et al., 2015). It is possible that conduction slowing in the atrium underlies the association between *MYH6* and abnormal function of the sinus node. That genes expressed in the atrium but not in the sinus node can affect sinus is further illustrated by Cx40 knock-out mice in which the dominant pacemaker is not always the SAN (Bagwe et al., 2005). Moreover, mutations in *SCN5A* can result in sick sinus syndrome (Benson et al., 2003) despite the lack of *SCN5A* expression in the sinus node.

GWAS LOCI RELATED TO PR INTERVAL

The PR interval is mainly determined by conduction through the atrioventricular junction (Meijler and Janse, 1988). The atrioventricular junction is a complex anatomical structure which was first described in 1906 by Sunao Tawara, who found cells forming a compact complex network but also small cells that joined into bundles (Tawara, 1906). These cells were later called compact nodal cells and transitional cells, respectively, and both have distinct electrophysiological properties (de Carvalho and de Almeida, 1960; Greener et al., 2011). A layer of transitional cells can be found in rings around the orifices of the AV valves where expression of Cx40 and SCN5A is low (Aanhaanen et al., 2010; Fedorov et al., 2011). This transitional ring lies on top of an atrioventricular nodal ring providing two conducting pathways with different electrophysiological characteristics both connecting the atria with the His bundle (Denes et al., 1973; **Figure 1B**). The presence of two conduction pathways illustrates the challenge of relating gene expression of single atrioventricular nodal cells to the electrophysiological phenotype of the atrioventricular node. Moreover, in the atrioventricular junction, not only the compact atrioventricular node contributes to atrioventricular delay but also all other cells present within the AV junction – e.g., transitional cells, fibroblasts and macrophages (Hulsmans et al., 2017). Similar to the sinus node, the function of the atrioventricular node depends on the interaction with these different cell-types.

The cells of the atrioventricular junction find their origin in the atrioventricular canal of the embryonic heart. Impulse conduction delay occurs in both the transitional cells and the compact atrioventricular node, therefore, normal development of the atrioventricular canal is crucial for atrioventricular delay in adult hearts (Meijler and Janse, 1988). Accordingly, GWAS for PR interval showed association with 18 of 44 loci which are related to heart development (van Setten et al., 2018), indicating that proper embryonic development is a crucial factor for adult AV conduction. Some of these loci are located near *TBX2* and *TBX3* – essential transcription factors controlling patterning of the atrioventricular canal during development (Holm et al., 2010; Pfeufer et al., 2010; Aanhaanen et al., 2011; van Setten et al., 2018; **Table 1**). Other loci are located nearby genes related to electrical function of the adult cardiomyocyte, like *SCN5A* and *CAMK2D* or cardiomyocyte contraction, like *TTN* and *MYH6*, however, the significance of these associations with PR interval await further investigation (Holm et al., 2010; van Setten et al., 2018).

GWAS LOCI RELATED TO QRS DURATION

Total ventricular activation time is visualized on the ECG as the duration of the QRS complex, which comprises conduction in the His-Purkinje system and in the ventricular myocardium. The cardiac sodium channel $Na_V1.5$ – encoded by *SCN5A* – is the major determinant of conduction in these tissues and, accordingly, QRS duration is associated with loci near *SCN5A* (Papadatos et al., 2002; Sotoodehnia et al., 2010). Variants in the *SCN10A* gene – encoding the neuronal sodium channel $Na_V1.8$ – associate with QRS duration as well (Sotoodehnia et al., 2010). These variants are located within an enhancer region that modulates expression of *SCN5A* which could explain a relation with QRS duration (Sotoodehnia et al., 2010; van den Boogaard et al., 2014). Although variants in these region do not always associate with QRS prolongation (Behr et al., 2015). Other variants related to QRS duration are those near or within genes involved in bundle branch development and working myocardial phenotype, like *TBX3*, *TBX5*, *TBX20*, *HAND1*, *DKK1*, and *NFIA* (Moskowitz et al., 2007; Bakker et al., 2008; Singh et al., 2009; Sotoodehnia et al., 2010). In addition variants in calcium handling genes such as *PLN*, *CACNA1D*, *STRN*, *PRKCA*, and *CASQ2*, *ATP2A2/ANAPC7* are associated with QRS duration (Sotoodehnia et al., 2010; van Setten et al., 2019). These variants could affect calcium homeostasis resulting in reduced sodium current and slow conduction and thereby prolong QRS duration (King et al., 2013).

The Purkinje network activates the ventricular myocardium via Purkinje muscle junctions composed of transitional cells connecting the Purkinje fibers to ventricular cardiomyocytes (**Figure 1B**; Martinez-Palomo et al., 1970; Tranum-Jensen et al., 1991). Similar to the AV node and the SAN, the connection of Purkinje cardiomyocytes with ventricular cardiomyocytes requires high resistance – preventing current-to-load mismatch (Rohr et al., 1997). We expect that reduction of electrical coupling in these junctions – by e.g., lower expression of CX40 – will delay ventricular activation, which prolongs QRS duration. Purkinje fibers develop from embryonic trabeculae (Jensen et al., 2012) where e.g., Cx40, *Scn5a*, *CnTn2* are abundantly present. The primordial Purkinje trabeculae require further specialization

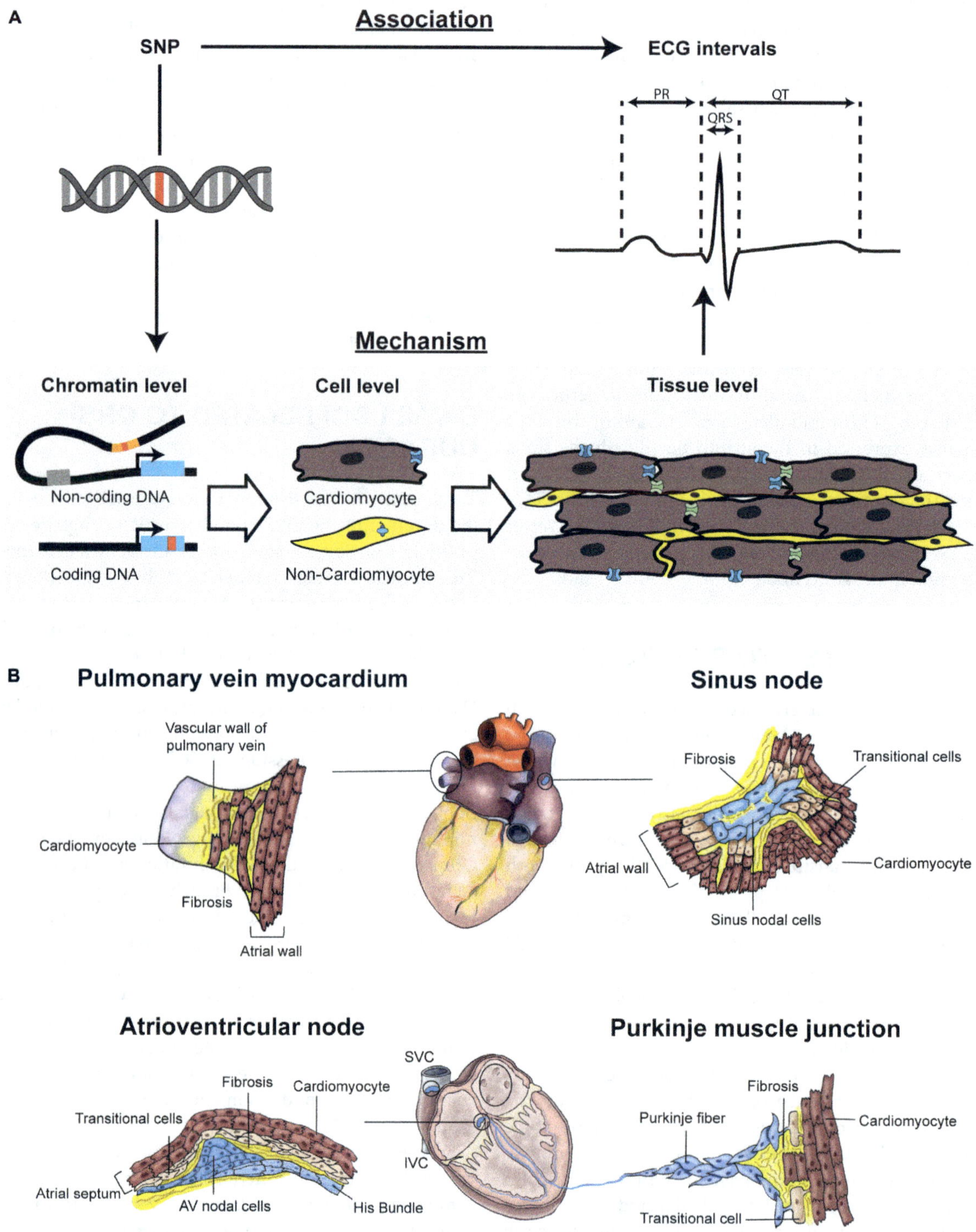

FIGURE 1 | In GWAS, **(A)** SNPs are associated with ECG intervals, like PR interval, QRS complex, and QT interval. To understand physiological relevance of a SNP three biological levels of organization should be studied (1) Chromatin level: Determine which gene(s) is affected by the SNP. The SNP (red mark) can be located in non-coding or coding DNA. For SNPs in non-coding DNA, it is important to determine which coding genes are affected. (2) Cell level: Determine in which cell types the gene is expressed. The cell type in which the affected gene is expressed is relevant for cellular function of the gene. (3) Tissue level: Determine how gene expression in a cell type affects tissue electrophysiology. Tissue electrophysiology can be related to ECG intervals. **(B)** Tissue structure is essential for proper conduction. The pulmonary vein has an outer sleeve of cardiomyocytes. These pulmonary vein cardiomyocytes are not as densely packed as the atrial cardiomyocytes – resulting in less coupling. Small reentry circuits or ectopic activity can therefore occur in pulmonary vein myocardium. The sinus node – where it is not insulated by fibrosis – connects with the atrial cardiomyocytes through transitional cells. In the atrioventricular junction, AV nodal cells are electrically connected with the atrial myocardium through a layer of transitional cells. In the Purkinje muscle junction, Purkinje cells connect with ventricular cardiomyocytes through transitional cells. AV, atrioventricular; IVC, inferior vena cava; SNP, Single nucleotide polymorphism; SVC, superior vena cava.

after birth under influence of *Nkx2-5* and *Irx3* expression and Notch signaling (Zhang et al., 2011; Rentschler et al., 2012). Homozygous *Irx3* loss-of-function mice have slowed conduction in Purkinje fibers (Koizumi et al., 2016). We expect that genetic variations affecting expression of these factors – that are involved in development and maturation of the Purkinje fibers – will relate to total ventricular activation time and thereby QRS duration in GWAS.

GWAS LOCI RELATED TO QT INTERVAL

The QT interval is a measure of ventricular repolarization and reflects the time between the first moment of activation to the last moment of repolarization. Accordingly, the QT interval relates to action potential duration (APD) but also to differences in regional conduction velocity. Conduction slowing in regions that repolarize late prolongs QT interval whereas conduction slowing in areas that repolarize early may not affect QT interval. The QT interval has an inverse relation with heart rate. This inverse relation results from shortening of the APD at higher rates due to activation of the slowly delayed rectifier current I_{Ks} (Boyett and Jewell, 1978; Carmeliet, 2006). QT intervals corrected for heart rate – QTc – or QT interval measured at similar heart rates may increase sensitivity for finding variants related to repolarization (Bazett, 1920). In mice, however, QT interval does not depend on heart rate. Therefore, QT interval – not QTc – should be used as measure for ventricular repolarization in mice (Speerschneider and Thomsen, 2013).

Genome Wide Association Studies for QT interval identified 22 loci (**Table 1**) of which many are in or near genes encoding for potassium channels or involved in calcium handling (Arking et al., 2014). Increased potassium current shortens QT interval whereas increased calcium current prolongs QT interval (Wemhöner et al., 2015; Landstrom et al., 2016). Nitric Oxide Synthase 1 Adaptor Protein (*NOS1AP*) – regulating calcium current – is associated with QT interval in GWAS (Arking et al., 2006, 2014). Genetic variation within the *NOS1AP* gene affects QT interval and is related to arrhythmogenesis in patients with the long QT syndrome (Crotti et al., 2009; Tomás et al., 2010). The effect of *NOS1AP* on QT interval, however, could also have an extracardiac pathway as its expression is high in brain (Xu et al., 2005) providing the possibility of *NOS1AP* to affect autonomic modulation of the QT interval (Yagishita et al., 2015).

GWAS LOCI RELATED TO ARRHYTHMIAS

Atrial Arrhythmias

Atrial fibrillation (AF) is the most common arrhythmia and the prevalence increases with age (Krijthe et al., 2013). AF results from an interplay between electrical (triggers and reentry), structural and hemodynamic remodeling (Schotten et al., 2011). The combination of these pathophysiological changes sets the stage for AF.

The trigger for AF is commonly near the connection between the left atrium and pulmonary veins (PVs) (Haïssaguerre et al., 1998). In humans – at this connection – the four PVs are enclosed by an outer sleeve of myocardium (Saito et al., 2000). PV cardiomyocytes are morphologically similar to atrial cardiomyocytes, but have a different developmental history (Verheule et al., 2002; Mommersteeg et al., 2007a). The formation of PV myocardium in mice highly depends on expression of *Pitx2* and *Nkx2-5* during development (Mommersteeg et al., 2007a). GWAS in more than 65 thousand AF patients identified 97 loci (Roselli et al., 2018) – including *PITX2* and *NKX2-5*, suggesting a relation of AF with PV formation during development. The myocardial sleeves of the PVs are thinner distal to the left atrium and end in single cardiomyocyte protrusions in the PV (**Figure 1B**; Verheule et al., 2002). These PV myocytes have a high resting membrane potential and low expression of inward rectifier channels (Ehrlich et al., 2003; Melnyk et al., 2005), setting the stage for spontaneous activity. Accordingly, variants near genes encoding inward rectifier channels – e.g., *KCNJ2, KCNJ5* – are associated with AF (Christophersen et al., 2017; Roselli et al., 2018).

Electrical remodeling is a cause and effect of reentry circuits that maintain AF. Reentry is facilitated by slow conduction and short APD (Wiener and Rosenblueth, 1946). Accordingly, GWAS for AF identified six genes encoding for potassium channels all involved in atrial APD: *KCND3, KCNH2, KCNN2*, and *KCNN3* (Roselli et al., 2018). Genes encoding channels involved in conduction – e.g., *GJA1, GJA5, SCN5A*, and *SCN10A* are also associated with AF (Christophersen et al., 2017; Roselli et al., 2018). Moreover, transcription factors involved in spatiotemporal expression of these ion channels – *TBX3, TBX5*, and *PITX2* – associate with AF as well (Tao et al., 2014; Nadadur et al., 2016). Novel findings have indicated that not only genes encoding ion channel are related to AF. Titin (TTN) – a large sarcomere protein – is associated with early onset AF (Choi et al., 2018). TTN dysfunction may predispose to AF by increasing myocardial fibrosis and prolonging PR interval, which are both associated with increased risk for AF (Ahlberg et al., 2018).

Ventricular Arrhythmias

Up to 80% of sudden cardiac arrests (SCA) are caused by acute ischemia resulting from coronary artery disease (Huikuri et al., 2001; Fishman et al., 2010). GWAS in patients with coronary artery disease identified 11 variants related to SCA of which eight were near or within genes related to long QT syndrome (Marsman et al., 2014). It is unclear whether these variants predispose to arrhythmias in general or only in the setting of coronary artery disease. A gene that does specifically relate to arrhythmias in the setting of acute myocardial ischemia is *CXADR* which encodes the CXADR Ig-like cell adhesion molecule (previously named Coxsackie and adenovirus receptor, CAR) (Bezzina et al., 2010). Reduced expression of CAR lowers sodium channel availability – thereby reducing conduction velocity – and facilitates reentry arrhythmias in the setting of ischemia (Marsman et al., 2014). Non-ischemia induced arrhythmias explain 20% of SCA and comprise a variety of arrhythmogenic syndromes which can be related to structural abnormal myocardium or genetic mutations (John et al., 2012). GWAS for SCA identified several genes which all associate with risk factors for SCA such as QRS duration and QT interval (Adabag et al., 2010; Arking et al., 2011; Milano et al., 2016; Ashar et al., 2018).

Genome Wide Association Studies for syncope – which is a common symptom of many arrhythmogenic syndromes – identified a genetic variant close in proximity to the gene zinc finger protein 804a (*ZNF804A*) (Hadji-Turdeghal et al., 2020). Whether a role of *ZNF804A* in cardiac arrhythmias or e.g., blood pressure regulation explains this association remains to be investigated.

Ventricular fibrillation is associated with IRX3 (Koizumi et al., 2016), which plays a role in conduction in Purkinje fibers. Ablation of Purkinje muscle junctions is a successful treatment for a subset of patients with idiopathic ventricular fibrillation indicating a role of Purkinje cells in these arrhythmias (Haïssaguerre et al., 2002).

Understanding arrhythmogenic mechanisms can guide interpretation of GWAS derived data. This is exemplified by the Brugada syndrome, which is characterized by ST segment elevation in the right precordial leads and ventricular arrhythmias. Initially, the Brugada syndrome was considered an ion channel disease mainly resulting from dysfunction of the cardiac sodium channel. However, only 20% of patients present with mutations in *SCN5A* (Antzelevitch et al., 2005). A GWAS in Brugada syndrome patients identified several variants in regulatory DNA controlling SCN5A expression (Bezzina et al., 2013). In order to discover causal variants in GWAS with limited number of patients, knowledge on the arrhythmogenic mechanism of the disease is helpful. Mechanistic studies in hearts from Brugada syndrome patients have suggested that arrhythmias occur due to conduction block in the presence of subtle structural abnormalities (Coronel et al., 2005; Hoogendijk et al., 2010). This suggests that variants near genes involved in the formation of fibrosis (*TGFB2)* or genes affecting safety factor of cardiac conduction (e.g., *SCN5A*, *GJA1*, *KCHIP1*) are important variants to further investigate.

CONCLUSION

Most of the variants provided by GWAS lie near or within expected candidate genes potentially explaining the phenotype they are associated with. However, the electrophysiological characterization of the vast majority of associated genes has not shown direct effects on ECG intervals nor on arrhythmia susceptibility. In this review, we emphasize that mechanistic knowledge of the structure-function relations underlying ECG intervals and arrhythmias should be considered when interpreting experimental characterization of these variants, in order to guide clinical applicability of GWAS data.

AUTHOR CONTRIBUTIONS

KS and BB designed and wrote the manuscript. VM, CG-M, and EL critically revised the manuscript.

REFERENCES

Aanhaanen, W. T. J., Mommersteeg, M. T. M., Norden, J., Wakker, V., de Gier-de Vries, C., Anderson, R. H., et al. (2010). Developmental origin, growth, and three-dimensional architecture of the atrioventricular conduction axis of the mouse heart. *Circ. Res.* 107, 728–736. doi: 10.1161/CIRCRESAHA.110.222992

Aanhaanen, W. T. J. J., Boukens, B. J. D. D., Sizarov, A., Wakker, V., de Gier-de Vries, C., van Ginneken, A. C., et al. (2011). Defective Tbx2-dependent patterning of the atrioventricular canal myocardium causes accessory pathway formation in mice. *J. Clin. Invest.* 121, 534–544. doi: 10.1172/JCI44350

Adabag, A. S., Luepker, R. V., Roger, V. L., and Gersh, B. J. (2010). Sudden cardiac death: epidemiology and risk factors. *Nat. Rev. Cardiol.* 7, 216–225. doi: 10.1038/nrcardio.2010.3

Ahlberg, G., Refsgaard, L., Lundegaard, P. R., Andreasen, L., Ranthe, M. F., Linscheid, N., et al. (2018). Rare truncating variants in the sarcomeric protein titin associate with familial and early-onset atrial fibrillation. *Nat. Commun.* 9:4316. doi: 10.1038/s41467-018-06618-y

Allah, E. A., Tellez, J. O., Yanni, J., Nelson, T., Monfredi, O., Boyett, M. R., et al. (2011). Changes in the expression of ion channels, connexins and Ca2+-handling proteins in the sino-atrial node during postnatal development. *Exp. Physiol.* 96, 426–438. doi: 10.1113/expphysiol.2010.055780

Amend, N., Thiermann, H., Worek, F., and Wille, T. (2019). The arrhythmogenic potential of nerve agents and a cardiac safety profile of antidotes – A proof-of-concept study using human induced pluripotent stem cells derived cardiomyocytes (hiPSC-CM). *Toxicol. Lett.* 308, 1–6. doi: 10.1016/j.toxlet.2019.03.003

Antzelevitch, C., Brugada, P., Borggrefe, M., Brugada, J., Brugada, R., Corrado, D., et al. (2005). Brugada syndrome: report of the second consensus conference: endorsed by the heart rhythm society and the European heart rhythm association. *Circulation* 111, 659–670. doi: 10.1161/01.CIR.0000152479.54298.51

Arking, D. E., Junttila, M. J., Goyette, P., Huertas-Vazquez, A., Eijgelsheim, M., Blom, M. T., et al. (2011). Identification of a sudden cardiac death susceptibility locus at 2q24.2 through genome-wide association in European ancestry individuals. *PLoS Genet.* 7:e1002158. doi: 10.1371/journal.pgen.1002158

Arking, D. E., Pfeufer, A., Post, W., Kao, W. H. L., Newton-Cheh, C., Ikeda, M., et al. (2006). A common genetic variant in the NOS1 regulator NOS1AP modulates cardiac repolarization. *Nat. Genet.* 38, 644–651. doi: 10.1038/ng1790

Arking, D. E., Pulit, S. L., Crotti, L., van der Harst, P., Munroe, P. B., Koopmann, T. T., et al. (2014). Genetic association study of QT interval highlights role for calcium signaling pathways in myocardial repolarization. *Nat. Genet.* 46, 826–836. doi: 10.1038/ng.3014

Ashar, F. N., Mitchell, R. N., Albert, C. M., Newton-Cheh, C., Brody, J. A., Müller-Nurasyid, M., et al. (2018). A comprehensive evaluation of the genetic architecture of sudden cardiac arrest. *Eur. Heart J.* 39, 3961–3969. doi: 10.1093/eurheartj/ehy474

Bagwe, S., Berenfeld, O., Vaidya, D., Morley, G. E., and Jalife, J. (2005). Altered right atrial excitation and propagation in connexin40 knockout mice. *Circulation* 112, 2245–2253. doi: 10.1161/CIRCULATIONAHA.104.527325

Bai, Y., Jones, P. P., Guo, J., Zhong, X., Clark, R. B., Zhou, Q., et al. (2013). Phospholamban knockout breaks arrhythmogenic Ca^{2+} waves and suppresses catecholaminergic polymorphic ventricular tachycardia in mice. *Circ. Res.* 113, 517–526. doi: 10.1161/CIRCRESAHA.113.301678

Bakker, M. L., Boukens, B. J., Mommersteeg, M. T. M. M., Brons, J. F., Wakker, V., Moorman, A. F. M. M., et al. (2008). Transcription factor Tbx3 is required for the specification of the atrioventricular conduction system. *Circ. Res.* 102, 1340–1349. doi: 10.1161/CIRCRESAHA.107.169565

Barbuti, A., Scavone, A., Mazzocchi, N., Terragni, B., Baruscotti, M., and Difrancesco, D. (2012). A caveolin-binding domain in the HCN4 channels mediates functional interaction with caveolin proteins. *J. Mol. Cell. Cardiol.* 53, 187–195. doi: 10.1016/j.yjmcc.2012.05.013

Barefield, D. Y., Puckelwartz, M. J., Kim, E. Y., Wilsbacher, L. D., Vo, A. H., Waters, E. A., et al. (2017). Experimental modeling supports a role for MyBP-HL as a novel myofilament component in arrhythmia and dilated cardiomyopathy. *Circulation* 136, 1477–1491. doi: 10.1161/CIRCULATIONAHA.117.028585

Barwe, S. P., Jordan, M. C., Skay, A., Inge, L., Rajasekaran, S. A., Wolle, D., et al. (2009). Dysfunction of ouabain-induced cardiac contractility in mice with heart-specific ablation of Na,K-ATPase beta1-subunit. *J. Mol. Cell. Cardiol.* 47, 552–560. doi: 10.1016/j.yjmcc.2009.07.018

Bazett, H. C. (1920). An analysis of the time-relations of electrocardiograms. *Heart* 7, 353–370. doi: 10.1111/j.1542-474X.1997.tb00325.x

Behr, E. R., Savio-Galimberti, E., Barc, J., Holst, A. G., Petropoulou, E., Prins, B. P., et al. (2015). Role of common and rare variants in SCN10A: results from the Brugada syndrome QRS locus gene discovery collaborative study. *Cardiovasc. Res.* 106, 520–529. doi: 10.1093/cvr/cvv042

Bender, K., Wellner-Kienitz, M. C., Inanobe, A., Meyer, T., Kurachi, Y., and Pott, L. (2001). Overexpression of monomeric and multimeric GIRK4 subunits in rat atrial myocytes removes fast desensitization and reduces inward rectification of muscarinic K(+) current (I(K(ACh))). Evidence for functional homomeric GIRK4 channels. *J. Biol. Chem.* 276, 28873–28880. doi: 10.1074/jbc.M102328200

Benson, D. W., Wang, D. W., Dyment, M., Knilans, T. K., Fish, F. A., Strieper, M. J., et al. (2003). Congenital sick sinus syndrome caused by recessive mutations in the cardiac sodium channel gene (SCN5A). *J. Clin. Invest.* 112, 1019–1028. doi: 10.1172/JCI200318062

Berecki, G., Wilders, R., de Jonge, B., van Ginneken, A. C. G., and Verkerk, A. O. (2010). Re-evaluation of the action potential upstroke velocity as a measure of the Na+ current in cardiac myocytes at physiological conditions. *PLoS One* 5:e15772. doi: 10.1371/journal.pone.0015772

Bezzina, C. R., Barc, J., Mizusawa, Y., Remme, C. A., Gourraud, J.-B., Simonet, F., et al. (2013). Common variants at SCN5A-SCN10A and HEY2 are associated with Brugada syndrome, a rare disease with high risk of sudden cardiac death. *Nat. Genet.* 45, 1044–1049. doi: 10.1038/ng.2712

Bezzina, C. R., Pazoki, R., Bardai, A., Marsman, R. F., de Jong, J. S. S. G., Blom, M. T., et al. (2010). Genome-wide association study identifies a susceptibility locus at 21q21 for ventricular fibrillation in acute myocardial infarction. *Nat. Genet.* 42, 688–691. doi: 10.1038/ng.623

Bleeker, W. K., Mackaay, A. J. C., Masson-Pevet, M., Bouman, L. N., and Becker, A. E. (1980). Functional and morphological organization of the rabbit sinus node. *Circ. Res.* 46, 11–22. doi: 10.1161/01.RES.46.1.11

Boukens, B. J., Rivaud, M. R., Rentschler, S., and Coronel, R. (2014). Misinterpretation of the mouse ECG: "Musing the waves of Mus musculus. *J. Physiol.* 592, 4613–4626. doi: 10.1113/jphysiol.2014.279380

Boyett, M. R., and Jewell, B. R. (1978). A study of the factors responsible for rate-dependent shortening of the action potential in mammalian ventricular muscle. *J. Physiol.* 285, 359–380. doi: 10.1113/jphysiol.1978.sp012576

Caballero, R., Utrilla, R. G., Amorós, I., Matamoros, M., Pérez-Hernández, M., Tinaquero, D., et al. (2017). Tbx20 controls the expression of the KCNH2 gene and of hERG channels. *Proc. Natl. Acad. Sci. U.S.A.* 114, E416–E425. doi: 10.1073/pnas.1612383114

Carmeliet, E. (2006). Action potential duration, rate of stimulation, and intracellular sodium. *J. Cardiovasc. Electrophysiol.* 17(Suppl. 1), S2–S7. doi: 10.1111/j.1540-8167.2006.00378.x

Chandler, N., Aslanidi, O., Buckley, D., Inada, S., Birchall, S., Atkinson, A., et al. (2011). Computer three-dimensional anatomical reconstruction of the human sinus node and a novel paranodal area. *Anat. Rec. (Hoboken).* 294, 970–979. doi: 10.1002/ar.21379

Chandler, N. J., Greener, I. D., Tellez, J. O., Inada, S., Musa, H., Molenaar, P., et al. (2009). Molecular architecture of the human sinus node insights into the function of the cardiac pacemaker. *Circulation* 119, 1562–1575. doi: 10.1161/CIRCULATIONAHA.108.804369

Cheng, W.-L., Kao, Y.-H., Chao, T.-F., Lin, Y.-K., Chen, S.-A., and Chen, Y.-J. (2019). MicroRNA-133 suppresses ZFHX3-dependent atrial remodelling and arrhythmia. *Acta Physiol. (Oxf).* 227:e13322. doi: 10.1111/apha.13322

Choi, S. H., Weng, L.-C., Roselli, C., Lin, H., Haggerty, C. M., Shoemaker, M. B., et al. (2018). Association between titin loss-of-function variants and early-onset atrial fibrillation. *JAMA* 320, 2354–2364. doi: 10.1001/jama.2018.18179

Christophersen, I. E., Rienstra, M., Roselli, C., Yin, X., Geelhoed, B., Barnard, J., et al. (2017). Large-scale analyses of common and rare variants identify 12 new loci associated with atrial fibrillation. *Nat. Genet.* 49, 946–952. doi: 10.1038/ng.3843

Coronel, R., Casini, S., Koopmann, T. T., Wilms-Schopman, F. J. G., Verkerk, A. O., de Groot, J. R., et al. (2005). Right ventricular fibrosis and conduction delay in a patient with clinical signs of Brugada syndrome: a combined electrophysiological, genetic, histopathologic, and computational study. *Circulation* 112, 2769–2777. doi: 10.1161/CIRCULATIONAHA.105.532614

Crotti, L., Monti, M. C., Insolia, R., Peljto, A., Goosen, A., Brink, P. A., et al. (2009). NOS1AP is a genetic modifier of the long-QT syndrome. *Circulation* 120, 1657–1663. doi: 10.1161/CIRCULATIONAHA.109.879643

Csepe, T. A., Kalyanasundaram, A., Hansen, B. J., Zhao, J., and Fedorov, V. V. (2015). Fibrosis: a structural modulator of sinoatrial node physiology and dysfunction. *Front. Physiol.* 6:37. doi: 10.3389/fphys.2015.00037

Dai, W., Laforest, B., Tyan, L., Shen, K. M., Nadadur, R. D., Alvarado, F. J., et al. (2019). A calcium transport mechanism for atrial fibrillation in Tbx5-mutant mice. *eLife* 8:e41814. doi: 10.7554/eLife.41814

de Carvalho, A., and de Almeida, D. (1960). Spread of activity through the atrioventricular node. *Circ. Res.* 8, 801–809. doi: 10.1161/01.RES.8.4.801

den Hoed, M., Eijgelsheim, M., Esko, T., Brundel, B. J. J. M., Peal, D. S., Evans, D. M., et al. (2013). Identification of heart rate-associated loci and their effects on cardiac conduction and rhythm disorders. *Nat. Genet.* 45, 621–631. doi: 10.1038/ng.2610

Denes, P., Wu, D., Dhingra, R. C., Chuquimia, R., and Rosen, K. M. (1973). Demonstration of dual A-V nodal pathways in patients with paroxysmal supraventricular tachycardia. *Circulation* 48, 549–555. doi: 10.1161/01.CIR.48.3.549

DiFrancesco, D., and Borer, J. S. (2007). The funny current: cellular basis for the control of heart rate. *Drugs* 67(Suppl. 2), 15–24. doi: 10.2165/00003495-200767002-00003

Drici, M. D., Arrighi, I., Chouabe, C., Mann, J. R., Lazdunski, M., Romey, G., et al. (1998). Involvement of IsK-associated K+ channel in heart rate control of repolarization in a murine engineered model of Jervell and Lange-Nielsen syndrome. *Circ. Res.* 83, 95–102. doi: 10.1161/01.res.83.1.95

Dustrude, E. T., Wilson, S. M., Ju, W., Xiao, Y., and Khanna, R. (2013). CRMP2 protein SUMOylation modulates NaV1.7 channel trafficking. *J. Biol. Chem.* 288, 24316–24331. doi: 10.1074/jbc.M113.474924

Ehrlich, J. R., Cha, T.-J., Zhang, L., Chartier, D., Melnyk, P., Hohnloser, S. H., et al. (2003). Cellular electrophysiology of canine pulmonary vein cardiomyocytes: action potential and ionic current properties. *J. Physiol.* 551, 801–813. doi: 10.1113/jphysiol.2003.046417

Eijgelsheim, M., Newton-Cheh, C., Sotoodehnia, N., de Bakker, P. I. W., Müller, M., Morrison, A. C., et al. (2010). Genome-wide association analysis identifies multiple loci related to resting heart rate. *Hum. Mol. Genet.* 19, 3885–3894. doi: 10.1093/hmg/ddq303

Eldabah, N., Nembo, E. N., Penner, M., Semmler, J., Swelem, R., Hassab, A., et al. (2018). Altered functional expression of β-Adrenergic receptors in rhesus monkey embryonic stem cell-derived cardiomyocytes. *Stem Cells Dev.* 27, 336–346. doi: 10.1089/scd.2017.0053

Fedorov, V. V., Ambrosi, C. M., Kostecki, G., Hucker, W. J., Glukhov, A. V., Wuskell, J. P., et al. (2011). Anatomic localization and autonomic modulation of atrioventricular junctional rhythm in failing human hearts. *Circ. Arrhythm. Electrophysiol.* 4, 515–525. doi: 10.1161/CIRCEP.111.962258

Fedorov, V. V., Glukhov, A. V., Chang, R., Kostecki, G., Aferol, H., Hucker, W. J., et al. (2010). Optical mapping of the isolated coronary-perfused human sinus node. *J. Am. Coll. Cardiol.* 56, 1386–1394. doi: 10.1016/j.jacc.2010.03.098

Fedorov, V. V., Schuessler, R. B., Hemphill, M., Ambrosi, C. M., Chang, R., Voloshina, A. S., et al. (2009). Structural and functional evidence for discrete exit pathways that connect the canine sinoatrial node and atria. *Circ. Res.* 104, 915–923. doi: 10.1161/CIRCRESAHA.108.193193

Fishman, G. I., Chugh, S. S., Dimarco, J. P., Albert, C. M., Anderson, M. E., Bonow, R. O., et al. (2010). Sudden cardiac death prediction and prevention: report from a national heart, lung, and blood institute and heart rhythm society workshop. *Circulation* 122, 2335–2348. doi: 10.1161/CIRCULATIONAHA.110.976092

Glukhov, A. V., Hage, L. T., Hansen, B. J., Pedraza-Toscano, A., Vargas-Pinto, P., Hamlin, R. L., et al. (2013). Sinoatrial node reentry in a canine chronic left ventricular infarct model: role of intranodal fibrosis and heterogeneity of refractoriness. *Circ. Arrhythm. Electrophysiol.* 6, 984–994. doi: 10.1161/CIRCEP.113.000404

Goldfarb, R. D., Glock, D., Johnson, K., Creasey, A. A., Carr, C., McCarthy, R. J., et al. (1998). Randomized, blinded, placebo-controlled trial of tissue factor pathway inhibitor in porcine septic shock. *Shock* 10, 258–264. doi: 10.1097/00024382-199810000-00005

Greener, I. D., Monfredi, O., Inada, S., Chandler, N. J., Tellez, J. O., Atkinson, A., et al. (2011). Molecular architecture of the human specialised atrioventricular conduction axis. *J. Mol. Cell. Cardiol.* 50, 642–651. doi: 10.1016/j.yjmcc.2010.12.017

GTEx Consortium (2013). The genotype-tissue expression (GTEx) project. *Nat. Genet.* 45, 580–585. doi: 10.1038/ng.2653

Hadji-Turdeghal, K., Andreasen, L., Hagen, C. M., Ahlberg, G., Ghouse, J., Bækvad-Hansen, M., et al. (2020). Genome-wide association study identifies locus at chromosome 2q32.1 associated with syncope and collapse. *Cardiovasc. Res.* 116, 138–148. doi: 10.1093/cvr/cvz106

Haïssaguerre, M., Jaïs, P., Shah, D. C., Takahashi, A., Hocini, M., Quiniou, G., et al. (1998). Spontaneous initiation of atrial fibrillation by ectopic beats originating in the pulmonary veins. *N. Engl. J. Med.* 339, 659–666. doi: 10.1056/NEJM199809033391003

Haïssaguerre, M., Shah, D. C., Jaïs, P., Shoda, M., Kautzner, J., Arentz, T., et al. (2002). Role of Purkinje conducting system in triggering of idiopathic ventricular fibrillation. *Lancet* 359, 677–678. doi: 10.1016/S0140-6736(02)07807-8

Hattori, T., Makiyama, T., Akao, M., Ehara, E., Ohno, S., Iguchi, M., et al. (2012). A novel gain-of-function KCNJ2 mutation associated with short-QT syndrome impairs inward rectification of Kir2.1 currents. *Cardiovasc. Res.* 93, 666–673. doi: 10.1093/cvr/cvr329

Heinig, M. (2018). Using gene expression to annotate cardiovascular GWAS loci. *Front. Cardiovasc. Med.* 5:59. doi: 10.3389/fcvm.2018.00059

Herron, T. J., Devaney, E., Mundada, L., Arden, E., Day, S., Guerrero-Serna, G., et al. (2010). Ca2+-independent positive molecular inotropy for failing rabbit and human cardiac muscle by alpha-myosin motor gene transfer. *FASEB J.* 24, 415–424. doi: 10.1096/fj.09-140566

Holm, H., Gudbjartsson, D. F., Arnar, D. O., Thorleifsson, G., Thorgeirsson, G., Stefansdottir, H., et al. (2010). Several common variants modulate heart rate, PR interval and QRS duration. *Nat. Genet.* 42, 117–122. doi: 10.1038/ng.511

Holm, H., Gudbjartsson, D. F., Sulem, P., Masson, G., Helgadottir, H. T., Zanon, C., et al. (2011). A rare variant in MYH6 is associated with high risk of sick sinus syndrome. *Nat. Genet.* 43, 316–323. doi: 10.1038/ng.781

Hoogendijk, M. G., Potse, M., Linnenbank, A. C., Verkerk, A. O., den Ruijter, H. M., van Amersfoorth, S. C. M., et al. (2010). Mechanism of right precordial ST-segment elevation in structural heart disease: excitation failure by current-to-load mismatch. *Hear. Rhythm* 7, 238–248. doi: 10.1016/j.hrthm.2009.10.007

Howden, R., Cooley, I., Van Dodewaard, C., Arthur, S., Cividanes, S., Leamy, L., et al. (2013). Cardiac responses to 24 hrs hyperoxia in Bmp2 and Bmp4 heterozygous mice. *Inhal. Toxicol.* 25, 509–516. doi: 10.3109/08958378.2013.808287

Huang, X., Li, Z., Hu, J., Yang, Z., Liu, Z., Zhang, T., et al. (2019). Knockout of Wdr1 results in cardiac hypertrophy and impaired cardiac function in adult mouse heart. *Gene* 697, 40–47. doi: 10.1016/j.gene.2019.02.023

Huikuri, H. V., Castellanos, A., and Myerburg, R. J. (2001). Sudden death due to cardiac arrhythmias. *N. Engl. J. Med.* 345, 1473–1482. doi: 10.1056/NEJMra000650

Hulsmans, M., Clauss, S., Xiao, L., Aguirre, A. D., King, K. R., Hanley, A., et al. (2017). Macrophages facilitate electrical conduction in the heart. *Cell* 169, 510–522.e20. doi: 10.1016/j.cell.2017.03.050

Inoue, T., Lin, X., Kohlmeier, K. A., Orr, H. T., Zoghbi, H. Y., and Ross, W. N. (2001). Calcium dynamics and electrophysiological properties of cerebellar Purkinje cells in SCA1 transgenic mice. *J. Neurophysiol.* 85, 1750–1760. doi: 10.1152/jn.2001.85.4.1750

Ishikawa, T., Jou, C. J., Nogami, A., Kowase, S., Arrington, C. B., Barnett, S. M., et al. (2015). Novel mutation in the α-myosin heavy chain gene is associated with sick sinus syndrome. *Circ. Arrhythmia Electrophysiol.* 8, 400–408. doi: 10.1161/CIRCEP.114.002534

Jensen, B., Boukens, B. J. D., Postma, A. V., Gunst, Q. D., van den Hoff, M. J. B., Moorman, A. F. M., et al. (2012). Identifying the evolutionary building blocks of the cardiac conduction system. *PLoS One* 7:e44231. doi: 10.1371/journal.pone.0044231

John, R. M., Tedrow, U. B., Koplan, B. A., Albert, C. M., Epstein, L. M., Sweeney, M. O., et al. (2012). Ventricular arrhythmias and sudden cardiac death. *Lancet* 380, 1520–1529. doi: 10.1016/S0140-6736(12)61413-5

Joyner, R. W., and van Capelle, F. J. (1986). Propagation through electrically coupled cells. How a small SA node drives a large atrium. *Biophys. J.* 50, 1157–1164. doi: 10.1016/S0006-3495(86)83559-7

Kao, Y.-H., Hsu, J.-C., Chen, Y.-C., Lin, Y.-K., Lkhagva, B., Chen, S.-A., et al. (2016). ZFHX3 knockdown increases arrhythmogenesis and dysregulates calcium homeostasis in HL-1 atrial myocytes. *Int. J. Cardiol.* 210, 85–92. doi: 10.1016/j.ijcard.2016.02.091

Kapoor, A., Sekar, R. B., Hansen, N. F., Fox-Talbot, K., Morley, M., Pihur, V., et al. (2014). An enhancer polymorphism at the cardiomyocyte intercalated disc protein NOS1AP locus is a major regulator of the QT interval. *Am. J. Hum. Genet.* 94, 854–869. doi: 10.1016/j.ajhg.2014.05.001

Kelly, R. G., Buckingham, M. E., and Moorman, A. F. (2014). Heart fields and cardiac morphogenesis. *Cold Spring Harb. Perspect. Med.* 4:a015750. doi: 10.1101/cshperspect.a015750

King, J. H., Wickramarachchi, C., Kua, K., Du, Y., Jeevaratnam, K., Matthews, H. R., et al. (2013). Loss of Nav1.5 expression and function in murine atria containing the RyR2-P2328S gain-of-function mutation. *Cardiovasc. Res.* 99, 751–759. doi: 10.1093/cvr/cvt141

Kirchhof, C. J., Bonke, F. I., Allessie, M. A., and Lammers, W. J. (1987). The influence of the atrial myocardium on impulse formation in the rabbit sinus node. *Pflugers Arch.* 410, 198–203. doi: 10.1007/bf00581916

Kléber, A. G., and Rudy, Y. (2004). Basic mechanisms of cardiac impulse propagation and associated arrhythmias. *Physiol. Rev.* 84, 431–488. doi: 10.1152/physrev.00025.2003

Knollmann, B. C., Casimiro, M. C., Katchman, A. N., Sirenko, S. G., Schober, T., Rong, Q., et al. (2004). Isoproterenol exacerbates a long QT phenotype in Kcnq1-deficient neonatal mice: possible roles for human-like Kcnq1 isoform 1 and slow delayed rectifier K+ current. *J. Pharmacol. Exp. Ther.* 310, 311–318. doi: 10.1124/jpet.103.063743

Koizumi, A., Sasano, T., Kimura, W., Miyamoto, Y., Aiba, T., Ishikawa, T., et al. (2016). Genetic defects in a His-Purkinje system transcription factor, IRX3, cause lethal cardiac arrhythmias. *Eur. Heart J.* 37, 1469–1475. doi: 10.1093/eurheartj/ehv449

Krijthe, B. P., Kunst, A., Benjamin, E. J., Lip, G. Y. H., Franco, O. H., Hofman, A., et al. (2013). Projections on the number of individuals with atrial fibrillation in the European Union, from 2000 to 2060. *Eur. Heart J.* 34, 2746–2751. doi: 10.1093/eurheartj/eht280

Lakatta, E. G., and DiFrancesco, D. (2009). What keeps us ticking: a funny current, a calcium clock, or both? *J. Mol. Cell. Cardiol.* 47, 157–170. doi: 10.1016/j.yjmcc.2009.03.022

Landstrom, A. P., Boczek, N. J., Ye, D., Miyake, C. Y., De la Uz, C. M., Allen, H. D., et al. (2016). Novel long QT syndrome-associated missense mutation, L762F, in CACNA1C-encoded L-type calcium channel imparts a slower inactivation tau and increased sustained and window current. *Int. J. Cardiol.* 220, 290–298. doi: 10.1016/j.ijcard.2016.06.081

Li, A., Ahsen, O. O., Liu, J. J., Du, C., McKee, M. L., Yang, Y., et al. (2013). Silencing of the *Drosophila* ortholog of SOX5 in heart leads to cardiac dysfunction as detected by optical coherence tomography. *Hum. Mol. Genet.* 22, 3798–3806. doi: 10.1093/hmg/ddt230

Li, H., Li, D., Wang, Y., Huang, Z., Xu, J., Yang, T., et al. (2019). Nkx2-5 defines a subpopulation of pacemaker cells and is essential for the physiological function of the sinoatrial node in mice. *Development* 146:dev178145. doi: 10.1242/dev.178145

Li, N., Hansen, B. J., Csepe, T. A., Zhao, J., Ignozzi, A. J., Sul, L. V., et al. (2017). Redundant and diverse intranodal pacemakers and conduction pathways protect the human sinoatrial node from failure. *Sci. Transl. Med.* 9:eaam5607. doi: 10.1126/scitranslmed.aam5607

Li, N., Timofeyev, V., Tuteja, D., Xu, D., Lu, L., Zhang, Q., et al. (2009). Ablation of a Ca2+-activated K+ channel (SK2 channel) results in action potential prolongation in atrial myocytes and atrial fibrillation. *J. Physiol.* 587, 1087–1100. doi: 10.1113/jphysiol.2008.167718

Liu, G.-Z., Hou, T.-T., Yuan, Y., Hang, P.-Z., Zhao, J.-J., Sun, L., et al. (2016). Fenofibrate inhibits atrial metabolic remodelling in atrial fibrillation through

PPAR-α/sirtuin 1/PGC-1α pathway. *Br. J. Pharmacol.* 173, 1095–1109. doi: 10.1111/bph.13438

Liu, Z., Hutt, J. A., Rajeshkumar, B., Azuma, Y., Duan, K. L., and Donahue, J. K. (2017). Preclinical efficacy and safety of KCNH2-G628S gene therapy for postoperative atrial fibrillation. *J. Thorac. Cardiovasc. Surg.* 154, 1644–1651.e8. doi: 10.1016/j.jtcvs.2017.05.052

Lübkemeier, I., Requardt, R. P., Lin, X., Sasse, P., Andrié, R., Schrickel, J. W., et al. (2013). Deletion of the last five C-terminal amino acid residues of connexin43 leads to lethal ventricular arrhythmias in mice without affecting coupling via gap junction channels. *Basic Res. Cardiol.* 108:348. doi: 10.1007/s00395-013-0348-y

Lugenbiel, P., Govorov, K., Rahm, A.-K., Wieder, T., Gramlich, D., Syren, P., et al. (2018). Inhibition of histone deacetylases induces K+ channel remodeling and action potential prolongation in HL-1 atrial cardiomyocytes. *Cell. Physiol. Biochem.* 49, 65–77. doi: 10.1159/000492840

Mahida, S., Mills, R. W., Tucker, N. R., Simonson, B., Macri, V., Lemoine, M. D., et al. (2014). Overexpression of KCNN3 results in sudden cardiac death. *Cardiovasc. Res.* 101, 326–334. doi: 10.1093/cvr/cvt269

Marsman, R. F. J., Bezzina, C. R., Freiberg, F., Verkerk, A. O., Adriaens, M. E., Podliesna, S., et al. (2014). Coxsackie and adenovirus receptor is a modifier of cardiac conduction and arrhythmia vulnerability in the setting of myocardial ischemia. *J. Am. Coll. Cardiol.* 63, 549–559. doi: 10.1016/j.jacc.2013.10.062

Martinez-Palomo, A., Alanis, J., and Benitez, D. (1970). Transitional cardiac cells of the conductive system of the dog heart, distinguishing morphological and electrophysiological features. *J. Cell Biol.* 47, 1–17. doi: 10.1083/jcb.47.1.1

Masuda, Y., and Kawamura, A. (2003). Acetylcholinesterase inhibitor (donepezil hydrochloride) reduces heart rate variability. *J. Cardiovasc. Pharmacol.* 41(Suppl. 1), S67–S71.

Mazhari, R., Nuss, H. B., Armoundas, A. A., Winslow, R. L., and Marbán, E. (2002). Ectopic expression of KCNE3 accelerates cardiac repolarization and abbreviates the QT interval. *J. Clin. Invest.* 109, 1083–1090. doi: 10.1172/JCI15062

Meijler, F. L., and Janse, M. J. (1988). Morphology and electrophysiology of the mammalian atrioventricular node. *Physiol. Rev.* 68, 608–647. doi: 10.1152/physrev.1988.68.2.608

Melnyk, P., Ehrlich, J. R., Pourrier, M., Villeneuve, L., Cha, T.-J., and Nattel, S. (2005). Comparison of ion channel distribution and expression in cardiomyocytes of canine pulmonary veins versus left atrium. *Cardiovasc. Res.* 65, 104–116. doi: 10.1016/j.cardiores.2004.08.014

Milano, A., Blom, M. T., Lodder, E. M., van Hoeijen, D. A., Barc, J., Koopmann, T. T., et al. (2016). Sudden cardiac arrest and rare genetic variants in the community. *Circ. Cardiovasc. Genet.* 9, 147–153. doi: 10.1161/CIRCGENETICS.115.001263

Mommersteeg, M. T. M., Brown, N. A., Prall, O. W. J., De Gier-De Vries, C., Harvey, R. P., Moorman, A. F. M., et al. (2007a). Pitx2c and Nkx2-5 are required for the formation and identity of the pulmonary myocardium. *Circ. Res.* 101, 902–909. doi: 10.1161/CIRCRESAHA.107.161182

Mommersteeg, M. T. M., Hoogaars, W. M. H., Prall, O. W. J., de Gier-de Vries, C., Wiese, C., Clout, D. E. W., et al. (2007b). Molecular pathway for the localized formation of the sinoatrial node. *Circ. Res.* 100, 354–362. doi: 10.1161/01.RES.0000258019.74591.b3

Montefiori, L. E., Sobreira, D. R., Sakabe, N. J., Aneas, I., Joslin, A. C., Hansen, G. T., et al. (2018). A promoter interaction map for cardiovascular disease genetics. *eLife* 7:e35788. doi: 10.7554/eLife.35788

Moreno, C., Oliveras, A., de la Cruz, A., Bartolucci, C., Muñoz, C., Salar, E., et al. (2015). A new KCNQ1 mutation at the S5 segment that impairs its association with KCNE1 is responsible for short QT syndrome. *Cardiovasc. Res.* 107, 613–623. doi: 10.1093/cvr/cvv196

Moskowitz, I. P. G., Kim, J. B., Moore, M. L., Wolf, C. M., Peterson, M. A., Shendure, J., et al. (2007). A molecular pathway including Id2, Tbx5, and Nkx2-5 required for cardiac conduction system development. *Cell* 129, 1365–1376. doi: 10.1016/j.cell.2007.04.036

Myers, E. J., Yuan, L., Felmlee, M. A., Lin, Y.-Y., Jiang, Y., Pei, Y., et al. (2016). A novel mutant Na+ /HCO3- cotransporter NBCe1 in a case of compound-heterozygous inheritance of proximal renal tubular acidosis. *J. Physiol.* 594, 6267–6286. doi: 10.1113/JP272252

Nadadur, R. D., Broman, M. T., Boukens, B., Mazurek, S. R., Yang, X., Van Den Boogaard, M., et al. (2016). Pitx2 modulates a Tbx5-dependent gene regulatory network to maintain atrial rhythm. *Sci. Transl. Med.* 8: 354ra115. doi: 10.1126/scitranslmed.aaf4891

Newton-Cheh, C., Eijgelsheim, M., Rice, K. M., De Bakker, P. I. W., Yin, X., Estrada, K., et al. (2009). Common variants at ten loci influence QT interval duration in the QTGEN Study. *Nat. Genet.* 41, 399–406. doi: 10.1038/ng.364

Nolte, I. M., Munoz, M. L., Tragante, V., Amare, A. T., Jansen, R., Vaez, A., et al. (2017). Genetic loci associated with heart rate variability and their effects on cardiac disease risk. *Nat. Commun.* 8:15805. doi: 10.1038/ncomms15805

Noureldin, M., Chen, H., and Bai, D. (2018). Functional characterization of novel atrial fibrillation-linked GJA5 (Cx40) mutants. *Int. J. Mol. Sci.* 19:977. doi: 10.3390/ijms19040977

Opthof, T., VanGinneken, A. C., Bouman, L. N., and Jongsma, H. J. (1987). The intrinsic cycle length in small pieces isolated from the rabbit sinoatrial node. *J. Mol. Cell. Cardiol.* 19, 923–934. doi: 10.1016/s0022-2828(87)80621-1

Orvos, P., Kohajda, Z., Szlovák, J., Gazdag, P., Árpádffy-Lovas, T., Tóth, D., et al. (2019). Evaluation of possible proarrhythmic potency: comparison of the effect of dofetilide, cisapride, sotalol, terfenadine, and verapamil on hERG and native IKr currents and on cardiac action potential. *Toxicol. Sci.* 168, 365–380. doi: 10.1093/toxsci/kfy299

Papadatos, G. A., Wallerstein, P. M. R., Head, C. E. G., Ratcliff, R., Brady, P. A., Benndorf, K., et al. (2002). Slowed conduction and ventricular tachycardia after targeted disruption of the cardiac sodium channel gene Scn5a. *Proc. Natl. Acad. Sci. U.S.A.* 99, 6210–6215. doi: 10.1073/pnas.082121299

Park, D. S., Woodman, S. E., Schubert, W., Cohen, A. W., Frank, P. G., Chandra, M., et al. (2002). Caveolin-1/3 double-knockout mice are viable, but lack both muscle and non-muscle caveolae, and develop a severe cardiomyopathic phenotype. *Am. J. Pathol.* 160, 2207–2217. doi: 10.1016/S0002-9440(10)61168-6

Pfeiffer, M. J., Quaranta, R., Piccini, I., Fell, J., Rao, J., Röpke, A., et al. (2018). Cardiogenic programming of human pluripotent stem cells by dose-controlled activation of EOMES. *Nat. Commun.* 9:440. doi: 10.1038/s41467-017-02812-6

Pfeufer, A., van Noord, C., Marciante, K. D., Arking, D. E., Larson, M. G., Smith, A. V., et al. (2010). Genome-wide association study of PR interval. *Nat. Genet.* 42, 153–159. doi: 10.1038/ng.517

Posokhova, E., Ng, D., Opel, A., Masuho, I., Tinker, A., Biesecker, L. G., et al. (2013). Essential role of the m2R-RGS6-IKACh pathway in controlling intrinsic heart rate variability. *PLoS One* 8:e76973. doi: 10.1371/journal.pone.0076973

Posokhova, E., Wydeven, N., Allen, K. L., Wickman, K., and Martemyanov, K. A. (2010). RGS6/Gβ5 complex accelerates IKACh gating kinetics in atrial myocytes and modulates parasympathetic regulation of heart rate. *Circ. Res.* 107, 1350–1354. doi: 10.1161/CIRCRESAHA.110.224212

Pott, C., Ren, X., Tran, D. X., Yang, M.-J., Henderson, S., Jordan, M. C., et al. (2007). Mechanism of shortened action potential duration in Na+-Ca2+ exchanger knockout mice. *Am. J. Physiol. Cell Physiol.* 292, C968–C973. doi: 10.1152/ajpcell.00177.2006

Purohit, A., Rokita, A. G., Guan, X., Chen, B., Koval, O. M., Voigt, N., et al. (2013). Oxidized Ca(2+)/calmodulin-dependent protein kinase II triggers atrial fibrillation. *Circulation* 128, 1748–1757. doi: 10.1161/CIRCULATIONAHA.113.003313

Rentschler, S., Yen, A. H., Lu, J., Petrenko, N. B., Lu, M. M., Manderfield, L. J., et al. (2012). Myocardial Notch signaling reprograms cardiomyocytes to a conduction-like phenotype. *Circulation* 126, 1058–1066. doi: 10.1161/CIRCULATIONAHA.112.103390

Rocher, A. B., Crimins, J. L., Amatrudo, J. M., Kinson, M. S., Todd-Brown, M. A., Lewis, J., et al. (2010). Structural and functional changes in tau mutant mice neurons are not linked to the presence of NFTs. *Exp. Neurol.* 223, 385–393. doi: 10.1016/j.expneurol.2009.07.029

Roder, K., Werdich, A. A., Li, W., Liu, M., Kim, T. Y., Organ-Darling, L. E., et al. (2014). RING finger protein RNF207, a novel regulator of cardiac excitation. *J. Biol. Chem.* 289, 33730–33740. doi: 10.1074/jbc.M114.592295

Rohr, S., Kucera, J. P., Fast, V. G., and Kléber, A. G. (1997). Paradoxical improvement of impulse conduction in cardiac tissue by partial cellular uncoupling. *Science* 275, 841–844. doi: 10.1126/science.275.5301.841

Roselli, C., Chaffin, M. D., Weng, L.-C., Aeschbacher, S., Ahlberg, G., Albert, C. M., et al. (2018). Multi-ethnic genome-wide association study for atrial fibrillation. *Nat. Genet.* 50, 1225–1233. doi: 10.1038/s41588-018-0133-9

Roder, K., Werdich, A. A., Li, W., Liu, M., Kim, T. Y., Organ-Darling, L. E., et al. (2014). RING finger protein RNF207, a novel regulator of cardiac excitation. *J. Biol. Chem.* 289, 33730–33740. doi: 10.1074/jbc.M114.592295

Rohr, S., Kucera, J. P., Fast, V. G., and Kléber, A. G. (1997). Paradoxical improvement of impulse conduction in cardiac tissue by partial cellular uncoupling. *Science* 275, 841–844. doi: 10.1126/science.275.5301.841

Roselli, C., Chaffin, M. D., Weng, L.-C., Aeschbacher, S., Ahlberg, G., Albert, C. M., et al. (2018). Multi-ethnic genome-wide association study for atrial fibrillation. *Nat. Genet.* 50, 1225–1233. doi: 10.1038/s41588-018-0133-9

Sah, R., Mesirca, P., Van den Boogert, M., Rosen, J., Mably, J., Mangoni, M. E., et al. (2013). Ion channel-kinase TRPM7 is required for maintaining cardiac automaticity. *Proc. Natl. Acad. Sci. U.S.A.* 110, E3037–E3046. doi: 10.1073/pnas.1311865110

Saito, T., Waki, K., and Becker, A. E. (2000). Left atrial myocardial extension onto pulmonary veins in humans: anatomic observations relevant for atrial arrhythmias. *J. Cardiovasc. Electrophysiol.* 11, 888–894. doi: 10.1111/j.1540-8167.2000.tb00068.x

Sapra, G., Tham, Y. K., Cemerlang, N., Matsumoto, A., Kiriazis, H., Bernardo, B. C., et al. (2014). The small-molecule BGP-15 protects against heart failure and atrial fibrillation in mice. *Nat. Commun.* 5:5705. doi: 10.1038/ncomms6705

Sato, P. Y., Musa, H., Coombs, W., Guerrero-Serna, G., Patiño, G. A., Taffet, S. M., et al. (2009). Loss of plakophilin-2 expression leads to decreased sodium current and slower conduction velocity in cultured cardiac myocytes. *Circ. Res.* 105, 523–526. doi: 10.1161/CIRCRESAHA.109.201418

Schotten, U., Verheule, S., Kirchhof, P., and Goette, A. (2011). Pathophysiological mechanisms of atrial fibrillation: a translational appraisal. *Physiol. Rev.* 91, 265–325. doi: 10.1152/physrev.00031.2009

Shin, J.-H., Bostick, B., Yue, Y., Hajjar, R., and Duan, D. (2011). SERCA2a gene transfer improves electrocardiographic performance in aged mdx mice. *J. Transl. Med.* 9:132. doi: 10.1186/1479-5876-9-132

Singh, R., Horsthuis, T., Farin, H. F., Grieskamp, T., Norden, J., Petry, M., et al. (2009). Tbx20 interacts with smads to confine tbx2 expression to the atrioventricular canal. *Circ. Res.* 105, 442–452. doi: 10.1161/CIRCRESAHA.109.196063

Sinner, M. F., Tucker, N. R., Lunetta, K. L., Ozaki, K., Smith, J. G., Trompet, S., et al. (2014). Integrating genetic, transcriptional, and functional analyses to identify 5 novel genes for atrial fibrillation. *Circulation* 130, 1225–1235. doi: 10.1161/CIRCULATIONAHA.114.009892

Smith, J. G., Magnani, J. W., Palmer, C., Meng, Y. A., Soliman, E. Z., Musani, S. K., et al. (2011). Genome-wide association studies of the PR interval in African Americans. *PLoS Genet.* 7:e1001304. doi: 10.1371/journal.pgen.1001304

Song, L., Alcalai, R., Arad, M., Wolf, C. M., Toka, O., Conner, D. A., et al. (2007). Calsequestrin 2 (CASQ2) mutations increase expression of calreticulin and ryanodine receptors, causing catecholaminergic polymorphic ventricular tachycardia. *J. Clin. Invest.* 117, 1814–1823. doi: 10.1172/JCI31080

Sotoodehnia, N., Isaacs, A., de Bakker, P. I. W., Dörr, M., Newton-Cheh, C., Nolte, I. M., et al. (2010). Common variants in 22 loci are associated with QRS duration and cardiac ventricular conduction. *Nat. Genet.* 42, 1068–1076. doi: 10.1038/ng.716

Speerschneider, T., and Thomsen, M. B. (2013). Physiology and analysis of the electrocardiographic T wave in mice. *Acta Physiol. (Oxf).* 209, 262–271. doi: 10.1111/apha.12172

Stroud, D. M., Yang, T., Bersell, K., Kryshtal, D. O., Nagao, S., Shaffer, C., et al. (2016). Contrasting Nav1.8 activity in Scn10a-/- ventricular myocytes and the intact heart. *J. Am. Heart Assoc.* 5:e002946. doi: 10.1161/JAHA.115.002946

Suarez, J., Gloss, B., Belke, D. D., Hu, Y., Scott, B., Dieterle, T., et al. (2004). Doxycycline inducible expression of SERCA2a improves calcium handling and reverts cardiac dysfunction in pressure overload-induced cardiac hypertrophy. *Am. J. Physiol. Heart Circ. Physiol.* 287, H2164–H2172. doi: 10.1152/ajpheart.00428.2004

Sugiyama, K., Sasano, T., Kurokawa, J., Takahashi, K., Okamura, T., Kato, N., et al. (2016). Oxidative stress induced ventricular arrhythmia and impairment of cardiac function in Nos1ap deleted mice. *Int. Heart J.* 57, 341–349. doi: 10.1536/ihj.15-471

Syeda, F., Holmes, A. P., Yu, T. Y., Tull, S., Kuhlmann, S. M., Pavlovic, D., et al. (2016). PITX2 modulates atrial membrane potential and the antiarrhythmic effects of sodium-channel blockers. *J. Am. Coll. Cardiol.* 68, 1881–1894. doi: 10.1016/j.jacc.2016.07.766

Tao, Y., Zhang, M., Li, L., Bai, Y., Zhou, Y., Moon, A. M., et al. (2014). Pitx2, an atrial fibrillation predisposition gene, directly regulates ion transport and intercalated disc genes. *Circ. Cardiovasc. Genet.* 7, 23–32. doi: 10.1161/CIRCGENETICS.113.000259

Tawara, S. (1906). *Das Reizleitungssystem des Säugetierherzens*. Jena: Fisher.

Tomás, M., Napolitano, C., De Giuli, L., Bloise, R., Subirana, I., Malovini, A., et al. (2010). Polymorphisms in the NOS1AP gene modulate QT interval duration and risk of arrhythmias in the long QT syndrome. *J. Am. Coll. Cardiol.* 55, 2745–2752. doi: 10.1016/j.jacc.2009.12.065

Tranum-Jensen, J., Wilde, A. A. M., Vermeulen, J. T., and Janse, M. J. (1991). Morphology of electrophysiologically identified junctions between Purkinje fibers and ventricular muscle in rabbit and pig hearts. *Circ. Res.* 69, 429–437. doi: 10.1161/01.RES.69.2.429

Tucker, N. R., Dolmatova, E. V., Lin, H., Cooper, R. R., Ye, J., Hucker, W. J., et al. (2017). Diminished PRRX1 expression is associated with increased risk of atrial fibrillation and shortening of the cardiac action potential. *Circ. Cardiovasc. Genet.* 10:e001902. doi: 10.1161/CIRCGENETICS.117.001902

Tuomi, J. M., Tyml, K., and Jones, D. L. (2011). Atrial tachycardia/fibrillation in the connexin 43 G60S mutant (Oculodentodigital dysplasia) mouse. *Am. J. Physiol. Heart Circ. Physiol.* 300, H1402–H1411. doi: 10.1152/ajpheart.01094.2010

Unudurthi, S. D., Wolf, R. M., and Hund, T. J. (2014). Role of sinoatrial node architecture in maintaining a balanced source-sink relationship and synchronous cardiac pacemaking. *Front. Physiol.* 5:446. doi: 10.3389/fphys.2014.00446

van den Boogaard, M., Smemo, S., Burnicka-Turek, O., Arnolds, D. E., van de Werken, H. J. G., Klous, P., et al. (2014). A common genetic variant within SCN10A modulates cardiac SCN5A expression. *J. Clin. Invest.* 124, 1844–1852. doi: 10.1172/JCI73140

van den Hoogenhof, M. M. G., Beqqali, A., Amin, A. S., van der Made, I., Aufiero, S., Khan, M. A. F., et al. (2018). RBM20 mutations induce an arrhythmogenic dilated cardiomyopathy related to disturbed calcium handling. *Circulation* 138, 1330–1342. doi: 10.1161/CIRCULATIONAHA.117.031947

van Duijvenboden, K., de Boer, B. A., Capon, N., Ruijter, J. M., and Christoffels, V. M. (2016). EMERGE: a flexible modelling framework to predict genomic regulatory elements from genomic signatures. *Nucleic Acids Res.* 44:e42. doi: 10.1093/nar/gkv1144

van Eif, V. W. W., Stefanovic, S., van Duijvenboden, K., Bakker, M., Wakker, V., de Gier-de Vries, C., et al. (2019). Transcriptome analysis of mouse and human sinoatrial node cells reveals a conserved genetic program. *Development* 146:dev173161. doi: 10.1242/dev.173161

van Ouwerkerk, A. F., Bosada, F. M., van Duijvenboden, K., Hill, M. C., Montefiori, L. E., Scholman, K. T., et al. (2019). Identification of atrial fibrillation associated genes and functional non-coding variants. *Nat. Commun.* 10:4755. doi: 10.1038/s41467-019-12721-5

van Setten, J., Brody, J. A., Jamshidi, Y., Swenson, B. R., Butler, A. M., Campbell, H., et al. (2018). PR interval genome-wide association meta-analysis identifies 50 loci associated with atrial and atrioventricular electrical activity. *Nat. Commun.* 9:2904. doi: 10.1038/s41467-018-04766-9

van Setten, J., Verweij, N., Mbarek, H., Niemeijer, M. N., Trompet, S., Arking, D. E., et al. (2019). Genome-wide association meta-analysis of 30,000 samples identifies seven novel loci for quantitative ECG traits. *Eur. J. Hum. Genet.* 27, 952–962. doi: 10.1038/s41431-018-0295-z

Veerman, C. C., Mengarelli, I., Guan, K., Stauske, M., Barc, J., Tan, H. L., et al. (2016). hiPSC-derived cardiomyocytes from Brugada syndrome patients without identified mutations do not exhibit clear cellular electrophysiological abnormalities. *Sci. Rep.* 6:30967. doi: 10.1038/srep30967

Verheule, S., Wilson, E. E., Arora, R., Engle, S. K., Scott, L. R., and Olgin, J. E. (2002). Tissue structure and connexin expression of canine pulmonary veins. *Cardiovasc. Res.* 55, 727–738. doi: 10.1016/S0008-6363(02)00490-X

Vikram, A., Lewarchik, C. M., Yoon, J.-Y., Naqvi, A., Kumar, S., Morgan, G. M., et al. (2017). Sirtuin 1 regulates cardiac electrical activity by deacetylating the cardiac sodium channel. *Nat. Med.* 23, 361–367. doi: 10.1038/nm.4284

Wang, H., Qin, J., Gong, S., Feng, B., Zhang, Y., and Tao, J. (2014). Insulin-like growth factor-1 receptor-mediated inhibition of A-type K(+) current induces sensory neuronal hyperexcitability through the phosphatidylinositol 3-kinase and extracellular signal-regulated kinase 1/2 pathways, independently of Akt. *Endocrinology* 155, 168–179. doi: 10.1210/en.2013-1559

Wemhöner, K., Friedrich, C., Stallmeyer, B., Coffey, A. J., Grace, A., Zumhagen, S., et al. (2015). Gain-of-function mutations in the calcium channel CACNA1C (Cav1.2) cause non-syndromic long-QT but not Timothy syndrome. *J. Mol. Cell. Cardiol.* 80, 186–195. doi: 10.1016/j.yjmcc.2015.01.002

West, T. C. (1955). Ultramicroelectrode recording from the cardiac pacemaker. *J. Pharmacol. Exp. Ther.* 115, 283–290.

Wiener, N., and Rosenblueth, A. (1946). The mathematical formulation of the problem of conduction of impulses in a network of connected excitable elements, specifically in cardiac muscle. *Arch. Inst. Cardiol. Mex* 16, 205–265.

Xu, B., Wratten, N., Charych, E. I., Buyske, S., Firestein, B. L., and Brzustowicz, L. M. (2005). Increased expression in dorsolateral prefrontal cortex of CAPON in schizophrenia and bipolar disorder. *PLoS Med.* 2:e263. doi: 10.1371/journal.pmed.0020263

Yagishita, D., Chui, R. W., Yamakawa, K., Rajendran, P. S., Ajijola, O. A., Nakamura, K., et al. (2015). Sympathetic nerve stimulation, not circulating norepinephrine, modulates T-peak to T-end interval by increasing global dispersion of repolarization. *Circ. Arrhythm. Electrophysiol.* 8, 174–185. doi: 10.1161/CIRCEP.114.002195

Yamaguchi, T., Suzuki, T., Sato, T., Takahashi, A., Watanabe, H., Kadowaki, A., et al. (2018). The CCR4-NOT deadenylase complex controls Atg7-dependent cell death and heart function. *Sci. Signal.* 11:eaan3638. doi: 10.1126/scisignal.aan3638

Yang, J.-M., Shen, C.-J., Chen, X.-J., Kong, Y., Liu, Y.-S., Li, X.-W., et al. (2019). erbb4 deficits in chandelier cells of the medial prefrontal cortex confer cognitive dysfunctions: implications for schizophrenia. *Cereb. Cortex* 29, 4334–4346. doi: 10.1093/cercor/bhy316

Yang, K.-C., Breitbart, A., De Lange, W. J., Hofsteen, P., Futakuchi-Tsuchida, A., Xu, J., et al. (2018). Novel adult-onset systolic cardiomyopathy due to MYH7 E848G mutation in patient-derived induced pluripotent stem cells. *JACC Basic Transl. Sci.* 3, 728–740. doi: 10.1016/j.jacbts.2018.08.008

Yi, F., Ling, T.-Y., Lu, T., Wang, X.-L., Li, J., Claycomb, W. C., et al. (2015). Down-regulation of the small conductance calcium-activated potassium channels in diabetic mouse atria. *J. Biol. Chem.* 290, 7016–7026. doi: 10.1074/jbc.M114.607952

Zaritsky, J. J., Redell, J. B., Tempel, B. L., and Schwarz, T. L. (2001). The consequences of disrupting cardiac inwardly rectifying K(+) current (I(K1)) as revealed by the targeted deletion of the murine Kir2.1 and Kir2.2 genes. *J. Physiol.* 533, 697–710. doi: 10.1111/j.1469-7793.2001.t01-1-00697.x

Zhang, S., Kim, K., Rosen, A., Smyth, J. W., Sakuma, R., Delgado-Olguín, P., et al. (2011). Iroquois homeobox gene 3 establishes fast conduction in the cardiac His-Purkinje network. *Proc. Natl. Acad. Sci. U.S.A.* 108, 13576–13581. doi: 10.1073/pnas.1106911108

Zhang, T., Yong, S. L., Tian, X.-L., and Wang, Q. K. (2007). Cardiac-specific overexpression of SCN5A gene leads to shorter P wave duration and PR interval in transgenic mice. *Biochem. Biophys. Res. Commun.* 355, 444–450. doi: 10.1016/j.bbrc.2007.01.170

Zhang, X.-D., Timofeyev, V., Li, N., Myers, R. E., Zhang, D.-M., Singapuri, A., et al. (2014). Critical roles of a small conductance Ca^{2+}-activated K^{+} channel (SK3) in the repolarization process of atrial myocytes. *Cardiovasc. Res.* 101, 317–325. doi: 10.1093/cvr/cvt262

Zhang, Z., He, Y., Tuteja, D., Xu, D., Timofeyev, V., Zhang, Q., et al. (2005). Functional roles of Cav1.3(alpha1D) calcium channels in atria: insights gained from gene-targeted null mutant mice. *Circulation* 112, 1936–1944. doi: 10.1161/CIRCULATIONAHA.105.540070

Zheng, Z., Wang, Z.-M., and Delbono, O. (2002). Charge movement and transcription regulation of L-type calcium channel alpha(1S) in skeletal muscle cells. *J. Physiol.* 540, 397–409. doi: 10.1113/jphysiol.2001.013464

Zhou, X., Wang, Z., Huang, B., Yuan, S., Sheng, X., Yu, L., et al. (2018). Regulation of the NRG1/ErbB4 pathway in the intrinsic cardiac nervous system is a potential treatment for atrial fibrillation. *Front. Physiol.* 9:1082. doi: 10.3389/fphys.2018.01082

14

Novel Optics-Based Approaches for Cardiac Electrophysiology

M. Caroline Müllenbroich[1], Allen Kelly[2], Corey Acker[3], Gil Bub[4], Tobias Bruegmann[5], Anna Di Bona[6], Emilia Entcheva[7], Cecilia Ferrantini[8], Peter Kohl[9], Stephan E. Lehnart[10,11,12], Marco Mongillo[13,14], Camilla Parmeggiani[8], Claudia Richter[15], Philipp Sasse[16], Tania Zaglia[13,14], Leonardo Sacconi[8,9,17†] and Godfrey L. Smith[2†]*

[1] School of Physics and Astronomy, University of Glasgow, Glasgow, United Kingdom, [2] Institute of Cardiovascular and Medical Sciences, University of Glasgow, Glasgow, United Kingdom, [3] Center for Cell Analysis and Modeling, UConn Health, Farmington, CT, United States, [4] Department of Physiology, McGill University, Montréal, QC, Canada, [5] Institute for Cardiovascular Physiology, University Medical Center Goettingen, Goettingen, Germany, [6] Department of Cardiac, Thoracic, Vascular Sciences and Public Health, University of Padova, Padova, Italy, [7] Department of Biomedical Engineering, The George Washington University, Washington, DC, United States, [8] European Laboratory for Nonlinear Spectroscopy, Sesto Fiorentino, Italy, [9] Institute for Experimental Cardiovascular Medicine, University Heart Center and Medical Faculty, University of Freiburg, Freiburg, Germany, [10] Heart Research Center Göttingen, University Medical Center Göttingen, Göttingen, Germany, [11] Department of Cardiology and Pneumology, Georg-August University Göttingen, Göttingen, Germany, [12] Cluster of Excellence "Multiscale Bioimaging: from Molecular Machines to Networks of Excitable Cells" (MBExC), University of Göttingen, Göttingen, Germany, [13] Department of Biomedical Sciences, University of Padova, Padova, Italy, [14] Veneto Institute of Molecular Medicine, Padova, Italy, [15] German Primate Center - Leibniz Institute for Primate Research, Göttingen, Germany, [16] Institute of Physiology I, Medical Faculty, University of Bonn, Bonn, Germany, [17] National Institute of Optics, National Research Council, Florence, Italy

***Correspondence:**
Godfrey L. Smith
godfrey.smith@glasgow.ac.uk

† These authors have contributed equally to this work

Optical techniques for recording and manipulating cellular electrophysiology have advanced rapidly in just a few decades. These developments allow for the analysis of cardiac cellular dynamics at multiple scales while largely overcoming the drawbacks associated with the use of electrodes. The recent advent of optogenetics opens up new possibilities for regional and tissue-level electrophysiological control and hold promise for future novel clinical applications. This article, which emerged from the international NOTICE workshop in 2018[1], reviews the state-of-the-art optical techniques used for cardiac electrophysiological research and the underlying biophysics. The design and performance of optical reporters and optogenetic actuators are reviewed along with limitations of current probes. The physics of light interaction with cardiac tissue is detailed and associated challenges with the use of optical sensors and actuators are presented. Case studies include the use of fluorescence recovery after photobleaching and super-resolution microscopy to explore the micro-structure of cardiac cells and a review of two photon and light sheet technologies applied to cardiac tissue. The emergence of cardiac optogenetics is reviewed and the current work exploring the potential clinical use of optogenetics is also described. Approaches which combine optogenetic manipulation and optical voltage measurement are discussed, in terms of platforms that allow real-time manipulation of whole heart electrophysiology in open and closed-loop systems to study optimal ways to terminate spiral arrhythmias. The

[1] http://www.notice.cnr.it/

design and operation of optics-based approaches that allow high-throughput cardiac electrophysiological assays is presented. Finally, emerging techniques of photo-acoustic imaging and stress sensors are described along with strategies for future development and establishment of these techniques in mainstream electrophysiological research.

Keywords: electrophysiology, optogenetics, heart, arrhythmia, fluorescence

INTRODUCTION

Electrodes vs. Light

Our current understanding of myocardial tissue electrophysiology is derived from measurements of action potential features i.e., activation, repolarization, and conduction velocity in myocardial tissue. It has been long known that the 3-dimensional (3D) structure of the tissue and regional differences in cell type composition are key determinants of electrophysiological behavior. Therefore, tools to allow interrogation and control of the electrophysiological state at various sites within myocardial tissue have high value for both research and therapy. Electrode based approaches offer the most direct way of measuring the electrical properties of the heart. However, these techniques present significant technical limitations. The gold standard for transmembrane measurements is the sharp microelectrode that gives high-resistance access to the intracellular medium at a single point to allow transmembrane voltage recording. This is in routine use in isolated tissue preparations (Hicks and Cobbe, 1991; Sicouri and Antzelevitch, 1991; Di Diego et al., 2013) but has limitations including: (i) maintenance of the delicate high-resistance intracellular access in an actively contracting tissue; (ii) the technical challenge associated with maintaining multiple simultaneous intracellular measurements to follow propagation; (iii) the difficulty in applying this technique to record transmural electrophysiology in an intact ventricular wall that in larger mammals can reach 1–2 cm thick. Despite these limitations, this technique has done much to inform scientists and clinicians of details of cardiac physiology, with work on cardiac tissue slices allowing insight into the changes in electrophysiology deep within large animal/ human myocardium (Camelliti et al., 2011). A technically simpler alternative is to use extracellular electrodes to measure potential differences between two points either on the epicardial surface, or within a solution-filled volume containing the heart. At one level this can be in the form of an electrocardiogram (ECG) used routinely for diagnostics in medicine. The most sophisticated version of this technique is body surface mapping which consists of simultaneous recordings from 300-400 points on the human chest and back. This technology, along with significant progress in solving the mathematical "inverse problem," allows the surface body mapping to be used to create and project a 3D electrogram (Rudy, 2013) onto a 3D image of the patient's heart obtained by other clinical imaging modalities. This approach requires a very large investment in facilities and clinical expertise that currently can only be achieved in a few selected centers and cannot be easily used in experimental investigations. Furthermore, while this technique delivers 3D activation maps of the heart, a transmembrane potential signal cannot be extracted from the data. Clinically, activation mapping provides the most accurate way to diagnose conduction defects within the human heart. More routinely across clinical cardiac electrophysiology, catheter electrodes are used to detect local activation timings. These local extracellular recordings include electrode designs to provide a monophasic action potential signal using a signal from a limited depolarized region to represent the "intracellular electrode" (Franz, 1999) and needle electrodes that penetrate the myocardium to different levels to map transmural activation (Pogwizd and Corr, 1987). Cardiac stimulation in parallel with the intrinsic sinus rate activation is a necessary tool for both diagnostic and therapeutic purposes in the clinical setting and an experimental tool in research. Conventional electrodes have the same constraints as voltage measurement systems in terms of accessible surfaces of the heart chambers and the inability to stimulate discrete volumes of myocardium within the ventricle. One additional complication occurs when electrode voltage measurement and stimulation systems are used in parallel; depending on the relative positions of each, the electric fields generated by stimulating electrodes will induce transient voltages in the measurement electrodes which interfere with recording the underlying tissue response during and shortly after stimulation. As will be described in the subsequent sections of this review, many of the constraints associated with electrodes can be overcome with the use of optical probes to measure and actuate electrical signals in cardiac tissue. These optical techniques come with their own limitations, often due to the way light interacts with biological tissues. Therefore, significant sections of this review are devoted to the basic physical principles associated with light/tissue interaction.

Fluorescent Dyes as Indicators of Cardiac Activity

Voltage-Sensitive Dyes

Voltage-sensitive dyes (VSD) are small fluorescent molecules that incorporate into cell membranes and report changes in transmembrane potential through changes in fluorescence. Ideally, the dye molecules should not change any "normal" functional or structural properties of the cell membrane and only integrate into the plasmalemma as opposed to intracellular membranes which are not involved in electrical activity. Furthermore, the fluorophore should ideally exhibit a high dynamic range, and respond rapidly (circa 1 ms) to any membrane potential changes.

Classic electrochromic VSD such as di-4-ANEPPS (excited in the blue-green band) have been used for decades in optical mapping experiments for detailed measurements of electrical propagation across tissues or whole organs. Since then, improved VSD have been engineered which feature increased overall brightness and voltage sensitivities through fluorination (Acker et al., 2011). Fluorination of VSD provides a tool for spectral tuning of probes, which is important for compatibility with two-photon imaging techniques (see **Box 2**) and facilitates the combination of optogenetic stimulation with optical recording (Yan et al., 2012; Crocini et al., 2016a). Another class of recently developed VSD, which relies on molecular wire photo-electron transfer (PeT), is becoming popular, thanks to their rapid response kinetics, photostability and relatively high dynamic range of fluorescence changes (20–27 %) (Miller et al., 2012). Originally developed for neuronal studies, PeT-based VSD have been used successfully in cardiac single cell and whole heart studies, proving particularly useful for deep-tissue electrophysiological measurements using two-photon imaging (Ghouri et al., 2018; Salerno et al., 2019; Klimas et al., 2020).

A common issue with dye loading is that the resulting fluorescence may display spatiotemporal variations. Uneven distribution of the probe within the tissue, heterogeneous tissue structure, non-uniform excitation light intensity, probe bleaching, motion artifacts and local changes in cell membrane structure might all contribute to time-dependent changes in detected signal. These variations then need to be removed by scaling the signal at each pixel to have the same range by calculating a $\Delta F/F$ transient.

These confounding signals can be reduced or eliminated using ratiometric approaches, where two separate signals with different responses are divided, canceling shared features while preserving or even amplifying the desired signal components. Ratiometry requires a VSD that undergoes a shift in the emission or excitation spectra depending on membrane voltage and can be employed to account for motion of cardiomyocytes (CM) and the beating heart. PeT-based VSD lack this property and therefore are unsuitable for ratiometric imaging. Care must therefore be taken in experimental design if confounding signals such as motion artifacts are thought to be a major issue. Successful use of a dye isobestic point to provide a ratiometric method that corrects for

BOX 1 | Light penetration in tissue

Physical Basis for Light Scattering in Tissue

Light of a given wavelength can be described as an electromagnetic wave in which the electric and magnetic components oscillate at a particular frequency. It is the vibration of the electric component of light (typically at $\approx 10^{15}$ Hz for red light) which is responsible for scattering: the wave's vibrational energy causes valence electrons in surrounding media to vibrate transiently. The energy absorbed by the electron is quickly released in its entirety again to generate a spherical wavelet of the same frequency (energy conserving elastic scattering). The repetitive absorption and re-emission of energy, typically in the order of femtoseconds for visible light, causes a cumulative delay, which is directly proportional to the number of molecules and hence of electrons the light can interact with per unit volume. The degree to which light slows while propagating through a medium is quantified by the refractive index of the media, which reports the ratio of speed of light in a vacuum (the only place where zero scattering occurs) divided by the speed of light in the medium. Apart from molecule density, the susceptibility of electrons to interact with light also affects the refractive index, which explains why lipid-rich structures such as cell membranes have a higher refractive index than surrounding water (1.45 vs. 1.33) even though they have a lower density (Richardson and Lichtman, 2015).

Scattering

Scattering occurs everywhere light enters a medium, even in transparent media like air, glass or water. In contrast to opaque media, transparent media have two important properties. Firstly, the density of scatterers is so high that many scatterers exist over distances much smaller than the wavelength of light. Secondly, the scatterers are homogeneously distributed which means that lateral scattering is effectively canceled out by destructive interference of secondary wavelets and no light propagates perpendicular to the impinging light wave. In the forward direction, scatterers are activated sequentially and their excitations sum constructively, leading to attenuation-free propagation of light. When a medium is not homogeneous but instead contains structures whose size is comparable with the wavelength of the light (300–700 nm for visible light), strong Rayleigh scattering occurs. The magnitude of Rayleigh scattering is inversely proportional to the fourth power of the wavelength which means that longer wavelengths are scattered less than shorter wavelengths. In biological tissue heterogeneous structures include cellular constituents, such as ribosomes, nuclei, nucleoli, mitochondria, lipid droplets, membranes, myelin, cytoskeletal components, and extracellular matrix constituents such as collagen and elastin. These scatterers are inhomogenously distributed and give rise to substantial lateral scattering which no longer cancels out entirely due to destructive interference. Multiple scattering over a sufficient tissue thickness leads to tissue opacity.

Light Penetration in Tissue

Light can be described as an electromagnetic wave characterized by its wavelength, its power (watts W = Joule/second) and its irradiance (intensity, W/m^2). Only in homogeneous media does light propagate along a straight line. In this case, the energy of light is mostly lost through absorption of the medium and is converted to thermal energy, fluorescence or photobiochemical reactions. In elastic scattering events, the energy of the light is not lost but the direction of light propagation changes. Consequently, irradiance decreases in the direction of propagation in the measure that scattering causes lateral spreading of the light.

The intensity of light passing through a scattering and reflecting sample is given by

$$I_\lambda(d) = (1 - R)I_0 \exp(-\epsilon_\lambda d) \tag{1}$$

where d is the distance traveled in the medium, R is the reflectance, and ϵ_λ is the extinction coefficient which is the sum of the medium's absorption and scattering coefficients (Deng et al., 2014). Using this framework, light scattering can be quantified by a single number; the penetration depth I which describes the depth at which light decays to $1/e$ (about one third) of its incident intensity I_0 and is given by the inverse of the extinction coefficient of the medium: $I = 1/\epsilon_\lambda$.

Absorption

Hemoglobin, myoglobin, and melanin are the primary molecules responsible for visible light absorption in heart tissue. The "near-infrared window" is a section of the electromagnetic spectrum in which biological tissue only weakly absorbs, usually using light with wavelengths of 650–1.350 nm for example in near-infrared (IR) fluorophore excitation or with two-photon microscopy (see **Box 2**).

movement artifact has been successfully implemented (Bachtel et al., 2011). Ratiometric imaging has been employed for optical mapping experiments during open heart surgery (Lee et al., 2012a, 2019). Recent improvements and optimization efforts, including for ratiometric imaging, were described in a recent review article (Acker et al., 2020).

Despite remaining challenges, VSD combined with appropriate imaging methods can provide easy access to high quality voltage recordings from cell culture, tissue, or whole heart preparations with high speed and spatial resolution. Constraints continue to exist in the form of light-tissue interactions (see **Box 1**) which limit the precise spatio-temporal delivery of light patterns in 3D, especially at depth. This may be overcome somewhat through invasive methods, including stimulation through intramural light delivery using optrodes or implantable micro-LEDs (Byars et al., 2003; Caldwell et al., 2005; Zgierski-Johnston et al., 2020). Red-shifting of probes additionally allows one to use longer wavelengths for excitation and emission which experience less scattering and absorption in biological tissues and therefore enable extraction of signals from deeper tissue layers. Examples of such red-shifted VSD include di-4-ANBDQPQ (electrochromic; 620–660 nm excitation) and BeRST (PeT; 630 nm excitation) (Huang et al., 2015). The latter has recently been used in all-optical cardiac electrophysiology platforms for drug screening to accommodate spectrally blue-light induced optogenetic pacing and simultaneous calcium and voltage imaging (Klimas et al., 2020). For ratiometric imaging, the additional spectral bandwidth required to perform emission or excitation ratiometry may impose constraints on multi-modal acquisition. Additionally, to detect action potential features of 1 ms duration (e.g., action potential upstroke) with a fast impulse response, the sampling rate of the optical system must exceed 1 kHz. These demands require the development of sophisticated multi-modal optical imaging systems. Common issues remain across all VSD that still limit their applicability in cardiac electrophysiology; the most prominent of these being the inability to measure absolute voltages with high precision. This combined with the lack of an option for optical measurement of transmembrane current or an easy way to inject either inward or outward current optically means that an all-optical voltage clamp is not yet feasible. However, a successful implementation of an optical dynamic clamp to boost I_{K1} in human inducible pluripotent stem cell (iPSC)-derived CM has been demonstrated (Quach et al., 2018).

Calcium Sensitive Dyes

Due to the fundamental importance of Ca^{2+} in the excitation contraction coupling process in CM, we briefly touch upon calcium (Ca^{2+}) imaging which optically quantifies Ca_i^{2+} transients. Still extensively used since their development in the 1980s, fluorescent probes developed in the Tsien lab combine a Ca^{2+} chelator with a fluorophore, for example fluorescein, stilbene or rhodamine, within the same molecule. A variety of probes are now available which display a range of quantum efficiencies, photobleaching stabilities, sensitivities, and selectivities for Ca^{2+}, as well as differences in excitation spectra and temporal resolution. Some probes shift in emission wavelength upon Ca^{2+} binding to enable ratiometric quantitative measurements of the intracellular free Ca^{2+} concentration (Fura-2, Grynkiewicz et al., 1985), while others are non-ratiometric (Rhod-2). A recent review on ratiometric and non-ratiometric Ca_i^{2+} probes including probes for imaging of sarcoplasmic reticulum Ca^{2+} and probes compatible with potentiometric voltage dyes for multi-modal optical mapping is provided elsewhere (Jaimes III et al., 2016). As with VSD, careful consideration must be given to Ca^{2+} probe compartmentalization and how it could be influenced by probe concentration and loading conditions, especially duration and temperature. Measuring intracellular Ca^{2+} also offers a set of considerations which strongly influence the choice of indicator. Molecule binding affinity determines the Ca^{2+} concentration range within which the indicator is useful. High affinity indicators such as Fluo-3 and Fura-2 are appropriate for cardiac cytosolic Ca^{2+} measurements. However, many intracellular compartments contain much higher concentrations (such as the sarcoplasmic reticulum where Ca^{2+} levels approach 1 mM range) and require low affinity indicators, for example Fluo-5N (Wu and Bers, 2006). It is also important to remember that indicators themselves act as Ca^{2+} ion buffers. Therefore, minimizing the influence of the indicator on physiological processes requires a trade-off between keeping intracellular dye concentration as low as possible while maintaining good signal-to-noise ratio (Paredes et al., 2008).

Optogenetics: From Genetically Expressed Indicators to Light-Sensitive Ion Channels

Optogenetics, in its broadest sense, describes a set of tools which perform complementary functions: light-driven actuators impose targeted perturbations of either electrophysiological signals (Nagel et al., 2002) or activate intracellular signaling pathways e.g., G-protein coupled receptors (Makowka et al., 2019), while light emitting reporters reveal them (Miesenböck, 2009). This powerful combination of active interrogation and passive observation affords one the ability to infer spatiotemporal dynamics of complex systems that cannot be easily elucidated from the activity of their individual components (Entcheva and Bub, 2016). The genes coding for optogenetic proteins, be they light-emitting reporters or light-driven actuators, are encoded in DNA vectors and introduced under the control of a (potentially cell type-specific) promoter into the genome of the host organism. This causes selected cells to produce the optogenetic proteins with the cell's endogenous synthesizing machinery. Using the cell itself to express the reporter (or actuator) overcomes some of the aforementioned limitations of intracellular loading associated with exogenous probes. The combination of cell-selectivity in gene expression and wavelength-specificity of protein activation, provide the outstanding scientific value of optogenetics. The possibility to spectrally combine optical actuators and reporters allows for completely contact-free all-optical interrogation and control. Recent comprehensive reviews details cardiac applications of optogenetics over the last decade (Koopman et al., 2017; Entcheva and Kay, 2021).

Optogenetic reporters translate CM electrophysiological signals into optical signals. Virtually all genetically-encoded Ca^{2+} indicators (GECI, reviewed in Kotlikoff, 2007; Whitaker, 2010), are derivatives of the green fluorescent protein (GFP). For example, G-CaMP modulates its output signal through Ca^{2+}-dependent conformational changes that allow or restrict solvent access to the chromophore, which causes increased brightness with Ca^{2+} binding (Chen et al., 2013).

Genetically-encoded voltage indicators (GEVI) report changes in membrane potential from individual cells or populations using voltage-sensitive fluorescent proteins. Current GEVI are limited by the brightness and photostability of fluorescent proteins. The electric field decreases exponentially with distance from the cell membrane, which means the available volume for voltage indicators is restricted to the cell membrane, i.e., a very small fraction of the total cell volume. Additionally, because membrane potential changes can occur over very short timescales, only a few photons are emitted from a restricted volume over a restricted time making their detection statistically difficult. Expressing more reporter molecules bears the risk of observation interfering with the very quantity of interest, electrical excitability, because the mobile charges of voltage probes sensing the cellular membrane potential add a capacitive load to the cell membrane. Whether this increased membrane capacitance influences action potential characteristics is unclear, and seems to depend on the target system, the specific GEVI being used and its overall expression levels (Yang and St-Pierre, 2016). The most commonly used GEVI in cardiac *in vitro* applications so far is ArcLight (Jin et al., 2012), a bright GEVI with relatively slow kinetics, limiting its ability to capture detailed action potential morphology. A new chemigenetic GEVI, Voltron, combines the specificity of genetically encoded reagents with the superior photophysics of synthetic rhodamine dyes like the Janelia Fluor instead of protein-based fluorophores. In a hybrid approach, a genetically expressed scaffold, composed of a voltage-sensitive microbial rhodopsin domain with a dye-capture protein domain, irreversibly binds the synthetic dye (Abdelfattah et al., 2019). Changes in membrane potential alter the absorption spectrum of the rhodopsin domain in Voltron which in turn reversibly modulates the degree of fluorescence quenching of the dye through Förster resonance energy transfer (FRET), yielding a GEVI with increased photon output.

In addition to being used as reporters, optogenetics also includes a suite of genetically-expressed photosensitive actuators which alter the ionic flux through cellular membranes in response to light of specific wavelengths (Nagel et al., 2002). For example, upon illumination with 465 nm, Channelrhodopsin-2 (ChR2) (Nagel et al., 2003; Boyden et al., 2005) a light-sensitive cation channel opens and depolarizes the cell, which can be used to elicit action potentials in excitable cells such as neurons and CM. These channels have been extensively color-tuned (Prigge et al., 2012) and ion pumps expand the toolset to bi-directional control of transmembrane voltage. For example, light-activated potassium channels have been used to inhibit activation by hyperpolarizing the cell (Sierra et al., 2018). Optogenetic actuation allows one to conduct light stimulation or inhibition of cells that do not normally respond to light, supporting the investigation of causal relationships within networks of cells. An exciting development in optogenetics is the possibility of optically controlling exogenous gene expression itself (De Mena et al., 2018). Further manipulation of natural photo switches has expanded the toolkit from light-activated membrane channels to non-channel proteins designed to induce protein-protein interactions (Deisseroth, 2011). These new interaction tools include light-activated enzymes and transcription factors which permit expression of genes in locally defined tissue regions. An important consideration when using optical approaches is the amount of light required to either create sufficient fluorescence signal to be detected or to activate a light-driven protein function. This value is usually a balance between the need to maximize excitation/ photo-conversion and need to minimize photo-bleaching and cellular photo-damage. **Table 1** indicates the light irradiance needed at the sample/ tissue/ cell used in the study of cardiac tissue using a range of light sources and optics. For single photon applications approximately 10–100 mW μm^{-2} is commonly used, while two-photon applications require approximately 10,000 higher power but at approximately double the wavelength.

MULTIMODAL IMAGING OF INTRACELLULAR Ca^{2+} AND MEMBRANE POTENTIAL

Cardiac excitation-contraction coupling is governed by the complex and dynamic interplay between membrane ion fluxes and intracellular Ca^{2+} handling processes and manifested in the action potential and intracellular Ca^{2+} transient, respectively. Multimodal acquisitions, i.e., the simultaneous monitoring of calcium and voltage at high spatiotemporal resolution, are important because they provide insight into excitation contraction coupling and arrhythmia mechanism (Salama and Hwang, 2009). The prevailing technique of concurrent

TABLE 1 | Values in this table indicate the approximate irradiance required from different light sources at the sample to image Ca^{2+} or activate ChR2.

Light sources	Wavelength (typical) (nm)	Illumination optics (typical)	Irradiance
Light emitting diodes/ Xe lamps	400–700	Macro/microscope objective	10 mW mm^{-2} Funken et al., 2019, 2020
Continuous wave laser (single photon)	400–700	Microscope (1 μm × 1 μm spot)	5–10 μW μm^{-2} Centonze and White, 1998
Ultrashort pulsed laser (two photon)	700–1100	Microscope (1 μm × 1 μm spot)	5–10 mW μm^{-2} Bush et al., 2007

The wavelengths are chosen to represent common voltage/ Ca^{2+} fluorescent indicators and optogenetic applications.

tracking of fluorescent reporters of either membrane voltage or cytoplasmic Ca^{2+} is optical mapping (Jaimes III et al., 2016).

Optical Mapping

In optical mapping the most basic fluorescent microscope, a wide-field microscope (or macroscope for large field of view), is employed to flood-illuminate the sample and detect the fluorescence of indicators across the entire field of view. For the heart, in particular Langendorff setups, different geometries can be used that can be based on photodiode arrays (Efimov et al., 1994; Qu et al., 2007) or camera(s) with suitable lenses. This can be single-view (Lee et al., 2011), multiple-camera / multiple-view (Cathey et al., 2019) or single-camera/ multiple-view (Lee et al., 2012b). The wide-field illumination and detection scheme has the advantage of being fast and simple, and it can obtain both topographical and dynamic information. Usually, mercury lamps or LEDs are used for fluorescence excitation and if functional data are to be acquired, a high-speed imaging system is needed to capture and visualize small changes in fluorescence intensity. Considering the minimum sampling frequency necessary, according to the Nyquist sampling theorem, to achieve a temporal resolution suitable for tracking action potential propagation (*ms*) the camera employed in optical mapping must operate at a minimum frame rate of $\sim 2\,kHz$. Frame rate requirements for Ca^{2+} imaging, where Ca^{2+} release from the sarcoplasmic reticulum is the fastest part of the transient and time to peak is in the order of $\sim$ 10–30 ms, are more relaxed. The high costs associated with setups capable of high frame rates can be circumvented by "temporal pixel multiplexing" techniques that embed temporal information in still images to enhance the temporal resolution of imaging methods (Bub et al., 2010). Further requirements for the camera, typically a charge coupled device (CCD) or scientific complementary metal-oxide semiconductor (sCMOS) camera, are very low read-out noise, high quantum efficiency and high well depth to capture the small fluorescence variations associated with action potential or Ca^{2+} release with enough dynamic range and signal-to-noise ratio. Multimodal acquisition can be achieved in several ways. Certain combinations of Ca^{2+} indicators and VSD can be excited by a single light source due to overlapping excitation spectra but distinct emission bands, thereby minimizing signal cross talk (for example the Ca^{2+} indicator Rhod-2 and VSD RH-237, Salama and Hwang, 2009). Separation of the emitted fluorescence signal into different detectors (or different areas of the same sensor) can be achieved with dichroic mirrors and emission filters (Yan et al., 2012). Multiplexing can also occur by excitation, albeit at a reduced temporal resolution, by turning different LEDs on and off sequentially during synchronized image acquisition to excite spectrally-separable voltage and calcium probes during synchronized image acquisition (Lee et al., 2011; Klimas et al., 2020). Low-magnification cardiac optical mapping *in vitro* presents higher demands on the imaging systems compared to whole heart imaging due to the very thin layer of cells generating a signal (Entcheva and Bien, 2006). Hence the need for high-numerical aperture (NA) lenses borrowed from photography, more sensitive detectors and better fluorescent reporters to map voltage and Ca^{2+} excitation in human induced pluripotent stem-cell-derived CM, for example.

One issue that has featured in the majority of optical mapping studies is the requirement that the underlying epicardium does not move substantially during the imaging process over the contraction/relaxation cycle. In early studies, this was achieved by gently pressing the right ventricle/ left ventricle (LV/RV) surface against an optical surface during image capture (Kanai and Salama, 1995). This procedure requires care to prevent the development of ischaemic areas when physically restraining the heart. More commonly, contraction related movement is minimized by chemical electro-mechanical uncouplers such as the myosin inhibitors butanedione monoxime (Kettlewell et al., 2004) or blebbistatin (Fedorov et al., 2007). These compounds block contraction by direct inhibition of the myofilaments, thus limiting motion artifacts whilst preserving electrophysiological function. Though there is published evidence for direct effects of most of the common uncouplers on electrophysiology (Kettlewell et al., 2004; Brack et al., 2013; Kappadan et al., 2020), the magnitude and importance of this limitations is debated. Derivatives of blebbistatin, i.e., para-nitro blebbistatin (Képiró et al., 2014) and para-amino blebbistatin (Várkuti et al., 2016) have chemical features that facilitate their use as uncouplers but similarly require rigorous testing for non-specific effects on cardiac electrophysiology.

In addition to the potential direct effects of chemical uncouplers on cardiac electrophysiology there is also the physiological influence of muscle length and contraction on electrophysiology via a series of mechano-electric feedback (MEF) systems (Quinn and Kohl, 2021). This issue can be circumvented by the application of processing algorithms to the moving isolated heart to track epicardial regions during contraction, thereby minimizing movement artifact (Christoph and Luther, 2018). These approaches are not system-specific and their use is restricted to the few labs able to support the complex post-acquisition analysis. The outcome of these approaches is not just the electrical map of the imaged surface, but the mechanical behavior of the myocardium, by itself an important physiological feature and one which informs the study of phenomena associated with MEF.

Myocardial motion alone can be used to infer activation timings and patterns in the absence of probes to monitor electrical activity (Christoph et al., 2018). When applied to the whole heart during the cardiac cycle, this approach has the complication of interpretation as movement depends on a number of factors including preload and afterload. With this caveat, computationally streamlined image analysis techniques have been developed to track motion of contracting tissue (Burton et al., 2015; Sala et al., 2018). Among other advantages, dye-free imaging works at all wavelengths, which simplifies its integration with spectrally-restricted opsins used for actuation (Burton et al., 2015) and in mechanically similar muscle systems such as cultured CM monolayers these techniques can map patterns of contraction over long periods of time. Furthermore, recently developed random access parallel imaging, inspired by a Newtonian telescope-based addressing of samples without moving parts, demonstrated high-throughput dye-free imaging in 96-well format (Ashraf et al., 2021). An important consideration when analyzing optical mapping data from thick tissue or whole heart preparations is that this technique lacks optical sectioning. Since illuminating light penetrates several millimeters into highly scattering cardiac tissue, the resultant electrophysiological signals arise from a volume below the tissue surface. As a result, signal features such as transient upstroke morphology and duration are prolonged (Girouard et al., 1996), particularly in optical action potentials. This also has implications for multimodal imaging setups utilizing distinct wavelength excitation light sources, since the longer wavelength light will penetrate deeper, exciting a larger volume of tissue. These features appear at first disadvantageous, however the fact that optical action potentials carry information about the electrophysiology of a tissue volume has been used to reveal subepicardial fiber orientation based on action potential upstroke shape (Hyatt et al., 2005). Dual excitation of spectrally separated VSD has also been used successfully to reveal unique information about transmural heterogeneities and endocardial electrophysiology in rat hearts (Walton et al., 2010). Looking to the future, with the emergence of low-cost high-speed cameras, volumetric optical mapping in small-size hearts has been shown to be possible with multi-plane multi-camera parallel imaging (Sacconi et al., 2020).

Two-Photon Microscopy for Deep Tissue Access

While optical mapping has proven to be a powerful and versatile tool, in its classic implementation, lack of depth discrimination limits the degree of information on transmural electrophysiology. The increasing need to investigate biological specimens in 3D has driven the development of optical techniques capable of volumetric imaging. As opposed to physical sectioning, these techniques, most notably confocal, two-photon (TPM) and light-sheet microscopy, use optical sectioning to obtain depth-specific information.

In confocal microscopy the sample is sequentially illuminated by a diffraction limited spot, typically employing single photon excitation, and the signal from this spot is registered using a point detector masked by a small pinhole. Similar to TPM, confocal microscopy is a serial sampling instrument which uses the same objective for excitation and detection (epi-configuration). The pinhole gives confocal microscopy its optical sectioning capability because it prevents or at least severely attenuates the detection of light emitted from areas outside of the focal volume. The pinhole is placed in an image plane and typically has a diameter of 1-2 Airy units. The image of the pinhole in the object plane restricts the volume from which photons will be collected, thereby increasing image contrast.

In confocal and wide-field microscopy, contrast is generated from light-matter interactions in which the elementary process (absorption, scattering, etc.) only involves a single photon and which therefore depends linearly on the incident light intensity. Non-linear microscopy methods, such as TPM (Denk et al., 1990) rely on higher-order light matter interactions involving two or more photons for contrast generation. This fundamental difference is the source of numerous new imaging properties. TPM is especially well-suited for deep tissue imaging as it supports imaging scattering samples non-invasively with sub-micrometer resolution in 3D. Moreover, due to the excitation process, which results from the simultaneous absorption of two photons, there are a number of unique advantages such as reduced specimen photodamage and enhanced penetration depth.

Optical Sectioning Microscopy in the Intact Heart

Optical sectioning techniques like confocal and two-photon microscopy enable one to look beneath the sample surface to resolve cellular processes and structures within discrete volumes of tissue. A wealth of information can therefore be gained from measurement of cardiac cellular electrophysiology deep beneath the epicardium of the intact heart. Cardiac TPM allows for both *in vivo* and *ex vivo* cellular and cell layer-scale electrophysiological and intracellular Ca^{2+} measurements across the myocardial wall (Rubart et al., 2003; Kelly et al., 2013, 2018; Ghouri et al., 2018). Cardiac TPM has been critical in defining the importance of structural features for transmural conduction, both in healthy tissue and in models of reduced tissue excitability (Kelly et al., 2013, 2018) including confirmation of heterocellular electrical coupling of cardiac myocytes and fibroblasts (Rubart et al., 2018), previously established by optical mapping (Quinn et al., 2016). This is aided significantly by the ability to perform simultaneous two-photon fluorescence and second harmonic generation microscopy, enabling label-free imaging and quantification of collagen in live tissue, an important marker of pathological remodeling in cardiac disease (Martin et al., 2013). For *in vivo* TPM, the motion of the heart becomes a significant technical challenge which cannot be overcome with chemical uncouplers. However, several publications have detailed methodological considerations to allow this type of imaging (Lee et al., 2012c; Vinegoni et al., 2015), which has aided in better understanding of cardiac immune cell motility and trafficking (Kreisel et al., 2010; Li et al., 2013). Here we describe several avenues of cardiac electrophysiological research which continue to benefit from developments in TPM.

Transmural Imaging

Electrical propagation under normal circumstances adopts a significant transmural axis, from the endocardium toward the epicardial surface. Within the intramural space, this electrical wavefront encounters an array of physical discontinuities; blood vessels, extracellular clefts and regions of heterogeneous fibrotic distribution. The laminar arrangement of CM within the ventricle shift and rotate at right angles to each other, sometimes abruptly (within 2–3 cell layers of thickness) (Hooks et al., 2007). These factors have a measurable impact on electrophysiology, even in healthy hearts. In combination with optical mapping, *ex vivo* whole heart recordings yield a wealth of information about ventricular electrophysiology across a wide region, which can then be examined at the cellular scale within the transmural wall, affording greater detail about the influence of microscopic myocardial wall tissue features (cell orientation, cell distribution, microarchitecture, including the influence of scar tissue in disease) on electrophysiology and transmural conduction. As with optical mapping, electrophysiology can be tracked with rapid scanning TPM in conjunction with VSD such as di-4-ANEPPS, albeit over a restricted field of view using a high-NA objective. The optical sectioning power of TPM however, allows for action potential characteristics at a given transmural depth to be faithfully captured, with 2 kHz scanning rates capable of resolving action potential rise time characteristics in multiple small animal species with similar fidelity to sharp microelectrodes (Ghouri et al., 2015). Serial scanning necessitates slow volumetric rates, which requires electrical stimulation of the heart to generate a repeated sequence of activation, a common approach in isolated perfused heart experiments. This carries the added caveat however that beat-to-beat variability, an important property of whole heart electrophysiology, cannot be examined. Thus, an average profile of transmural electrical conduction can be constructed from sequential volumetric measurements using the electrical stimulus as a timing reference. This approach revealed that surface boundary conditions measurably increase action potential upstroke velocity as the wavefront approaches the epicardial surface transmurally, demonstrating the strong electrotonic load influence on CM action potential properties (Kelly et al., 2013). This technique was also key in describing conduction abnormality in a model of Brugada syndrome, an inherited arrhythmic disorder often characterized by slow conduction, right ventricular arrhythmias and higher risk of sudden death. Combining TPM with computational simulations, it was found that the less compact structural arrangement of the right ventricle made it uniquely susceptible to conduction slowing when myocyte excitability is reduced, particularly at higher heart rates (Kelly et al., 2018).

Electrical Coupling of Implanted iPSC-Derived CM Grafts After MI

The intrinsic regenerative capacity of the heart is limited; estimates place cell turnover in adult humans at 0.5–1 % *per annum* (Bergmann et al., 2009). As a result, ischemic insults (myocardial infarction) activate inflammation-mediated signaling cascades which replace necrotic tissue with a vascularized infarct scar, reducing the overall contractile capacity of the heart and forming a substrate for ventricular arrhythmias. One of the promising repair strategies to emerge in recent years involves implantation of engineered heart tissue (EHT) constructs, grown from iPSC-CM, directly over the infarct to restore function. This has met with some success in both small (Matsuo et al., 2015; Pecha et al., 2019) and large animal models (Gao et al., 2017), but questions remain over the extent of EHT coupling to native myocardium, as well as the long-term survival of the originally-implanted cells. Addressing these questions has generated a number of technical challenges that TPM can help overcome (Weinberger et al., 2016). Electrophysiological assessment via optical mapping of voltage sensitive dyes alone struggles to fully distinguish between electrical activity of the EHT and normal myocardium. It has been known for some time that fluorescent "bleed-through" from surviving endocardial tissue (or, if the infarct is thin enough, septal tissue) will contaminate the optical map of the infarct with implanted EHT, giving the appearance of relatively healthy looking action potentials from largely-free scar. Gene-silencing of G-CaMP indicators expressed in the EHT was also observed to occur when hearts were explanted 4 weeks post-surgery. TPM helped to overcome these setbacks by allowing delineation of EHT and infarct electrophysiology through serial optical sectioning, demonstrating that electrical coupling of EHT and native myocardium can occur, albeit with a relatively low success rate (Weinberger et al., 2016). While the above patches were developed with the aim of aiding contractile function, another exciting application of engineered tissue is to serve as electrical conduction tracts. This has been shown to efficiently bridge atrio-ventricular conduction in a murine model of atrio-ventricular node failure (Cingolani et al., 2014), and shows that electrical integration of engineered tissue constructs can indeed be achieved with potentially far-reaching consequences for translation (Kohl, 2014). In any case, the further development of EHT-based organ repair is uniquely poised to benefit from the discriminating power that TPM optical sectioning provides.

Origin of the Electrical Conduction Through Myocardial Infarct Scar

Questions remain over electrical interaction between the infarct scar and healthy myocardium. Surviving islands of myocardium and remnant electrical activity within the infarct are well-documented (Walker et al., 2007), with myofibroblasts implicated in permitting electrical propagation between the border zone and surviving myocardium within the scar itself (Quinn et al., 2016). Several studies using TPM have sought to elucidate the mechanism of infarct conduction. Combined optical mapping-TPM systems and dual voltage and Ca^{2+} labeling has been used to distinguish between myocyte and non-myocyte electrical propagation within the infarct zone in rat hearts, using the absence of an intracellular Ca^{2+} transient as an indicator of non-myocyte electrotonic interaction (Ghouri et al., 2018). A similar analysis of the peri-infarct zone in mice expressing CM-specific GFP, identified non-myocyte electrical activity attributed to myofibroblasts exhibiting markedly slowed action potential upstrokes (Rubart et al., 2018). Engraftment of Connexin-43 (Cx43) expressing non-myocytes (Roell et al., 2007), or over-expression of Cx43 in murine infarct tissue (Roell et al., 2018), aided trans-scar conduction, implicating heterocellular contributions to electrical propagation in the heart. A thorough investigation of myocyte-fibroblast interaction within mouse infarct using a similar CM-specific labeling approach is currently being undertaken.

Random Access Multiphoton Microscopy in the T-Tubular System

Random access multiphoton microscopy (RAMP) (Sacconi et al., 2012) based on acousto-optic deflectors (AODs) was recently used in combination with novel VSD with improved photostability (Yan et al., 2012) to measure T-tubular action potentials at multiple sites with high spatio-temporal resolution. The authors observed that a tight electrical coupling between distinct membrane domains (i.e., surface sarcolemma and

T-tubules) is guaranteed only in healthy cells. Conversely, experiments on disease models showed that action potential propagation in the structurally remodeled T-tubular system can fail and local spontaneous depolarizations can occur in the electrically disconnected T-tubules (Sacconi et al., 2012). A simultaneous recording of the action potential and local Ca^{2+} release was used to dissect the consequences of electrical defects on intracellular Ca^{2+} dynamics. Specifically, the authors implemented a double staining approach, combining a Ca^{2+} reporter (FluoForte GFP-certified) with a fluorinated VSD. Two-photon excitation features were exploited to simultaneously excite both dyes, while band-pass filters were used to select the two distinct spectral ranges of the overlapping fluorescence spectra. A spectral unmixing procedure was applied to properly uncouple voltage and Ca^{2+} signals. Employing this approach in combination with the random access modality, the authors were able to optically record action potentials in several T-tubules and, simultaneously, the corresponding local Ca^{2+} transients (Crocini et al., 2014). **Figure 1** shows an example of an optical recording of voltage and Ca^{2+} release in six different positions across the sarcolemma. The signal-to-noise ratio of the proposed method was sufficient to detect the presence of an action potential and to assess the temporal features of Ca^{2+} dynamic in single shot recordings, without averaging sequential trials. The utility of the system in detecting electrical activity and local Ca^{2+} release simultaneously in multiple sites was used to solve unanswered questions about the spatio-temporal relationship between sub-cellular alterations of Ca^{2+} release and T-tubular electrical and structural defects in several cardiac diseases including ischemic heart failure (Crocini et al., 2014), spontaneously hypertensive rats in overt heart failure (Scardigli et al., 2018a), and hypertrophic cardiomyopathy (Crocini et al., 2016b).

Enhancing the Utility of Two-Photon Optical Sectioning Microscopy for Cardiac Applications

Non-linear imaging (**Box 2**) is uniquely applicable to transmural cardiac studies and combined with several adjacent technologies, including optical mapping and emerging optogenetic tools, provides a powerful and versatile analytical tool for cardiac electrophysiology. Despite this, significant challenges remain to prevent its widespread adoption which are intrinsic both to the technology itself and cardiac muscle in particular. Understanding

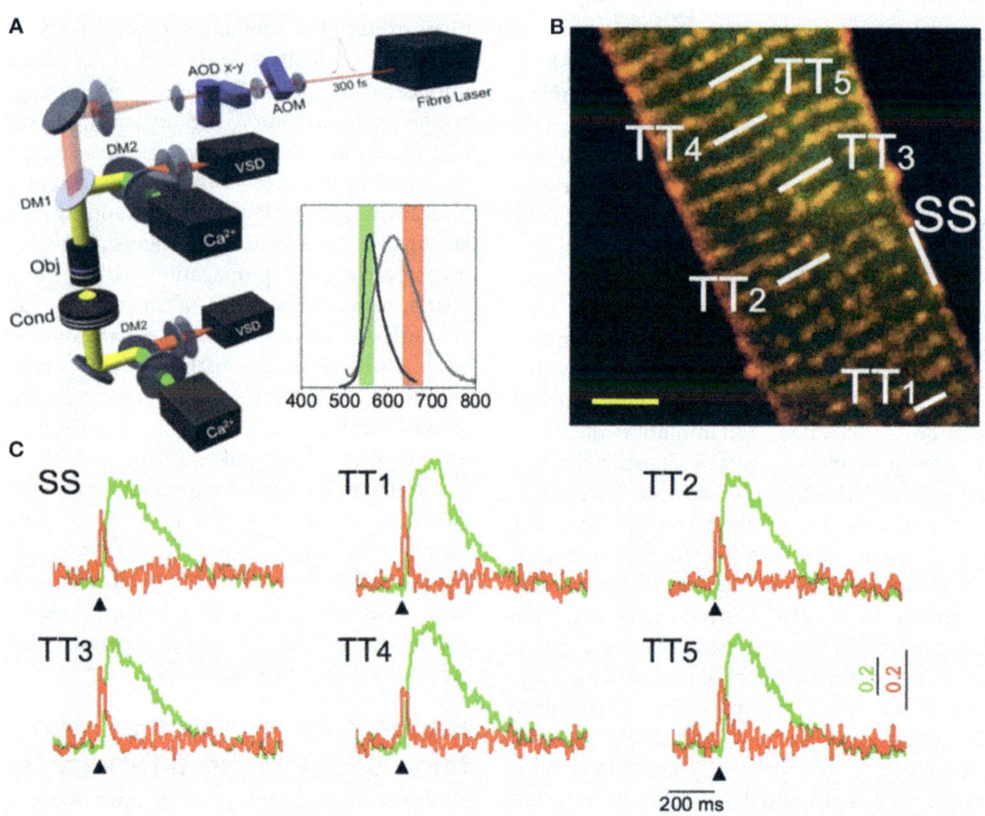

FIGURE 1 | Multi-site voltage and Ca^{2+} recording. **(A)** Scheme of the Random Access Multi-Photon (RAMP) microscope based on two orthogonally-mounted acousto-optical deflectors (AODs -x and -y) for laser scanning. Inset shows the emission spectra of the Ca^{2+} indicator (in dark gray) and voltage sensitive dye (in light gray) together with their fluorescence filter acquisition band. **(B)** Image of a stained rat ventricular cardiac cell: di-4-ANE(F)PPTEA in red and GFP-certified Fluoforte in green. Scale bar: 5 μm **(C)** Real time fluorescence traces collected from the scanned sites indicated in white in **(B)**: surface sarcolemma (SS) and five T-tubules (TTi). Membrane voltage is shown in red and Ca^{2+} in green. Reproduced and modified from Crocini et al. (2014).

BOX 2 | Two-photon microscopy

Physical Background

In conventional fluorescence spectroscopy, a fluorescent molecule is excited by absorption of one photon whose energy corresponds to the energy gap between the ground state and the excited state of the molecule. However, the same excitation is also possible by the near-simultaneous absorption, i.e., within 1e−16 s, of two photons of approximately double the wavelength via a short-lived, virtual intermediate state. The combined energy of the two long-wavelength, low-energy photons produce an excitation equivalent to the absorption of a single photon possessing twice the energy. The emitted fluorescence generated by the simultaneous absorption of two photons is indistinguishable to single photon excitation fluorescence emission. The simultaneous absorption of two photons is the origin of the quadratic dependence on the light intensity: in TPM, doubling the excitation intensity produces four times the fluorescence. This non-linear dependence of two-photon absorption is the basis for the intrinsic localization of fluorescence generation and therefore the optical sectioning capability, i.e., the imaging of specific planes within the sample without the need for physical slicing.

Requirements

Like most non-linear processes, the excitation probability in two-photon excitation fluorescence is extremely low but can be optimized to generate enough signal by concentrating the excitation light in space and time. Spatial compression is achieved by tight focusing with high-NA objective lenses. This increases the local intensity at the focal point and with it the probability for two-photon excitation. Away from the 3D focal spot the probability for simultaneous absorption drops off drastically such that virtually no fluorescence is generated outside the focal volume (Zipfel et al., 2003). Scattered excitation light is too dilute to excite by two-photon absorption and too long in wavelength to be absorbed otherwise. Owing to the low two-photon absorption cross-section inherent to non-linear processes, a useful fluorescence signal can only be achieved with ultrashort pulses which compress excitation intensity in the time domain. Ultrafast pulsed lasers concentrate photons into very short (pulse width τ), high peak intensity pulses separated by e−8 intervals (repetition rate R), keeping the average power relatively low. This increases the signal by a factor of $1/(\tau * R)^{n-1}$ compared to continuous-wave illumination, where n is the number of photons involved in the elementary process (Helmchen and Denk, 2005). At present, the most commonly used lasers in TPM setups are mode-locked titanium sapphire (Ti:Sa) which typically generate pulses with τ = 100–150 fs at τ = 80–100 MHz. They are tunable from 680 to 1, 080 nm.

Image Formation

The laser is focused onto the sample and scanned through the specimen in a raster fashion by a scanner, most commonly a pair of galvanometer mirrors (one for each image axis). The image is reconstructed from digitizing the point measurements of the fluorescence intensity at each position in the sample. Emission collection can be efficient and simple because all photons generated are signal and there is virtually no background: even multiply-scattered fluorescence photons can be assigned to their origin due to the localized nature of signal generation. To increase efficiency of fluorescence collection, non-descanned detectors are employed, most commonly large area photomultiplier tubes (PMTs) positioned close to the back aperture of the microscope objective. PMTs allow for the detection of multiply scattered fluorescence photons that may leave the objective lens at randomly divergent angles and are also favored for their high gain and low readout noise.

Advantages

A key advantage of TPM over confocal microscopy is reduced attenuation in biological specimens due to reduced scattering and absorption of near infrared light when compared to UV and visible light. Even though Rayleigh scattering is just an approximation in biological imaging, the inverse relationship ($\sim \lambda^{-4}$) between scattering and excitation wavelength remains valid. This results in deeper penetration of the pulsed laser source into scattering samples compared to conventional microscopy. Also, the "optical window," placed at 700–1.000 nm where tissue absorbance is orders of magnitude less than the absorption in the UV or visible region, falls conveniently into the spectral excitation window of TPM. Lower photon absorption in the tissue additionally means lower levels of phototoxicity and sample heating. However it should be noted that within the focal volume, the possibility of bleaching, damage and reduced viability remains.

Increasing Excitation Efficiency

Since the fluorescence signal in TPM scales with $1/(\tau^*R)$, an increase in signal can be achieved with a reduction in the duty cycle $\tau * R$. A reduction of the repetition rate R increases pulse energy, however, a limit is given by the repetition rate since at least one laser pulse must be delivered per image pixel. The reduction of pulse duration τ also leads to increased signal but accurate dispersion correction in the optical train becomes essential. As pulsed laser light traverses the beam path of a microscope, the optical elements slow the shorter wavelength components of the pulse relative to the longer wavelengths, consequently broadening the pulse; a phenomenon known as (positive) group velocity dispersion (GVD). Positive GVD compensation is achieved by introducing optical elements which exhibit negative GVD, introducing an equal but opposite dispersion on the pulse prior to entering the microscope, thus maintaining the shortest pulse duration at the sample plane. Dispersion compensation is often achieved using prisms (Akturk et al., 2006) or chirped mirrors where multiple layers of dielectric material with increasing layer spacing vary the distance traveled by different wavelengths of the pulse and compensate for GVD (Szipöcs et al., 1994). Importantly, GVD worsens the shorter the pulse since the spectral bandwidth of the pulse increases with decreasing pulse duration. A limit to the benefits of shorter pulses is reached when the spectral width of the laser excitation approaches or exceeds the width of the excitation spectrum of the dye ~ 30–40 nm (full width at half maximum).

The Fundamental Depth Limit

The imaging depth in TPM cannot be increased indefinitely by increasing the excitation efficiency of the laser. A fundamentally constrained penetration depth restricts investigations in cardiac tissue to a few hundreds of micrometers in mouse left ventricle tissue (Salerno et al., 2019). In turbid media, the ballistic (unscattered) fraction of photons reaching the focal spot decays exponentially with depth. The total power of light reaching a certain depth decays more slowly, approximately as 1/depth. Due to these different decay rates, at depths depending on the scattering mean free path length and anisotropy of the tissue, the peak intensity of ballistic light will fall below that of scattered light, effectively rendering imaging impossible. Even before this depth limit is reached, background fluorescence generated partially by ballistic and mostly by scattered light near the surface will dominate the signal (Theer and Denk, 2006). The fundamental imaging depth in TPM is reached when this out-of-focus (background) fluorescence equals the fluorescence signal emanating from the focal spot; the signal-to-background ratio reaches unity. This fundamental limit to achievable tissue penetration depth is a direct consequence of light scattering by tissue and irrespective of available laser power or potential photodamage.

these limitations and available options for overcoming them is critical for informing the next generation of 3D cardiac imaging studies based on TPM.

The ubiquity of optical mapping in cardiac electrophysiological research owes its popularity not only to the high quality and throughput of the data generated, but also the relative simplicity of the setup, particularly with regards to excitation light sources. In contrast, TPM has a relatively high cost and perceived complexity barrier which has restricted its widespread adoption in cardiac electrophysiology. Full commercial microscope systems remain expensive platforms, often bundled with tuneable Ti-sapphire lasers which do not deliver sufficient power to the sample plane for deep tissue imaging at wavelengths within the second IR imaging window ($> 1000nm$). Data throughput, particularly for whole heart imaging is also relatively low. Owing to the need for tight spatial focusing, it is technically challenging to combine the high spatial resolution of TPM with larger fields of view and/ or fast volumetric imaging rates. Axial focusing remains slow and limited to the speed of a resonant objective piezo scanner, though remote refocusing (Botcherby et al., 2008; Alfred Millett-Sikking and York, 2018) increases axial scan speed and has been used for fast measurements of sarcomere length and cell orientation in Langendorff-perfused hearts (Botcherby et al., 2013). The following sections discuss these aspects in more detail.

Increasing Imaging Depth

As highlighted in **Box 2**, a fundamental imaging depth limit exists for a given system, independent of the excitation efficiency of the laser. This is due primarily to tissue scattering effects and increasing background fluorescence generated near the tissue surface (assuming tissue staining is homogeneous throughout the sample thickness). Several optical techniques have been proposed to overcome the TPM depth limit, while retaining scanning rates necessary for optical electrophysiology measurements. Temporal focusing, primarily used to allow video-rate optical sectioning, images a scan line across a blazed diffraction grating to spatially separate the spectral components of the laser pulse, effectively broadening the pulse width. The grating is imaged onto the sample plane via a high-NA objective lens and scanned in one axis to form an image. In theory this should reduce surface background fluorescence because the broadened pulse entering the sample only becomes short enough to permit non-linear interactions at the objective focal plane (Tal et al., 2005). While this approach is successful for rapid-scanning, improved depth imaging is questionable. This is because while point-scanning systems can use all scattered photons to detect an image, only ballistic or weakly scattered photons are useful for image formation with temporal focusing. A direct comparison of temporal focusing microscopy and TPM estimated the latter has up to 2X the penetration depth in highly scattering biological material (Rowlands et al., 2015). Alternatively, differential aberration correction was designed specifically to reduce background fluorescence contamination by placing a deformable mirror into the beam path of a raster scanning TPM which periodically (every second line or frame) introduces an optical aberration pattern to defocus the laser pulse. This preferentially reduces focal excitation while preserving the background. Subtracting the defocused image from the original produces an enhanced contrast image (Leray and Mertz, 2006; Leray et al., 2008). Contrast at a given depth is improved by up to 6X, a potentially significant gain in TPM depth imaging. It should be noted however, that because two images must be formed, the frame rate is effectively halved. A variant of this approach using a delay line and a fixed aberration optic allows near-simultaneous acquisition of two images in separate channels (Xiao and Mertz, 2019). Differential aberration shows promise as a powerful, lightweight approach for deeper TPM imaging and a thorough quantitative evaluation of its usefulness using cardiac muscle is warranted.

The Red Shift

A different approach to increasing the penetration depth of non-linear microscopy techniques is to decrease the effects of scattering itself. Novel engineered fluorophores, whose absorption and emission spectra are shifted toward the IR, take advantage of the decreased scattering of longer wavelengths. However, to image deeper into highly scattering samples, 3PM, the simultaneous absorption of three photons (of 1,300 or 1.700 nm wavelength) to excite fluorescence, has emerged as a promising technique which outperforms two-photon excitation of a different fluorophore at the same wavelength. Due to the higher non-linearity of the 3-photon absorption process, its cross section is several orders of magnitude smaller compared to TPM and this leads to virtually background-free deep imaging and highly improved signal-to-background ratio. However, the extremely low 3PA cross-sections (for example resulting in absorption rates $\sim$ 20 orders of magnitude lower than 2PA), necessitate higher pulse energies, usually obtained by low repetition rate (2–4 MHz) lasers. The higher peak energy results in higher peak power and therefore an increased risk of non-linear tissue damage whereas the longer wavelength leads to higher absorption and therefore more sample heating.

CORRELATION OF STRUCTURE AND FUNCTION

A major current technical challenge in optical cardiac imaging is the deterministic correlation between structural features and functional performance at different hierarchical levels, from subcellular components such as individual Ryanodine receptors (RyR) using DNA-PAINT techniques (Hurley et al., 2020) to single isolated CM and intact heart tissue. Assessing the structure and the corresponding local function in a correlative manner is particularly relevant in pathological settings where structural and ultra-structural alterations occur e.g., alteration of excitation-contraction coupling machinery, myofilament disarray or extracellular fibrosis. In the subsequent two sections, two case studies are described to demonstrate the power of optical techniques to measure and assess the function of sub-resolution membrane structures within cardiac muscle cells.

Super-Resolution Techniques Applied to Cardiac Muscle Electrophysiology

The function, morphology, and proteome of atrial (ACM) vs. ventricular (VCM) CM differ significantly (Brandenburg et al., 2016a). Compared to VCM, the ACM's triangle-shaped action potential and phase-2 plateau are markedly shorter, yet followed by a more gradual phase-3 repolarization and a less negative resting membrane potential (Fatkin et al., 2007). In contrast, intracellular Ca^{2+} release in ACM is highly heterogeneous and is frequently described as a slow inward-propagating U-shaped Ca^{2+} gradient (Thul et al., 2012; Greiser et al., 2014). However, contractile activation of atrial compared to ventricular muscle strips occurs significantly faster (Lüss et al., 1999). This results in a conceptual paradox: how is atrial excitation and contraction rapidly coupled, if cell-wide Ca^{2+} release is 1–2 orders of magnitude slower in ACM compared to VCM (Thul et al., 2012; Greiser et al., 2014)? The case study described below demonstrates the use of super-resolution techniques to investigate the details of sub-micron structures in cardiac cells.

In rodent ACM typically no or only few residual T-tubules are reported (Kirk et al., 2003). In contrast, VCM are characterized by a high density of T-tubules, where each may rapidly propagate electrical signals (see also section 2.4). To combine cell isolation with high-resolution imaging workflows for ACM, fluorescent dyes that selectively intercalate in the extracellular membrane leaflet are highly attractive to assess the local membrane structure and integrity (Wagner et al., 2014; Brandenburg et al., 2018). Surprisingly, when implementing stringent cell quality and confocal imaging workflows, 100% of ACM isolated from mouse hearts were shown to exhibit a unique cell-wide transverse-axial-tubule (TAT) membrane network (**Figure 2A**, left) (Brandenburg et al., 2016b). Importantly, analysis of the TAT components revealed that axially oriented A-tubules dominate the ACM membrane network, whereas T-tubules are far less abundant (**Figure 2A**, right).

Interestingly, confocal imaging failed to locally resolve di-8-ANEPPS stained A-tubule cross-sections, whereas STimulated Emission Depletion (STED) superresolution nanoscopy improved local contrast sufficiently to determine the width (δ)

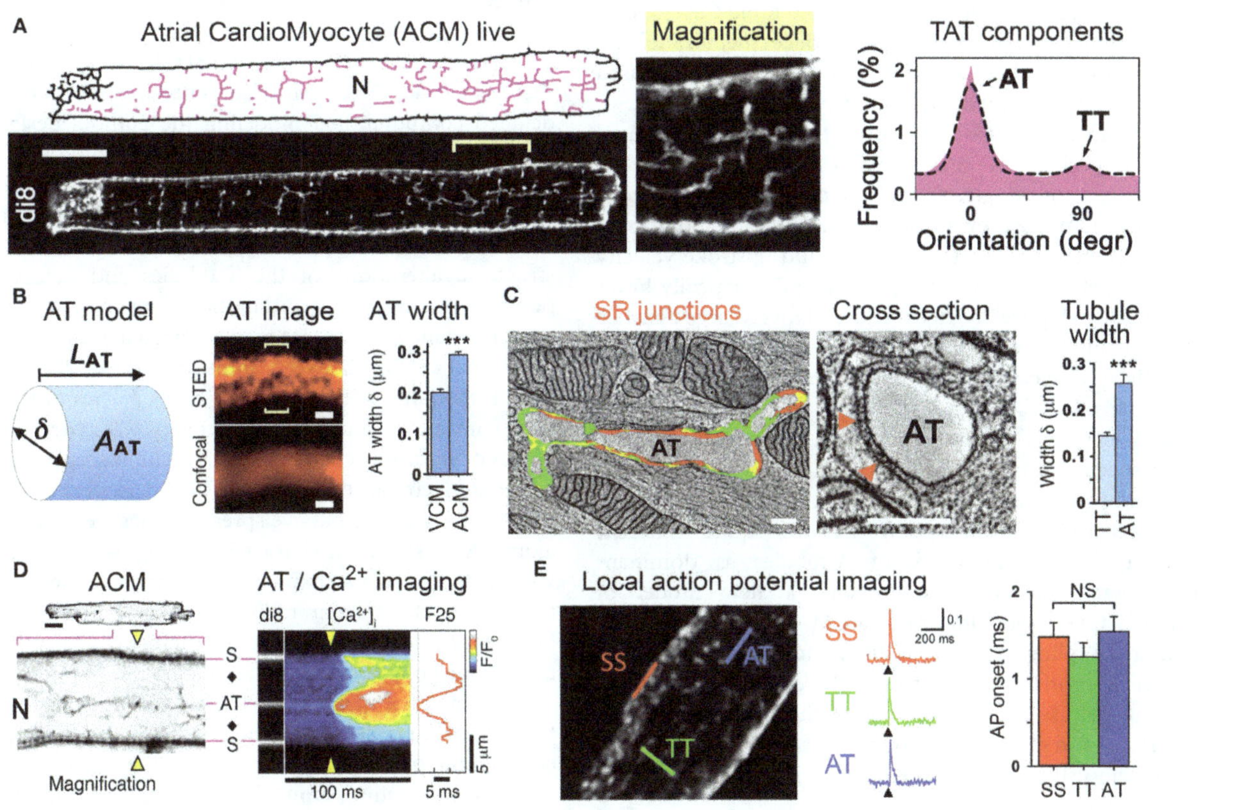

FIGURE 2 | A-tubules provide Ca^{2+} signaling super-hubs for atrial excitation-contraction coupling. **(A)** Confocal live imaging of di-8-ANEPPS stained (di8) TAT structures visualized as skeleton (pink). N, nucleus. Scale bar 10 µm. Histogram showing the TAT component orientations and Gaussian fit. Abundant AT (0°) vs. sparse TT (90°) components. **(B)** Cartoon of a cylindrical AT model. AT width (δ) measurements were used to estimate the surface area (AAT); LAT, AT component length. AT width was determined from optical cross sections (brackets) using the local STED signal distribution and compared between VCM vs. ACM as bar graph. Scales 200 nm. **(C)** Electron tomography images and segmentation of a longitudinally sectioned and a cross-sectioned AT structure. Scales 200 nm. Red color indicating AT-SR junctions ≤ 15 nm in gap width containing RyR2 densities. Red triangles mark two exemplary electron densities compatible with RyR2 channels. **(D)** Confocal negative contrast visualization of intracellular AT structures and transversal line scanning (yellow triangles) of intracellular Ca^{2+} imaging (fluo-4). A field potential-evoked Ca^{2+} transient is activated at AT and subsurface (S) structures; black diamonds, off-membrane cytosolic sites; F25, Ca^{2+} signal onset at 25% signal amplitude; $\Delta F/F_0$, normalized fluorescence intensity ratio as indicated by look-up-table; N, nucleus. **(E)** Two-photon action potential recordings from specific TAT components labeled with the voltage-sensitive dye di-4-ANE(F)PTEA (2 µM). Normalized fluorescence traces ($\Delta F/F_0$) were recorded from the scan regions indicated by color. At AT, TT, and SS membranes structures the simultaneous action potential activation upon pacing (black arrowheads) is apparent. Grouped bar graph showing no significant difference for action potential onset (the time interval between the end of the stimulus and the rise of the fluorescence signal above a threshold of 4% $\Delta F/F_0$. AT, A-tubule; TT, T-tubule; SS, subsurface membrane site. NS, not significant. Adapted from Brandenburg et al. (2016b).

of intact A-tubules in living ACM (**Figure 2B**). On average, the A-tubule width was significantly larger in ACM compared to VCM (**Figure 2B**) (Brandenburg et al., 2016b), suggesting that A-tubules exhibit a much larger cytosolic membrane surface area (AAT). Indeed, electron tomography of high-pressure frozen ACM showed that A-tubules exist as large cylindrical membrane structures that form extensive SR junctions densely filled with RyR2 Ca^{2+} release channels (**Figure 2C**, left) (Brandenburg et al., 2016b). Finally, quantitative analysis confirmed that A-tubules exhibit approximately 100 nm larger diameters than T-tubules in ACM (**Figure 2C**, right).

Using immunostaining of ACM, voltage-dependent L-type Ca^{2+} channels were identified in A-tubules: Cav1.2 clusters were shown to occur at a higher density in A-tubules compared to T-tubules (Brandenburg et al., 2016b), and additionally Cav1.3 clusters were localized in A-tubules (Brandenburg et al., 2018). Consistent with abundant L-type Ca^{2+} channel clusters in A-tubules, intracellular Ca^{2+} imaging combined with di-8-ANEPPS staining showed field pacing-evoked rapid Ca^{2+} release gradients around A-tubules, whereas surface membrane and particularly cytosolic sites each showed a significantly increased Ca^{2+} release latency (**Figure 2D**) (Brandenburg et al., 2016b).

Finally, RAMP was used for local *in situ* action potential recording at specific TAT sites in living ACM (**Figure 2E**, left and section 2.4). Strikingly, action potentials recorded locally at A-tubules, T-tubules, or subsurface sites showed the same rapid onset (**Figure 2E**, right), amplitude and upstroke velocity (Brandenburg et al., 2016b). Thus, despite a dramatically lower T-tubule density (**Figure 2A**, right) and a relatively large distance from the cell surface, voluminous A-tubules appear to function very effectively as electrical conduits for rapid action potential spread deep inside ACM.

While the physiological and clinical relevance of these new atria-specific A-tubule findings is still emerging, several important implications are obvious: (1) ACM express a cell-specific electrically excitable TAT network quite different from VCM; (2) the discovery of A-tubules as dominant excitable membrane conduits provides a new model of "super-hub" Ca^{2+} signaling and ACM-specific excitation-contraction coupling; (3) in addition to Cav1.3 channels thousands of proteins are differentially expressed in ACM (Brandenburg et al., 2016a), yet none of the clinically relevant ion channels and G-Protein coupled receptors have been mechanistically established in the context of A-tubule membrane organelles so far.

As functional L-type Ca^{2+} channel changes represent a disease mechanism of atrial fibrillation, major future questions are how Cav1.2 and Cav1.3 clusters are organized locally and relatively to RyR2 channel Ca^{2+} release sites, and which specific voltage-dependent roles the atrial L-type Ca^{2+} channel isoforms exert in A-tubules. Interestingly, while the Cav1.2 interacting protein junctophilin-2 is expressed five-fold less in the atria compared to the ventricles, it is highly abundant inside sarcoplasmic reticulum (SR) junctions along A-tubules (Brandenburg et al., 2019). Thus, non-invasive superresolution optical methods are not only essential for establishing differential Cav1.2 and Cav1.3 functions in ACM, but they will be instrumental for identifying early disease-causative mechanisms of atrial cardiomyopathy preceding atrial fibrillation and stroke (Goette et al., 2016).

Fluorescence Recovery After Photobleaching to Probe Structure and Function of the T-Tubular System

The optical technique of fluorescence recovery after photobleaching (FRAP) microscopy is a useful method for examining the diffusion of probes within limited structures within the cell (Bers and Shannon, 2013). In relation to examining the diffusion within the TAT structure, FRAP has been used to demonstrate marked species differences in the tortuously and therefore lumenal diffusion of solutes within these membrane structures (Kong et al., 2018). In this study the authors used FRAP microscopy to probe the diffusion properties of TAT: fluorescent dextran within the TAT system lumen was photo bleached and signal recovery by diffusion of unbleached dextran from the extracellular space was monitored. Remarkable is how an optical-based imaging approach can support or implement structural data hitherto achievable only with 3D electron tomography (Rog-Zielinska et al., 2018). More in general, combining FRAP with detailed computational modeling the authors designed a new pathway to understanding how TAT remodeling may contribute to altered cellular function. In this respect, the combination of FRAP with optical voltage measurements from TAT membranes has also offered the opportunity to study the relationship between structural alterations of the T-tubules and defects of action potential propagation found in the failing heart.

For instance, in a recent study, Scardigli et al. (2017) exploited the formal analogy between diffusion and electrical conductivity to link the latter with the diffusion properties of the TAT. The time constant of fluorescence recovery was correlated with the apparent diffusion coefficient of the fluorescent molecules and linked to electrical conductivity. These data were used to evaluate the efficiency of the passive spread of membrane depolarization along TAT system. The characteristic length constant of T-tubules was calculated as approximately 300 μm: an order of magnitude larger than the cellular radius, indicating a remarkable safety factor of the normal TAT system structure in passively conveying membrane potential changes across the cell.

Further refinement of the FRAP technique was then employed to address the role of the mechanical activity associated with contraction in the cardiac cell with the enhanced movement of solutes including ions through the tortuous TAT system driven by advection-assisted diffusion (Rog-Zielinska et al., 2021). This phenomena is thought to offset the accumulation of solutes within the TAT system as a result of changes in heart rate (Rog-Zielinska et al., 2021). This novel finding provides another potential mechanism for dysfunction, namely the reduced capacity for solute exchange that may result from a remodeled TAT system in failing hearts.

Light-Sheet Microscopy for Mesoscale Structural Imaging

Taking correlative work to another order of magnitude, extremely challenging current experiments aim to dissect morpho-functional relationships between cellular organization and functional abnormalities at the whole organ level. At the tissue level, current studies generally associate structural alterations with the corresponding electromechanical dysfunction without showing real cause-effect relations. What is missing is a direct link between the functional study and quantification of tissue disorganization performed on the same tissue. The main limitation is the inefficacy of standard imaging methods and staining approaches in performing high resolution imaging (cellular or sub-cellular resolution) in tissue. During the past years, different methods have been developed for clearing fixed tissue. Most of them, however, present several limitations such as tissue shrinkage, structural alteration, fluorescence quenching and incompatibility with immunostaining (Silvestri et al., 2016). The challenge of producing large, transparent and fluorescently-labeled volumes has been overcome recently by applying a tissue transformation approach, CLARITY, and it's related derivatives (Chung et al., 2013; Pianca et al., 2019; Olianti et al., 2020, 2021). These methods allow high transparency, immunolabeling and structural and molecular preservation. One drawback with the current techniques is the poor penetration rates of the tissue by antibodies, to the extent that many months of incubation are sometimes required depending on tissue dimensions.

Clearing methods render biological tissue transparent by equilibrating the refractive index throughout a sample to reduce inhomogeneities in light scatterers (Richardson and Lichtman, 2015). Different approaches have been proposed based on organic solvents, high-refractive index aqueous solutions, hyperhydrating solutions and tissue transformation (Silvestri et al., 2016). Most notable amongst the latter approaches, CLARITY (Chung et al., 2013) employs hydrogel embedding of the sample by perfusing tissue with a fixative, a temperature-sensitive crosslinker and the hydrogel monomer which forms covalent links with native proteins. After fixation, the tissue of interest is warmed to induce cross-linking of the monomers into a nanoporous hydrogel mesh. Lipids are then removed from the sample with a detergent solution either passively, or actively through electrophoresis. The lipid-free samples are then incubated in refractive index matching solutions for clearing. This method in combination with advanced imaging techniques such as light-sheet or two-photon microscopy (see **Box 2**) allows 3D reconstruction of substantial heart tissues at high resolution.

Light-sheet microscopy, originally described in 1903 (Siedentopf and Zsigmondy, 1903) and re-invigorated in the early 2000s (Huisken et al., 2004), achieves optical sectioning over the entire field of view by selectively illuminating a thin slice of tissue with a sheet of light which is positioned to coincide with the focal plane of a perpendicularly placed microscope objective for fluorescence detection. In contrast to point-scanning epi-illumination methods like confocal or TPM, this uncoupled illumination—detection scheme has two major advantages. Firstly, the detection scheme is essentially that of a wide-field microscope and hence affords much faster acquisition rates through the registration of multiple points in parallel rather than sequentially. Secondly, the selective illumination greatly reduces unnecessary photoactivation and bleaching of fluorophores above and below the focal plane. However, this very same uncoupling of excitation and detection makes light-sheet microscopy particularly sensitive to tissue scattering and the technique thus requires samples that are either intrinsically transparent (e.g., Zebrafish larvae) or else an opaque tissue that has been made transparent through tissue clearing. If tissue is intrinsically transparent, it is possible to combine structural observations in live tissue, even over extended periods of time (for example to track every single cardiac cell during early ontogenetic development in the Zebrafish heart) with functional Ca^{2+} imaging (Weber et al., 2017; Taylor et al., 2019).

This mesoscopic imaging may help to elucidate the role of cellular organization in cardiac electro-mechanical (dys)function and pave the way for a unifying approach which integrates functional and structural data. Such an experimental model would enable a comprehensive investigation of the morphological changes that lead to electrical and mechanical alterations after disease-associated structural remodeling.

THE USE OF LIGHT TO MANIPULATE AND MEASURE CARDIAC ELECTROPHYSIOLOGY

Extending the application of optical techniques in cardiac applications, optogenetics has added the capability to manipulate cardiac function by light (see review Entcheva and Kay, 2021). Optogenetics combines targeted light stimulation and the genetic expression of light-sensitive ion channels or pumps to enable cell-specific, non-contact stimulation with sub-millisecond temporal and micrometer spatial resolution. The characterization of the non-selective cation channel Channelrhodopsin2 (ChR2) in the early 2000s (Nagel et al., 2002) initiated the explosive growth of field of optogenetics. Compared to electrical stimulation, in excitable cells expressing ChR2, pulsed illumination induces inward currents which not only trigger excitation but can also precisely modify the shape of action potentials (Park et al., 2014; Williams and Entcheva, 2015). Light responsive Cl^- and H^+ pumps, as well as K^+ and Cl^- ion channels allow light-induced hyperpolarization of cardiac tissue. Direct optogenetic hyperpolarization with patterned light has been used to provide mechanistic information about circuits involved in cardiac pacemaking (Arrenberg et al., 2010), or to affect cardiac arrhythmias by selective expression in sympathetic neurons in a canine model of post-ischemic electrophysiological remodeling (Yu et al., 2017). The ability to bi-directionally manipulate cardiac function (to excite and to inhibit) using light, and the possibility to combine these newer optical tools with optical mapping have afforded new means to address mechanistic and translational questions related to cardiac arrhythmias (Entcheva and Bub, 2016).

Optogenetic Cardioversion/Defibrillation: Progress and Challenges

Beyond optogenetic pacing demonstrated in early cardiac studies (Arrenberg et al., 2010; Bruegmann et al., 2010;

Jia et al., 2011), proof-of-concept studies for optogenetic cardioversion/defibrillation have been shown in transgenic mice and wild type mice and rats after AAV-mediated expression of ChR2 (Bruegmann et al., 2016, 2018; Crocini et al., 2016a; Nyns et al., 2016). The light parameters (light intensity, pulse duration, etc.) required for successful termination have been determined using many different approaches for illumination (optical fiber/global LED, DMD, and μLED) and computational modeling. Using this range of techniques, different excitation patterns are possible, opening the way for the investigation of a range of defibrillation approaches including: (i) targeted pacing to fill the excitable gap or (ii) continuous illumination for prolonged phases of depolarization with the aim of a complete conduction block. Interestingly, conduction block seemed to be more effective but required higher light intensities compared to targeted pacing when illumination was performed randomly without analysis of the underlying arrhythmia pattern (Bruegmann et al., 2018). However, knowing the underlying reentry wavefronts including the spatial extent of excitation gaps or global illumination of the whole ventricular surface might enable a reduction in the light intensity requirements (Crocini et al., 2016a). For targeted pacing, feedback loops between sensing electrodes or optical mapping and light stimulation have been developed which permit testing numerical hypotheses for more effective, gentle cardioversion/ defibrillation (Hussaini et al., 2021). The translation to larger animals including humans has been investigated using, *in silico* modeling. This work indicates that in principle, the optogenetic route is feasible and suggests defibrillation mechanisms distinct from that achieved by conventional chest paddles (Bruegmann et al., 2016; Hussaini et al., 2021). However, there are considerable technical issues to overcome including: (i) the need for gene transfer, (ii) the expression of non-mammalian opsins in humans and (iii) implantation of light sources. Nevertheless, the gain would be pain-free, tissue-sparing and efficient arrhythmia termination in the clinic.

Real-Time Manipulation of Cardiac Electrical Activity in a Closed-Loop System

All-optical cardiac electrophysiology is a powerful contactless interrogation and manipulation technique (Entcheva and Bub, 2016; Scardigli et al., 2018b). A recent example of the capability of optical voltage reporters combined with optogenetic actuators at the whole heart level is the development of a wide-field mesoscope to simultaneously optically map and manipulate action potential propagation in whole mouse hearts (Scardigli et al., 2018b) (**Figure 3A**). A computer-controlled digital micromirror device (DMD, see **Box 3**) capable of drawing arbitrarily-chosen illumination patterns was used to create precise spatial and temporal patterns of optogenetic stimulation on the epicardial surface of isolated hearts (**Figure 3B**). Operating in closed-loop with a feedback-control strategy, this system can react in real-time to ongoing electrophysiology as revealed by optical mapping, opening the prospect for real-time resynchronization therapy and cardiac defibrillation. These techniques can serve as a "biological stimulator" (for example by optical stimulation of ChR2), or as a "biological inhibitor" (when using optically-activated K^+ flux systems) to inform new *in vivo* strategies for controlling arrhythmias. Such a system is an ideal test-bed to investigate strategies to defibrillate or interrupt tachyarrhythmias using the minimal power and area of illumination with a view to advancing our knowledge of the electrophysiology of arrhythmias that may be translatable to the clinics.

Wave Control to Improve Arrhythmia Management and Termination

Present-day electronic cardiac devices include cardiac pacemakers (to maintain normal rhythm) and cardioverter-defibrillators to terminate arrhythmias and restore normal rhythm. With newer optical technologies, including optogenetic modulation of cardiac function, conceptually new strategies for control have been proposed that are not possible with classic

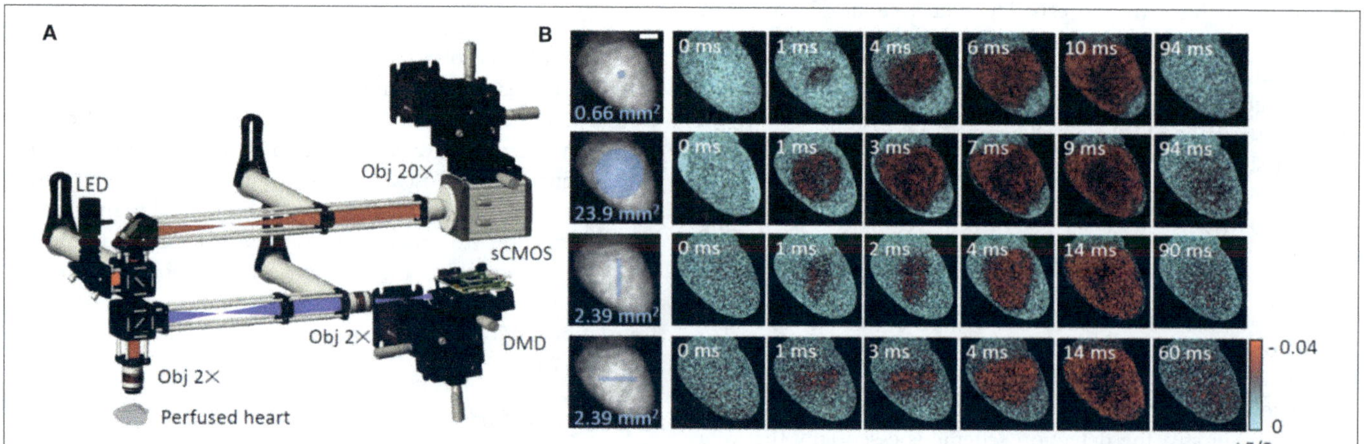

FIGURE 3 | (A) Optical setup for real-time closed-loop optogenetic stimulation with a digital micromirror device (DMD) in response to ongoing cardiac activity, simultaneously optically mapped with a sCMOS camera. **(B)** Exemplary customizable stimulation pattern and cardiac excitation wavefronts. Modified from Scardigli et al. (2018b).

BOX 3 | Digital Micromirror Devices

A digital micromirror device, or DMD, is a micro-opto-electromechanical system comprised of millions of microscopically small moving mirrors to create a video display of the type now found in digital projectors. The mirrors on the DMD are arranged on a μm diamond pixel geometry and by applying a tilt angle of ±12°, each micro-mirror can be switched on or off individually. A high numerical aperture relay system can be used to project the DMD pattern onto the sample. DMDs have been employed for controlling cardiac activity at fine spatial and temporal scales using light in cultured cardiac monolayers and whole-heart preparations. These light projectors offer sub-millisecond temporal resolution and have been used to demonstrate fine control of tissue functional properties, including wave velocity (Burton et al., 2015), or to embed high temporal resolution "small" images into larger but more slowly acquired still image sequences (temporal pixel multiplexing, Bub et al., 2010).

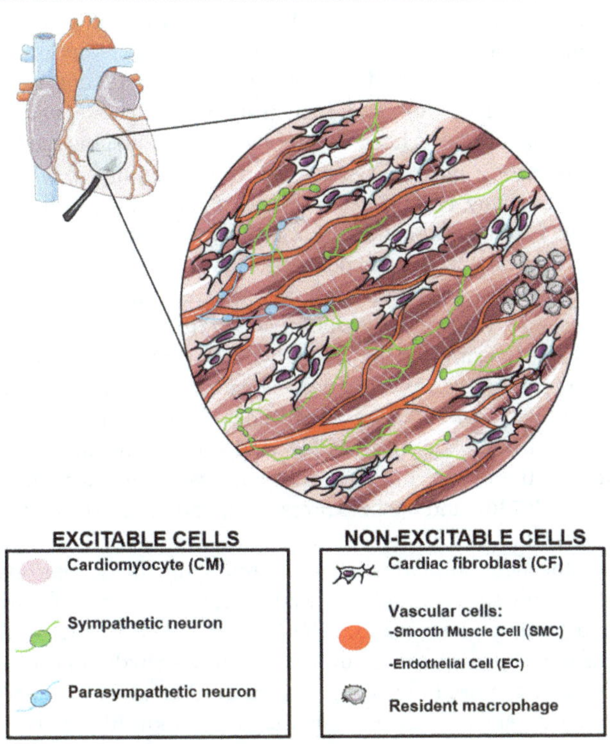

FIGURE 4 | The heart is a multicellular network of excitable and non-excitable cells, which have been targeted with various opsins for optogenetic investigation. Modified from Zaglia et al. (2019).

electrical means. Using optogenetic actuation and dye-free optical mapping, it was demonstrated that the direction, speed and chirality of cardiac excitation waves can be modulated by light (Burton et al., 2015). To achieve this, a quasi-real time feedback was applied with dynamically-modulated light patterns using a DMD. Space-time varying illumination enables "wave steering" (Entcheva and Bub, 2016) and can bring insights for finer arrhythmia control in the clinic with lower-energy approaches and devices. Until recently, the only options for wave control have been pharmacological (adding exogenous compounds that alter cardiac channel function) or electrical (using an electrode or an array of electrodes to stimulate the tissue). These approaches have limitations as they either change wave properties in the entire tissue or at a limited number of locations due to physical limits on the density and number of electrodes in an electrode array. All-optical electrophysiology offers the ability to deliver dynamic space-time patterns of light for stimulation/suppression, and the possibility for real-time feedback control of macroscopic emergent properties, i.e., cardiac waves of excitation. Wave control goes beyond the simple initiation and termination of excitation waves (pacing and defibrillation/cardioversion) and the associated frequency modulation. Instead, using all-optical means, one can focus on manipulation of the macroscopic (emergent) properties. Recent examples include termination of arrhythmias through re-entrant wave drift induced by longer low-light pulses (Hussaini et al., 2021). While high spatial and temporal resolution optogenetic manipulation in the intact heart *in vivo* is still not feasible, optogenetic tools yield, for the first time, an experimental platform to rapidly test anti-arrhythmic strategies in *ex-vivo* preparations. This offers the flexibility to manipulate the electrophysiological variables within the heart hitherto only possible in computational models.

Cell Specific Optogenetics to Interrogate the Myocardial Network

Different from conventional electrophysiological approaches, optogenetics, by its nature, is cell type specific, as sensitivity to photostimulation or optical reporting of function are achieved by transgene expression. This feature was immediately exploited in neuroscience, as it enabled the functional dissection of neuronal circuits in the multiplexed network forming the central nervous system. An emerging concept of the heart as an interconnected multicellular system is a prerequisite to formulate the appropriate physiological questions optogenetics can answer (**Figure 4**). Heart function is based on the anatomical and functional interaction between excitable (i.e., working and conducting CM), non-excitable conductive [e.g., cardiac fibroblasts (Quinn et al., 2016) and macrophages (Hulsmans et al., 2017)], and extrinsic excitable (i.e., cardiac autonomic neurons) cells, and non-excitable modulators (i.e., endothelial and smooth muscle cells) (Zaglia et al., 2019). Cell-specific optogenetic stimulation within intact heart has first been demonstrated in a proof-of-principle study by Bruegmann and colleagues (Bruegmann et al., 2010), and subsequently this approach was used to infer the contribution of working and conducting CM to arrhythmias in the normal and ischemic myocardium. While alterations in the Purkinje Fiber (PF) network, including both PF cell dysfunction and PF coupling to the working CM have been suggested in several acquired or genetic cardiovascular diseases, assessment of PF function is only indirect and non-specific with conventional electrophysiological techniques. Cardiac optogenetics has allowed direct investigation of the source-sink relation in the conduction system vs. working myocardium, and by combining it with a 3D morphological study of the PF network, to determine that the high arrhythmogenicity of the right ventricular outflow tract depends on the peculiar displacement of the terminal PF network (Zaglia et al., 2015).

Another excitable cell population, critical for regulating cardiac function, is represented by autonomic neurons, which densely innervate the myocardium, including extracardiac sympathetic and parasympathetic neurones and a dense network of cardiac ganglia (Julian et al., 2021), influencing potentially all cardiac cell types (Franzoso et al., 2016). It is increasingly evident that neuronal remodeling (i.e., changes in distribution and function of cardiac innervation) takes place upon physiological (e.g., exercise, pregnancy, aging) and pathological (e.g., ischemic damage, heart failure) conditions. *In vivo* assessment of cardiac autonomic neuron function is technically challenging and non-selective. Several groups have used optogenetics to achieve control of cardiac sympathetic (Wengrowski et al., 2015; Yu et al., 2017; Prando et al., 2018; Burton et al., 2020) or parasympathetic (Moreno et al., 2019; Rajendran et al., 2019) neurons, to assess their effects on heart function, to study the biophysics of neuro-cardiac communication and to prevent sympathetic neurons from triggering arrhythmias in post-ischemic electrophysiological remodeling.

Furthermore, in addition to the studies of excitable cells, the method has recently been used in approaches to investigate non-myocyte cell populations. Non-CM cells in the myocardium are mostly inexcitable, and they have classically been relegated to forming the cardiac vascular bed (i.e., endothelial cells, smooth muscle cells) or regulating the extracellular compartment (e.g., fibroblasts). Rapidly accruing evidence has shown that these cell types play additional roles in paracrine and endocrine signaling, and may influence cardiac activity. In addition, some 25 years ago, it had been suggested that cardiac fibroblasts may potentially couple to CM via connexins, affecting cardiac electrophysiology (Kohl et al., 1994). This hypothesis was eventually confirmed in native tissue, using optogenetic expression of GEVI in cardiac non-myocytes (Quinn et al., 2016). Furthermore, expression of Channelrhodpsin-2 (ChR2) or Archaerhodopsin (ArchT) was achieved in primary cardiac fibroblasts, and heterocellular coupling with CM was further investigated (Yu and Entcheva, 2016; Funken et al., 2020; Simone et al., 2020; Boyle et al., 2021; Kostecki et al., 2021). ChR2 expression in smooth muscle cells of the coronary vessels has shown to be a potent tool to control vascular tone, demonstrating local and rapidly induced light-activated vasospasm (Wu et al., 2015). In parallel, selective expression of ChR2 in endothelial cells has shown that modulation of endothelial cell membrane potential can also trigger local vasospasm (Zhang et al., 2015), suggesting heterocellular coupling between the two important cellular components of the vessel wall. Optogenetics was exploited to study the biology of resident heart macrophages, which were shown to electrically communicate via connexins with atrio-ventricular node cells and to influence conduction (Hulsmans et al., 2017). Thus optogenetics revealed novel functions, especially related to heterocellular coupling, of smooth muscle cells, endothelial cells and macrophages.

Long term cardiac studies or experiments in conscious, freely moving animals are technically more demanding than in brain research, due to obvious differences in anatomical constraints. In particular, continuous movement of the heart hampers the stable implantation of light-emitting devices (for example, optrodes which have been developed for deep brain stimulation have limited use in the heart) (sta, 0000). These limitations can be overcome by progress in bioengineering aimed at the development of biocompatible and flexible light emitting tools to be positioned on the epicardial surface or around cardiac neurons (Gutruf et al., 2019). Collaboration with medical physicists would also allow simultaneous optogenetic stimulation of CM or cardiac neurons with the assessment of cardiac function by echocardiography or other imaging methods such as cardiac magnetic resonance. Another limitation, which will presumably be resolved in the next few years, is that, up to now, cardiac optogenetics has mainly been used in rodents, while very little has been performed in bigger animal models (e.g., pigs, sheep), which may be more informative for their closeness to human electrophysiology. In general terms, the clinical or experimental applicability in humans is not immediate, as it requires expression of an exogenous gene in the heart, and implantation of a light emitting source. Rapid progress in molecular biology has yielded viral vectors encoding opsins suited to the use in humans (FDA-approved, ClinicalTrials.gov NCT02556736), and opsin expression in patient hearts may thus be foreseen.

Optogenetic inhibition of autonomic sympathetic neurons is theoretically suited to ablate the adrenergic component favoring or sustaining arrhythmias. The further development of this concept will presumably be utilized to study arrhythmogenesis in genetic or acquired cardiovascular diseases in which adrenergic stress has a key role (catecholaminergic polymorphic ventricular tachycardia, arrhythmogenic cardiomyopathy, Takotsubo cardiomyopathy). While several opsin variants with specific advantages have been used in neurosciences (sta, 0000), cardiac optogenetics has thus far, exploited almost exclusively ChR2 with some exceptions (Kopton et al., 2018; Sierra et al., 2018). It is to be expected that in the next years many newly developed photoactivatable tools will be used in heart studies. In addition to channel-forming opsins, signaling opsins have been developed for spatially and temporally accurate photo-interrogation of signaling pathways in cells/ *in vivo*.

Proof of concept examples have shown light-modulation of G_q and G_s signaling pathways (Beiert et al., 2014; Makowka et al., 2019). Specifically, optogenetic stimulation of the adrenergic G_s signaling cascade using JellyFish Opsin in cultured CM and in the heart of transgenic animals was shown to have a very high light sensitivity, fast kinetics and high spatial resolution (Makowka et al., 2019). The precise time point of activation by triggered illumination allowed to identify differential downstream kinetics of cAMP/PKA effects on pacemaking (positive chronotropy), sarco/endoplasmic reticulum Ca^{2+}-ATPase activation (positive lusitropy) and Ca^{2+} induced Ca^{2+} release mechanism (positive inotropy). Furthermore, local illumination allowed to identify regions in the heart which are more sensitive to pathological adrenergic effects such as the left atrium, in which arrhythmogenic premature contractions were induced by localized optogenetic G_s stimulation (Makowka et al., 2019). Importantly, in this special issue of Frontiers in Physiology, Cokic et al. show that long wave opsin enables control of the inhibitory G_i signaling pathway in CM using red light (625 nm), which is spectrally compatible with a blue light sensitive (450–550 nm) optogenetic actuators or reporters (Cokic et al., Optogenetic stimulation of G_i signaling enables instantaneous modulation of CM pacemaking, Cokic et al., this issue). Thus, the combination of Jellyfish Opsin with long wave cone Opsin will allow alternating activation of G_s and G_i signaling to study the effect of dysbalanced sympathetic and parasympathetic vegetative nerve input on the heart which may be involved in cardiac pathologies. Using implantable light emitting devices and optogenetic G protein-coupled receptors it will be possible to study acute and chronic effects of G_s, G_i or G_q stimulation on cardiac remodeling and electrophysiology including arrhythmia, hypertrophy or heart failure.

Immediate Translational Application of All-Optical Cardiac Electrophysiology

The pharmaceutical industry and associated regulatory authorities require that all drugs are tested for their cardiotoxic effects before being released for human testing. Early, comprehensive and inexpensive detection of pro-arrhythmic effects based on inhibition of ion channels that control excitability and action potential duration can save the industry considerable costs (Gintant et al., 2019). The CIPA (Comprehensive *In vitro* Pro-arrhythmia Assay) initiative has stimulated the development of newer testing platforms that can provide better predictive value for drug development. The features of an assay required by this sector are: (i) standardized cardiac cells/ tissue and protocols, (ii) scalability and medium-high throughput, i.e., hundreds of assays/ system/ day, and (iii) excellent predictive value relevant to human use. Over the last 10 years commercial sources of human iPSC-CM have become available as a source of standardized human myocardial material. Currently the electrophysiology of monolayer cultures human hiPSC-CM is the most common preparation with electrical activity of the monolayer assessed from an array of monopolar extracellular electrodes (micro-electrode array) embedded into the base of the culture dish. A limitation of these field potentials generated by the intrinsic spontaneous electrical activity of the coupled monolayer of cells is the poor capture of the repolarization dynamics, including action potential duration and shape, which are perceived as some of the most predictive indicators of pro-arrhythmic responses. Alternatively, ion channel responses are tested with planar automated patch clamp systems that offer scalability compared to the traditional gold standard to quantify electrophysiology. Both approaches, used by the pharmaceutical industry, have limitations stemming from the requirement for close contact between the cells and the

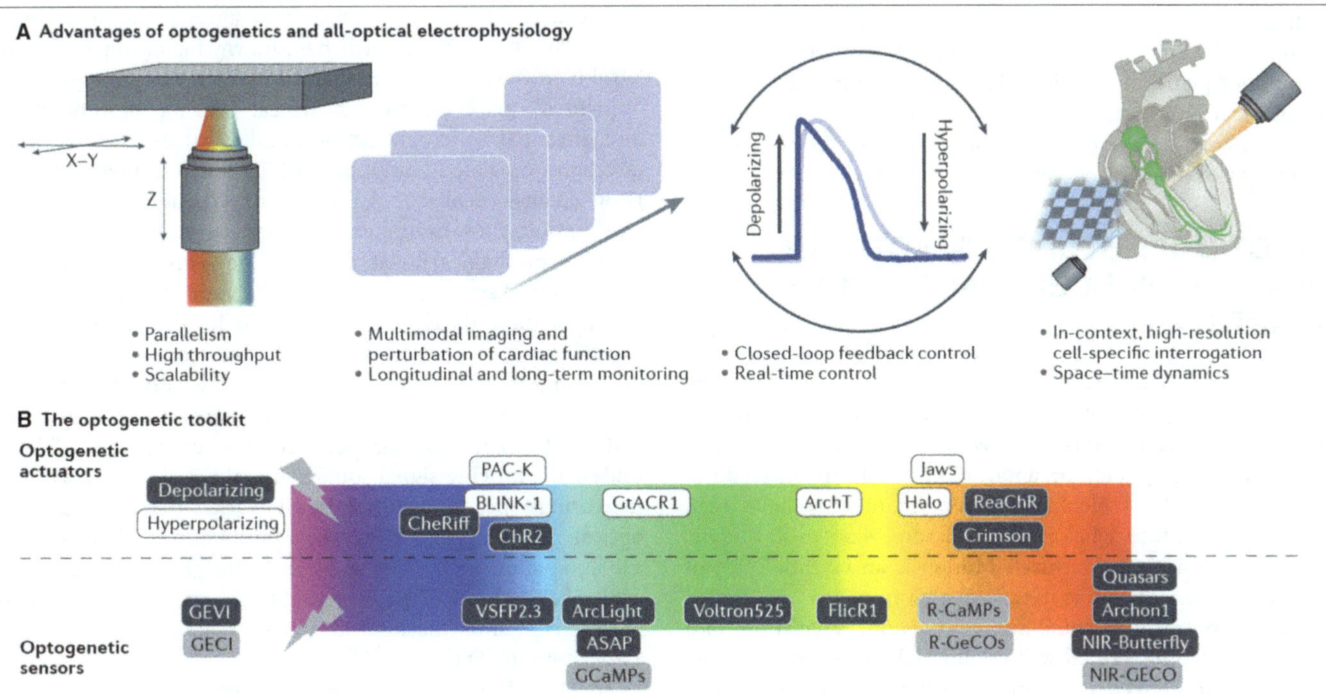

FIGURE 5 | All-optical cardiac electrophysiology and the toolkit of optogenetic actuators and reporters. **(A)** Advantages of all-optical cardiac electrophysiology using optogenetic tools. **(B)** Spectral compatibility of optogenetic actuators and reporters for voltage (GEVI) and calcium (GECI) with the possibility for bi-directional control (depolarization and hyperpolarization) of cardiac excitation. Reproduced with permission from Entcheva and Kay (2021).

electrodes for generating meaningful signals, which makes their use with iPSC-CM somewhat problematic.

Optical technologies for recording and for stimulation offer several advantages to address these challenges. As shown in **Figure 5A**, these advantages include built-in scalability and high-throughput due to: (i) contactless nature, (ii) high-content functional information through multi-modal imaging and control, (iii) longitudinal observations and (iv) the ability for closed-loop control within multicellular context. Optogenetic pacing has been combined with microelectrode array recordings for better control of the frequency (restitution) responses to drugs of human iPSC-CM (Lapp et al., 2017). Voltage-sensitive and calcium-sensitive dyes have been used in commercial pre-clinical assay platforms to quantify pro-arrhythmic responses to drugs (Hortigon-Vinagre et al., 2016; Pfeiffer-Kaushik et al., 2019).

Optogenetics-inspired developments of automated high-throughput platforms for drug testing using all-optical cardiac electrophysiology have been deployed in conjunction with human iPSC-CM (Dempsey et al., 2016; Klimas et al., 2016, 2020; Werley et al., 2017; Credi et al., 2021). These platforms incorporate spectrally-compatible optogenetic actuators with optogenetic and/or optical reporters for voltage and calcium (**Figure 5B**) to provide comprehensive characterization of electromechanical responses to drugs. Some of these systems have already found their way into the industrial setting. The immense information content from such high-throughput platforms, combined with machine learning algorithms can yield new hybrid *in vitro* - *in silico* methods for drug development and for better mechanistic understanding of cardiac arrhythmias. Furthermore, dye-free, completely non-invasive approaches (Ashraf et al., 2021), together with microfluidics-enabled high-throughput platforms (Wei et al., 2020) can allow the chronic longitudinal monitoring of human iPSC-CM. These techniques will facilitate studies on maturation processes, cardiac disease modeling and tissue regeneration.

FUNCTIONAL STUDIES IN ACTIVELY CONTRACTING CELLS AND WHOLE HEARTS

As pointed out before (e.g., section 4.3), imaging of "a moving target" poses significant challenges. In cardiac research, use of mechanical constraints that reduce tissue motion relative to the imaging system, or application of electro-mechanical uncouplers (such as blebbistatin, see section 2.1) have been employed to reduce what is often, if somewhat misleadingly, referred to as a motion artifact. Motion is an essential part of cardiac function, of course. Electrical activation, Ca^{2+}-mediated excitation-contraction coupling, contraction, relaxation and diastolic stretching, are all well-established targets for imaging. They are closely linked, over timescales from near-instantaneous beat-by-beat responses (e.g., stretch-activation of ion channels, Quinn and Kohl, 2021), over metabolic feedback to electro-mechanical function over minutes and hours (e.g., activation of K^+-channels that open in response to a reduction in ATP Van Wagoner and Lamorgese, 1994, on to tissue remodeling over years (e.g., during aging and in disease, Lyon et al., 2020). By restricting motion for the sake of functional observation, we alter the very system we wish to study (Kappadan et al., 2020).

Increasingly, therefore, attempts are being made to image cardiac structure and function while keeping the mechanical environment as close to *in vivo* conditions as possible. For cardiac cells and cultures, this involves tools to stretch single cells (Iribe et al., 2007) or cell cultures (Zhang et al., 2008). These have given rise to otherwise "hidden" physiological responses, such as the discovery of stretch-induced Ca^{2+} release from the sarcoplasmic reticulum (Iribe et al., 2009), or the mechanistic explanation of stretch-induced conduction slowing by surface membrane integration of caveolae (Pfeiffer et al., 2014). Optical voltage mapping in actively contracting Langendorff-perfused hearts, using ratiometry and software motion correction, reveals more physiologically relevant information about the electromechanical and energetic performance of the heart (Kuzmiak-Glancy et al., 2018; Kappadan et al., 2020).

It remains more difficult to take "motion" as an input parameter to ultrastructural research. Electron microscopy, for example, is conducted on fixed samples—so motion as such is excluded. Efforts have been made to control the mechanical state of cells or tissue, prior to fixation, and to use sarcomere length as a qualifier of the mechanical state of CM when exploring ultrastructural cell properties (Kohl et al., 2003). However, chemical tissue fixation is slow compared to beat-by-beat dynamics. This can be addressed by high pressure freezing, where recent commercial systems have built-in optical and electrical stimulation capacity so that CM may be preserved for electron microscopy at predefined states in their mechanical cycle. This type of approach has shown, for example, that the T-tubular system of ventricular CM (see section 2/**Figure 2**) is "squeezed" twice on every heartbeat (during diastolic stretch and during systolic contraction), and that this gives rise to an advection-mediated component of T-tubular content exchange (Rog-Zielinska et al., 2021). Over the next decade this direction of work should allow examination of the cross-talk between cardiac electrics, mechanics, metabolics, (epi-)genetics and structure in a time-resolved spatial manner as part of basic cardiac research.

All of these developments will also benefit from improved algorithms for "motion tracking"—i.e., computational post-processing that allows one to maintain the association between parameters recorded on fixed detectors (from optical mapping systems to echo and magnetic resonance imaging) with the underlying moving signal source (Inagaki et al., 2004). This can increasingly be done in a fiducial marker-free manner, using optical mapping data (Christoph and Luther, 2018), or even a combination of optical and echo data gathering (Christoph et al., 2018). The latter paper superbly illustrates the interrelation of electrical and mechanical waves, highlighting their close association in 3D myocardium.

In the clinical setting, tracking of cardiac motion not only provides important information of the ultimate function of the heart - its ability to pump blood - but it conveys insight into regional differences of activation and relaxation of ventricular myocardium. "Dys-synchrony" is problematic for cardiac function, and mechanical mapping may provide insight into spatial heterogeneities, even of underlying electrical properties. In long QT syndrome, for example, disease diagnosis can be improved if mechanical properties are tracked (Lang et al., 2016). The benefit here is that it is comparatively straightforward to track motion non-invasively in 3D, and certainly easier to do so than to track electrical activity in 3D within the whole heart. A remaining caveat is that structural imaging to discern motion only offers direct insight into strain amplitudes and dynamics: thus far, there is no non-invasive technique to measure stress within the myocardium. In basic science, fluorescent reporters of stress are being developed (Meng et al., 2008; Grashoff et al., 2010; Meng and Sachs, 2012) which may pave the way toward—at least experimentally—tracking of both strain and stress in the heart. Metabolic optical imaging using native tissue fluorophores, e.g., NADH, is yet another clinically-translatable optical approach to quantifying cardiac function in health and disease with high spatial resolution (Wengrowski et al., 2014).

An exciting current development in dynamic cardiac 3D imaging is photoacoustic (or optoacoustic) imaging (Lin et al., 2018; Karlas et al., 2019). This uses a pulsed laser to deliver light into tissue. There, photons interact with suitable reporters, causing their transient thermoelastic expansion. The ultrasonic waves generated by this can be detected using ultrasonic transducers and analyzed to produce images of structure and function. Reporters can be native molecules, such as hemoglobin (whose photo-acoustic signature changes with oxygenation—for example allowing one to detect cancer in patients, Zalev et al., 2019), transgenically expressed probes such as GCaMP in experimental animals (Gottschalk et al., 2019), or dyes such as indocyanine green (Deán-Ben et al., 2015). The latter approach has been used for tomographic imaging of the beating, isolated mouse heart *in situ*. If this technique could be used in combination with recently developed photoacoustic voltage-sensitive dyes that allow one to "listen to voltage" (Zhang et al., 2017). This would represent a break-through for measuring transmural electro-mechanical dynamics in the heart.

CONCLUSIONS

This article highlights recent developments in the technical areas of optical voltage measurements and optogenetic applications to cardiac electrophysiology. While similar techniques are being developed in neuroscience, cardiac tissue presents a series of additional challenges related to the highly scattering nature of the myocardium and movement associated with contraction. In the past, progress in electrophysiology has relied on developments in physics and engineering. This article describes some of the fundamentals of physics that underlie optical techniques used to measure and manipulate the electrical activity of the heart. The prospect of translation of these research techniques to the clinic is also discussed as is their recent use in the industrial setting of toxicology screening for adverse effects on cardiac electrophysiology. In all of these situations, the use of optical tools to measure and manipulate cardiac electrophysiology is a rapidly advancing topic that promises to yield new insights and techniques to address the treatment of cardiac arrhythmias.

AUTHOR CONTRIBUTIONS

MCM, PK, LS, and GS planned the content. MCM and GS organized the writing. AK edited the initial submission. All authors contributed to the article and approved the submitted version.

ACKNOWLEDGMENTS

MCM acknowledges a Marie Sklodowska-Curie fellowship (MSCA-IF-EF-ST Grant Agreement No. 842893). AK was supported by the British Heart Foundation through project Grant PG/17/12/32847. EE acknowledges NIH Grant R01-HL144157 and NSF Grant EFMA 1830941. PK and LS are members of the German Centre of Research Excellence SFB1425 (DFG #422681845). SEL was supported by Deutsche Forschungsgemeinschaft through SFB1190 (project P03), and under Germanys Excellence Strategy 793 (EXC2067/1-390729940). SEL is an investigator of DZHK (German Centre for Cardiovascular Research). TZ acknowledges STARS-SKoOP (UNIPD). The authors would like to thank Dr. Remi Peyronnet, Dr. Eva Rog-Zielinska, Dr. Franziska Schneider-Warme, Dr. Viviane Timmermann, and Dr. Callum Zgierski-Johnston from the Institute for Experimental Cardiovascular Medicine, University of Freiburg for their critical reading of and editorial comments on a revised form of this manuscript.

REFERENCES

Optogenetics at Stanford. Available online at: https://web.stanford.edu/group/dlab/optogenetics (accessed March 11, 2020).

Abdelfattah, A. S., Kawashima, T., Singh, A., Novak, O., Liu, H., Shuai, Y., et al. (2019). Bright and photostable chemigenetic indicators for extended *in vivo* voltage imaging. *Science* 365, 699–704. doi: 10.1126/science.aav6416

Acker, C. D., Yan, P., and Loew, L. M. (2011). Single-voxel recording of voltage transients in dendritic spines. *Biophys. J.* 101, L11–L13. doi: 10.1016/j.bpj.2011.06.021

Acker, C. D., Yan, P., and Loew, L. M. (2020). Recent progress in optical voltage-sensor technology and applications to cardiac research: from single cells to whole hearts. *Prog. Biophys. Mol. Biol.* 154, 3–10. doi: 10.1016/j.pbiomolbio.2019.07.004

Akturk, S., Gu, X., Kimmel, M., and Trebino, R. (2006). Extremely simple single-prism ultrashort-pulse compressor. *Optics Express* 14, 10101–10108. doi: 10.1364/OE.14.010101

Alfred Millett-Sikking, N. H., Thayer, A. B., and York, A. G. (2018). *Remote Refocus Enables Class-Leading Spatiotemporal Resolution in 4D optical Microscopy*. Github.

Arrenberg, A., Stainier, D., Baier, H., and Huisken, J. (2010). Optogenetic control of cardiac function. *Science* 330, 971–974. doi: 10.1126/science.1195929

Ashraf, M., Mohanan, S., Sim, B., Tam, A., Rahemipour, K., Brousseau, D., et al. (2021). Random access parallel microscopy. *eLife* 10:e56426. doi: 10.7554/eLife.56426

Bachtel, A. D., Gray, R. A., Stohlman, J. M., Bourgeois, E. B., Pollard, A. E., and Rogers, J. M. (2011). A novel approach to dual excitation ratiometric optical mapping of cardiac action potentials with di-4-ANEPPS using pulsed led excitation. *IEEE Trans. Biomed. Eng.* 58, 2120–2126. doi: 10.1109/TBME.2011.2148719

Beiert, T., Bruegmann, T., and Sasse, P. (2014). Optogenetic activation of GQ signalling modulates pacemaker activity of cardiomyocytes. *Cardiovasc. Res.* 102, 507–516. doi: 10.1093/cvr/cvu046

Bergmann, O., Bhardwaj, R. D., Bernard, S., Zdunek, S., Barnabé-Heider, F., Walsh, S., et al. (2009). Evidence for cardiomyocyte renewal in humans. *Science* 324, 98–102. doi: 10.1126/science.1164680

Bers, D. M., and Shannon, T. R. (2013). Calcium movements inside the sarcoplasmic reticulum of cardiac myocytes. *J. Mol. Cell. Cardiol.* 58, 59–66. doi: 10.1016/j.yjmcc.2013.01.002

Botcherby, E. J., Corbett, A., Burton, R. A., Smith, C. W., Bollensdorff, C., Booth, M. J., et al. (2013). Fast measurement of sarcomere length and cell orientation in Langendorff-perfused hearts using remote focusing microscopy. *Circ. Res.* 113, 863–870. doi: 10.1161/CIRCRESAHA.113.301704

Botcherby, E. J., Juškaitis, R., Booth, M. J., and Wilson, T. (2008). An optical technique for remote focusing in microscopy. *Optics Commun.* 281, 880–887. doi: 10.1016/j.optcom.2007.10.007

Boyden, E. S., Zhang, F., Bamberg, E., Nagel, G., and Deisseroth, K. (2005). Millisecond-timescale, genetically targeted optical control of neural activity. *Nat. Neurosci.* 8, 1263–1268. doi: 10.1038/nn1525

Boyle, P., Yu, J., Klimas, A., Williams, J., Trayanova, N., and Entcheva, E. (2021). Optogap is an optogenetics-enabled assay for quantification of cell-cell coupling in multicellular cardiac tissue. *Sci. Rep.* 11:9310. doi: 10.1038/s41598-021-88573-1

Brack, K. E., Narang, R., Winter, J., and Ng, A. (2013). The mechanical uncoupler blebbistatin is associated with significant electrophysiological effects in the isolated heart. *Exp. Physiol.* 98, 1009–1027. doi: 10.1113/expphysiol.2012.069369

Brandenburg, S., Arakel, E. C., Schwappach, B., and Lehnart, S. E. (2016a). The molecular and functional identities of atrial cardiomyocytes in health and disease. *Biochim. Biophys. Acta Mol. Cell Res.* 1863, 1882–1893. doi: 10.1016/j.bbamcr.2015.11.025

Brandenburg, S., Kohl, T., Williams, G. S., Gusev, K., Wagner, E., Rog-Zielinska, E. A., et al. (2016b). Axial tubule junctions control rapid calcium signaling in atria. *J. Clin. Investig.* 126, 3999–4015. doi: 10.1172/JCI 88241

Brandenburg, S., Pawlowitz, J., Eikenbusch, B., Peper, J., Kohl, T., Mitronova, G. Y., et al. (2019). Junctophilin-2 expression rescues atrial dysfunction through polyadic junctional membrane complex biogenesis. *JCI Insight* 4:127116. doi: 10.1172/jci.insight.127116

Brandenburg, S., Pawlowitz, J., Fakuade, F. E., Kownatzki-Danger, D., Kohl, T., Mitronova, G. Y., et al. (2018). Axial tubule junctions activate atrial Ca^{2+} release across species. *Front. Physiol.* 9:1227. doi: 10.3389/fphys.2018.01227

Bruegmann, T., Beiert, T., Vogt, C., Schrickel, J., and Sasse, P. (2018). Optogenetic termination of atrial fibrillation in mice. *Cardiovasc. Res.* 114, 713–723. doi: 10.1093/cvr/cvx250

Bruegmann, T., Boyle, P., Christoph, C., Vogt, V., Karathanos, T., Hermenegild, A., et al. (2016). Optogenetic defibrillation terminates ventricular arrhythmia in mouse hearts and human simulations. *J. Clin. Investig.* 126, 3894–3904. doi: 10.1172/JCI88950

Bruegmann, T., Malan, D., Hesse, M., Beiert, T., Fuegemann, C. J., Fleischmann, B. K., et al. (2010). Optogenetic control of heart muscle *in vitro* and *in vivo*. *Nature Methods* 7:897. doi: 10.1038/nmeth.1512

Bub, G., Tecza, M., Helmes, M., Lee, P., and Kohl, P. (2010). Temporal pixel multiplexing for simultaneous high-speed, high resolution imaging. *Nature Methods* 7, 209–211. doi: 10.1038/nmeth.1429

Burton, R., Tomek, J., Ambrosi, C., Larsen, H., Sharkey, A., Capel, R., et al. (2020). Optical interrogation of sympathetic neuronal effects on macroscopic cardiomyocyte network dynamics. *iScience* 23:101334. doi: 10.1016/j.isci.2020.101334

Burton, R. A., Klimas, A., Ambrosi, C. M., Tomek, J., Corbett, A., Entcheva, E., et al. (2015). Optical control of excitation waves in cardiac tissue. *Nat. Photon.* 9:813. doi: 10.1038/nphoton.2015.196

Bush, P. G., Wokosin, D. L., and Hall, A. C. (2007). Two-versus one photon excitation laser scanning microscopy: critical importance of excitation wavelength. *Front. Biosci.* 12:2646. doi: 10.2741/2261

Byars, J. L., Smith, W. M., Ideker, R. E., and Fast, V. G. (2003). Development of an optrode for intramural multisite optical recordings of VM in the heart. *J. Cardiovasc. Electrophysiol.* 14, 1196–1202. doi: 10.1046/j.1540-8167.2003.03203.x

Caldwell, B. J., Legrice, I. J., Hooks, D. A., Tai, D. C.-S., Pullan, A. J., and Smaill, B. H. (2005). Intramural measurement of transmembrane potential in the isolated pig heart: validation of a novel technique. *J. Cardiovasc. Electrophysiol.* 16, 1001–1010. doi: 10.1111/j.1540-8167.2005.40558.x

Camelliti, P., Abou Al-Saud, S., Smolenski, R. T., Al-Ayoubi, S., Bussek, A., Wettwer, E., et al. (2011). Adult human heart slices are a multicellular system suitable for electrophysiological and pharmacological studies. *J. Mol. Cell. Cardiol.* 51, 390–398. doi: 10.1016/j.yjmcc.2011.06.018

Cathey, B., Obaid, S., Zolotarev, A. M., Pryamonosov, R. A., Syunyaev, R. A., George, S. A., et al. (2019). Open-source multiparametric optocardiography. *Sci. Rep.* 9, 1–12. doi: 10.1038/s41598-018-36809-y

Centonze, V. E., and White, J. G. (1998). Multiphoton excitation provides optical sections from deeper within scattering specimens than confocal imaging. *Biophys. J.* 75, 2015–2024. doi: 10.1016/S0006-3495(98)77643-X

Chen, T.-W., Wardill, T. J., Sun, Y., Pulver, S. R., Renninger, S. L., Baohan, A., et al. (2013). Ultrasensitive fluorescent proteins for imaging neuronal activity. *Nature* 499, 295–300. doi: 10.1038/nature12354

Christoph, J., Chebbok, M., Richter, C., Schröder-Schetelig, J., Bittihn, P., Stein, S., et al. (2018). Electromechanical vortex filaments during cardiac fibrillation. *Nature* 555, 667–672. doi: 10.1038/nature26001

Christoph, J., and Luther, S. (2018). Marker-free tracking for motion artifact compensation and deformation measurements in optical mapping videos of contracting hearts. *Front. Physiol.* 9:1483. doi: 10.3389/fphys.2018.01483

Chung, K., Wallace, J., Kim, S.-Y., Kalyanasundaram, S., Andalman, A. S., Davidson, T. J., et al. (2013). Structural and molecular interrogation of intact biological systems. *Nature* 497, 332–337. doi: 10.1038/nature12107

Cingolani, E., Ionta, V., Cheng, K., Giacomello, A., Cho, H. C., and Marbán, E. (2014). Engineered electrical conduction tract restores conduction in complete heart block: from *in vitro* to *in vivo* proof of concept. *J. Am. Coll. Cardiol.* 64, 2575–2585. doi: 10.1016/j.jacc.2014.09.056

Credi, C., Balducci, V., Munagala, U., Cianca, C., Bigiarini, S., De Vries, A. A., et al. (2021). Fast optical investigation of cardiac electrophysiology by parallel detection in multiwell plates. *Front. Physiol.* 12:692496. doi: 10.3389/fphys.2021.692496

Crocini, C., Coppini, R., Ferrantini, C., Yan, P., Loew, L. M., Tesi, C., et al. (2014). Defects in t-tubular electrical activity underlie local alterations of calcium release in heart failure. *Proc. Natl. Acad. Sci. U.S.A.* 111, 15196–15201. doi: 10.1073/pnas.1411557111

Crocini, C., Ferrantini, C., Coppini, R., Scardigli, M., Yan, P., Loew, L. M., et al. (2016a). Optogenetics design of mechanistically-based stimulation patterns for cardiac defibrillation. *Sci. Rep.* 6:35628. doi: 10.1038/srep35628

Crocini, C., Ferrantini, C., Scardigli, M., Coppini, R., Mazzoni, L., Lazzeri, E., et al. (2016b). Novel insights on the relationship between t-tubular defects and contractile dysfunction in a mouse model of hypertrophic cardiomyopathy. *J. Mol. Cell. Cardiol.* 91, 42–51. doi: 10.1016/j.yjmcc.2015.12.013

De Mena, L., Rizk, P., and Rincon-Limas, D. E. (2018). Bringing light to transcription: the optogenetics repertoire. *Front. Genet.* 9:518. doi: 10.3389/fgene.2018.00518

Deán-Ben, X. L., Ford, S. J., and Razansky, D. (2015). High-frame rate four dimensional optoacoustic tomography enables visualization of cardiovascular dynamics and mouse heart perfusion. *Sci. Rep.* 5, 1–9. doi: 10.1038/srep13240

Deisseroth, K. (2011). Optogenetics. *Nat. Methods* 8, 26–29. doi: 10.1038/nmeth.f.324

Dempsey, G., Chaudhary, K., Atwater, N., Nguyen, C., Brown, B., McNeish, J., et al. (2016). Cardiotoxicity screening with simultaneous optogenetic pacing, voltage imaging and calcium imaging. *J. Pharmacol. Toxicol. Methods* 81, 240–250. doi: 10.1016/j.vascn.2016.05.003

Deng, W., Goldys, E. M., Farnham, M. M., and Pilowsky, P. M. (2014). Optogenetics, the intersection between physics and neuroscience: light stimulation of neurons in physiological conditions. *Am. J. Physiol. Regul. Integr. Comp. Physiol.* 307, R1292–R1302. doi: 10.1152/ajpregu.00072.2014

Denk, W., Strickler, J. H., and Webb, W. W. (1990). Two-photon laser scanning fluorescence microscopy. *Science* 248, 73–76. doi: 10.1126/science.2321027

Di Diego, J. M., Sicouri, S., Myles, R. C., Burton, F. L., and Smith, G. L. (2013). Optical and electrical recordings from isolated coronary-perfused ventricular wedge preparations. *J. Mol. Cell. Cardiol.* 54, 53–64. doi: 10.1016/j.yjmcc.2012.10.017

Efimov, I. R., Huang, D. T., Rendt, J. M., and Salama, G. (1994). Optical mapping of repolarization and refractoriness from intact hearts. *Circulation* 90, 1469–1480. doi: 10.1161/01.CIR.90.3.1469

Entcheva, E., and Bien, H. (2006). Macroscopic optical mapping of excitation in cardiac cell networks with ultra-high spatiotemporal resolution. *Prog. Biophys. Mol. Biol.* 92, 232–257. doi: 10.1016/j.pbiomolbio.2005.10.003

Entcheva, E., and Bub, G. (2016). All-optical control of cardiac excitation: combined high-resolution optogenetic actuation and optical mapping. *J. Physiol.* 594, 2503–2510. doi: 10.1113/JP271559

Entcheva, E., and Kay, M. W. (2021). Cardiac optogenetics: a decade of enlightenment. *Nat. Rev. Cardiol.* 18, 349–367. doi: 10.1038/s41569-020-00478-0

Fatkin, D., Otway, R., and Vandenberg, J. I. (2007). Genes and atrial fibrillation: a new look at an old problem. *Circulation* 116, 782–792. doi: 10.1161/CIRCULATIONAHA.106.688889

Fedorov, V. V., Lozinsky, I. T., Sosunov, E. A., Anyukhovsky, E. P., Rosen, M. R., Balke, C. W., et al. (2007). Application of blebbistatin as an excitation-contraction uncoupler for electrophysiologic study of rat and rabbit hearts. *Heart Rhythm* 4, 619–626. doi: 10.1016/j.hrthm.2006.12.047

Franz, M. (1999). Current status of monophasic action potential recording: theories, measurements and interpretations. *Cardiovasc. Res.* 41, 25–40. doi: 10.1016/S0008-6363(98)00268-5

Franzoso, M., Zaglia, T., and Mongillo, M. (2016). Putting together the clues of the everlasting neuro-cardiac liaison. *Biochim. Biophys. Acta Mol Cell Res.* 1863, 1904–1915. doi: 10.1016/j.bbamcr.2016.01.009

Funken, M., Bruegmann, T., and Sasse, P. (2020). Selective optogenetic stimulation of fibroblasts enables quantification of hetero-cellular coupling to cardiomyocytes in a three-dimensional model of heart tissue. *Europace* 22, 1590–1599. doi: 10.1093/europace/euaa128

Funken, M., Malan, D., Sasse, P., and Bruegmann, T. (2019). Optogenetic hyperpolarization of cardiomyocytes terminates ventricular arrhythmia. *Front. Physiol.* 10:498. doi: 10.3389/fphys.2019.00498

Gao, L., Kupfer, M. E., Jung, J. P., Yang, L., Zhang, P., Da Sie, Y., et al. (2017). Myocardial tissue engineering with cells derived from human-induced pluripotent stem cells and a native-like, high-resolution, 3-dimensionally printed scaffold. *Circ. Res.* 120, 1318–1325. doi: 10.1161/CIRCRESAHA.116.310277

Ghouri, I. A., Kelly, A., Burton, F. L., Smith, G. L., and Kemi, O. J. (2015). 2-photon excitation fluorescence microscopy enables deeper high-resolution imaging of voltage and Ca^{2+} in intact mice, rat, and rabbit hearts. *J. Biophoton.* 8, 112–123. doi: 10.1002/jbio.201300109

Ghouri, I. A., Kelly, A., Salerno, S., Garten, K., Stølen, T., Kemi, O.-J., et al. (2018). Characterization of electrical activity in post-myocardial infarction scar tissue in rat hearts using multiphoton microscopy. *Front. Physiol.* 9:1454. doi: 10.3389/fphys.2019.00364

Gintant, G., Burridge, P., Gepstein, L., Harding, S., Herron, T., Hong, C., et al. (2019). Use of human induced pluripotent stem cell-derived cardiomyocytes in preclinical cancer drug cardiotoxicity testing: a scientific statement from the american heart association. *Circ. Res.* 125, e75–e92. doi: 10.1161/RES.0000000000000291

Girouard, S., Laurita, K., and Rosenbaum, D. (1996). Unique properties of cardiac action potentials recorded with voltage-sensitive dyes. *J. Cardiovasc. Electrophysiol.* 7, 1024–1038. doi: 10.1111/j.1540-8167.1996.tb00478.x

Goette, A., Kalman, J. M., Aguinaga, L., Akar, J., Cabrera, J. A., Chen, S. A., et al. (2016). EHRA/HRS/APHRS/SOLAECE expert consensus on atrial cardiomyopathies: definition, characterization, and clinical implication. *Europace* 18, 1455–1490. doi: 10.1093/europace/euw161

Gottschalk, S., Degtyaruk, O., Mc Larney, B., Rebling, J., Hutter, M. A., Deán-Ben, X. L., et al. (2019). Rapid volumetric optoacoustic imaging of neural dynamics across the mouse brain. *Nat. Biomed. Eng.* 3, 392–401. doi: 10.1038/s41551-019-0372-9

Grashoff, C., Hoffman, B. D., Brenner, M. D., Zhou, R., Parsons, M., Yang, M. T., et al. (2010). Measuring mechanical tension across vinculin reveals regulation of focal adhesion dynamics. *Nature* 466, 263–266. doi: 10.1038/nature 09198

Greiser, M., Kerfant, B.-G., Williams, G. S., Voigt, N., Harks, E., Dibb, K. M., et al. (2014). Tachycardia-induced silencing of subcellular Ca^{2+} signaling in atrial myocytes. *J. Clin. Investig.* 124, 4759–4772. doi: 10.1172/JCI70102

Grynkiewicz, G., Poenie, M., and Tsien, R. Y. (1985). A new generation of Ca^{2+} indicators with greatly improved fluorescence properties. *J. Biol. Chem.* 260, 3440–3450. doi: 10.1016/S0021-9258(19)83641-4

Gutruf, P., Yin, R. T., Lee, K. B., Ausra, J., Brennan, J. A., Qiao, Y., et al. (2019). Wireless, battery-free, fully implantable multimodal and multisite pacemakers for applications in small animal models. *Nat. Commun.* 10, 1–10. doi: 10.1038/s41467-019-13637-w

Helmchen, F., and Denk, W. (2005). Deep tissue two-photon microscopy. *Nat. Methods* 2, 932–940. doi: 10.1038/nmeth818

Hicks, M., and Cobbe, S. (1991). Effect of glibenclamide on extracellular potassium accumulation and the electrophysiological changes during myocardial ischaemia in the arterially perfused interventricular septum of rabbit. *Cardiovasc. Res.* 25, 407–413. doi: 10.1093/cvr/25.5.407

Hooks, D. A., Trew, M. L., Caldwell, B. J., Sands, G. B., LeGrice, I. J., and Smaill, B. H. (2007). Laminar arrangement of ventricular myocytes influences electrical behavior of the heart. *Circ. Res.* 101, e103–e112. doi: 10.1161/CIRCRESAHA.107.161075

Hortigon-Vinagre, M., Zamora, V., Burton, F., Green, J., Gintant, G., and Smith, G. (2016). The use of ratiometric fluorescence measurements of the voltage sensitive dye Di-4-ANEPPS to examine action potential characteristics and drug effects on human induced pluripotent stem cell-derived cardiomyocytes. *Toxicol. Sci.* 154, 320–331. doi: 10.1093/toxsci/kfw171

Huang, Y., Walker, A. S., and Miller, E. W. (2015). A photostable silicon rhodamine platform for optical voltage sensing. *J. Am. Chem. Soc.* 137, 10767–10776. doi: 10.1021/jacs.5b06644

Huisken, J., Swoger, J., Del Bene, F., Wittbrodt, J., and Stelzer, E. H. (2004). Optical sectioning deep inside live embryos by selective plane illumination microscopy. *Science* 305, 1007–1009. doi: 10.1126/science.1100035

Hulsmans, M., Clauss, S., Xiao, L., Aguirre, A. D., King, K. R., Hanley, A., et al. (2017). Macrophages facilitate electrical conduction in the heart. *Cell* 169, 510–522. doi: 10.1016/j.cell.2017.03.050

Hurley, M. E., Sheard, T. M., Norman, R., Kirton, H. M., Shah, S. S., Pervolaraki, E., et al. (2020). A correlative super-resolution protocol to visualise structural underpinnings of fast second-messenger signalling in primary cell types. *Methods*. 193, 27–37. doi: 10.1016/j.ymeth.2020.10.005

Hussaini, S., Venkatesan, V., Biasci, V., Romero Sepúlveda, J. M., Quinonez Uribe, R. A., Sacconi, L., et al. (2021). Drift and termination of spiral waves in optogenetically modified cardiac tissue at sub-threshold illumination. *eLife* 10:e59954. doi: 10.7554/eLife.59954

Hyatt, C. J., Mironov, S. F., Vetter, F. J., Zemlin, C. W., and Pertsov, A. M. (2005). Optical action potential upstroke morphology reveals near-surface transmural propagation direction. *Circ. Res.* 97, 277–284. doi: 10.1161/01.RES.0000176022.74579.47

Inagaki, M., Hidaka, I., Aiba, T., Tatewaki, T., Sunagawa, K., and Sugimachi, M. (2004). "High resolution optical mapping of cardiac action potentials in freely beating rabbit hearts," in *26th Annual International Conference of the IEEE Engineering in Medicine and Biology Society* (IEEE), 3578–3580. doi: 10.1109/IEMBS.2004.1404006

Iribe, G., Helmes, M., and Kohl, P. (2007). Force-length relations in isolated intact cardiomyocytes subjected to dynamic changes in mechanical load. *Am. J. Physiol. Heart Circ. Physiol.* 292, H1487–H1497. doi: 10.1152/ajpheart.00909.2006

Iribe, G., Ward, C. W., Camelliti, P., Bollensdorff, C., Mason, F., Burton, R. A., et al. (2009). Axial stretch of rat single ventricular cardiomyocytes causes an acute and transient increase in Ca^{2+} spark rate. *Circ. Res.* 104, 787–795. doi: 10.1161/CIRCRESAHA.108.193334

Jaimes, I. I. I., R., Walton, R. D., Pasdois, P., Bernus, O., Efimov, I. R., et al. (2016). A technical review of optical mapping of intracellular calcium within myocardial tissue. *Am. J. Physiol. Heart Circ. Physiol.* 310, H1388–H1401. doi: 10.1152/ajpheart.00665.2015

Jia, Z., Valiunas, V., Lu, Z., Bien, H., Liu, H., Wang, H., et al. (2011). Stimulating cardiac muscle by light: cardiac optogenetics by cell delivery. *Circ. Arrhythmia Electrophysiol.* 4, 753–760. doi: 10.1161/CIRCEP.111.964247

Jin, L., Han, Z., Platisa, J., Wooltorton, J. R., Cohen, L. B., and Pieribone, V. A. (2012). Single action potentials and subthreshold electrical events imaged in neurons with a fluorescent protein voltage probe. *Neuron* 75, 779–785. doi: 10.1016/j.neuron.2012.06.040

Julian, K., Prichard, B., Raco, J., Jain, R., and Jain, R. (2021). A review of cardiac autonomics: from pathophysiology to therapy. *Future Cardiol.* doi: 10.2217/fca-2021-0041. [Epub ahead of print].

Kanai, A., and Salama, G. (1995). Optical mapping reveals that repolarization spreads anisotropically and is guided by fiber orientation in guinea pig hearts. *Circ. Res.* 77, 784–802. doi: 10.1161/01.RES.77.4.784

Kappadan, V., Telele, S., Uzelac, I., Fenton, F., Parlitz, U., Luther, S., et al. (2020). High-resolution optical measurement of cardiac restitution, contraction, and fibrillation dynamics in beating vs. blebbistatin-uncoupled isolated rabbit hearts. *Front. Physiol.* 11:464. doi: 10.3389/fphys.2020.00464

Karlas, A., Fasoula, N.-A., Paul-Yuan, K., Reber, J., Kallmayer, M., Bozhko, D., et al. (2019). Cardiovascular optoacoustics: from mice to men-a review. *Photoacoustics* 14, 19–30. doi: 10.1016/j.pacs.2019.03.001

Kelly, A., Ghouri, I. A., Kemi, O. J., Bishop, M. J., Bernus, O., Fenton, F. H., et al. (2013). Subepicardial action potential characteristics are a function of depth and activation sequence in isolated rabbit hearts. *Circ. Arrhythmia Electrophysiol.* 6, 809–817. doi: 10.1161/CIRCEP.113.000334

Kelly, A., Salerno, S., Connolly, A., Bishop, M., Charpentier, F., Stølen, T., et al. (2018). Normal interventricular differences in tissue architecture underlie right ventricular susceptibility to conduction abnormalities in a mouse model of brugada syndrome. *Cardiovasc. Res.* 114, 724–736. doi: 10.1093/cvr/cvx244

Képiró, M., Várkuti, B. H., Végner, L., Vörös, G., Hegyi, G., Varga, M., et al. (2014). para-nitroblebbistatin, the non-cytotoxic and photostable myosin ii inhibitor. *Angew. Chem. Int. Ed.* 53, 8211–8215. doi: 10.1002/anie.201403540

Kettlewell, S., Walker, N., Burton, F., and Smith, G. (2004). The electrophysiological and mechanical effects of 2,3-butanedione monoxime and cytochalasin-d in the Langendorff perfused rabbit heart. *Exp. Physiol.* 89, 163–172. doi: 10.1113/expphysiol.2003.026732

Kirk, M. M., Izu, L. T., Chen-Izu, Y., McCulle, S. L., Wier, W. G., Balke, C. W., et al. (2003). Role of the transverse-axial tubule system in generating calcium sparks and calcium transients in rat atrial myocytes. *J. Physiol.* 547, 441–451. doi: 10.1113/jphysiol.2002.034355

Klimas, A., Ambrosi, C. M., Yu, J., Williams, J. C., Bien, H., and Entcheva, E. (2016). Optodyce as an automated system for high-throughput all-optical dynamic cardiac electrophysiology. *Nat. Commun.* 7, 1–12. doi: 10.1038/ncomms11542

Klimas, A., Ortiz, G., Boggess, S., Miller, E., and Entcheva, E. (2020). Multimodal on-axis platform for all-optical electrophysiology with near-infrared probes in human stem-cell-derived cardiomyocytes. *Prog. Biophys. Mol. Biol.* 154, 62–70. doi: 10.1016/j.pbiomolbio.2019.02.004

Kohl, P. (2014). Structural and functional recoupling of atrial and ventricular myocardium. *J. Am. Coll. Cardiol.* 64, 2586–2588. doi: 10.1016/j.jacc.2014.09.055

Kohl, P., Cooper, P. J., and Holloway, H. (2003). Effects of acute ventricular volume manipulation on *in situ* cardiomyocyte cell membrane configuration. *Prog. Biophys. Mol. Biol.* 82, 221–227. doi: 10.1016/S0079-6107(03)00024-5

Kohl, P., Kamkin, A., Kiseleva, I., and Noble, D. (1994). Mechanosensitive fibroblasts in the sino-atrial node region of rat heart: interaction with cardiomyocytes and possible role. *Exp. Physiol. Transl. Integr.* 79, 943–956. doi: 10.1113/expphysiol.1994.sp003819

Kong, C. H., Rog-Zielinska, E. A., Kohl, P., Orchard, C. H., and Cannell, M. B. (2018). Solute movement in the t-tubule system of rabbit and mouse cardiomyocytes. *Proc. Natl. Acad. Sci.* 115, E7073–E7080. doi: 10.1073/pnas.1805979115

Koopman, C. D., Zimmermann, W. H., Knöpfel, T., and de Boer, T. P. (2017). Cardiac optogenetics: using light to monitor cardiac physiology. *Basic Res. Cardiol.* 112, 1–13. doi: 10.1007/s00395-017-0645-y

Kopton, R. A., Baillie, J. S., Rafferty, S. A., Moss, R., Zgierski-Johnston, C. M., Prykhozhij, S. V., et al. (2018). Cardiac electrophysiological effects of light-activated chloride channels. *Front. Physiol.* 9:1806. doi: 10.3389/fphys.2018.01806

Kostecki, G., Shi, Y., Chen, C., Reich, D., Entcheva, E., and Tung, L. (2021). Optogenetic current in myofibroblasts acutely alters electrophysiology and conduction of co-cultured cardiomyocytes. *Sci. Rep.* 11:4430. doi: 10.1038/s41598-021-83398-4

Kotlikoff, M. I. (2007). Genetically encoded Ca^{2+} indicators: using genetics and molecular design to understand complex physiology. *J. Physiol.* 578, 55–67. doi: 10.1113/jphysiol.2006.120212

Kreisel, D., Nava, R. G., Li, W., Zinselmeyer, B. H., Wang, B., Lai, J., et al. (2010). *In vivo* two-photon imaging reveals monocyte-dependent neutrophil extravasation during pulmonary inflammation. *Proc. Natl. Acad. Sci. U.S.A.* 107, 18073–18078. doi: 10.1073/pnas.1008737107

Kuzmiak-Glancy, S., Covian, R., Femnou, A., Glancy, B., Jaimes, R., Wengrowski, A. W., et al. (2018). Cardiac performance is limited by oxygen delivery to the mitochondria in the crystalloid-perfused working heart. *Am. J. Physiol. Heart Circ. Physiol.* 314, H704–H715. doi: 10.1152/ajpheart.00321.2017

Lang, C., Menza, M., Jochem, S., Franke, G., Feliz, S. P., Brunner, M., et al. (2016). Electro-mechanical dysfunction in long qt syndrome: role for arrhythmogenic risk prediction and modulation by sex and sex hormones. *Prog. Biophys. Mol. Biol.* 120, 255–269. doi: 10.1016/j.pbiomolbio.2015.12.010

Lapp, H., Bruegmann, T., Malan, D., Friedrichs, S., Kilgus, C., Heidsieck, A., et al. (2017). Frequency-dependent drug screening using optogenetic stimulation of human iPSC-derived cardiomyocytes. *Sci. Rep.* 7, 1–12. doi: 10.1038/s41598-017-09760-7

Lee, P., Bollensdorff, C., Quinn, T. A., Wuskell, J. P., Loew, L. M., and Kohl, P. (2011). Single-sensor system for spatially resolved, continuous, and multiparametric optical mapping of cardiac tissue. *Heart Rhythm* 8, 1482–1491. doi: 10.1016/j.hrthm.2011.03.061

Lee, P., Quintanilla, J. G., Alfonso-Almazan, J. M., Galán-Arriola, C., Yan, P., Sánchez-González, J., et al. (2019). *In vivo* ratiometric optical mapping enables high-resolution cardiac electrophysiology in pig models. *Cardiovasc. Res.* 115, 1659–1671. doi: 10.1093/cvr/cvz039

Lee, P., Taghavi, F., Yan, P., Ewart, P., Ashley, E. A., Loew, L. M., et al. (2012a). *In situ* optical mapping of voltage and calcium in the heart. *PLoS ONE* 7:e42562. doi: 10.1371/journal.pone.0042562

Lee, P., Yan, P., Ewart, P., Kohl, P., Loew, L. M., and Bollensdorff, C. (2012b). Simultaneous measurement and modulation of multiple physiological parameters in the isolated heart using optical techniques. *Pflügers Arch. Eur. J. Physiol.* 464, 403–414. doi: 10.1007/s00424-012-1135-6

Lee, S., Vinegoni, C., Feruglio, P. F., Fexon, L., Gorbatov, R., Pivoravov, M., et al. (2012c). Real-time *in vivo* imaging of the beating mouse heart at microscopic resolution. *Nat. Commun.*3, 1–8. doi: 10.1038/ncomms2060

Leray, A., Lillis, K., and Mertz, J. (2008). Enhanced background rejection in thick tissue with differential-aberration two-photon microscopy. *Biophys. J.* 94, 1449–1458. doi: 10.1529/biophysj.107.111476

Leray, A., and Mertz, J. (2006). Rejection of two-photon fluorescence background in thick tissue by differential aberration imaging. *Optics Express* 14, 10565–10573. doi: 10.1364/OE.14.010565

Li, W., Goldstein, D. R., and Kreisel, D. (2013). Intravital 2-photon imaging, leukocyte trafficking, and the beating heart. *Trends Cardiovasc. Med.* 23, 287–293. doi: 10.1016/j.tcm.2013.04.002

Lin, H.-C. A., Déan-Ben, X. L., Reiss, M., Schöttle, V., Wahl-Schott, C. A., Efimov, I. R., et al. (2018). Ultrafast volumetric optoacoustic imaging of whole isolated beating mouse heart. *Sci. Rep.* 8, 1–7. doi: 10.1038/s41598-018-32317-1

Lüss, I., Boknik, P., Jones, L. R., Kirchhefer, U., Knapp, J., Linck, B., et al. (1999). Expression of cardiac calcium regulatory proteins in atrium v ventricle in different species. *J. Mol. Cell. Cardiol.* 31, 1299–1314. doi: 10.1006/jmcc.1999.0962

Lyon, A., Babalis, D., Morley-Smith, A., Hedger, M., Barrientos, A. S., Foldes, G., et al. (2020). Investigation of the safety and feasibility of AAV1/SERCA2a gene transfer in patients with chronic heart failure supported with a left ventricular assist device-the serca-lvad trial. *Gene Therapy* 27, 579–590. doi: 10.1038/s41434-020-0171-7

Makowka, P., Bruegmann, T., Dusend, V., Malan, D., Beiert, T., Hesse, M., et al. (2019). Optogenetic stimulation of G_s-signaling in the heart with high spatio-temporal precision. *Nat. Commun.* 10:1281. doi: 10.1038/s41467-019-09322-7

Martin, T. P., Norris, G., McConnell, G., and Currie, S. (2013). A novel approach for assessing cardiac fibrosis using label-free second harmonic generation. *Int. J. Cardiovasc. Imaging* 29, 1733–1740. doi: 10.1007/s10554-013-0270-2

Matsuo, T., Masumoto, H., Tajima, S., Ikuno, T., Katayama, S., Minakata, K., et al. (2015). Efficient long-term survival of cell grafts after myocardial infarction with thick viable cardiac tissue entirely from pluripotent stem cells. *Sci. Rep.* 5, 1–14. doi: 10.1038/srep16842

Meng, F., and Sachs, F. (2012). Orientation-based fret sensor for real-time imaging of cellular forces. *J. Cell Sci.* 125, 743–750. doi: 10.1242/jcs.093104

Meng, F., Suchyna, T. M., and Sachs, F. (2008). A fluorescence energy transfer-based mechanical stress sensor for specific proteins *in situ*. *FEBS J.* 275, 3072–3087. doi: 10.1111/j.1742-4658.2008.06461.x

Miesenböck, G. (2009). The optogenetic catechism. *Science* 326, 395–399. doi: 10.1126/science.1174520

Miller, E. W., Lin, J. Y., Frady, E. P., Steinbach, P. A., Kristan, W. B. J., and Tsien, R. Y. (2012). Optically monitoring voltage in neurons by photo-induced electron transfer through molecular wires. *Proc. Natl. Acad. Sci. U.S.A.* 109, 2114–2119. doi: 10.1073/pnas.1120694109

Moreno, A., Endicott, K., Skancke, M., Dwyer, M. K., Brennan, J., Efimov, I. R., et al. (2019). Sudden heart rate reduction upon optogenetic release of acetylcholine from cardiac parasympathetic neurons in perfused hearts. *Front. Physiol.* 10:16. doi: 10.3389/fphys.2019.00016

Nagel, G., Ollig, D., Fuhrmann, M., Kateriya, S., Musti, A. M., Bamberg, E., et al. (2002). Channelrhodopsin-1: a light-gated proton channel in green algae. *Science* 296, 2395–2398. doi: 10.1126/science.1072068

Nagel, G., Szellas, T., Huhn, W., Kateriya, S., Adeishvili, N., Berthold, P., et al. (2003). Channelrhodopsin-2, a directly light-gated cation-selective membrane channel. *Proc. Natl. Acad. Sci. U.S.A.* 100, 13940–13945. doi: 10.1073/pnas.1936192100

Nyns, E., Kip, A., Bart, C., Plomp, J., Zeppenfeld, K., Schalij, M., et al. (2016). Optogenetic termination of ventricular arrhythmias in the whole heart: towards biological cardiac rhythm management. *Eur. Heart J.* 38, 2132–2136. doi: 10.1093/eurheartj/ehw574

Olianti, C., Costantini, I., Giardini, F., Lazzeri, E., Crocini, C., Ferrantini, C., et al. (2020). 3d imaging and morphometry of the heart capillary system in spontaneously hypertensive rats and normotensive controls. *Sci. Rep.* 10, 1–9. doi: 10.1038/s41598-020-71174-9

Olianti, C., Giardini, F., Lazzeri, E., Costantini, I., Silvestri, L., Coppini, R., et al. (2021). Optical clearing in cardiac imaging: a comparative study. *Prog. Biophys. Mol. Biol.* doi: 10.1016/j.pbiomolbio.2021.07.012. [Epub ahead of print].

Paredes, R. M., Etzler, J. C., Watts, L. T., and Lechleiter, J. D. (2008). Chemical calcium indicators. *Methods* 46, 143–151. doi: 10.1016/j.ymeth.2008.09.025

Park, S., Lee, S., Tung, L., and Yue, D. (2014). Optical mapping of optogenetically shaped cardiac action potentials. *Sci. Rep.* 4:6125. doi: 10.1038/srep06125

Pecha, S., Yorgan, K., Röhl, M., Geertz, B., Hansen, A., Weinberger, F., et al. (2019). Human iPS cell-derived engineered heart tissue does not affect ventricular arrhythmias in a guinea pig cryo-injury model. *Sci. Rep.* 9, 1–12. doi: 10.1038/s41598-019-46409-z

Pfeiffer, E., Wright, A., Edwards, A., Stowe, J., McNall, K., Tan, J., et al. (2014). Caveolae in ventricular myocytes are required for stretch-dependent conduction slowing. *J. Mol. Cell. Cardiol.* 76, 265–274. doi: 10.1016/j.yjmcc.2014.09.014

Pfeiffer-Kaushik, E., Smith, G., Cai, B., Dempsey, G., Hortigon-Vinagre, M., Zamora, V., et al. (2019). Electrophysiological characterization of drug response in hsc-derived cardiomyocytes using voltage-sensitive optical platforms. *J. Pharmacol. Toxicol. Methods* 99:106612. doi: 10.1016/j.vascn.2019.106612

Pianca, N., Di Bona, A., Lazzeri, E., Costantini, I., Franzoso, M., Prando, V., et al. (2019). Cardiac sympathetic innervation network shapes the myocardium by locally controlling cardiomyocyte size through the cellular proteolytic machinery. *J. Physiol.* 597, 3639–3656. doi: 10.1113/JP276200

Pogwizd, S. M., and Corr, P. B. (1987). Reentrant and nonreentrant mechanisms contribute to arrhythmogenesis during early myocardial ischemia: results using three-dimensional mapping. *Circ. Res.* 61, 352–371. doi: 10.1161/01.RES.61.3.352

Prando, V., Da Broi, F., Franzoso, M., Plazzo, A. P., Pianca, N., Francolini, M., et al. (2018). Dynamics of neuroeffector coupling at cardiac sympathetic synapses. *J. Physiol.* 596, 2055–2075. doi: 10.1113/JP275693

Prigge, M., Schneider, F., Tsunoda, S. P., Shilyansky, C., Wietek, J., Deisseroth, K., et al. (2012). Color-tuned channelrhodopsins for multiwavelength optogenetics. *J. Biol. Chem.* 287, 31804–31812. doi: 10.1074/jbc.M112.391185

Qu, F., Ripplinger, C. M., Nikolski, V., Grimm, C., and Efimov, I. R. (2007). Three-dimensional panoramic imaging of cardiac arrhythmias in rabbit heart. *J. Biomed. Opt.* 12:044019. doi: 10.1117/1.2753748

Quach, B., Krogh-Madsen, T., Entcheva, E., and Christini, D. (2018). Light-activated dynamic clamp using iPSC-derived cardiomyocytes. *Biophys. J.* 115, 2206–2217. doi: 10.1016/j.bpj.2018.10.018

Quinn, T. A., Camelliti, P., Rog-Zielinska, E. A., Siedlecka, U., Poggioli, T., O'Toole, E. T., et al. (2016). Electrotonic coupling of excitable and nonexcitable cells in the heart revealed by optogenetics. *Proc. Natl. Acad. Sci.* 113, 14852–14857. doi: 10.1073/pnas.1611184114

Quinn, T. A., and Kohl, P. (2021). Cardiac mechano-electric coupling: acute effects of mechanical stimulation on heart rate and rhythm. *Physiol. Rev.* 101, 37–92. doi: 10.1152/physrev.00036.2019

Rajendran, P. S., Challis, R. C., Fowlkes, C. C., Hanna, P., Tompkins, J. D., Jordan, M. C., et al. (2019). Identification of peripheral neural circuits that regulate heart rate using optogenetic and viral vector strategies. *Nat. Commun.* 10, 1–13. doi: 10.1101/456483

Richardson, D. S., and Lichtman, J. W. (2015). Clarifying tissue clearing. *Cell* 162, 246–257. doi: 10.1016/j.cell.2015.06.067

Roell, W., Klein, A. M., Breitbach, M., Becker, T. S., Parikh, A., Lee, J., et al. (2018). Overexpression of cx43 in cells of the myocardial scar: correction of post-infarct arrhythmias through heterotypic cell-cell coupling. *Sci. Rep.* 8, 1–14. doi: 10.1038/s41598-018-25147-8

Roell, W., Lewalter, T., Sasse, P., Tallini, Y. N., Choi, B.-R., Breitbach, M., et al. (2007). Engraftment of connexin 43-expressing cells prevents post-infarct arrhythmia. *Nature* 450, 819–824. doi: 10.1038/nature06321

Rog-Zielinska, E. A., Kong, C. H. T., Zgierski-Johnston, C. M., Verkade, P., Mantell, J., Cannell, M. B., et al. (2018). Species differences in the morphology of transverse tubule openings in cardiomyocytes. *Europace* 20(Suppl_3), iii120–iii124. doi: 10.1093/europace/euy245

Rog-Zielinska, E. A., Scardigli, M., Peyronnet, R., Zgierski-Johnston, C. M., Greiner, J., Madl, J., et al. (2021). Beat-by-beat cardiomyocyte t-tubule deformation drives tubular content exchange. *Circ. Res.* 128, 203–215. doi: 10.1161/CIRCRESAHA.120.317266

Rowlands, C. J., Bruns, O. T., Bawendi, M. G., and So, P. T. (2015). Objective, comparative assessment of the penetration depth of temporal-focusing microscopy for imaging various organs. *J. Biomed. Opt.* 20:061107. doi: 10.1117/1.JBO.20.6.061107

Rubart, M., Tao, W., Lu, X.-L., Conway, S. J., Reuter, S. P., Lin, S.-F., et al. (2018). Electrical coupling between ventricular myocytes and myofibroblasts in the infarcted mouse heart. *Cardiovasc. Res.* 114, 389–400. doi: 10.1093/cvr/cvx163

Rubart, M., Wang, E., Dunn, K. W., and Field, L. J. (2003). Two-photon molecular excitation imaging of Ca^{2+} transients in Langendorff-perfused mouse hearts. *Am. J. Physiol. Cell Physiol.* 284, C1654–C1668. doi: 10.1152/ajpcell.00469.2002

Rudy, Y. (2013). Noninvasive electrocardiographic imaging of arrhythmogenic substrates in humans. *Circ. Res.* 112, 863–874. doi: 10.1161/CIRCRESAHA.112.279315

Sacconi, L., Ferrantini, C., Lotti, J., Coppini, R., Yan, P., Loew, L. M., et al. (2012). Action potential propagation in transverse-axial tubular system is impaired in heart failure. *Proc. Natl. Acad. Sci. U.S.A.* 109, 5815–5819. doi: 10.1073/pnas.1120188109

Sacconi, L., Silvestri, L., Rodriguez, E., Armstrong, G., Pavone, F., Shrier, A., et al. (2020). Khz-rate volumetric voltage imaging of the whole zebrafish heart. *bioRxiv*. doi: 10.1101/2020.07.13.196063

Sala, L., van Meer, B. J., Tertoolen, L. G., Bakkers, J., Bellin, M., Davis, R. P., et al. (2018). Musclemotion: a versatile open software tool to quantify cardiomyocyte and cardiac muscle contraction *in vitro* and *in vivo*. *Circ. Res.* 122, e5–e16. doi: 10.1101/160754

Salama, G., and Hwang, S.-,m. (2009). Simultaneous optical mapping of intracellular free calcium and action potentials from Langendorff perfused hearts. *Curr. Protoc. Cytometry* 49, 12–17. doi: 10.1002/0471142956.cy1217s49

Salerno, S., Garten, K., Smith, G. L., Stølen, T., and Kelly, A. (2019). Two-photon excitation of fluovolt allows improved interrogation of transmural electrophysiological function in the intact mouse heart. *Prog. Biophys. Mol. Biol.* 154, 11–20. doi: 10.1016/j.pbiomolbio.2019.08.007

Scardigli, M., Crocini, C., Ferrantini, C., Gabbrielli, T., Silvestri, L., Coppini, R., et al. (2017). Quantitative assessment of passive electrical properties of the cardiac t-tubular system by frap microscopy. *Proc. Natl. Acad. Sci. U.S.A.* 114, 5737–5742. doi: 10.1073/pnas.1702188114

Scardigli, M., Ferrantini, C., Crocini, C., Pavone, F. S., and Sacconi, L. (2018a). Interplay between sub-cellular alterations of calcium release and t-tubular defects in cardiac diseases. *Front. Physiol.* 9:1474. doi: 10.3389/fphys.2018.01474

Scardigli, M., Müllenbroich, C., Margoni, E., Cannazzaro, S., Crocini, C., Ferrantini, C., et al. (2018b). Real-time optical manipulation of cardiac conduction in intact hearts. *J. Physiol.* 596, 3841–3858. doi: 10.1113/JP276283

Sicouri, S., and Antzelevitch, C. (1991). A subpopulation of cells with unique electrophysiological properties in the deep subepicardium of the canine ventricle. The M cell. *Circ. Res.* 68, 1729–1741. doi: 10.1161/01.RES.68.6.1729

Siedentopf, H., and Zsigmondy, R. (1903). Visualization and size measurement of ultramicroscopic particles, with special application to gold-colored ruby glass. *Ann. Phys.* 10, 1–39.

Sierra, Y. A. B., Rost, B. R., Pofahl, M., Fernandes, A. M., Kopton, R. A., Moser, S., et al. (2018). Potassium channel-based optogenetic silencing. *Nat. Commun.* 9, 1–13. doi: 10.1038/s41467-018-07038-8

Silvestri, L., Costantini, I., Sacconi, L., and Pavone, F. S. (2016). Clearing of fixed tissue: a review from a microscopist's perspective. *J. Biomed. Opt.* 21:081205. doi: 10.1117/1.JBO.21.8.081205

Simone, S., Moyle, S., Buccarello, A., Dellenbach, C., Kucera, J., and Rohr, S. (2020). The role of membrane capacitance in cardiac impulse conduction: an optogenetic study with non-excitable cells coupled to cardiomyocytes. *Front. Physiol.* 11:194. doi: 10.3389/fphys.2020.00194

Szipöcs, R., Ferencz, K., Spielmann, C., and Krausz, F. (1994). Chirped multilayer coatings for broadband dispersion control in femtosecond lasers. *Opt. Lett.* 19, 201–203. doi: 10.1364/OL.19.000201

Tal, E., Oron, D., and Silberberg, Y. (2005). Improved depth resolution in video-rate line-scanning multiphoton microscopy using temporal focusing. *Opt. Lett.* 30, 1686–1688. doi: 10.1364/OL.30.001686

Taylor, J. M., Nelson, C. J., Bruton, F. A., Kaveh, A., Buckley, C., Tucker, C. S., et al. (2019). Adaptive prospective optical gating enables day-long 3d time-lapse imaging of the beating embryonic zebrafish heart. *Nat. Commun.* 10, 1–15. doi: 10.1038/s41467-019-13112-6

Theer, P., and Denk, W. (2006). On the fundamental imaging-depth limit in two-photon microscopy. *JOSA A* 23, 3139–3149. doi: 10.1364/JOSAA.23.003139

Thul, R., Coombes, S., Roderick, H. L., and Bootman, M. D. (2012). Subcellular calcium dynamics in a whole-cell model of an atrial myocyte. *Proc. Natl. Acad. Sci. U.S.A.* 109, 2150–2155. doi: 10.1073/pnas,.1115855109

Van Wagoner, D. R., and Lamorgese, M. (1994). Ischemia potentiates the mechanosensitive modulation of atrial atp-sensitive potassium channels A. *Ann. N. Y. Acad. Sci.* 723, 392–395. doi: 10.1111/j.1749-6632.1994.tb36755.x

Várkuti, B. H., Képiró, M., Horváth, I., Á., Végner, L., Ráti, S., et al. (2016). A highly soluble, non-phototoxic, non-fluorescent blebbistatin derivative. *Sci. Rep.* 6, 1–10. doi: 10.1038/srep26141

Vinegoni, C., Aguirre, A. D., Lee, S., and Weissleder, R. (2015). Imaging the beating heart in the mouse using intravital microscopy techniques. *Nat. Protoc.* 10:1802. doi: 10.1038/nprot.2015.119

Wagner, E., Brandenburg, S., Kohl, T., and Lehnart, S. E. (2014). Analysis of tubular membrane networks in cardiac myocytes from atria and ventricles. *J. Visual. Exp.* 92:e51823. doi: 10.3791/51823

Walker, N. L., Burton, F. L., Kettlewell, S., Smith, G. L., and Cobbe, S. M. (2007). Mapping of epicardial activation in a rabbit model of chronic myocardial infarction: response to atrial, endocardial and epicardial pacing. *J. Cardiovasc. Electrophysiol.* 18, 862–868. doi: 10.1111/j.1540-8167.2007.00858.x

Walton, R. D., Benoist, D., Hyatt, C. J., Gilbert, S. H., White, E., and Bernus, O. (2010). Dual excitation wavelength epifluorescence imaging of transmural electrophysiological properties in intact hearts. *Heart Rhythm* 7, 1843–1849. doi: 10.1016/j.hrthm.2010.08.019

Weber, M., Scherf, N., Meyer, A. M., Panakova, D., Kohl, P., and Huisken, J. (2017). Cell-accurate optical mapping across the entire developing heart. *eLife* 6:e28307. doi: 10.7554/eLife.28307

Wei, L., Li, W., Entcheva, E., and Li, Z. (2020). Microfluidics-enabled 96-well perfusion system for high-throughput tissue engineering and long-term all-optical electrophysiology. *Lab Chip* 20, 4031–4042. doi: 10.1039/D0LC00615G

Weinberger, F., Breckwoldt, K., Pecha, S., Kelly, A., Geertz, B., Starbatty, J., et al. (2016). Cardiac repair in guinea pigs with human engineered heart tissue from induced pluripotent stem cells. *Sci. Transl. Med.* 8:363ra148. doi: 10.1126/scitranslmed.aaf8781

Wengrowski, A., Kuzmiak-Glancy, S., Jaimes, R., c., and Kay, M. (2014). Nadh changes during hypoxia, ischemia, and increased work differ between isolated heart preparations. *Am. J. Physiol. Heart Circ. Physiol.* 306, H529–H537. doi: 10.1152/ajpheart.00696.2013

Wengrowski, A. M., Wang, X., Tapa, S., Posnack, N. G., Mendelowitz, D., and Kay, M. W. (2015). Optogenetic release of norepinephrine from cardiac sympathetic neurons alters mechanical and electrical function. *Cardiovasc. Res.* 105, 143–150. doi: 10.1093/cvr/cvu258

Werley, C., Chien, M., and Cohen, A. (2017). Ultrawidefield microscope for high-speed fluorescence imaging and targeted optogenetic stimulation. *Biomed. Opt. Express* 8, 5794–5813. doi: 10.1364/BOE.8.005794

Whitaker, M. (2010). "Genetically encoded probes for measurement of intracellular calcium," in *Methods in Cell Biology*, Michael Whitaker (ed), Vol. 99 (Elsevier), 153–182. doi: 10.1016/B978-0-12-374841-6.00006-2

Williams, J., and Entcheva, E. (2015). Optogenetic versus electrical stimulation of human cardiomyocytes: modelling insights. *Biophys. J.* 108, 1934–1945. doi: 10.1016/j.bpj.2015.03.032

Wu, X., and Bers, D. M. (2006). Sarcoplasmic reticulum and nuclear envelope are one highly interconnected Ca^{2+} store throughout cardiac myocyte. *Circ. Res.* 99, 283–291. doi: 10.1161/01.RES.0000233386.02708.72

Wu, Y., Li, S.-S., Jin, X., Cui, N., Zhang, S., and Jiang, C. (2015). Optogenetic approach for functional assays of the cardiovascular system by light activation of the vascular smooth muscle. *Vasc. Pharmacol.* 71, 192–200. doi: 10.1016/j.vph.2015.03.006

Xiao, S., and Mertz, J. (2019). Contrast improvement in two-photon microscopy with instantaneous differential aberration imaging. *Biomed. Opt. Express* 10, 2467–2477. doi: 10.1364/BOE.10.002467

Yan, P., Acker, C. D., Zhou, W.-L., Lee, P., Bollensdorff, C., Negrean, A., et al. (2012). Palette of fluorinated voltage-sensitive hemicyanine dyes. *Proc. Natl. Acad. Sci. U.S.A.* 109, 20443–20448. doi: 10.1073/pnas.1214850109

Yang, H. H., and St-Pierre, F. (2016). Genetically encoded voltage indicators: opportunities and challenges. *J. Neurosci.* 36, 9977–9989. doi: 10.1523/JNEUROSCI.1095-16.2016

Yu, J., and Entcheva, E. (2016). "Inscribing optical excitability to non-excitable cardiac cells: viral delivery of optogenetic tools in primary cardiac fibroblasts," *Methods Mol Biol.* 1408:303–317. doi: 10.1007/978-1-4939-3512-3_21

Yu, L., Zhou, L., Cao, G., Po, S. S., Huang, B., Zhou, X., et al. (2017). Optogenetic modulation of cardiac sympathetic nerve activity to prevent ventricular arrhythmias. *J. Am. Coll. Cardiol.* 70, 2778–2790. doi: 10.1016/j.jacc.2017.09.1107

Zaglia, T., Di Bona, A., and Mongillo, M. (2019). A light wand to untangle the myocardial cell network. *Methods Protoc.* 2:34. doi: 10.3390/mps2020034

Zaglia, T., Pianca, N., Borile, G., Da Broi, F., Richter, C., Campione, M., et al. (2015). Optogenetic determination of the myocardial requirements for extrasystoles by cell type-specific targeting of channelrhodopsin-2. *Proc. Natl. Acad. Sci. U.S.A.* 112, E4495–E4504. doi: 10.1073/pnas.1509380112

Zalev, J., Richards, L. M., Clingman, B. A., Harris, J., Cantu, E., Menezes, G. L., et al. (2019). Opto-acoustic imaging of relative blood oxygen saturation and total hemoglobin for breast cancer diagnosis. *J. Biomed. Opt.* 24:121915. doi: 10.1117/1.JBO.24.12.121915

Zgierski-Johnston, C., Ayub, S., Fernández, M., Rog-Zielinska, E., Barz, F., Paul, O., et al. (2020). Cardiac pacing using transmural multi-led probes in channelrhodopsin-expressing mouse hearts. *Prog. Biophys. Mol. Biol.* 154, 51–61. doi: 10.1016/j.pbiomolbio.2019.11.004

Zhang, H. K., Yan, P., Kang, J., Abou, D. S., Le, H. N., Jha, A. K., et al. (2017). Listening to membrane potential: photoacoustic voltage-sensitive dye recording. *J. Biomed. Opt.* 22:045006. doi: 10.1117/1.JBO.22.4.045006

Zhang, S., Cui, N., Wu, Y., Zhong, W., Johnson, C. M., and Jiang, C. (2015). Optogenetic intervention to the vascular endothelium. *Vasc. Pharmacol.* 74, 122–129. doi: 10.1016/j.vph.2015.05.009

Zhang, Y., Sekar, R. B., McCulloch, A. D., and Tung, L. (2008). Cell cultures as models of cardiac mechanoelectric feedback. *Prog. Biophys. Mol. Biol.* 97, 367–382. doi: 10.1016/j.pbiomolbio.2008.02.017

Zipfel, W. R., Williams, R. M., and Webb, W. W. (2003). Nonlinear magic: multiphoton microscopy in the biosciences. *Nat. Biotechnol.* 21, 1369–1377. doi: 10.1038/nbt899

Permissions

All chapters in this book were first published by Frontiers; hereby published with permission under the Creative Commons Attribution License or equivalent. Every chapter published in this book has been scrutinized by our experts. Their significance has been extensively debated. The topics covered herein carry significant findings which will fuel the growth of the discipline. They may even be implemented as practical applications or may be referred to as a beginning point for another development.

The contributors of this book come from diverse backgrounds, making this book a truly international effort. This book will bring forth new frontiers with its revolutionizing research information and detailed analysis of the nascent developments around the world.

We would like to thank all the contributing authors for lending their expertise to make the book truly unique. They have played a crucial role in the development of this book. Without their invaluable contributions this book wouldn't have been possible. They have made vital efforts to compile up to date information on the varied aspects of this subject to make this book a valuable addition to the collection of many professionals and students.

This book was conceptualized with the vision of imparting up-to-date information and advanced data in this field. To ensure the same, a matchless editorial board was set up. Every individual on the board went through rigorous rounds of assessment to prove their worth. After which they invested a large part of their time researching and compiling the most relevant data for our readers.

The editorial board has been involved in producing this book since its inception. They have spent rigorous hours researching and exploring the diverse topics which have resulted in the successful publishing of this book. They have passed on their knowledge of decades through this book. To expedite this challenging task, the publisher supported the team at every step. A small team of assistant editors was also appointed to further simplify the editing procedure and attain best results for the readers.

Apart from the editorial board, the designing team has also invested a significant amount of their time in understanding the subject and creating the most relevant covers. They scrutinized every image to scout for the most suitable representation of the subject and create an appropriate cover for the book.

The publishing team has been an ardent support to the editorial, designing and production team. Their endless efforts to recruit the best for this project, has resulted in the accomplishment of this book. They are a veteran in the field of academics and their pool of knowledge is as vast as their experience in printing. Their expertise and guidance has proved useful at every step. Their uncompromising quality standards have made this book an exceptional effort. Their encouragement from time to time has been an inspiration for everyone.

The publisher and the editorial board hope that this book will prove to be a valuable piece of knowledge for researchers, students, practitioners and scholars across the globe.

List of Contributors

Edison F. Carpio, Juan F. Gomez, Alejandro Lopez-Perez and Jose M. Ferrero
Centre for Research and Innovation in Bioengineering (Ci2B), Universitat Politècnica de València, Valencia, Spain

Rafael Sebastian
Computational Multiscale Simulation Lab (CoMMLab), Department of Computer Science, Universitat de València, Valencia, Spain

Eduardo Castellanos and Jesus Almendral
Electrophysiology Laboratory and Arrhythmia Unit, Grupo HM Hospitales, Hospital Monteprincipe, University CEU-San Pablo, Madrid, Spain

M. Izquierdo and Ricardo Ruiz
INCLIVA Health Research Institute, Valencia, Spain
Arrhythmia Unit, Cardiology Department, Hospital Clínico Universitario de Valencia, Valencia, Spain

Martin Bishop
Division of Imaging Sciences & Biomedical Engineering, Department of Biomedical Engineering, King's College London, London, United Kingdom

Ana Mincholé
Department of Computer Science, University of Oxford, Oxford, United Kingdom

Ernesto Zacur and Vicente Grau
Institute of Biomedical Engineering (IBME), University of Oxford, Oxford, United Kingdom

Rina Ariga
Division of Cardiovascular Medicine, Radcliffe Department of Medicine, University of Oxford, Oxford, United Kingdom

Erik Willemen, Rick Schreurs, John Walmsley, Tammo Delhaas and Frits W. Prinzen
Cardiovascular Research Institute Maastricht (CARIM), Maastricht University, Maastricht, Netherlands

Peter R. Huntjens and Joost Lumens
IHU-LIRYC Electrophysiology and Heart Modeling Institute, Pessac, France

Marc Strik and Kevin Vernooy
Department of Cardiology, Maastricht University Medical Center, Maastricht, Netherlands

Gernot Plank
Institute of Biophysics, Medical University of Graz, Graz, Austria

Edward Vigmond
Univeristy of Bordeaux, IMB UMR 5251, Talence, France

Ronald Wilders
Department of Medical Biology, Amsterdam University Medical Centers, Amsterdam, Netherlands

Jean Bragard
Department of Physics and Applied Mathematics, University of Navarra, Pamplona, Spain

Aparna C. Sankarankutty and Frank B. Sachse
Nora Eccles Harrison Cardiovascular Research and Training Institute, University of Utah, Salt Lake City, UT, United States
Department of Biomedical Engineering, University of Utah, Salt Lake City, UT, United States

Jorge Sánchez, Laura Martinez-Mateu, Lucia Romero, Javier Saiz and Beatriz Trenor
Centre for Research and Innovation in Bioengineering, Universitat Politècnica de València, Valencia, Spain

Dominic G. Whittaker
Faculty of Biological Sciences, School of Biomedical Sciences, University of Leeds, Leeds, United Kingdom
Biological Physics Group, School of Physics and Astronomy, The University of Manchester, Manchester, United Kingdom

Jules C. Hancox
Biological Physics Group, School of Physics and Astronomy, The University of Manchester, Manchester, United Kingdom
Cardiovascular Research Laboratories, Department of Physiology, Pharmacology and Neuroscience, School of Medical Sciences, University of Bristol, Bristol, United Kingdom

Henggui Zhang
Biological Physics Group, School of Physics and Astronomy, The University of Manchester, Manchester, United Kingdom
School of Computer Science and Technology, Harbin Institute of Technology, Harbin, China
Space Institute of Southern China, Shenzhen, China
Key Laboratory of Medical Electrophysiology of Ministry of Education and Medical Electrophysiological Key Laboratory of Sichuan Province, Institute of Cardiovascular Research, Southwest Medical University, Luzhou, China

Adityo Prakosa, Julie Shade, Plamen Nikolov and Natalia A. Trayanova
Department of Biomedical Engineering, Johns Hopkins University, Baltimore, MD, United States

Dongdong Deng
Department of Biomedical Engineering, Johns Hopkins University, Baltimore, MD, United States
School of Biomedical Engineering, Dalian University of Technology, Dalian, China

Xin Zhou and Alfonso Bueno-Orovio
Department of Computer Science, British Heart Foundation Centre of Research Excellence, University of Oxford, Oxford, United Kingdom

Blanca Rodriguez
Department of Computer Science, British Heart Foundation Centre of Research Excellence, University of Oxford, Oxford, United Kingdom
Department of Computer Science, University of Oxford, Oxford, United Kingdom

Richard J. Schilling and Claire Kirkby
St Bartholomew's Hospital, London, United Kingdom

Chris Denning and Divya Rajamohan
Department of Stem Cell Biology, Centre for Biomolecular Sciences, University of Nottingham, Nottingham, United Kingdom

Kevin Burrage
Department of Computer Science, British Heart Foundation Centre of Research Excellence, University of Oxford, Oxford, United Kingdom
Australian Research Council Centre of Excellence for Mathematical and Statistical Frontiers, Queensland University of Technology, Brisbane, QLD, Australia
School of Mathematical Sciences, Queensland University of Technology, Brisbane, QLD, Australia

Andrew Tinker and Stephen C. Harmer
The William Harvey Research Institute, Barts and The London School of Medicine and Dentistry, Queen Mary University of London, London, United Kingdom

Haibo Ni, Stefano Morotti and Eleonora Grandi
Department of Pharmacology, University of California, Davis, Davis, CA, United States

Dimitrios Poulikakos, Sofia Skampardoni, Darren Green and Philip Kalra
Renal Department, Salford Royal NHS Foundation Trust, Salford, United Kingdom
Centre for Cardiac Research, Institute of Cardiovascular Sciences, The University of Manchester, Manchester, United Kingdom

Katerina Hnatkova and Marek Malik
National Heart and Lung Institute, Imperial College London, London, United Kingdom

Koen T. Scholman
Department of Medical Biology, Amsterdam University Medical Centers, University of Amsterdam, Amsterdam, Netherlands

Elisabeth M. Lodder
Department of Experimental Cardiology, Amsterdam University Medical Centers, University of Amsterdam, Amsterdam, Netherlands

Bastiaan J. Boukens
Department of Medical Biology, Amsterdam University Medical Centers, University of Amsterdam, Amsterdam, Netherlands
Department of Experimental Cardiology, Amsterdam University Medical Centers, University of Amsterdam, Amsterdam, Netherlands

Veronique M. F. Meijborg
Department of Experimental Cardiology, Amsterdam University Medical Centers, University of Amsterdam, Amsterdam, Netherlands
Netherlands Heart Institute, Utrecht, Netherlands

Carolina Gálvez-Montón
ICREC Research Program, Germans Trias I Pujol Health Science Research Institute, Badalona, Spain
CIBERCV, Instituto de Salud Carlos III, Madrid, Spain

M. Caroline Müllenbroich
School of Physics and Astronomy, University of Glasgow, Glasgow, United Kingdom

Allen Kelly and Godfrey L. Smith
Institute of Cardiovascular and Medical Sciences, University of Glasgow, Glasgow, United Kingdom

Corey Acker
Center for Cell Analysis and Modeling, UConn Health, Farmington, CT, United States

Gil Bub
Department of Physiology, McGill University, Montréal, QC, Canada

Tobias Bruegmann
Institute for Cardiovascular Physiology, University Medical Center Goettingen, Goettingen, Germany

Anna Di Bona
Department of Cardiac, Thoracic, Vascular Sciences and Public Health, University of Padova, Padova, Italy

Emilia Entcheva
Department of Biomedical Engineering, The George Washington University, Washington, DC, United States

Cecilia Ferrantini and Camilla Parmeggiani
European Laboratory for Nonlinear Spectroscopy, Sesto Fiorentino, Italy

Peter Kohl
Institute for Experimental Cardiovascular Medicine, University Heart Center and Medical Faculty, University of Freiburg, Freiburg, Germany

Stephan E. Lehnart
Heart Research Center Göttingen, University Medical Center Göttingen, Göttingen, Germany
Department of Cardiology and Pneumology, Georg-August University Göttingen, Göttingen, Germany
Cluster of Excellence "Multiscale Bioimaging: from Molecular Machines to Networks of Excitable Cells" (MBExC), University of Göttingen, Göttingen, Germany

Marco Mongillo and Tania Zaglia
Department of Biomedical Sciences, University of Padova, Padova, Italy
Veneto Institute of Molecular Medicine, Padova, Italy

Claudia Richter
German Primate Center - Leibniz Institute for Primate Research, Göttingen, Germany

Philipp Sasse
Institute of Physiology I, Medical Faculty, University of Bonn, Bonn, Germany

Leonardo Sacconi
European Laboratory for Nonlinear Spectroscopy, Sesto Fiorentino, Italy
Institute for Experimental Cardiovascular Medicine, University Heart Center and Medical Faculty, University of Freiburg, Freiburg, Germany
National Institute of Optics, National Research Council, Florence, Italy

Index

www.ingramcontent.com/pod-product-compliance
Lightning Source LLC
LaVergne TN
LVHW060546210926
848485LV00005B/1267
* 9 7 8 1 6 3 9 2 7 9 5 9 3 *